Manual of
Middle Ear Surgery

Volume 1

Manual of Middle Ear Surgery

Volume 1:
Approaches,
Myringoplasty,
Ossiculoplasty
and Tympanoplasty

Mirko Tos

Foreword by
Michael E. Glasscock III

1103 illustrations

1993
Georg Thieme Verlag
Stuttgart · New York

Thieme Medical Publishers, Inc.
New York

Mirko Tos, M. D.
Professor and Chairman, Department of Otorhinolaryngology
Gentofte Hospital
University of Copenhagen
Niels Andersens Vej 65, 2000 Hellerup
Denmark

Library of Congress Cataloging-in-Publication Data

Tos, Mirko:
Manual of middle ear surgery / Mirko Tos, [Drawings by Regitze Steinbruch]. – Stuttgart ; New York : Thieme.

Vol. 1. Approaches, myringoplasty, ossiculoplasty and tympanoplasty / foreword by Michael E. Glasscock III. – 1993

Important Note: Medicine is an ever-changing science undergoing continual development. Research and clinical experience are continually expanding our knowledge, in particular our knowledge of proper treatment and drug therapy. Insofar as this book mentions any dosage or application, readers may rest assured that the authors, editors and publishers have made every effort to ensure that such references are in accordance with the state of knowledge at the time of production of the book. Nevertheless this does not involve, imply, or express any guarantee or responsibility on the part of the publishers in respect of any dosage instructions and forms of application stated in the book. Every user is requested to examine carefully the manufacturers' leaflets accompanying each drug and to check, if necessary in consultation with a physician or specialist, whether the dosage schedules mentioned therein or the contraindications stated by the manufacturers differ from the statements made in the present book. Such examination is particularly important with drugs that are either rarely used or have been newly released on the market. Every dosage schedule or every form of application used is entirely at the user's own risk and responsibility. The authors and publishers request every user to report to the publishers any discrepancies or inaccuracies noticed.

Drawings by Regitze Steinbruch
Cover drawing by Renate Stockinger

Some of the product names, patents and registered designs referred to in tis book are in fact registered trademarks or proprietary names even though specific reference to this fact is not always made in the text. Therefore, the appearance of a name without designation as proprietary is not to be construed as a representation by the publisher that it is in the public domain.

This book, including all parts thereof, is legally protected by copyright. Any use, exploitation or commercialization outside the narrow limits set by copyright legislation, without the publisher's consent, is illegal and liable to prosecution. This applies in particular to photostat reproduction, copying, mimeographing or duplication of any kind, translating, preparation of microfilms, and electronic data processing and storage.

© 1993 Georg Thieme Verlag, Rüdigerstraße 14, D-7000 Stuttgart 30, Germany
Thieme Medical Publishers, Inc., 381 Park Avenue South, New York, NY 10016

Typesetting by primustype R. Hurler, D-7311 Notzingen

Printed in Germany
by Karl Grammlich, D-7401 Pliezhausen

ISBN 3-13-112701-5 (GTV, Stuttgart)
ISBN 0-86577-498-6 (TMP, New York)

1 2 3 4 5 6

Foreword

Mirko Tos has written a splendid book on middle ear surgery. His thirty years of experience are evident in his broad knowledge of temporal bone anatomy and middle ear physiology and histology.

What makes this well-illustrated book unique is that the author himself made all the initial drawings. The pictures are simple and straightforward and, therefore, easy to follow and understand.

The manuscript covers every imaginable aspect of middle ear surgery from preoperative evaluation and management of middle ear disease through anesthesia and surgical technique. Incisions, graft materials, ossicular reconstruction, and many more topics are presented in an interesting and readable text.

Middle ear surgeons the world over will enjoy this book and residents will find it an excellent resource in their formative years.

May 1993

Michael E. Glasscock III,
M.D., F.A.C.S.
The Otology Group
Nashville, Tennessee, USA

Preface

One goal of this book is to teach young otologists various tympanoplasty procedures by guiding them through the operations with step-by-step illustrations.

Another important goal is to categorize the many modifications of approaches and tympanoplasty into related groups and subgroups. For this reason, I also include some abandoned methods. Also, I often refer to the methods by the names of the authors or surgeons who popularized or promoted them. The explosive, worldwide development of middle ear surgery in the 1960s makes it sometimes impossible to determine correctly the first author of a method, and I apologize for any errors in this respect.

It is a great privilege to have been an ear surgeon for more than 30 years in the fascinating pioneer period during which new methods and materials in tympanoplasty have constantly been developed. Doing clinical research on middle ear surgery during this period enabled me to meet practically all of the pioneers and masters in the field. Discussions with them during the many panels and symposia through the years have given me inside information that I could not have gotten just by reading their publications.

By way of the groundbreaking research done during the 1960s and 1970s on histopathology of the middle ear and on epidemiology, etiology, and pathogenesis of secretory otitis, I came into contact early on with a large group of scientists interested in the middle ear and eustachian tube, which greatly influenced my view of middle ear surgery.

All illustrations, except two, were made especially for this book in the following manner: I sketched each illustration in pencil on parchment paper, then gave it to the artist, Regitze Steinbruch, who copied it and redrew it in ink on another parchment.

We both learned a lot from each other during the year in which we worked together. It is well known that realistic, precise illustrations of the middle ear are extremely difficult to draw. Usually, I could see only after Ms. Steinbruch had finished an illustration that my initial drawing should have been different, more precise, or simply better. She made the many corrections cheerfully—a quality that, in addition to her skills, significantly contributed to the book. Helene Ryttersgaard and her staff at the Audiovisual Department of Gentofte Hospital was also extremely helpful.

I would like to thank Dr. Simon Bear, an otologist from Bristol, for providing assistance on questions of language during his three-month stay at the Gentofte Hospital as well as after returning home. I also thank Dr. Chia-Fong Liang, an otologist from Taiwan, for taking the time to read the manuscript during his nine-month stay in our department and after leaving for Glasgow. The staff of the Gentofte Hospital Library was extremely helpful by finding the literature I needed. My secretaries, Brigitte Hammershøy and Inge Joost, typed and corrected the manuscript. Without the extreme efficiency of Ms. Joost in particular, this book could not have been finished on time.

Last but not least, I thank my wife Nives for her patience during the many weekends at our home when the work has being done.

Copenhagen, February 1993 *Mirko Tos*

Contents

Part 1 Approaches   1

**1 Indications for Surgery
    and Preoperative Management** 2
   Cholesteatomas 2
   Noncholesteatomatous Chronic Otitis 3
      Middle Ear Mucosa 4
      Aural Polyps 4
   Preoperative Treatment 4
      Local Medicaments 4
   Surgical Treatment 5
   Introduction to Approaches
        to the Middle Ear 5
   Terminology of Canal-Skin Incisions 6

2 Anesthesia 7
   General or Local Anesthesia 7
   Local Anesthesia 7
      Preoperative Sedation 7
      Local Anesthetic Techniques 8
   General Anesthesia 10

3 Endaural Approach 11
   Ear Speculum 11
      Selfretaining Ear Speculum 11
      Fixed Ear Speculum 11
      Application 15
   Intercartilaginous (Heermann) A and B
        Incisions 15
      No Tympanomeatal Flap 18
      Small Tympanomeatal Flap 18
      Lateral Displacement
        of the Canal Skin 18
      Laterally-Based Skin Flap 20
      Large Tympanomeatal Flap 20
      Panse Flap 22
      Canal Skin Removal 23
   Heermann C Incision 24
   Shambaugh Incision 25
   Lempert Incision 26
   Farrior Incision 28
      Canal Skin Removal 29
      Inferior Vascular Strip 29
      Anterior Vascular Strip 30
      Superior Vascular Strip 31

4 Retroauricular Approach 34
   Retroauricular Fold Incision 35
      Lateral Circumferential Incision 35
      Plester Technique 35
      Palva's Swing-Door Technique 38
      Fisch Technique 39
      Farrior Technique 41
      Canal Skin Removal 41
      Medial Circumferential Incision 42
   Wullstein-Kley Technique 42
      Superolaterally-Based Flap 44
      Laterally-Based Flap 45
      Management
        of the Tympanomeatal Flap .. 45
   No Circumferential Incision 50
      Drum Remnant Epithelium
        Elevation (Morimitsu) 50
      Annulus and Drum
        Remnant Elevation 51
   Posterosuperior Incision (Portmann) 51
   Retroauricular Flap Incisions 55
   Posterior Vascular Strip Technique
   (Sheehy) 60

5 Superior Approach 63
   Osteoplastic Epitympanotomy
   (S. Wullstein) 63

6 Anterior Approach 68
   Popper Technique 68
   Goodhill Technique 68

7 Tympanotomies 70
   Posterior Tympanotomy 70
   Inferior Tympanotomy 75
      Hypotympanotomy 77
   Anterior Tympanotomy 81
   Superior Tympanotomy 83
      Atticotomy 84
      Aditotomy 85

Part II Myringoplasty — 87

8 Graft Materials — 88
- Terminology of Grafts — 88
- Autogenous Grafts — 88
- Temporalis Muscle Fascia — 88
  - Fascia in the Endaural Approach — 90
  - Fascia in the Retroauricular Approach — 95
- Tragal Perichondrium — 97
  - Tragal Cartilage — 100
- Conchal Perichondrium and Cartilage — 102
  - Cartilage Via a Separate Posterior Incision — 102
  - Cartilage Via Retroauricular Incisions — 103
  - Resection Lines of the Conchal Cartilage — 108
  - Cartilage Via an Endaural Approach — 109
- Periosteum — 111
  - Mastoid-Process Periosteum — 111
  - Temporal Squama Periosteum — 112
  - Periosteum Via an Endaural Approach — 114
- Vein Graft — 116
- Fatty Tissue — 117
  - Harvesting Fatty Tissue — 117
  - Myringoplasty with Fatty Tissue — 118
- Subcutaneous Tissue — 119
- Fascia Lata — 120
- Ear-Canal Skin — 120
  - Myringoplasty with Canal Skin — 121
- Heterotopic Skin — 124
  - Full-Thickness Grafts — 124
  - Split-Skin Grafts — 125
- Allogenous Grafts — 126
  - Allogenous Ear Drum — 126
  - Lyophilized Dura — 127
- Xenogenous Grafts — 127

9 Myringoplasty: General Aspects Definitions — 128
- Definitions — 128
- Classification of Perforations — 128
- Pathogenetic Aspects — 128
- Classification of Myringoplasty Techniques — 132
- General Principles of Myringoplasty Techniques — 133
- Excision of the Edges of the Perforation — 133
- Dissection on the Perforation Edge — 135
- Management of Drum-Remnant Epithelium — 139
- Removal of the Drum Epithelium — 139
- Epithelial Flaps — 141
- Fixation of the Underlay Graft under the Drum Remnant — 144
- Fibrin Glue in Tympanoplasty — 149
  - Autogenous Fibrin Glue — 149
  - Allogenous Fibrin Glue — 150

10 Onlay Techniques — 152
- Techniques with Removal of the Epithelium — 152
  - Anterior Perforation — 152
  - Inferior Perforation — 153
  - Total Perforation — 155
  - Posterior Perforation — 156
- Onlay Techniques with Epithelial Flaps — 157
  - Anterior Perforation — 157
  - Inferior Perforation — 164
  - Total Perforation — 169
  - Posterior Perforation — 179
- The Onlay Sandwich Technique — 181

11 Underlay Techniques — 184
- Techniques Without Tympanomeatal Flaps — 184
  - Anterior Perforation — 184
  - Inferior Perforation — 186
- Techniques with Tympanomeatal Flaps — 188
- Swing-Door Technique — 188
  - Posterior Perforation — 188
  - Total Perforation — 190
  - Inferior Perforation — 192
- The Large Tympanomeatal Flap Techniques — 194
  - Anterior Perforation — 194
  - Inferior Perforation — 196
  - Posterior Perforation — 199
  - Posterior Tympanotomy in Anterior Perforation — 200
- Total Elevation of the Fibrous Annulus — 202
- Underlay Sandwich Techniques — 205

12 Perichondrium and Cartilage in Myringoplasty — 208
- Perichondrium in Total Perforation — 208
- Combined Perichondrium-Cartilage Grafts — 210
- Tragal and Conchal Cartilage Plates — 212
- Microsliced Septal Cartilage — 212
- Palisade Cartilage Tympanoplasty (Heermann) — 214

13 Myringoplasty in a Curved Ear Canal 217

Endaural Approach with an Ear Speculum 217
Retroauricular Approach 225
Endaural Approach 226
Sheehy's Skin Removal Approach 228

14 Allogenous Ear Drum Transplantation 229

Dissection of Allogenous Drum 229
Allograft Drum in Small and Middle-Sized Perforations 231
Allogenous Drum in Total Perforation with Intact Malleus 231

Part III Ossiculoplasty and Tympanoplasty 237

15 Tympanoplasty–General 238

Classification of Tympanoplasty 238
Incidence of Ossicular-Chain Pathology ... 243

16 Type 2 Tympanoplasty, Stapes Present 245

Ossicles, Bone, Cartilage, Tooth 245
Interpositions 245
Use of Autogenous Incus 245
Extraction of the Incus 245
Disruption of the Incudostapedial Joint . 249
Disruption of the Intact Ossicular Chain 252
Interposition of the Incus 254
Incus Interpositions in Patients with a Retracted Malleus 260
Shaping the Incus 265
Shaping the Malleus Head 271
Shaping Cortical Bone 273
Allogenous Stapes 277
Cartilage 277
Allogenous Costal Cartilage Prostheses 282
Allogenous Dentin Prostheses 284

17 Type 2 Tympanoplasty with Biocompatible Materials 285

Synthetic Biomaterials Polyethylene, Teflon 285
Porous Plastic 286
Ceramics 289
Bioinert Ceramics 289
Bioactive Ceramics 292
Glass Ionomer Cement 297
Metals 298
Titanium Prostheses 298
The Gerlach Wire-Basket Prosthesis ... 298
Palva Two-Legged and Three-Legged Wire Prostheses 330
Gold Prostheses 330

18 Transposition and Pexis in Type 2 Tympanoplasty 302

Transposition 302
Malleostapedial Transposition 302
Pexis 305
Myringoincudopexy 305
Incudostapediopexy 308
Malleostapediopexy 320
Myringostapediopexy 323

19 Tympanoplasty in Partial Defects of the Stapedial Arch 325

20 Tympanoplasty with the Malleus Handle Missing 330

Myringoplasty in Total Perforation 331
Disruption of the Ossicular Chain and Interposition of the Incus 334
Interposition of Cartilage Plates 336
Cartilage Plates in a Disrupted Ossicular Chain 338
Interposition of Other Prostheses 340
Allogenous Drum-Malleus Graft 340
Malleoplasty of the Defective Malleus Handle 342
Malleomyringoplasty 344
Preservation of the Malleus Handle 346

21 Type 3 Tympanoplasty with the Stapes Absent 348

Prognosis with Columellae 348
Variations in Columella Placement 348
Autogenous Incus Columella 350
Allogenous Incus 354
Cortical Bone 356
Autogenous and Allogenous Malleus Columella 357

Allogenous Stapes Columella 358
Cartilage Columella 362
Tragal and Conchal Cartilage
          Columella 362
Smyth's Septal Cartilage Columellae . . 365
Allogenous Costal Cartilage 366
Allogenous Dentin Columellae 367
Columellae with Biocompatible Materials . 368
Compound Columellae 377

22 Type 4 and 5 Tympanoplasty 383

Type 4 Tympanoplasty 383
    Type 4 Tympanoplasty Techniques 383
Type 5 Tympanoplasty 386
    Type 5 A Tympanoplasty Techniques . . 386
    Type 5 B Tympanoplasty Techniques . . 387
Packing the Ear Canal and the Cavity 390

References 391

Index 397

Part I
Approaches

1 Indications for Surgery and Preoperative Management

The main goals of tympanoplasty are to remove an active disease or to repair a sequela condition, either to prevent the recurrence of active disease or to improve the hearing.

It is beyond the scope of this surgical manual to discuss the audiological indications for surgery and the diagnostic problems. Only routine investigations of the most common surgical middle-ear diseases will be mentioned. These are grouped into cholesteatomas and noncholesteatomatous chronic otitis.

Cholesteatomas

Cholesteatomas are divided into:

1. **Attic cholesteatoma,** defined as a retraction (or perforation) of the Shrapnell's membrane extending into the attic or aditus, and eventually into the antrum, mastoid process, or tympanic cavity.

2. **Sinus cholesteatoma,** defined as a posterosuperior retraction (or perforation) of the pars tensa extending into the tympanic sinus and posterior tympanum, and from here under the incus into the attic or aditus ad antrum. There is no involvement of the anterior part of the tympanic cavity in sinus cholesteatoma. One-third of sinus cholesteatomas are located in the tympanic cavitiy alone, and can be reached by a transcanal route without mastoidectomy.

3. **Tensa retraction cholesteatoma,** defined as a retraction and adhesion of the entire pars tensa involving the tympanic orifice of the Eustachian tube, and extending up to the attic under the malleus folds and under the incus bidy or malleus head. One-third of tensa retraction cholesteatomas are located in the tympanic cavity alone.

Cholesteatomatous ears may be dry or discharging. During the first outpatient visit, the history is taken, and a general ENT investigation, including audiological tests with air and bone conduction and speech audiometry measuring the speech reception threshold (SRT) and discrimination score (DS) are performed. Valsalva's maneuver, or possibly typanometry in attic cholesteatoma, as well as a fistula test, are performed. The diagnosis ist made by otomicroscopy after careful suction of the secretion or removal of the crust from the ear canal or tympanic cavity. Initial information is given to the patient about the character of the disease, especially with regard to the possibility of progression and eventual complications. Operative procedures are discussed, either with the canal wall up or the canal wall down. If the ear is infected, a bacteriological investigation is carried out, and local treatment is started twice a day as follows: 1) Valsalva's maneuver to push the secretion into the ear canal; 2) cleaning the ear canal by sterile water; 3) hydrocortisone and antibiotic drops, decreasing if the secretion is diminishing. The patient is placed on the waiting list for surgery, and the period of waiting should not exceed more than one month.

We carry out a CT scan in cases where there is any suspicion of a fistula of the semicircular canal, or suspicion of intracranial complications and asymmetric sensorineural hearing loss, to exclude an acoustic neuroma.

In addition to these typical cholesteatoma types, the following rare cholesteatomas may be referred for surgery:

4. **Ear canal cholesteatoma,** usually originating inferiorly in the ear canal, with resorption of the tympanic bone.

5. **Posttraumatic cholesteatoma,** with an obvious explosion trauma or other severe trauma displacing the keratinized squamous epithelium into the middle ear.

6. **Congenital cholesteatoma,** with an intact drum located either in the mesotympanum (congenital or inclusion cholesteatoma) or elsewhere in the temporal bone, with no contact to the tympanic cavity and a completely normal drum.

These conditions are rare, and need to be more carefully evaluated before surgery is planned.

Recurrent cholesteatomas are not as rare, and relate to a previous operation. These are subdivided into:

7. **Residual cholesteatoma,** defined as cholesteatoma left behind outside the drum or ear canal wall (bony or soft) or cavity wall during the previous

cholesteatoma operation. Residual cholesteatoma is usually located posteriorly in the tympanic cavity behind an intact drum as a white prominence, or in the attic region.

8. **Recurrent cholesteatoma,** defined as a cholesteatoma that appears in a retraction pocket after a previous operation in which an intact canal wall technique has usually been used. The retraction can extend into the tympanic sinus, but usually it extends behind the bridge, or behind an intact bony ear canal, into the aditus and attic.

9. **Iatrogenic cholesteatoma,** defined as a new cholesteatoma after previous surgery for noncholesteatomatous middle-ear disease, e.g., in tympanoplasty with removal of the fibrous annulus and graft failure with ingrowth of the keratinized squamous epithelium along denuded bone into the tympanic cavity.

Noncholesteatomatous Chronic Otitis

The most common diagnoses are a) chronic suppurative (or purulent or granulating) otitis media, indicating an active condition with a discharging ear; and b) sequelae of chronic otitis, indicating a nonactive condition and a dry ear.

The pathoanatomic and functional aspects of noncholesteatomatous chronic otitis can be classified in terms of the following criteria:

1. The degree of hearing loss
2. Presence of perforation
3. Location of the perforation
4. Size of the perforation
5. Status of the ossicular chain
6. Degree of mucosal changes
7. Tubal function
8. Degree of adhesive changes
9. Bacterial infection
10. Degree of pneumatization
11. Degree of tympanosclerosis
12. Degree of concomitant external otitis

These aspects should be taken into consideration in the preoperative assessment of the patient.

There is a gradual transition between the chronically infected ear, termed chronic suppurative otitis media, and a constantly dry ear, termed sequelae of chronic otitis media. The two conditions cannot be separated into two distinct disease entities. When the condition is accompanied by secretion, it is called active chronic suppurative otitis, but the ear may become dry either spontaneously or following conservative treatment. The condition is then called a sequela of chronic otitis. A dry ear with perforation may become infected and start secreting, and this is then called chronic suppurative otitis media. The following changes are common in patients with intermittent secretion: the patient can go from chronic suppurative otitis media (i.e., discharge in the ear), via a transitional stage to the sequelae of chronic otitis media (i.e., the dry ear). The process may also be reversed.

Clinically noncholestateomatous chronic otitis media can be divided into:

1. **Constantly discharging ears.** Causes of chronic discharge may seldom be malnutrition, anemia, hypovitaminosis, and immune deficiencies. Most often, the causes are local, such as ear-canal eczema, abnormal migration of the epithelium of the tympanic membrane and ear canal, deep nonselfcleansing retraction pockets, deep hypotympanic air cells with retention of secretion, mucosal polyps, blockage of the aditus, and abnormal clearance of the Eustachian tube in cases of adhesions of the tympanic orifice and tubal isthmus.

2. **Intermittently secreting ears.** The mucosa is infected either via the Eustachian tube, in upper respiratory tract infections, or through the ear canal when the patient goes swimming, diving, or cleans the ear. Abnormal migration of epithelium from the tympanic membrane, which is usually directed away from the perforation margin, can cause repeated infections. Although clinically the ear may be dry, detritus and discharge can be observed on the tympanic membrane remnant and along the margin of the perforation. The lateral margin of the perforation may be covered with thick, moist middle-ear mucosa, and there may be eczema of the keratinized epithelium.

3. **Constantly dry ear with perforation.**

When a chronic ear is being assessed, information about the otorrhea, including its onset, duration, chronic or periodic occurrence, in addition to other characteristics, make it possible to assign the patient to one of these above-mentioned three groups.

Middle Ear Mucosa

At otomicroscopy, pathological changes in the ear canal, Shrapnell's membrane, the pars tensa, and in the tympanic cavity are described. The middle-ear mucosa observed with the otomicroscope may have following appearances:

1. It may be thin and normal-looking, which is usually the case with dry ears. The prognosis is good.
2. The mucosa may be thick but dry. This is a frequent finding in a dry ear without infection. However, the prognosis for this type of ear is poorer.
3. The mucosa can appear moist and thickened. It may either be in the process of improving from infection, which would make for a good prognosis, or be permanently changed, in which case the prognosis is poor. Clinically, the ear is relatively dry.
4. The mucosa may appear to be moderately thickened and edematous and have a distinct mucous film on the surface. Such mucosa contain a histologically high density of secretory elements. There is often an accumulation of mucus in the hypotympanum, and the mucosa is called the secretory mucosa.
5. Chronically infected mucosa with granulations, edema, swelling, an irregular surface, and severe discharge. This picture is typical of active chronic suppurative (or purulent or granulating) otitis media.
6. Acutely infected mucosa which is edematous and has a pulsating secretion but no granulations.

Aural Polyps

Aural polyps can play an important role in the sustained secretion. They may occlude a perforation, or even an entire ear canal. They may constitute the main source of secretion, as they contain exudate from the epithelial surface and many mucus-secreting elements. Polyps appear in characteristic areas:

1. Attic polyps issue from the margin of a large attic retraction (or perforation) in attic cholesteatoma.
2. Herodium defined as a flat polyp arising from the posterosuperior wall of the tympanic cavity in the region of chorda tympani (Sadé 1976). Usually there is a deep posterosuperior retraction (Larsen and Tos 1992).
3. Eustachian tube orifice polyps may block the Eustachian tube completely. The polyps may grow through an anterior or inferior perforation.
4. Polyps or granulation tissue in areas with bony resorption, such as the long process of the incus, around the stapes and umbo.
5. Polyps or granulation tissue in the hypotympanum.
6. Granulation tissue in the ear canal is an indication of carcinoma.
7. Polyps in the ear canal seen in Hand-Schüller-Christian disease and in eosinophilic granuloma.

Ears with aural polyps produce discharge.

Preoperative Treatment

The goal of treatment must be to render a discharging ear dry by conservative treatment, and then perform either a myringoplasty or tympanoplasty and close the perforation. This is done to prevent the infection of the middle ear from the outside, and to reestablish the middle-ear function.

An acute exacerbation of a sequelae of chronic otitis media can be treated with penicillin or other appropriate antibiotics following culture. Local treatment is also instituted.

Chronic discharge can often be arrested by intensive local treatment, which includes removal of polyps blocking the drainage using a polyp snare under the microscope or a curved forceps. The place of origin may give an indication of how careful one should be during removal. Granulation in the posterior part of the tympanic cavity surrounding the stapes must be removed in small pieces with curved microforceps, and polyps must always be investigated histologically.

The local aural hygiene in discharging ears once or twice a day is the same as that described for cholesteatoma. Besides Ringer's solution for irrigation, mild disinfectants can be used, such as 3% boric acid, 0.02% chlorhexidine, 12% ethanol, or others.

Local Medicaments

Ear drops are applied in the ear canal, followed by tragus massage. The patient should be placed in a supine position, with the treated ear upwards. In principle, three types of eardrops are used:

1. **Antibacterial agents** include chloramphenicol, polymyxins, tetracycline and sulfamethizole. They may have side-effects on the inner ear due to absorption through the round window.
2. **Glucocorticosteroids** prevent edema of the ear-canal skin, ear drum, and middle-ear mucosa. The following agents are commonly used: dexa-

methasone, betamethasone, prednisolone, and triamcinolone (e.g., Kenalog with salicylate acid and Kenalog with ethanol).
3. Combinations of antibacterial agents and glucocorticosteroids are often used with success, and the side-effects are no worse than when antibacterial agents alone are used.

Local application of antibiotic drops in large concentrations has been demonstrated experimentally to cause hearing impairment. Although the risk of ototoxicity is small when one is using therapeutic concentrations, antibiotic drops should be used only for a limited period of time. The present author does not use antibiotic powders.

Surgical Treatment

If the ear is not rendered dry by conservative treatment, a canal wall–up mastoidectomy with tympanoplasty is indicated. There are no rules as to how long conservative treatment should be continued in the attempt to attain a dry ear; it depends on the duration of the discharge before treatment, previous attempts at treatment, the severity of the complications, the patient's attitude and expectations and—no less—the surgeon's attitude. The present author usually continues conservative treatment for at least three months, regardless of the duration of aural discharge and previous attempts at making the ear dry. Most ears respond to the local treatment described above. Surgical intervention on dry ears is less extensive, because mastoidectomy can be avoided. The results are better, and preoperative sensorineural hearing los is less frequent in dry ears with tympanoplasty alone than in ears with mastoidectomy (Tos et al. 1984).

The following common nonchelosteatomatous conditions require surgery:

1. Chronic granulating (or suppurative or purulent) otitis media with discharging ear. An intact canal wall mastoidectomy with tympanoplasty in the same stage is performed.
2. A chronic granulating otitits media with very little discharge can often be treated using tympanoplasty alone, without mastoidectomy. The mucosa may be secretory, and mastoidectomy is, in my opinion, not always necessary.
3. Sequelae of chronic otitis media in dry ears, or almost dry ears, and perforation, with or without ossicular-chain pathology. This group is the largest one.
4. Adhesive otitis media.
5. Tympanosclerosis of the middle ear with tympanosclerotic masses fixing the stapes and/or the incus and malleus in the attic.
6. Severe myringosclerosis fixing the malleus.
7. Bony fixations of the malleus or incus.
8. Traumatic incus luxations, or other posttraumatic conditions.
9. Obliterative otitis denotes a condition with a thick drum in normal position, without retraction, but where the entire tympanic cavity is filled with fibrous tissue and the tympanic orifice of the Eustachian tube is blocked (Tos 1979).
10. Revisions for various reasons: reperforation, hearing loss, ossicular fixations, adhesions, retractions, discharge, etc.
11. Reconstructions of old radical cavities.
12. Various pathologies in the ear canal, such as exostosis, acquired atresia, and diffuse or localized stenosis.

In ears with perforation, a myringoplasty has proved to be the best form of prophylaxis against infection from the ear canal. Closure of a perforation is therefore indicated in young people and children, even with normal hearing. Before hearing-aid treatment in patients with sensorineural hearing loss and perforation, a myringoplasty is indicated even if the air–bone gap is small and hearing cannot be improved. A hearing aid in the ear canal changes the internal milieu of the external auditory canal and increases infection, so that hearing-aid treatment is seldom recommended in patients with perforation before the perforation has been closed.

Introduction to Aproaches to the Middle Ear

Over the last thirty years, several modifications of the basic approaches to the middle ear have been developed, all of which are still in use today:

1. The endaural approach
2. The retroauricular approach
3. The superior approach
4. The anterior approach

In the first part of this book, all the numerous variations of the approaches are illustrated in detail, in many casis even up to the stage just before placement of the fascia graft. Since I believe that the approach is the most important stage in tympanoplasty, this part is the largest one. The many variations illustrate surgeon's various philosophies, extending from hardly any contact with the ear-canal skin, as seen in speculum techniques, to extensive removal of the canal skin, as in several techniques used by Farrior and others.

Terminology of Canal-Skin Incisions

The following terms for incisions of the ear-canal skin will be used (Fig. **1**):
1. **The intercartilaginous incision** of the external meatus at the 12 o'clock position.
2. **The vertical incision** indicates superior extension of the intercartilaginous incisions.
3. **The lateral circumferential (circular) incision,** extending along the circumference of the ear canal at any level lateral to the middle of the ear canal.
4. **The medial circumferential incision,** extending at any level between the middle of the ear canal and the drum. The circumferential incisions are denoted clockwise for the right ear: 12 o'clock, 3 o'clock (anterior), 6 o'clock, and 9 o'clock (posterior); and for the left ear in the opposite direction, with the 9 o'clock position anterior and the 3 o'clock one posterior (Fig. **2**). Circumferential incisions can also be denoted as posterior, anterior, superior, or inferior.
5. **The medial radial incision** runs from the circumferential incision inside the ear canal and towards the drum.
6. **The lateral radial incision** runs from the circumferential incision outwards along the ear canal, towards the meatus. The exact placement of the radial incision is denoted by the clock. The lateral radial incision at the 12 o'clock position is identical with the intercartilaginous incision.
7. **The radial conchal incision** runs from the lateral circumferential incision towards the concha.

To avoid confusion, all illustrations of step-by-step operations presented here are made for the right ear. Descriptions of incisions in the text that refer to the clock position will also refer to the right ear only. The corresponding incisions in the left ear can be identified using Figure **2**.

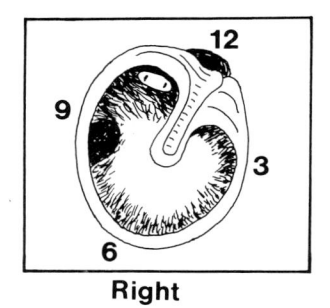

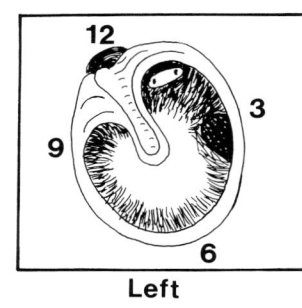

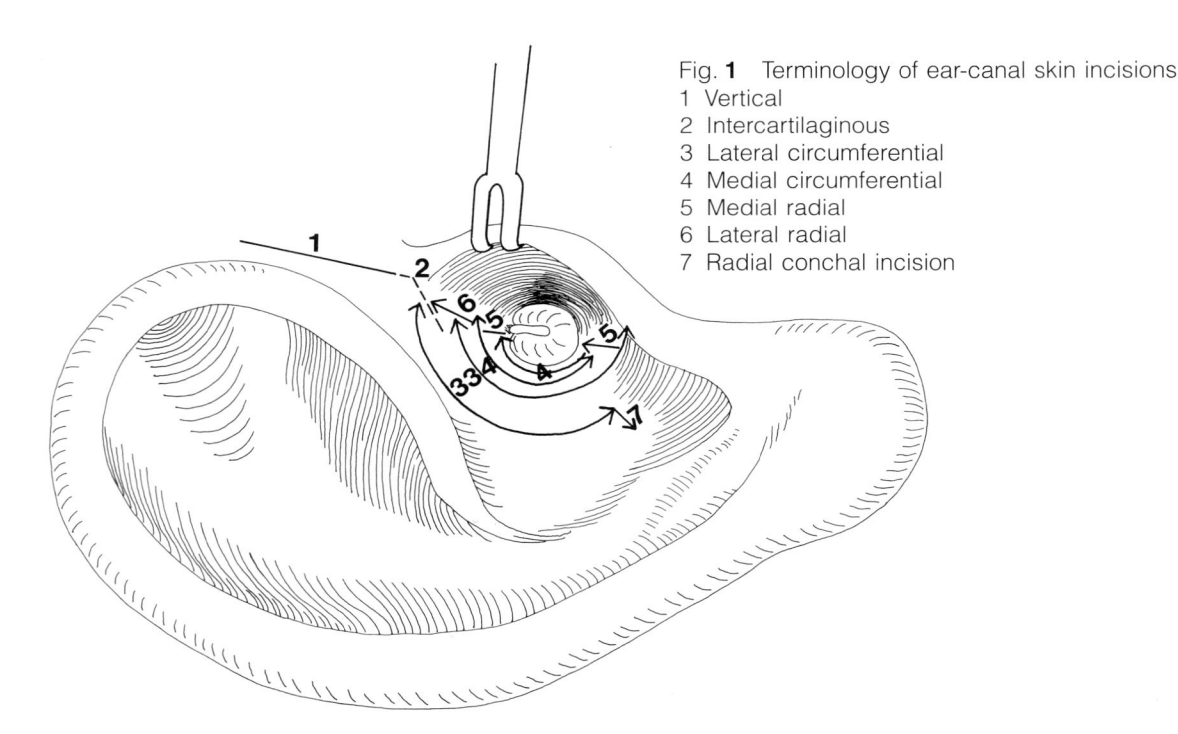

Fig. **2** Clock positions for canal-skin incisions on the right and left ears

Fig. **1** Terminology of ear-canal skin incisions
1 Vertical
2 Intercartilaginous
3 Lateral circumferential
4 Medial circumferential
5 Medial radial
6 Lateral radial
7 Radial conchal incision

2 Anesthesia

General or Local Anesthesia

Either general or local anesthesia can be used in middle-ear surgery. There are today, and have always been, considerable differences among otosurgeons in various clinics with regard to the use of general or local anestesia. Some surgeons exclusively use general anesthesia, even in stapedectomies, easy myringoplasties, and ossiculoplasties. Some use local anesthesia whenever possible, even in extensive mastoidectomies. The arguments for extensive use of local anesthesia relate to the risks associated with general anesthesia. Although casualties are statistically negligible in the hands of qualified and well-equipped anesthetists, anesthetic deaths do occasionally occur. A common argument is that in an elective procedure such as tympanoplasty, if it can be performed equally well under local anesthesia, no additional risk should be incurred by using general anesthesia. Other arguments for local anesthesia are the reduced bleeding involved, the ability to check alterations in hearing, and the greater effectiveness of the surgery.

The arguments for general anesthesia are that extensive removal of tympanic cavity mucosa or tympanic cavity cholesteatoma, as well as any surgery in the anterior tympanon or tympanic orifice of the Eustachian tube, are better done under general anesthesia than under local anesthesia. In addition, all cases requiring mastoidectomy or reconstruction of the ear canal are better done under general than under local anesthesia.

There is general agreements that the following categories of patients should have general anesthesia: children, uncooperative adults, apprehensive adults, and patients who spontaneously prefer or request general anesthesia. In the following procedures, the vast majority of surgeons will prefer general anesthesia: in teaching situations; in any surgery lasting more than $1^1/_2$–2 hours, in mastoidectomies, in cholesteatomas or actively infected middle ears, in reconstructions of old radical cavities, and in revision tympanoplasties where major pieces of temporal muscle fascia have already been harvested previously.

Local anesthesia is generally limited to cooperative adults with dry, noninfected ears and no evidence of mastoid disease.

During the first twenty years in which I carried out middle-ear surgery, I exclusively used general anesthesia in all cases; during the last ten years, however, I have increasingly used local anesthesia. Despite many revisions and difficult cases, local anesthesia is used in more than half of my adult patients. In addition the advantages mentioned above, local anesthesia makes it easier to plan the operative program, with greater independence of the hospital's anesthetics service and thus better resource utilization. Today's trend towards very short hospital stays, or even outpatient treatment, for middle-ear surgery favors the use of local anesthesia.

Local Anesthesia

Preoperative Sedation

With local anesthesia, surgeons themselves should usually order the medication for patients who are to undergo surgery under local anesthesia. There are many methods of premedication. For adults with a weight more than 40 kg we use morphine–scopolamine (0.4 mg scopolaminebromide, one 10 mg morphinechloride per mL) to be injected intramusculary one hour before the operation in a dosage correlating to the patient's weight and age:

41– 50 kg	0.7 mL
51– 60 kg	0.8 mL
61– 70 kg	0.9 mL
71– 80 kg	1.1 mL
81– 90 kg	1.2 mL
91–100 kg	1.4 mL

The dosage is reduced by 25% in those between 60 and 70 years of age and by 50% in those older than 70 years.

Plester uses 0.5 mg flunitrazepam + 0.5 mg atropine, injected intramuscularly 30–40 minutes before local anesthesia. Immediately before local anesthesia, possible additional sedation with 0.2 mg flunitrazepam can be given intravenously. Deep sedation should already be in effect at the start of the operation, since intraoperative sedation is difficult or even impossible in a patient who is in a state of excitement. Intravenous administration of

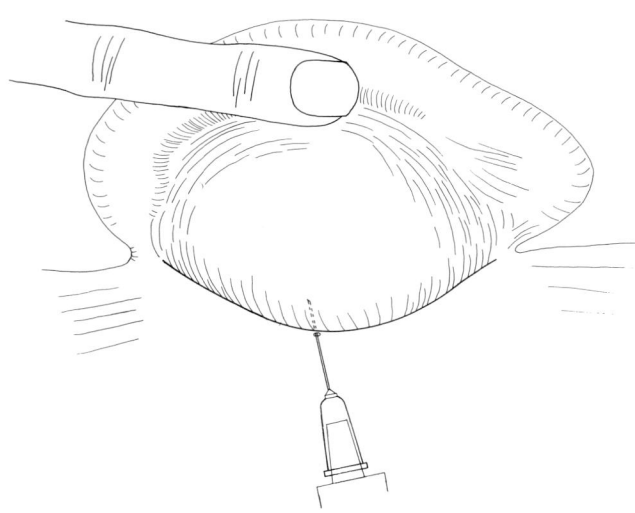

Fig. 3 **The Plester local anesthesia technique**, step 1: injecting lidocaine into the retroauricular fold

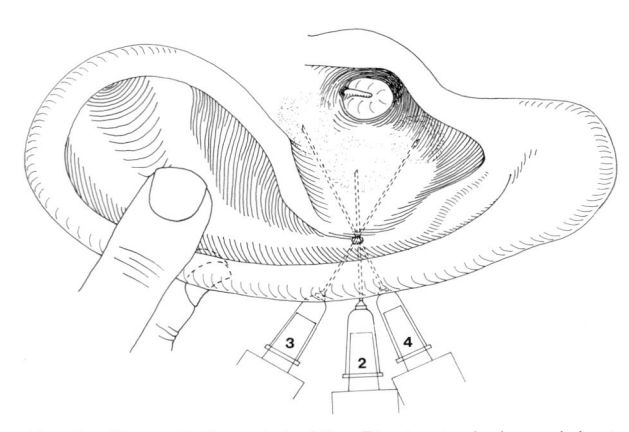

Fig. 4 Steps 2, 3, and 4 of the Plester technique, injecting lidocaine with the same needle posteriorly, inferiorly, and superiorly under the ear-canal skin

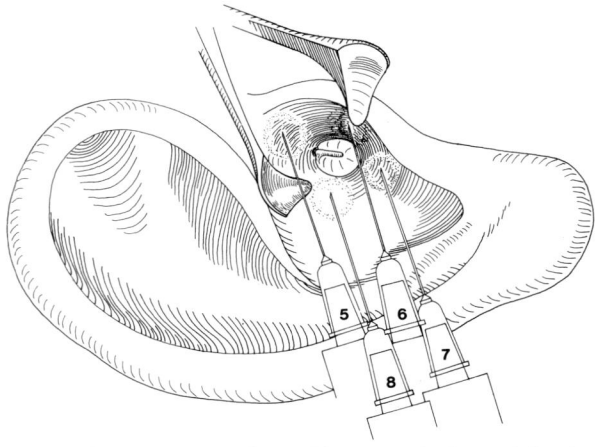

Fig. 5 Steps 5 to 8 of the Plester technique, injecting lidocaine through the ear canal subperiosteally at the 12-o'clock, 3-o'clock, 6-o'clock, and 9-o'clock positions

0.2 mg flunitrazepam can be repeated during the operation if necessary, but the maximal total dosage of 1.5 mg should not be exceeded without control of respiration.

Some other surgeons (Wolferman) use diazepam instead of flunitrazepam.

Complications of premedication are unexpected sedation and loss of consciousness, with a risk of respiratory depression. The patient should be checked during intraoperative and postoperative sedation, and particular attention should be given to the position of the jaw and the tongue.

Local Anesthetic Techniques

The majority of surgeons use 1% lidocaine (Xylocaine) with 5 µg epinephrine (adrenaline) per 1 mL 1% lidocaine. Plester uses a relatively high concentration of epinephrine (1:1000 per 1 mL 1% lidocaine), but the patient is continuously monitored using electrocardiography. Due to the high concentration of epinephrine, Plester uses maximally 3–5 mL of 1% lidocaine. Wolferman uses 2% lidocaine with ephedrine 1:100,000, usually no more than 8 mL. The techniques used to inject the local anesthetic vary between surgeons.

Plester technique. Very little anesthetic is used, but it should be introduced precisely in eight steps:

Step 1. The concha is pulled anteriorly, and 0.5 mL of 1% lignocaine is jected in the postauricular fold region (Fig. 3).

Step 2. The same needle is introduced subcutaneously under the posterior ear-canal skin, and 0.5 mL lidocaine is injected (Fig. 4). A pale prominence in the posterior canal skin wall will be visible.

Step 3. The same needle is introduced through the same original point in an inferior direction, towards the inferior wall of the ear canal, and 0.5 mL lidocaine is injected.

Step 4. The same needle is introduced towards the superior wall of the ear canal, and 0.5 mL lidocaine is injected (Fig. 4).

Steps 5–8. The external meatus is opened by the nose speculum, and 0.3 mL lidocaine is injected superiorly at the 12-o'clock position, anteriorly at the 3-o'clock position inferiorly at the 6-o'clock position, and posteriorly at the 9-o'clock position (Fig. 5). The lumen of the needle points towards the bone, and the lidocaine is injected subperiosteally

(Fig. **6**). The ear-canal skin becomes white and prominent around the injection point.

The infiltration of the anterior ear canal is especially important because of the anesthesia of the meatal nerve deriving from the auriculotemporal nerve. By infiltrating the posterior ear-canal skin, the ramus auricularis of the vagal nerve is anesthetized. The lidocaine injection should be carried out slowly, avoiding vesicles, hematomas, and ruptures of the canal skin.

If any pain occurs during work on the middle ear mucosa, supported by the tympanic plexus, the medial wall of the tympanic cavity can be anesthetized using Gelfoam balls moistened in a 4% tetracaine solution.

Wullstein technique. To anesthetize mastoid region Wullstein prefers an injection 2–3 cm behind the postauricular fold, infiltrating the mastoid surface subcutaneously. Using the same injection point the superior and inferior attachments of the auricle are anesthetized, as well as the region around the ear canal (Fig. **7**). Topical anesthesia of the mucosa using tetracaine can be repeated several times during the operation.

Jonkees technique. Jongkees (1982) prefers three injection points for a retroauricular approach (Fig. **8**). Lidocaine at 1%, with 1:1000 epinephrine, is infiltrated subcutaneously in the mastoid region and around the ear canal.

For the Heermann or Lempert endaural approach, Jongkees starts with an injection anteriorly to the tragus (Fig. **9**), followed by a second injection anteriorly to the helix, and then an injection around the ear canal at the 12, 9, 6, and 3-o'clock positions, respectively.

To harvest the temporalis muscle fascia in an endaural approach with the ear speculum, using a separate incision superiorly to the auricle, a separate local infiltration of the skin with 1% lidocaine is performed just before local anesthesia of the ear region starts.

To harvest conchal cartilage or conchal pericondrium in an endaural approach, separate local anesthesia of the posterior surface of the auricle is performed (Fig. **10**).

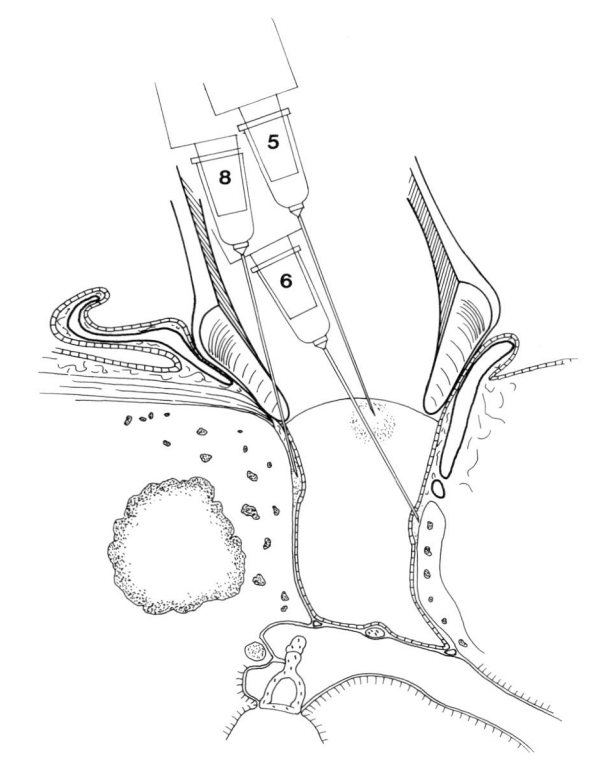

Fig. **6** Side view of the ear canal, illustrating the subperiosteal injections superiorly at the 12-o'clock position (step 5), anteriorly at the 3-o'clock position (step 6), and posteriorly at the 9-o'clock position (step 8)

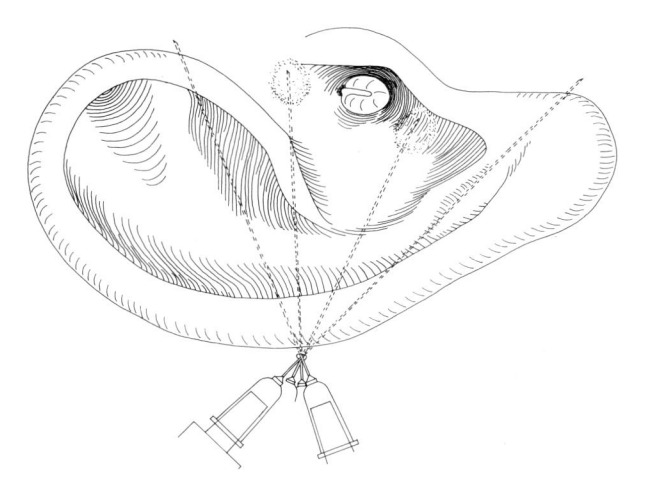

Fig. **7 The Wullstein local anesthesia technique** for mastoidectomy, with the injection point 2–3 cm behind the retroauricular fold

Fig. 8

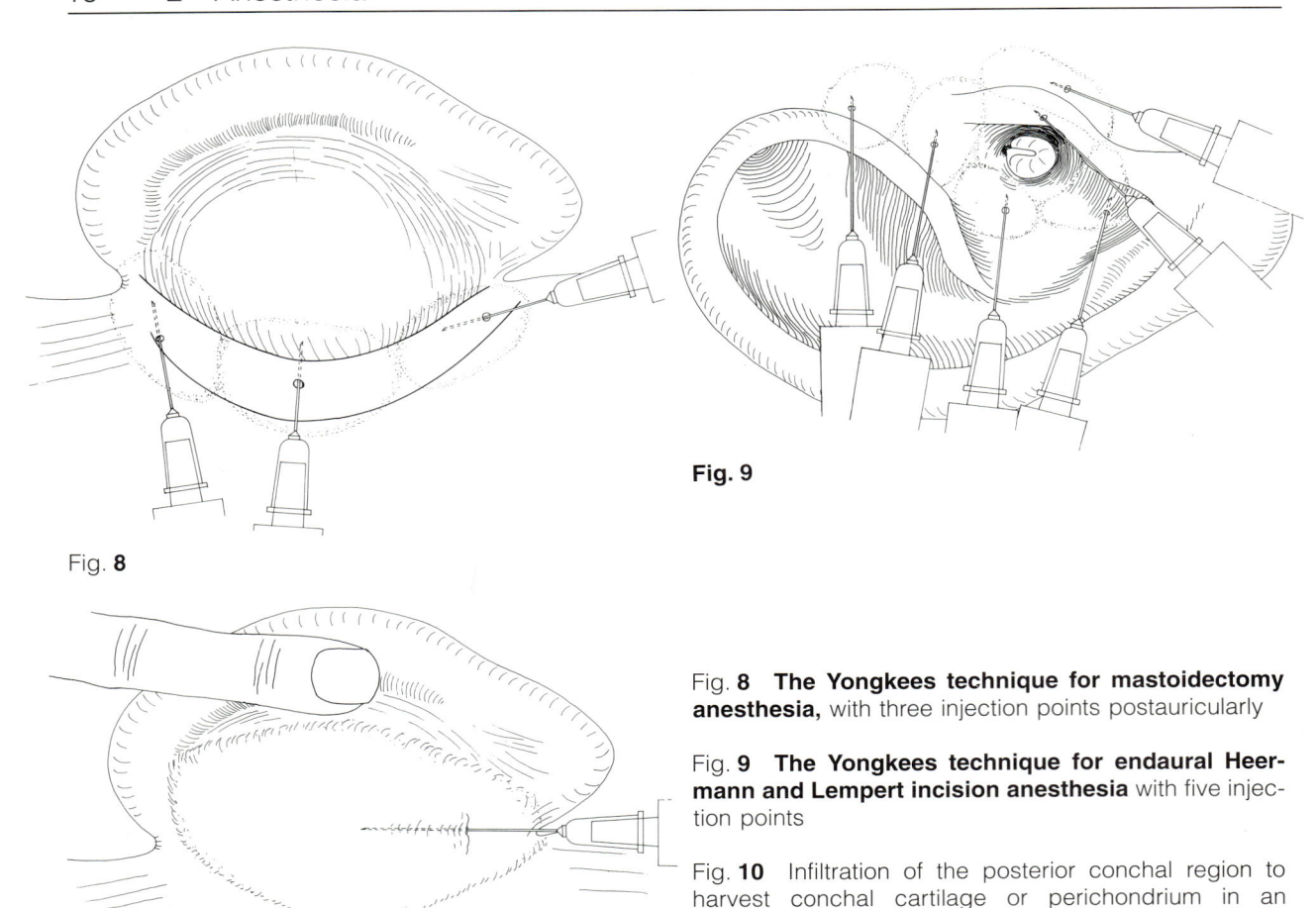

Fig. 9

Fig. 10

Fig. **8 The Yongkees technique for mastoidectomy anesthesia,** with three injection points postauricularly

Fig. **9 The Yongkees technique for endaural Heermann and Lempert incision anesthesia** with five injection points

Fig. **10** Infiltration of the posterior conchal region to harvest conchal cartilage or perichondrium in an endaural approach

General Anesthesia

As mentioned above, general anesthesia is used in our department for all mastoidectomies, for extensive and long-lasting procedures, and for children. Our anesthetics department uses the following method of general endotracheal anesthesia: if the patient is otherwise healthy, only routine preoperative tests are receommended. Oral diazepam is most often given for premedication. Following diazepam/ barbiturate induction and muscular relaxation with suxamethonium, the trachea is intubated. Anesthesia is maintained with nitrous oxide in oxygen and moderate dosage of a narcotic. A nondepolarizing neuromuscular blocker is used for muscular relaxation, and enflurane is given to secure sleep and maintain blood pressure at a low normal level. We do not use any hypotension anesthesia for middle-ear surgery. Usually, some local anesthesia with lidocaine and epinephrine is given at the beginning of the operation, and mucosal bleeding is controlled by Gelfoam balls moistened in an epinephrine solution.

When the drum is grafted, administration of nitrous oxide is stopped for a period, but this is seldom really necessary. Usually a slit can be left to let the gases escape during the fixation of the graft, and the slit is closed at the very end of the operation. After the operation, the patient is extubated in the operating room, and remains in the recovery room for a couple of hours.

3 Endaural Approach

In the endaural, or transmeatal, or transcanal approach, the instruments pass through the introitus and the lateral part of the external auditory meatus, which can either remain intact during the surgery, but has to be stretched by an ear speculum, or can be more or less widened using various incisions.

Widening of the external auditory meatus depends on pathological conditions, on the purpose of the surgery, on myringoplasty or tympanoplasty techniques, and on a need to open the attic, antrum, or mastoid process.

Ear Speculum

There are two types of ear speculum, selfretaining and fixed.

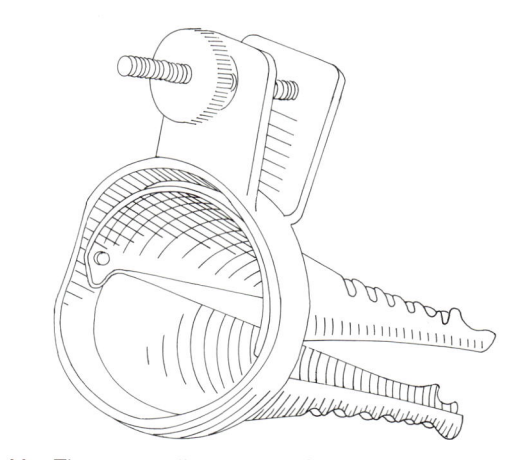

Fig. 11 The expanding and selfretaining ear speculum (Holmgreen-Plester)

Selfretaining Ear Speculum

After being placed in the external auditory meatus, the two blades of the selfretaining and expanding speculum (Holmgren-Plester, Fig. 11) are expanded by a screw arrangement, and thus fixing the speculum into place in the meatus.

The advantages of this speculum are that the tilting needed to change the visualization of the operating field is easy to do, and that it does not need any special arrangements for fixation. There is no external fixation of the speculum. The disadvantage of this speculum is that its intrameatal fixation is neither solid nor stable. During surgery and manipulation with instruments the speculum may tilt and mobilize, causing damage to the meatal skin, producing disturbing bleeding. Today, the expanding speculum is relatively seldom used in tympanoplasty.

Fixed Ear Speculum

The nonexpanding and fixed ear speculum is commonly used. A set of Richards specula ranging from the smallest, with a diameter of 4 mm, increasing by 0.5 mm to the largest, with a diameter of 8 mm, is commercially available through Smith and Nephew-Richards Company (Fig. 12). The speculum is held in place by various holders, which are fixed to the operating table. The Richards speculum

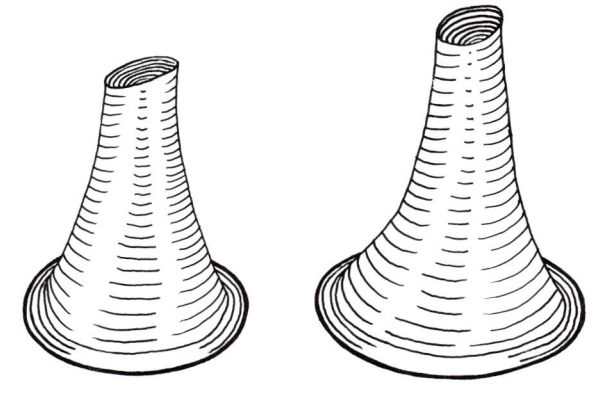

Fig. 12 The nonexpanding, fixed ear specula. Long speculum (right) and short speculum (left)

holder (Fig. 13) adapts to any standard ear speculum (Fig. 14) and fits into the sliding bar on the edge of the operating table. A special arrangement allows movement in the superoinferior and anteroposterior directions, and rotation as well. A modification of the Richards speculum holder is Schuknecht's speculum holder. Both holders allow the speculum to be fixed in any position. The holders mentioned are fixed at the operating table in front of the patient's head (Figs. 13–18).

Another type of speculum holder, the universal speculum holder, available from Xomed-Treace

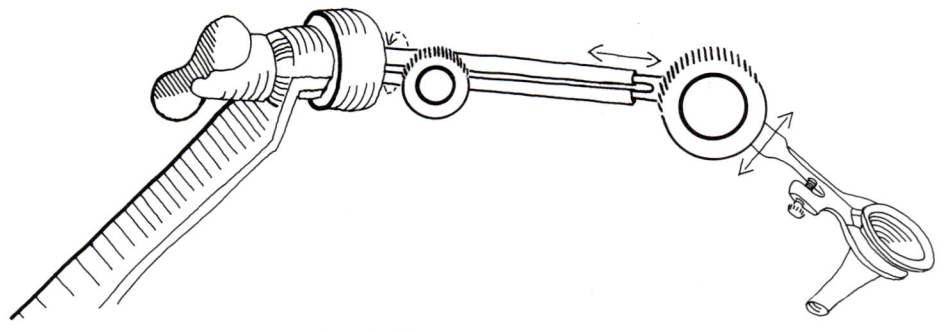

Fig. 13 The Richards speculum holder

company (Fig. **16**), is fixed to the operating table behind the patient's head. The holder arm is flexible, and is easily positioned in the desired configuration to retain the speculum in the ear canal. It can then be made semirigid by turning the large end knob. A slight amount of flexibility is left, to provide the surgeon with a limited amount of necessary adjustment.

After squeezing the largest possible ear speculum into the external auditory meatus and fixation of the speculum, a good overall view of the entire drum can be obtained in cases with a very wide and straight ear canal (Figs. **14, 18**), but often the position of the speculum has to be changed during myringoplasty of the subtotal or total perforation. When working superiorly in the tympanic cavity, the entire speculum holder can easily be tilted by pressing it towards the inferior meatal cartilage (the antitragus) (Fig. **19**). To visualize the hypotympanum, the speculum holder, with the speculum, is moved in the opposite direction (Fig. **20**).

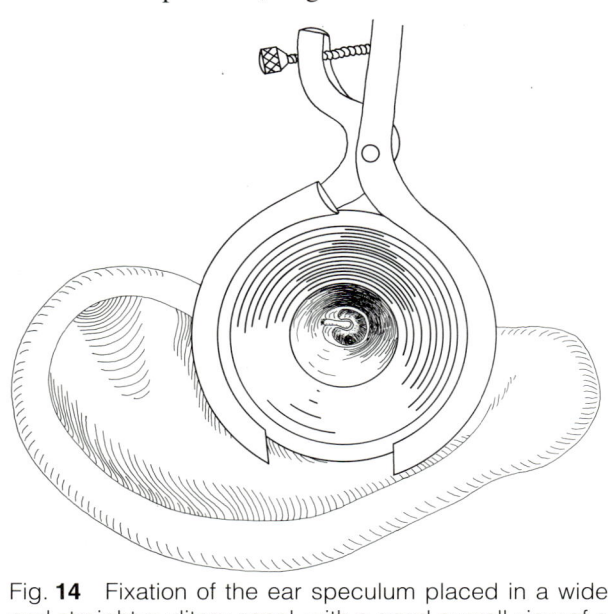

Fig. 14 Fixation of the ear speculum placed in a wide and straight auditory canal, with a good overall view of a subtotal ear-drum perforation

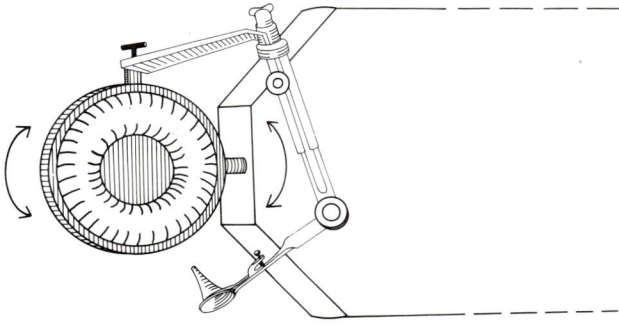

Fig. 15 Operating table, with fixation of the ear speculum holder to the table

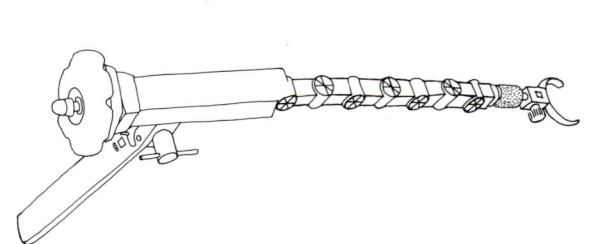

Fig. 16 The Treace speculum holder

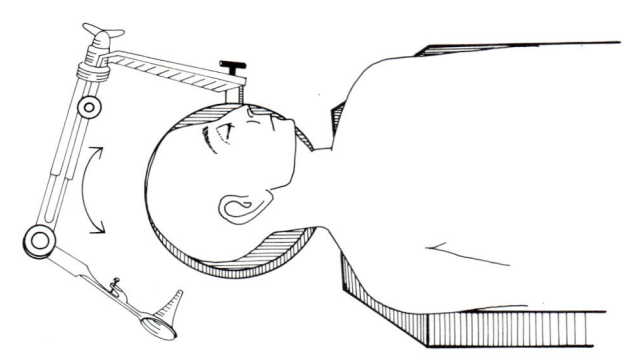

Fig. 17 Placement of the patient on the operating table

Fig. **18** Superoinferior cross-section through the ear canal with the ear speculum

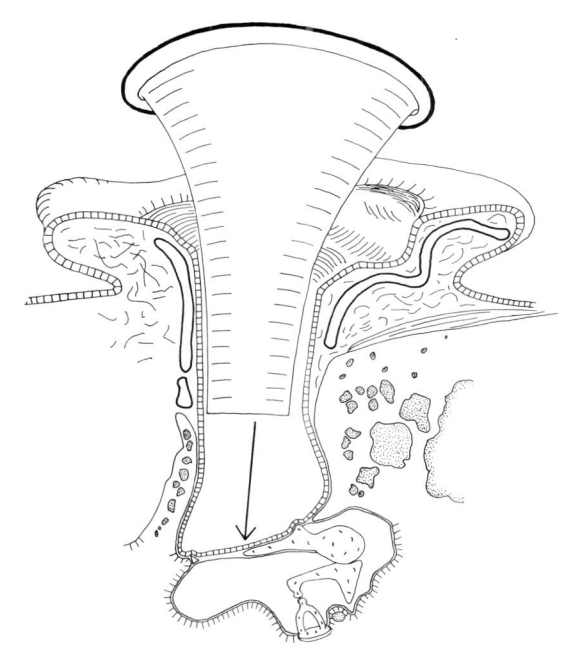

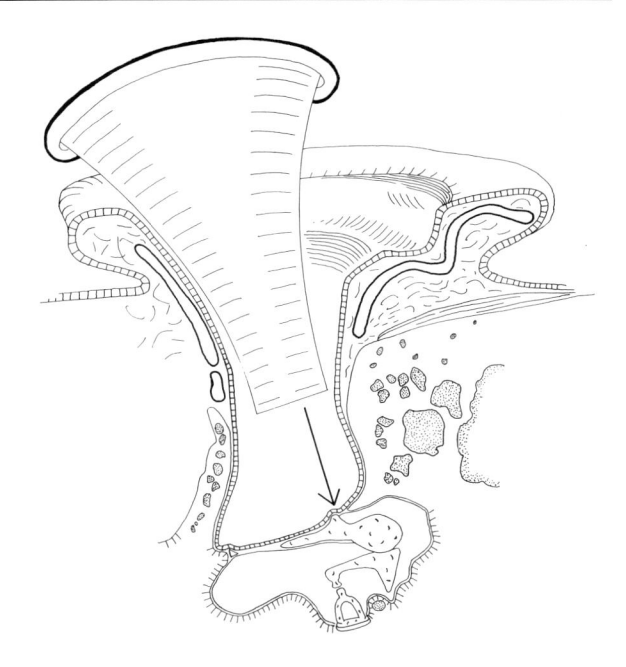

Fig. **19** The speculum is tilted toward the superior part of the drum

The speculum is of considerable value in surgery in the posterior tympanum, and none of the other approaches can provide a view of the posterior tympanum as good and convenient as that of the endaural approach using the ear speculum. By pressing the speculum on the very mobile tragal cartilage, it can be moved far anteriorly while the operating table is rotated towards the surgeon (Figs. **21, 22**). In cases with anterior pathology, an adequate view towards the anterior tympanomeatal angle can often—but not always—be obtained by tilting the speculum (Fig. **23**) an rotating the operating table away from the surgeon.

In some ears with an extremely narrow external meatus, a small intercartilaginous incision at the 12-o'clock position through the fibrous subcutaneous tissue to the temporalis muscle fascia is necessary in order to squeeze a sufficiently large speculum through the meatus (Fig. **24**).

The entire operating table should be able to rotate towards and away from the surgeon and move up and down as well as in the Trendelenburg or anti-Trendelenburg positions. The combination of rotation of the operating table and tilting of the speculum provides a good view of all regions of the tympanic cavity, including the tympanic orifice of the Eustachian tube (Figs. **15, 20**).

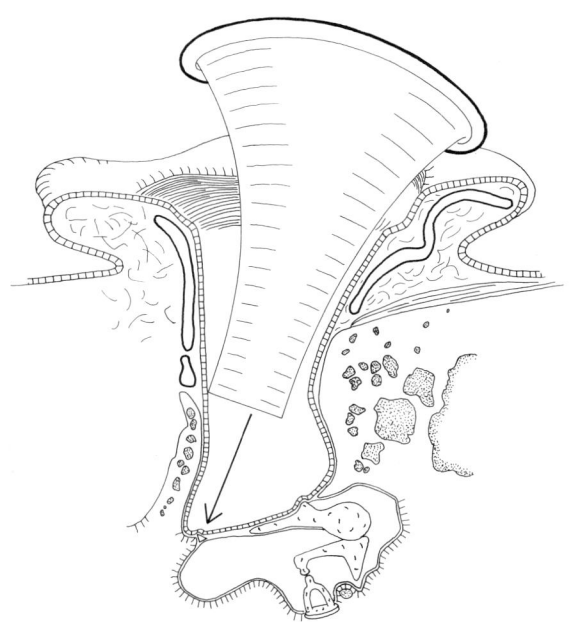

Fig. **20** The speculum is tilted toward the inferior half of the drum

14   3 Endaural Approach

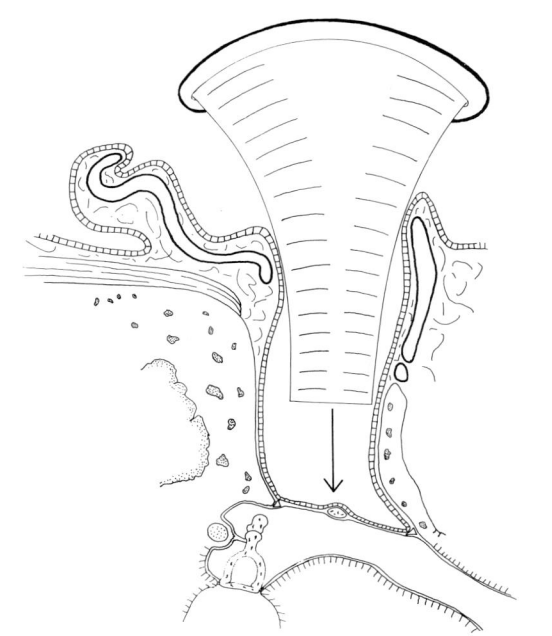

Fig. 21 Anteroposterior cross-section of the ear canal with the ear speculum

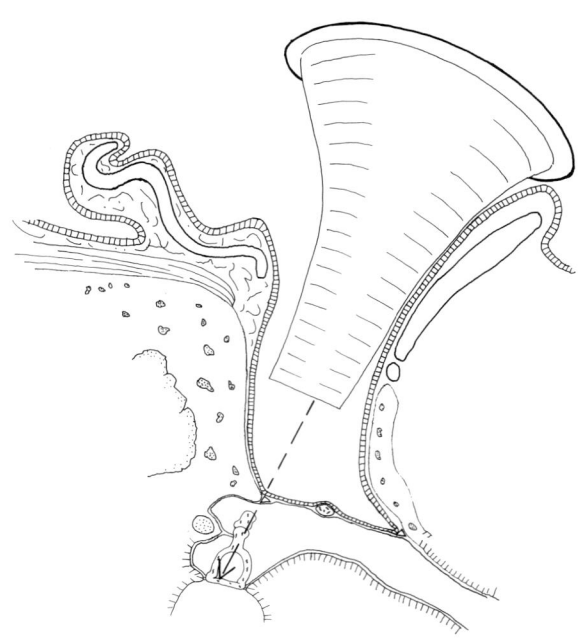

Fig. 22 The ear speculum is tilted toward the posterior part of the drum

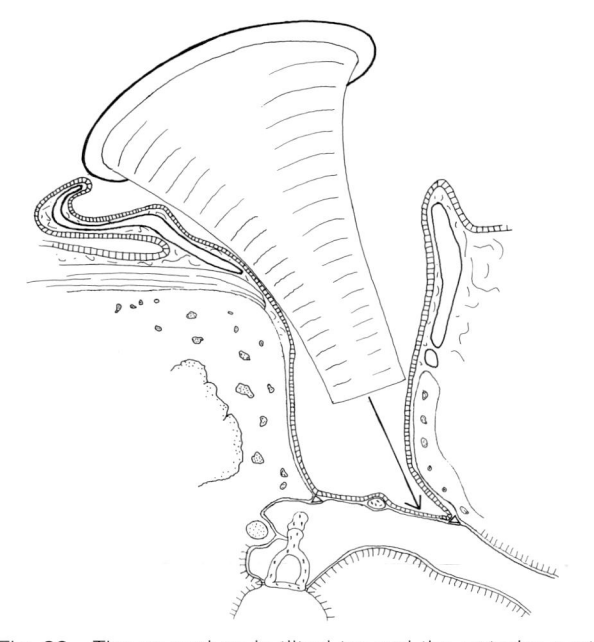

Fig. 23 The speculum is tilted toward the anterior part of the drum

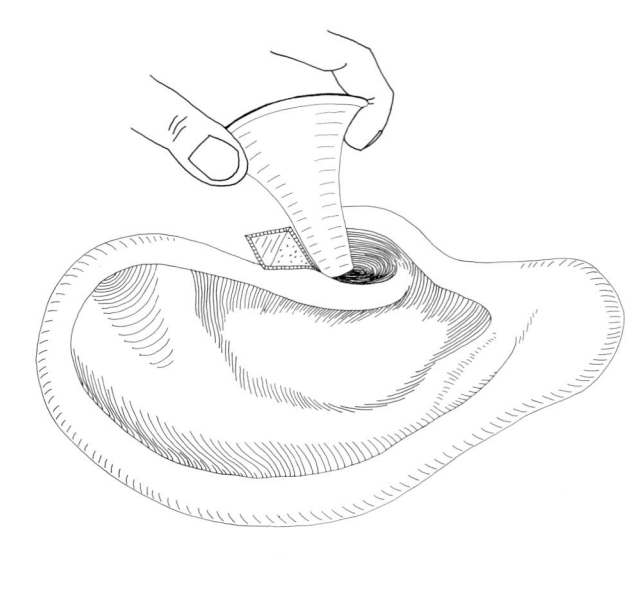

Fig. 24 A small intercartilaginous incision through the fibrous subcutaneous tissue in a extremely narrow ear canal, in order to squeeze the speculum through the meatus

Application

The endaural route through the ear speculum is highly recommended in all stapes surgery, all ears with posttraumatic or postinfectious conductive deafness with an intact drum, posterior perforation of the drum, posterior retraction and adhesive otitis, small sinus tympani cholesteatoma with posterosuperior perforation of the pars tensa, and also in ears with total and anterior perforations with a visible perforation edge.

The use of the ear speculum is highly recommended in tympanoplasty in children. Even if the auditory canal in children is narrow, it is worthwhile to operate through the speculum without incising the ear-canal skin, which may later lead to stenosis of the introitus of the meatus. The great *advantage* of surgery through the speculum is the excellent visibility of the posterior tympanum it provides, with no disturbing bleeding from the wound edges, no postoperative care of the auditory meatus, which remains intact, and no risk of any stenosis of the auditory meatus.

For patients who will still need a hearing aid after the operation, the endaural approach through the speculum is the approach of choice. With the increasing age of patients undergoing middle-ear surgery, the number of patients with a preoperative or postoperative hearing aid is increasing. The following categories of patients are candidates for a postoperative hearing aid: 1) Patients with preoperative sensorineural deafness due to various causes, including presbyacusis combined with some conductive hearing loss, with or without drum perforation. Some of these patients already have hearing aids before the operation, and will still need one oven after fully successful tympanoplasty. 2) Patients with insufficient hearing improvement of conductive hearing loss.

Any surgery of the meatus will delay fitting for a hearing-aid, and postoperative changes in the ear canal may later cause the ear mold to fail to seal.

The *disadvantage* of the endaural route through the speculum is the sense of restricted space during surgery, especially for beginners in middle-ear surgery. The need for frequent adjustment of the ear speculum, and poor access to the anterior tympanum and the bony part of the Eustachian tube in some cases, are additional disadvantages.

Intercartilaginous (Heermann) A and B Incisions

Instead of an ear speculum, the introitus of the auditory meatus is widened by a skin incision and a blunt selfretaining retractor. The intercartilaginous (anterior) incisura is located at the 12-o'clock position in the meatus, between the tragal cartilage and the helix cartilage (Fig. **25**). It can be widened considerably by pulling the auricle and concha cartilage posteriorly and the tragal cartilage anteriorly (Fig. **26**).

The intercartilaginous incision should be performed with accuracy under an operating microscope. The auricle is pulled posteriorly by the surgeon's fingers, and the tragus is pulled anteriorly with a blunt speculum held by a scrub nurse or the assistant. A nasal speculum can also be used to spread the meatal introitus before the Heermann incision.

The intercartilaginous incision starts with a scalpel in the bony part of the external auditory canal at the 12-o'clock position, at a point 6 mm lateral to Shrapnell's membrane, and continues laterally on the bone towards the meatus and through the stretched intercartilaginous (anterior) incisura (Fig. **27**). After leaving the introitus of the

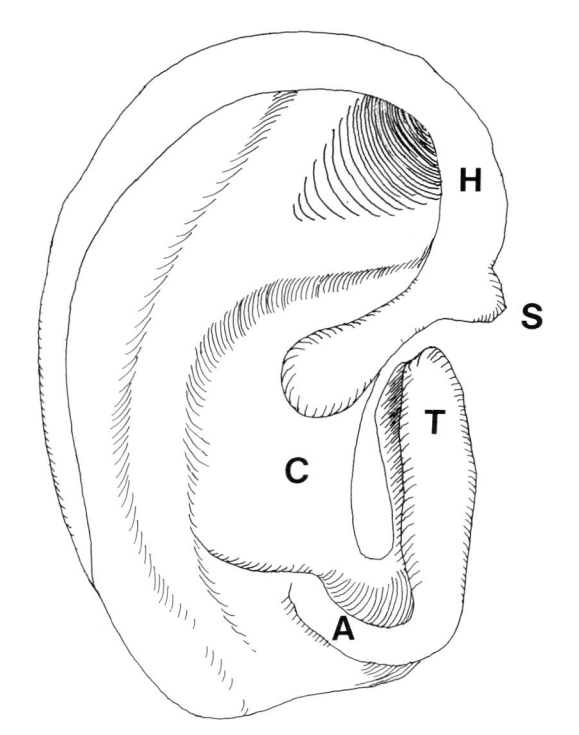

Fig. **25** The cartilaginous auricle, with the helix (H), the spine of the helix (S), the tragus (T) and antitragus, (A) and the conchal cartilage (C)

external auditory meatus, it follows the edge of the crus of the helix upwards for about 1.5 cm (Heermann A), or continues upwards another 1–1.5 cm (Heermann B) (Fig. 27), and it ends when the helix changes direction to become horizontal. If the incision is made correctly, cutting through the cartilage of the helix or the tragus will be avoided. Inside the bony canal, the incision should be brought down to the bone. Outside the canal, it should remain superficial, leaving the temporalis muscle fascia intact. However, the thin anterior auricular muscle has to be cut.

In the Heermann A incision, cutting of the anterior auricular vein and artery which arise from the superficial temporal vein and artery (Fig. 27) can be avoided, but the size of the fascia that can be obtained through this incision will be small. The Heermann A incision is therefore used only in myringoplasty for small perforations, in cases with an intact drum, and by some surgeons in stapedectomy (Figs. 28, 29).

In the majority of tympanoplasty cases with an endaural approach, the Heermann B incision has to be performed (Figs. 30, 31), and the anterior auricular vessels have to be coagulated by bipolor coagulation and divided.

In order to mobilize the auricle, allowing opening of the ear canal by the intercartilaginous incision, an incision along the lower edge of the tem-

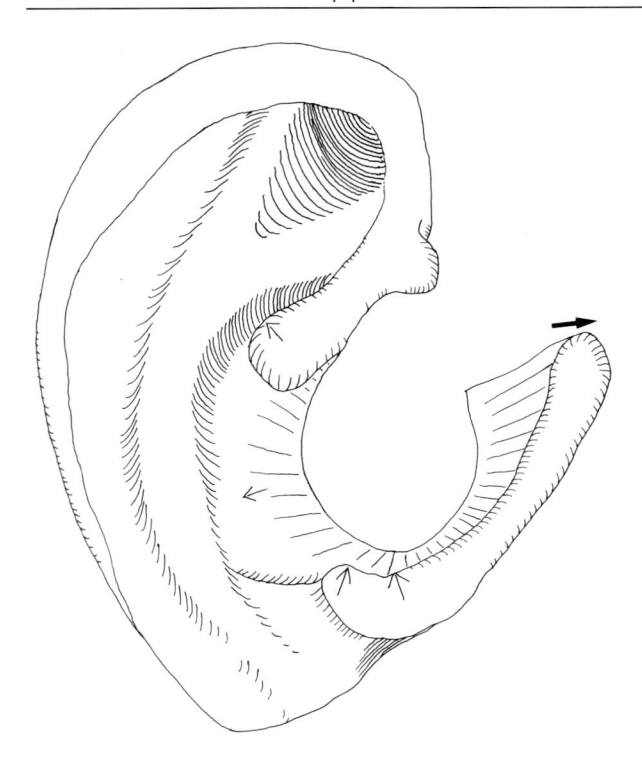

Fig. 26 Using traction with holders, the intercartilaginous incision is widened. The tragal and conchal cartilage move outwards, but the antitragal cartilage moves superiorly, often hampering the view (arrow)

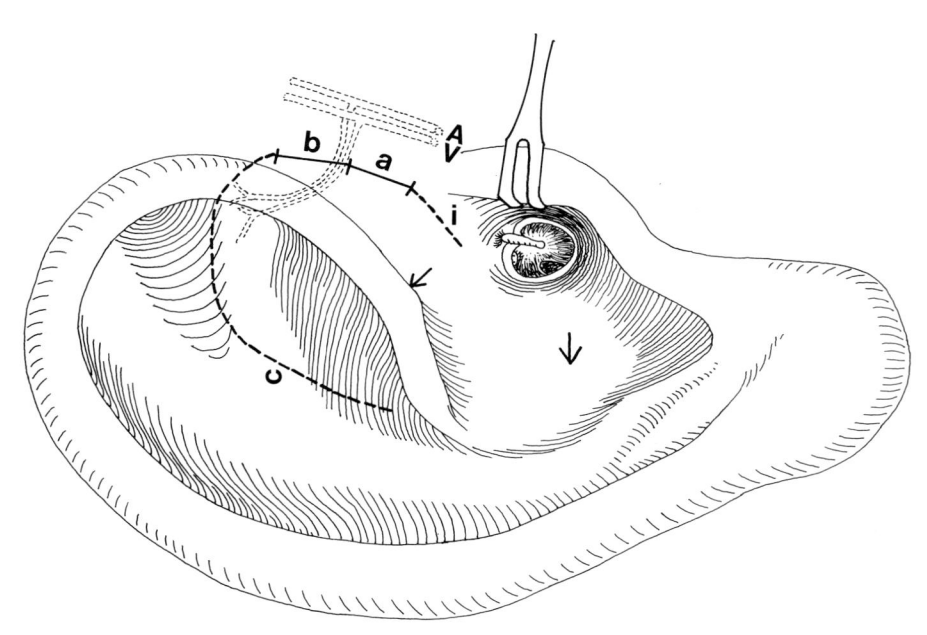

Fig. 27 **The Heermann A, B, and C endaural incisions** and placement of the intercartilaginous incision (i); posterior movement of the helix and the concha (arrows)
A Superficial temporal artery

Intercartilaginous (Heermann) A and B Incisions

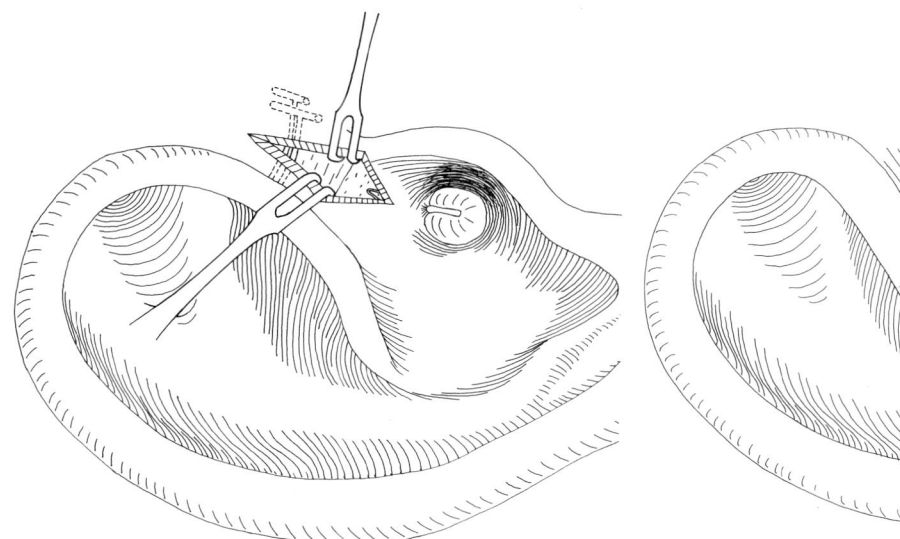

Fig. 28 **The Heermann A incision**

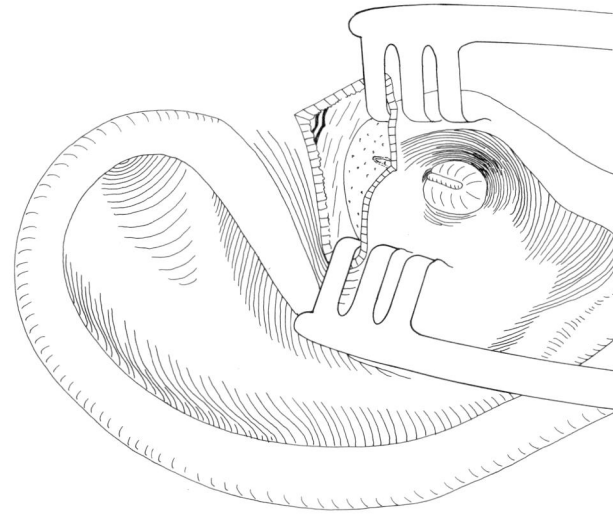

Fig. 29 A selfretaining speculum in place in a Heermann A incision

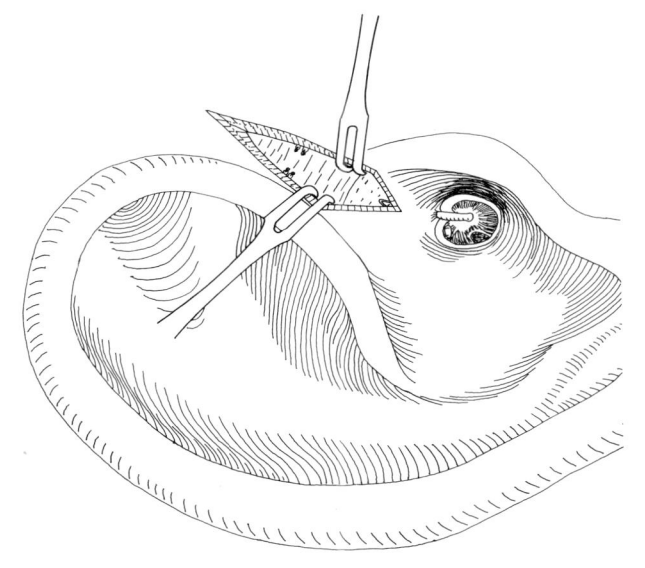

Fig. 30 **The Heermann B incision**

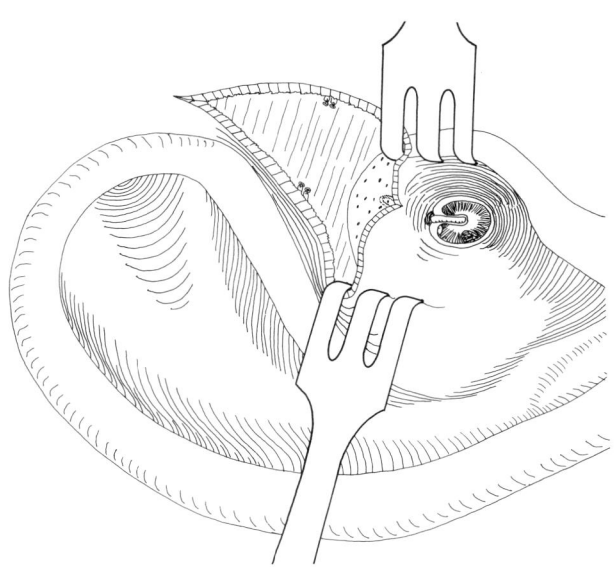

Fig. 31 Temporalis muscle fascia exposed in a Heermann B incision

poralis muscle has to be performed using a knife (Fig. **32**) or a pair of scissors.

There are several modifications of the endaural approach using the Heermann incision. These relate to:

1. The presence and placement of the circumferential incision of the posterior ear-canal skin, and the size of the tympanomeatal flap.
2. The management of the lateral part of the ear-canal skin (left in place, displaced inferiorly, laterally, or medially, and partially or totally removed).
3. The size and extension of the intercartilaginous incision outside the auditory meatus (vertical incision). Heermann divided the external skin incision into: incision A, extending 1.5 cm upwards, incision B, extending approximately 2.5 cm upwards, and incision C, continuing backwards around the attachment of the auricle (Fig. **27**).

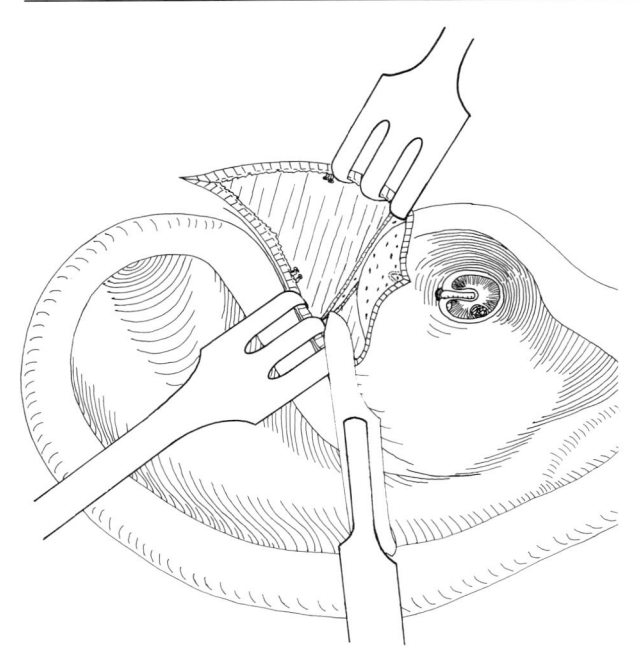

Fig. 32 The lower edge of the temporalis muscle has been cut by a knife

No Tympanomeatal Flap

No circumferential skin incision in the posterior canal-wall skin is performed, and there is no tympanomeatal flap (Fig. 29). The Heermann A incision is held in place by a blunt, selfretaining retractor. This type of approach can be used for myringoplasty in ears with minor central perforations when there is no intention of exploring the tympanic cavity.

Small Tympanomeatal Flap

Using a medially-placed circumferential (Rosen) incision from the 12 to 6-o'clock positions, a small tympanomeatal flap is created (Fig. 33). The circular incision is placed independently of the intercartilaginous incision. This approach is used in stapedectomy and in tympanoplasty cases with an intact drum. After tympanotomy, the tympanomeatal flap is pushed anteriorly. The size of the flap depends on the purpose of the tympanotomy. If the incudostapedial joint is visible, major removal of the bony annulus will not be necessary, and the flap can be small, approximately 4 mm. If there is deep posterior retraction or adhesive otitis, the tympanomeatal flap should be large, approximately 6–7 mm, to cover the defect of the posterior bony annulus that may arise ofter removal of the bony annulus.

In cases with closure of a drum perforation by endaural approach, either with onlay or underlay grafting techniques, the placement of the circumferential incision differs in various myringoplasty methods. The circular incision can be placed close to the annulus, and the small tympanomeatal flap with the annulus will be cut at the 9-o'clock position, making a small superior and inferior skin flap (Fig. 34).

All myringoplasties and tympanoplasties that do not require surgery in the attic, antrum, or mastoid process can be carried out using the endaural approach with an intercartilaginous incision and formation of a tympanomeatal flap.

Lateral Displacement of the Canal Skin

Circumferential incision with lateral dissection of the posterior canal wall skin without a radial incision at the 6-o'clock position is a common modification of the Heermann incision. For endaural surgery in the attic and antrum, the bone of the superoposterior wall of the auditory canal should be exposed. For mastoidectomy, more space will be needed. After completion of the Heermann B incision (Fig. 35), a medial circumferential incision of the posterior canal wall skin from the 12-o'clock to 6-o'clock positions, localized about 4 mm lateral to the annulus, is performed with a round, angled incision knife. The circumferential incision is connected to the intercartilaginous incision, and the skin flap with the periosteum is carefully dissected laterally, exposing the bone of the superior and posterior canal wall, the suprameatal spine (Henle's spine) and the tympanomastoid suture (Fig. 36). Some of the cortical bone of the mastoid process is exposed too. Along the lower border of the temporalis muscle, an incision going through the subcutaneous tissue and the periosteum is performed, to facilitate exposure of the mastoid process.

The size of the tympanomeatal flap, and the localization of the circular incision, depend on the purpose of the tympanoplasty. The flap can be as small as 2 mm, but also considerably larger.

Intercartilaginous (Heermann) A and B Incisions

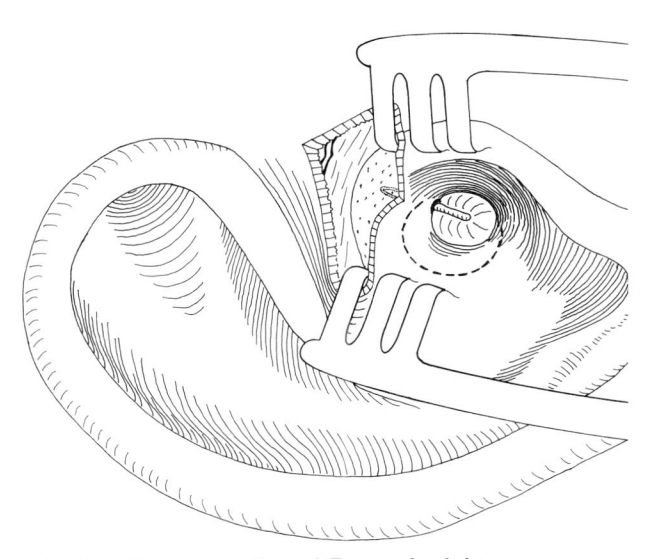

Fig. 33 **Heermann A and Rosen incisions**

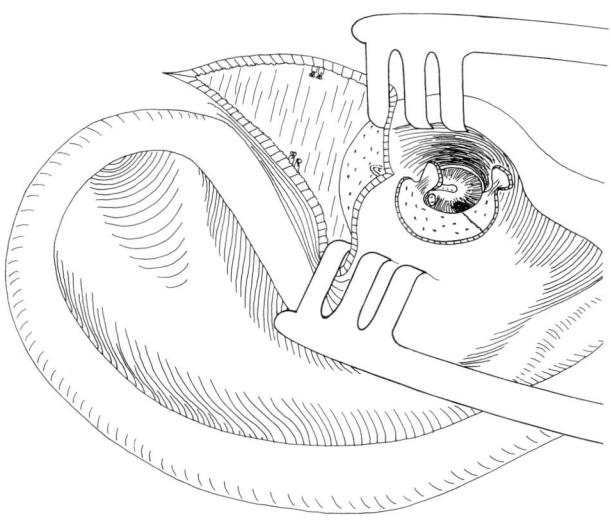

Fig. 34 **A Heermann B incision** with a small tympanomeatal flap created by a separate Rosen incision. The flap is divided by a radial incision at the 9-o'clock position into a superior and an inferior flap

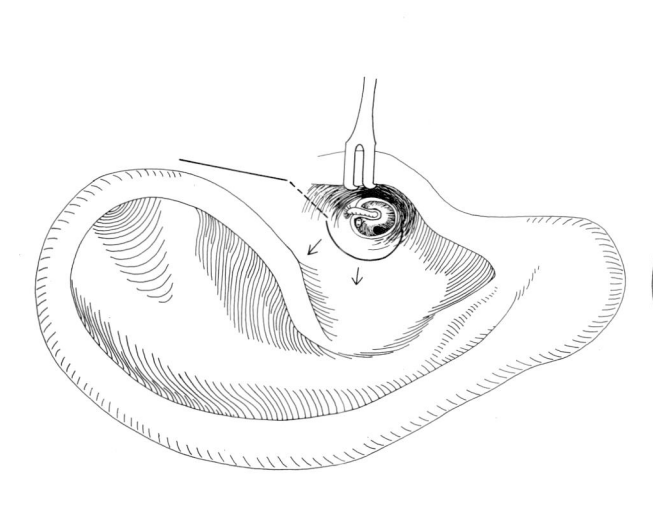

Fig. 35 **A Heermann B incision** with a medial circumferential incision and lateral displacement of the canal skin (arrows)

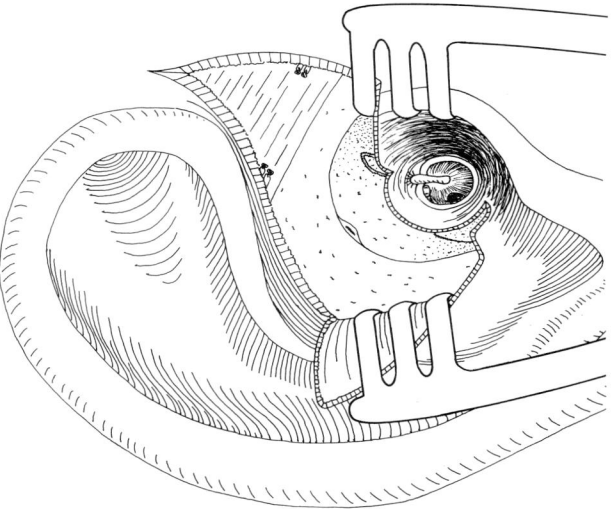

Fig. 36 Elevation of the canal skin outward, and exposure of the bone of the superior and posterior canal wall and mastoid process

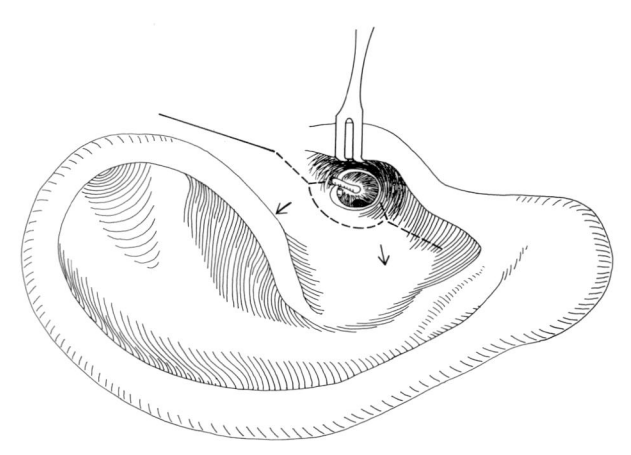

Fig. 37 Heermann B incision, medial circumferential incision, medial radial incision, and lateral radial incision, with displacement of the canal skin outwards (arrows)

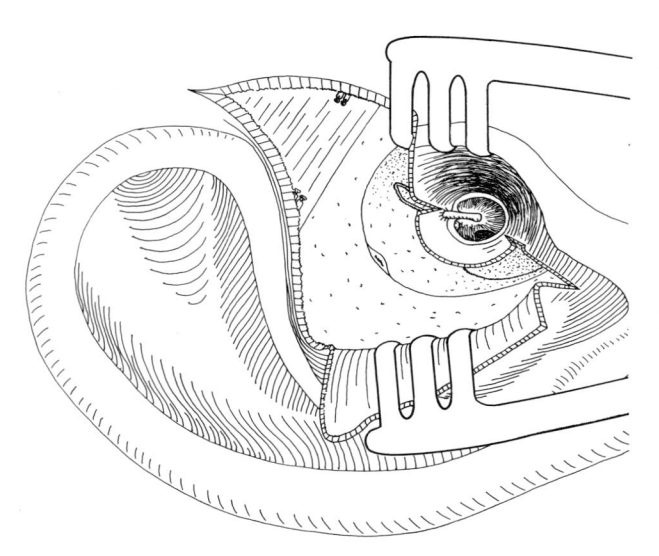

Fig. 38 The canal skin is elevated, and a laterally-based skin flap is held in place, exposing the bone of the ear canal and the mastoid process

Laterally-Based Skin Flap

After completion of the Heermann B incision and a circumferential incision, a medial radial incision at the 6-o'clock position in the ear-canal skin is performed (Fig. 37). The radial incision starts medially, close to the fibrous annulus, with a sickle knife, and continues outwards to the circumferential incision. The lateral radial incision continues towards the conchal cartilage, and from there on can be performed with a scalpel. The skin of the posterior ear-canal wall is carefully dissected outwards with an angled round knife or a curved elevator. After the suprameatal spine is reached, an incision through the subcutaneous tissue and periosteum along the lower border of the temporalis muscle is necessary in order to dissect the periosteum from the bone posteriorly to the suprameatal spine and expose as much of the cortical bone of the mastoid process as possible. The laterally-based skin flap is held in place with a strong selfretaining retractor (Fig. 38). At the superior part of the Heermann B incision, another selfretaining retractor may be needed. After the tympanoplasty, the lateral flap is replaced in the same position in the auditory canal. If the auditory canal wall bone has been removed, the flap will be a valuable part of the reconstruction of the new ear canal or epithelial lining of the cavity.

Large Tympanomeatal Flap

After the Heermann B incision is completed (Fig. 39), a laterally-placed circumferential incision in the posterior canal wall skin is performed with a scalpel. The incision is placed laterally along the bony cartilaginous junction (Fig. 39). This creates a large Surdille flap, which can be elevated towards the fibrous annulus and pushed anteriorly. The flap is still connected inferiorly to the canal-wall skin, which is untouched (Fig. 40), but this connection can be cut by a sickle knife or a scalpel, making the flap more mobile. This type of flap can be too large, and may have to be "hidden" in the anterior tympanomeatal angle during further surgery. The radial incision for the mobilization of the Surdille flap goes at the 6-o'clock position from the lateral circumferential incision towards the annulus.

An incision through the periosteum along the inferior border of the temporalis muscle allows elevation of the periosteum and subcutis, as well as elevating the posterior auricular muscles backwards, and the mastoid process is further exposed. The exposure can be held apart with two selfretaining retractors, one placed inferiorly and the other superiorly, or the temporalis muscle can be held away by one or more surgical stays (Fig. 41).

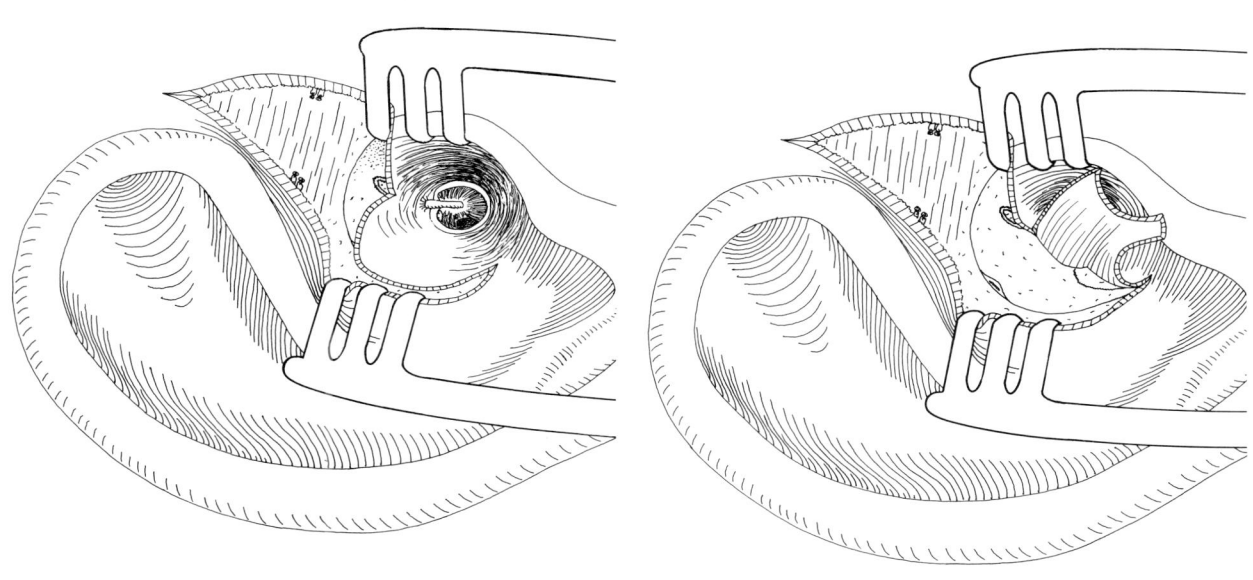

Intercartilaginous (Heermann) A and B Incisions

Fig. **39** A Heermann B incision and a lateral circumferential incision

Fig. **40** The canal skin is elevated, forming a large Surdille flap based inferiorly and medially

The subcutaneous tissue with the periosteum can be excised and used us the free flap for obliteration of the cavity, or as an inferior pedicled subcutis–periosteal flap.

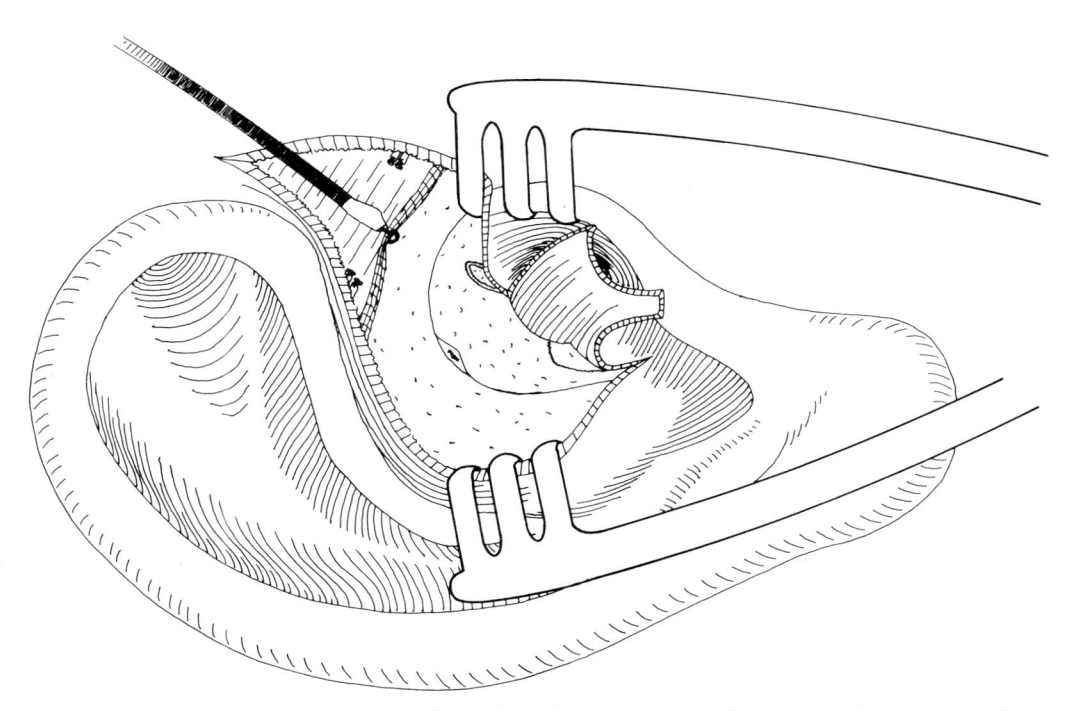

Fig. **41** An incision through the periosteum along the inferior border of the temporalis muscle, which is held in place with a surgical stay

Panse Flap

A large Surdille flap can be reduced in size by an additional circumferential incision running parallel and medial to the previous lateral incision (Fig. 42). By elevating the skin between the two circular incisions in the inferior direction, a small inferior pedicled Panse flap can be developed. Medially, a small Surdille tympanomeatal flap or a large Rosen flap is left behind (Fig. 43).

A large Panse flap can be achieved by a circumferential incision close to the annulus and a medial radial incision at the 12-o'clock position (Figs. 44, 45).

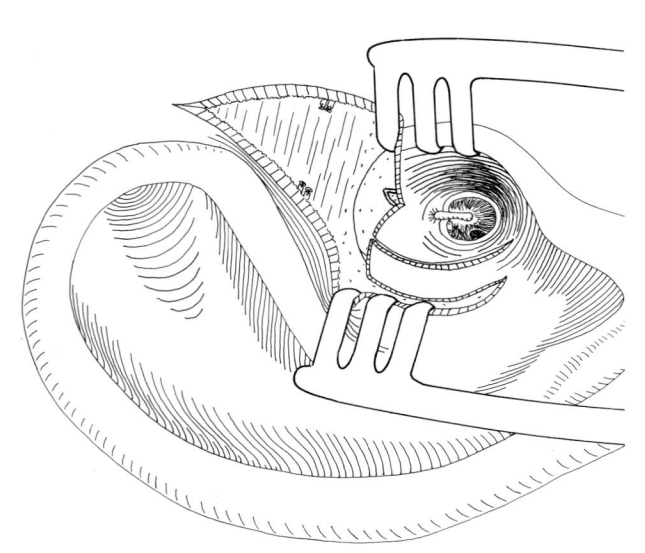

Fig. 42 Formation of a small Panse flap with parallel circumferential incisions

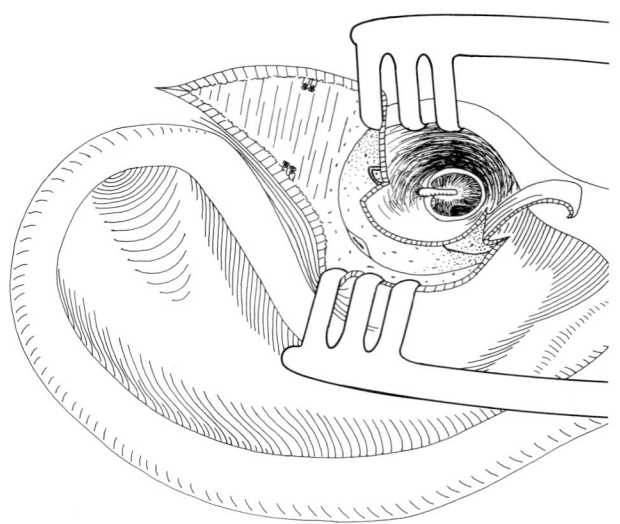

Fig. 43 The skin between the circumferential incisions is elevated, and the Panse flap is based inferiorly

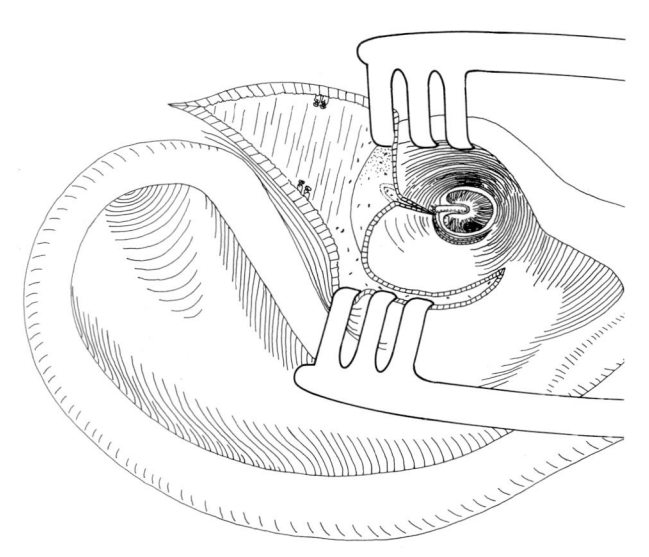

Fig. 44 Formation of large Panse flap using a radial incision at the 12-o'clock position and a circumferential incision close to the annulus

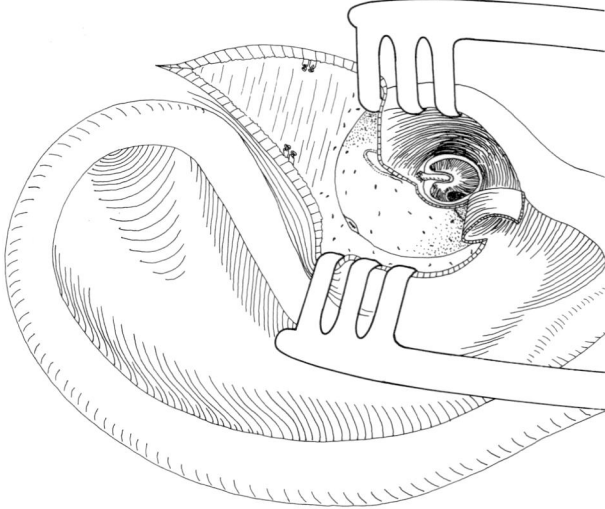

Fig. 45 The skin is elevated, and the large Panse flap is placed inferiorly

Canal Skin Removal

The small Panse flap can be removed by an incision at the 6-o'clock position and stored in Ringer's solution, to be reinserted at the end of the operation, either in the same position or elsewhere in the possible cavity or on the new drum (Fig. 45). The tympanomeatal flap is still attached to the drum.

The large Panse flap (Fig. 45) can easily be removed by scissors, leaving only a small strip of the canal skin along the annulus. After removal of the small Panse flap (Fig. 43), a relatively large tympanomeatal flap will remain in place (Fig. 46).

The Surdille flap can be removed in toto by a radial incision at the 6-o'clock position, elevation of the flap to the annulus, and a circumferential incision along the annulus with the sickle knife (Fig. 47).

In an endaural approach with the Heermann B incision, there is usually enough space to survey the tympanic cavity and, with the modifications described, enough exposure for the atticotomy, atticoantrotomy, conservative radical mastoidectomy or even an extensive radical mastoidectomy. In ears with a large mastoid-cell system, i.e., cells in the sinodural angle or behind the sigmoid sinus, as well as in the apex of the mastoid process, the pathological process cannot be reached using an endaural approach with the Heermann B incision. In such cases, a Heermann C incision is necessary.

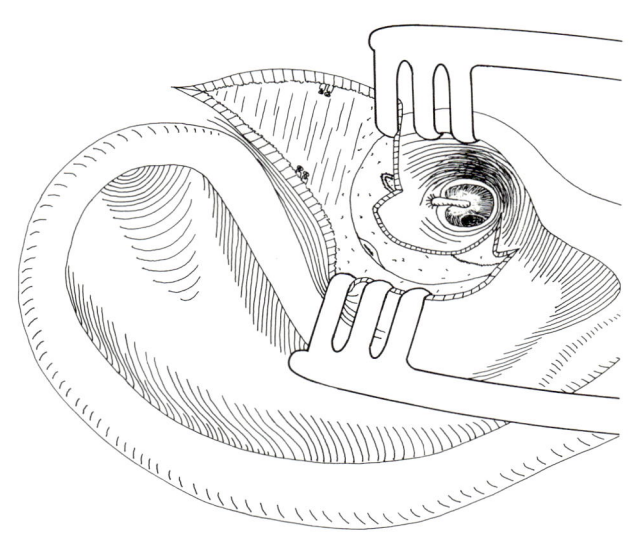

Fig. 46 The small Panse flap has been removed, but the tympanomeatal flap is still attached to the drum

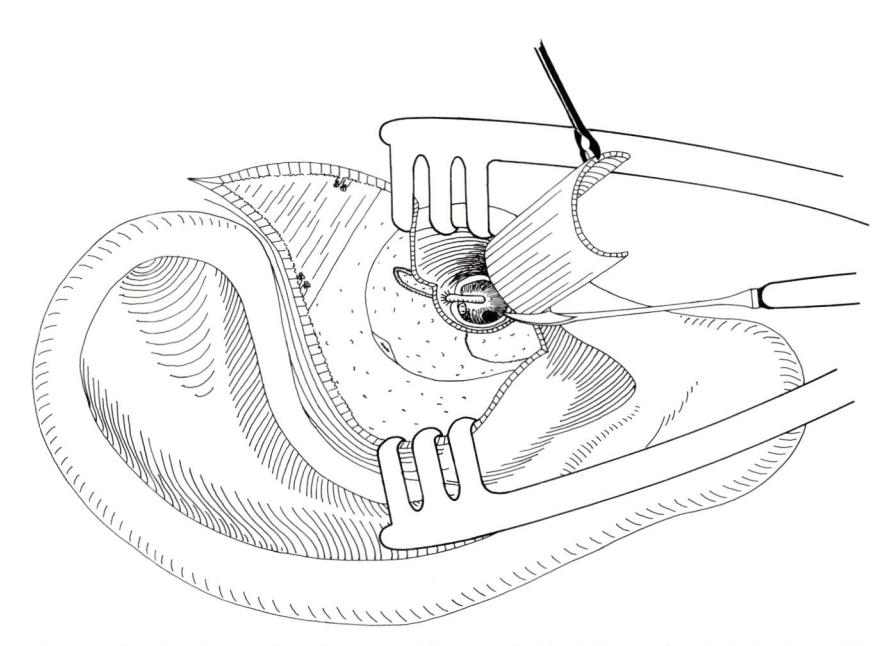

Fig. 47 An entire Surdille flap is elevated and removed by a radial incision at the 6-o'clock position and a circumferential incision along the annulus

Heermann C Incision

Usually a Heermann C incision (Fig. **35**) is performed after it has been recognized that the exposure provided by the Heermann B incision is insufficient. The Heermann C incision is therefore performed after the incisions of the auditory canal have been completed, and also after an incision along the inferior border of the temporalis muscle has been made and the mastoid process exposed. Situations of this sort may include:

1. A laterally displaced ear-canal skin without an inferior radial incision (Fig. **36**).
2. A laterally displaced ear-canal skin flap with an inferior radial incision (Figs. **37, 38**).
3. A circumferential incision laterally in the ear canal (Fig. **39**), either with the Panse flap preserved (Figs. **43, 45**) or removed (Fig. **46**).
4. A medially dissected (Figs. **40, 41**) or removed Surdille flap (Fig. **47**).

The Heermann C incision as an additional incision follows incision B (Fig. **27**). By pulling the auricle posteriorly and inferiorly with the retractor or with the fingers, the curved Heermann C incision starts at the top of the Heermann B incision and continues around the superior attachment of the auricle. With a Freer dissector or Metzenbaum scissors, the surgical plane on the temporalis muscle fascia is further established posteriorly and inferiorly under the auricle, as well as towards the tip of the mastoid process (Fig. **48**). The incision goes through the skin and superior auricular muscle, exposing a large area of the temporal muscle fascia. The skin incision is continued behind the auricle, and gradually the superior half of the auricle together with the subcutaneous tissue and posterior auricular muscles, are totally freed from the mastoid process and folded posteroinferiorly out of the operating field (Fig. **49**). The ear-canal skin attached to the concha is carefully preserved and folded away together with the auricle. The periosteum is freed posteriorly, exposing as much of the cortical bone of the mastoid process as possible. A selfretaining retractor holds the incisions in place (Fig. **49**). The skin covering the inferior ear canal wall and the inferior part of the concha, as well as the antitragus, is pulled and held away with hooks and elastic surgical stays (Fig. **49**).

We have found the commercially available hooks useful in otoneurosurgery and middle-ear surgery for holding the various flaps. In comparison to the selfretaining metal retractors, elastic surgical stays do not disturb the view of the middle ear when the patient is tilted.

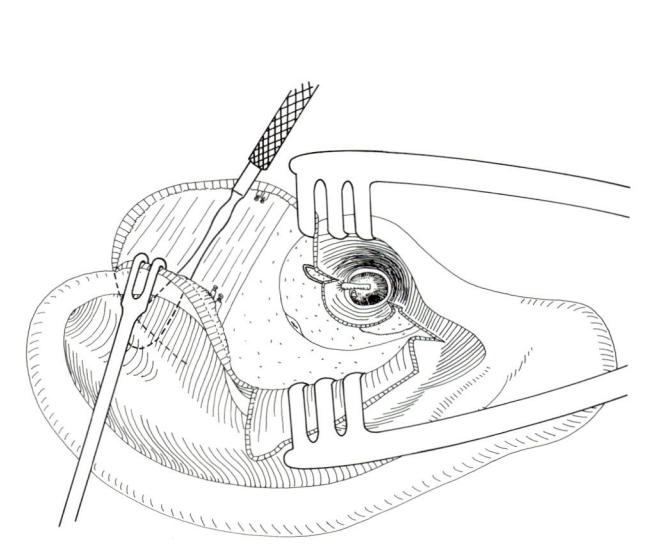

Fig. **48** **A Heermann C incision,** with elaboration of the surgical plane on the temporalis muscle fascia

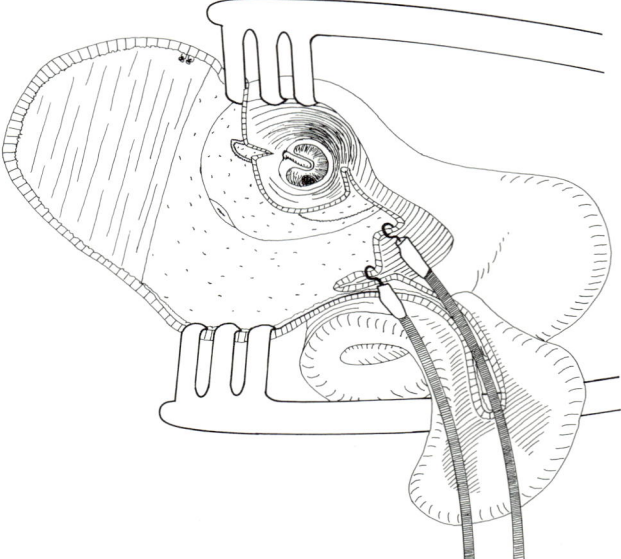

Fig. **49** The Heermann C incision is completed, and the mastoid process is widely exposed

Shambaugh Incision

There are small variations between Shambaugh's and Lempert's incisions. What the two procedures have in common both is an intercartilaginous incision at the 12-o'clock position and a laterally-placed circumferential incision along the bone-cartilage junction, resulting in a large Surdille flap.

The Shambaugh incision is made in two stages with a scalpel. The circumferential incision begins at the 12-o'clock position on the superior meatal wall, about 1 cm from the outer edge of the meatus along the bone-cartilage junction. The incision extends at about the same level to the posterior meatal wall at the 7-o'clock position on the right side and at the 5-o'clock position on the left side. It then angles outwards for 2–3 mm to the edge of the conchal cartilage, but not into the conchal cartilage itself (Fig. 50).

The second incision begins, like the first, at the 12-o'clock position at the superior meatal wall, and extends directly upwards in the anterior (intertragic) incisura, to a point about halfway between the meatus and the upper edge of the auricle (1.5 cm). If greater exposure is needed, the vertical incision can be extended upwards to the upper edge of the auricle. The incision goes through the skin and auricular muscles down to the temporal muscle fascia, which remains intact. The anterior auricular artery and vein, which cross over the incision, are coagulated and cut. The circumferential incision goes through the periosteum by holding the knife at an angle, so that it will not plunge into the bony meatus. With a broad periosteal elevator placed in the first incision, the periosteum of the entire mastoid process is elevated posteriorly (Fig. 51). The superior meatal-wall skin and periosteum is elevated anteriorly over the posterior root of the zygomatic bone.

The anterosuperior meatal spine of the tympanosquamous suture (notch of Rivinus) can often be prominent, hampering the elevation of the skin at the 12-o'clock region. The meatal skin should, in any endaural incision, be dissected off the notch of Rivinus and should be preserved intact. To get sufficient exposure medial to the anterior spine, the canal-wall skin is dissected from the bone as far anteriorly along the fibrous annulus as possible (Fig. 52).

An incision of the periosteum is made along the inferior border of the temporalis muscle to facilitate exposure of the mastoid process. One selfretaining retractor is inserted beneath the periosteum, to hold the auricle retracted and maintain the exposure of the mastoid process. Another selfretaining retrac-

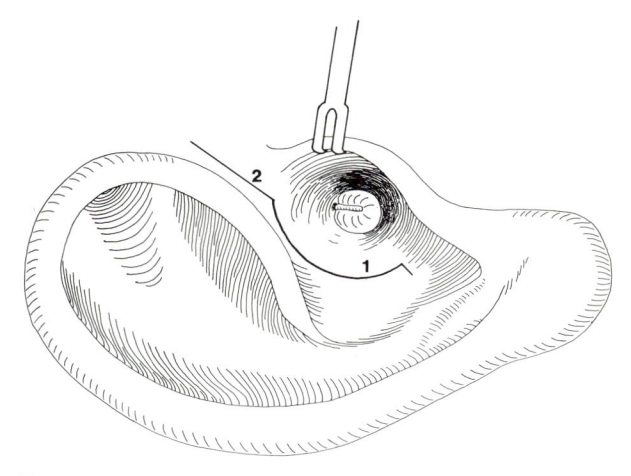

Fig. 50 **The Shambaugh endaural incision. 1** The circumferential incision with a small outward incision towards the concha. **2** The vertical incision

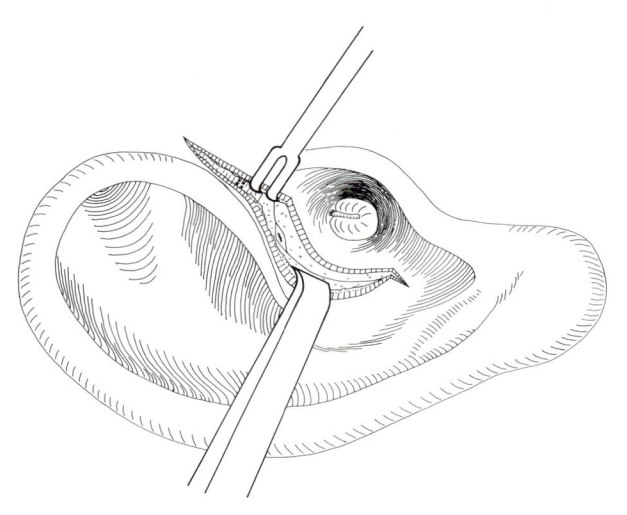

Fig. 51 The Shambaugh incision. Elevation of the periosteum

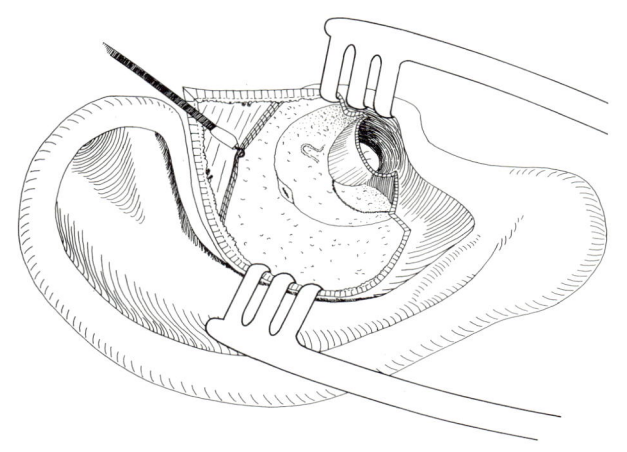

Fig. 52 Completed Shambaugh incision, with good exposure of the mastoid process. The posterior canal-wall skin is elevated to the fibrous annulus

tor may be used to retract the temporalis muscle and to achieve exposure superiorly, but a hook with an elastic stay elevating the muscle can also be useful (Fig. 52).

The original Shambaugh approach can be used for most temporal bone operations with canal-wall-down techniques, typically for Bondy's operation. It is less suitable for tympanoplastic procedures in the tympanic cavity, because of the large Surdille flap obstructing the view of the tympanic cavity.

Lempert Incision

After the surgeon has pulled the auricle backward with the fingers and the tragus has been pulled forward with a blunt retractor held by the scrub nurse, the anterior incisura is widened, and a vertical skin incision is started with a scalpel anteriorly to the helix, about 1.5 cm superior to the meatus, and continued down on the posterior wall of the bony meatus at the border between the conchal cartilage and bone. The incision continues around the circumference of the meatal introitus and ends at the 7-o'clock position. With a straight incision knife, a medial radial skin incision at the 7-o'clock position is performed (Fig. 53). The vertical incision is similar to Shambaugh's incision, going down to the fascia of the temporalis muscle, and the posterior circumferential incision goes through the periosteum. At the same level as the posterior circumferential incision, an anterior circumferential incision is performed up to the 4-o'clock position. From here, the

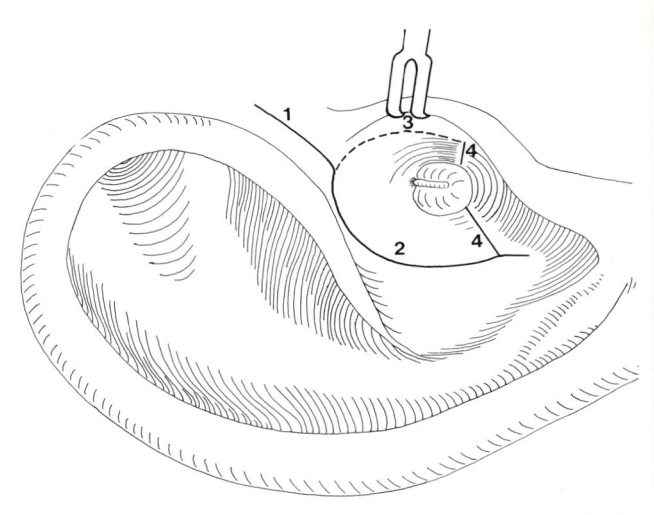

Fig. 53 **A Lempert incision,** consisting of a vertical incision (1), posterior (2) and anterior circumferential incisions (3), and a radial incision (4)

other radial incision goes medially towards the fibrous annulus. The radial incision is made with a straight incision knife. The periosteum of the mastoid process is elevated posteriorly (Fig. 54), and the mastoid process is exposed in the same way as that described for the Shambaugh incisions (Fig. 55).

The meatal skin is elevated, first posterosuperiorly at the suprameatal spine, then superiorly from the notch of Rivinus and tympanosquamous suture, and then posteroinferiorly from the tympanomastoid suture. Finally, the skin from the anterior meatal wall is elevated, and a large Surdille tym-

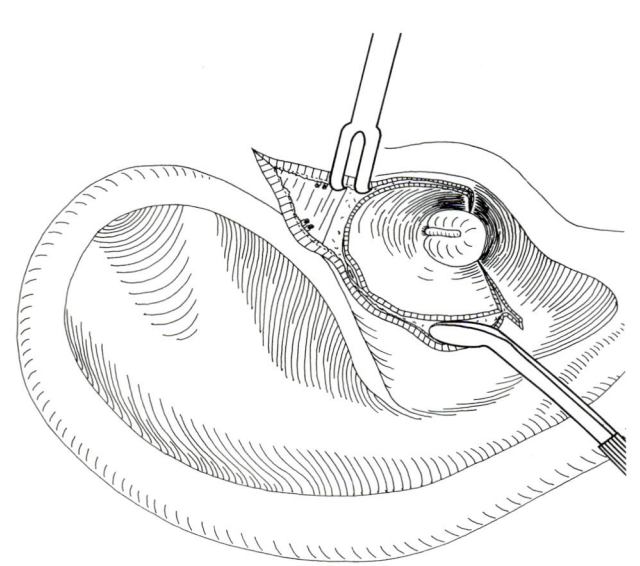

Fig. 54 Lempert incision, with elevation of the periosteum posteriorly

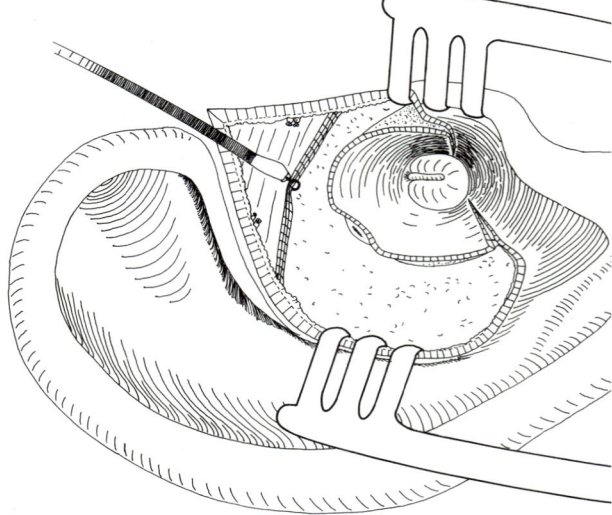

Fig. 55 Completed mastoid exposure in a Lempert incision

panomeatal flap is now formed. The flap dissection should be as delicate as possible, and it must not be unnecessarily traumatized. The Surdille flap is carefully elevated from the bone with a fine elevator, just as far as the tympanic membrane (Fig. **56**). The outer part of the Surdille flap is usually relatively thick and stiff. It should be thinned with scissors.

The Lempert incision with the large Surdille flap was the approach of choice in the fenestration operation for otosclerosis before the stapedectomy era. The large Surdille flap can cover the window made on the lateral semicircular canal, the attic region, and part of the cavity. After tympanotomy and elevation of Shrapnell's membrane, the fibrous annulus of the posterior part of the tympanic membrane, together with the attached flap, can be reflected forward and downward and held against the anteroinferior meatal wall with a retractor, proteecting the skin during further surgery (Fig. **57**).

Lempert's incision can be used in the same surgical procedures as Shambaugh's incision. After canal wall-down mastoidectomy, removal of the bridge anteriorly, resection of the head of the malleus, and further elevation of the anterior part of the anterior annulus, the tympanomeatal flap can be further enlarged and mobilized. The philosophy of such a large Surdille flap, originally applied in fenestration operations, is widely accepted in modern tympanoplasty with reconstruction of the ear canal, despite its many modifications, depending on the pathology. The Surdille flap is less suitable for tympanoplasty procedures in the tympanic cavity, because the large flap hampers visualization of the anterior and inferior regions.

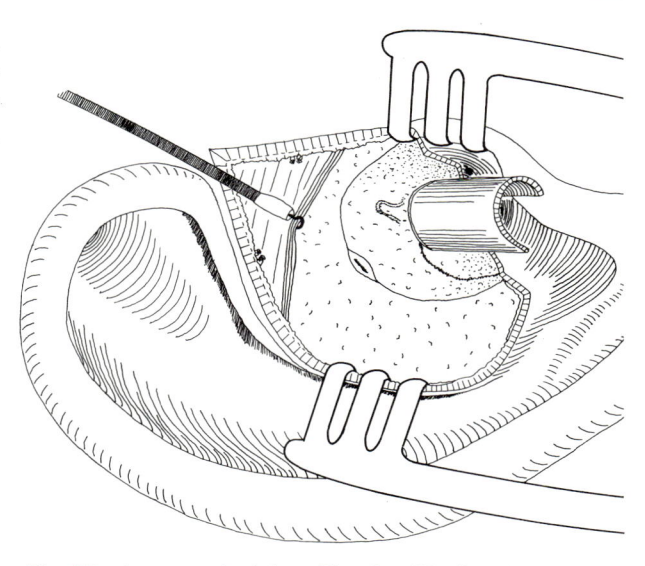

Fig. **56** Lempert incision. The Surdille flap is elevated to the fibrous annulus

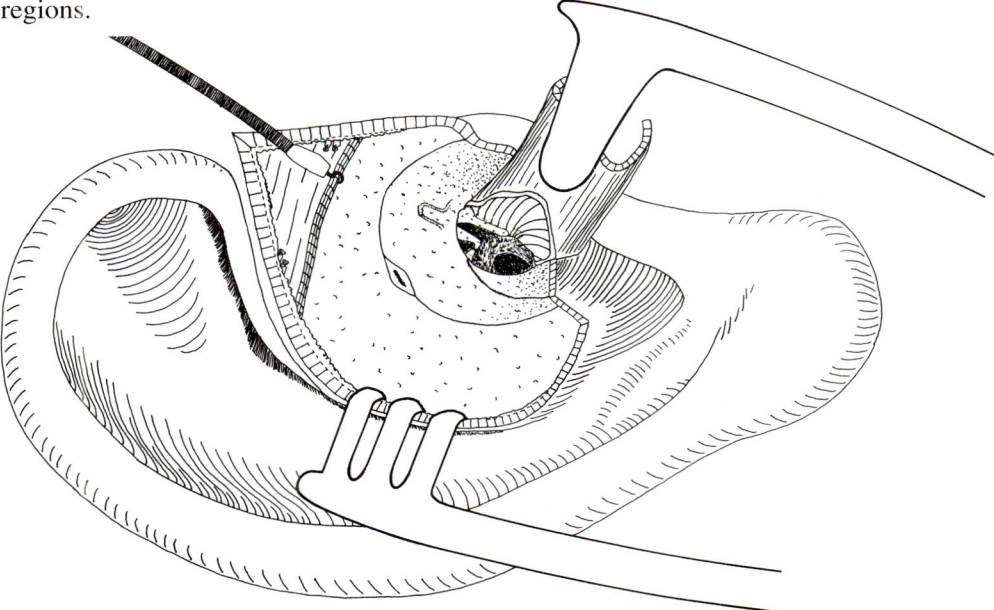

Fig. **57** A completed Lempert incision, with tympanotomy and protection of the Surdille flap

Farrior Incision

The Farrior endaural incision and the superior canal-skin graft are combinations and modifications of the Lempert and the Shambaugh endaural incisions. The Farrior circumferential incision begins anteriorly over the edge of the anterior bony canal wall at the 4-o'clock position on the right side, and extends circumferentially around the canal at a level medial to the spine of Henle. In the posterior canal wall, the circumferential incision continues 2–3 mm medial to the spine of Henle, resulting in a somewhat smaller Surdille flap than in the Lempert or Shambaugh incisions. As a consequence, the conchal canal skin flap is larger than in the Lempert or Shambaugh incisions, allowing dissection of a conchal flap (Fig. **58**). In the preparation of the conchal canal flap, all periosteum and subcutaneous tissue inferior to the temporalis muscle is primarily left attached to the conchal skin flap. Secondarily, the periosteum and subcutaneous tissue is dissected with a scalpel from the conchal skin away from the conchal cartilage (Fig. **59**). This mass of subcutaneous tissue and periosteum is left attached to the end of the undermined conchal canal skin flap, and serves to anchor the flap deep in the mastoid cavity, or partially obliterate the mastoid cavity. If conchal cartilage is prominent, or if a large ear canal is needed, a 2–3 mm strip of conchal cartilage can be resected. With a selfretaining retractor, the mastoid process is exposed widely (Fig. **60**).

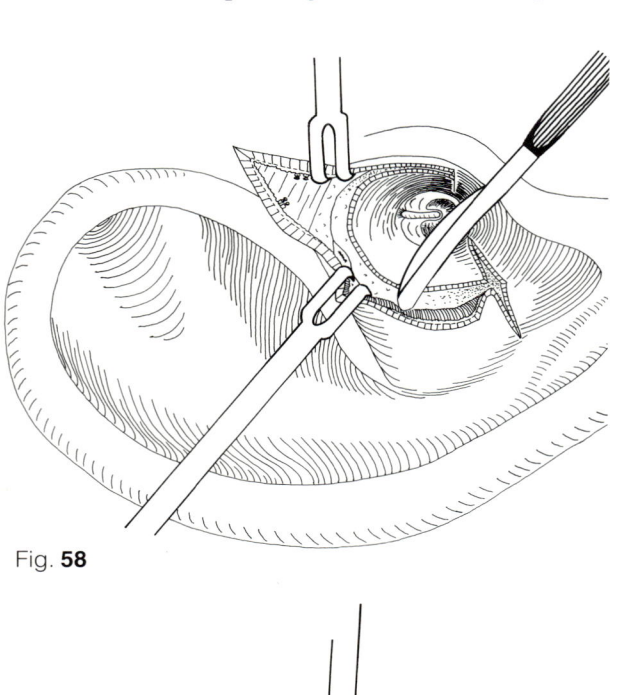

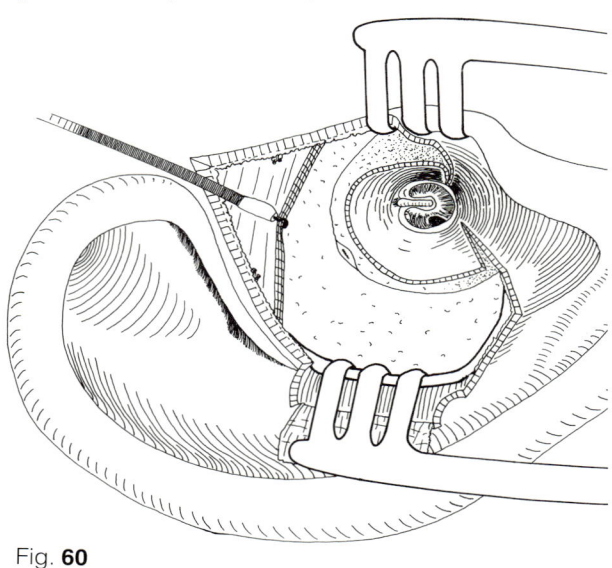

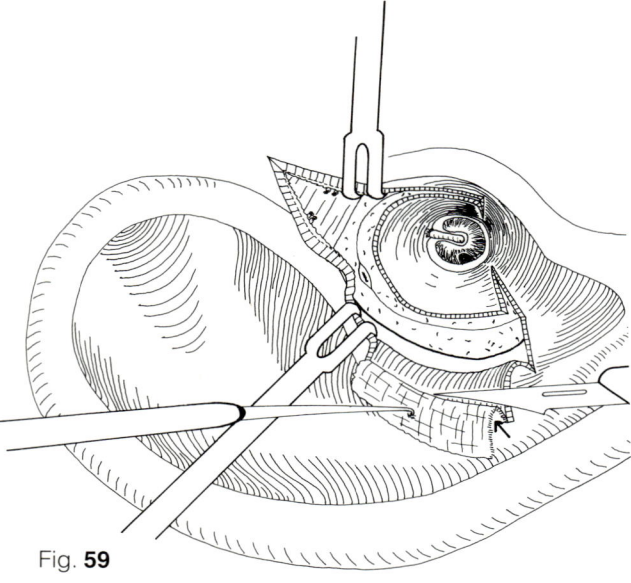

Fig. 58

Fig. 60

Fig. 59

Fig. **58** **The Farrior endaural incision.** The circumferential incision is placed medially to the spine of Henle, and a small conchal skin flap is folded outward. The periosteum is elevated posteriorly by a periosteal rugine

Fig. **59** Dissection of the conchal flap in a Farrior incision. The subcutaneous tissue and the periosteum is dissected from the conchal skin with a scalpel up to the last attachment, enlarging the length of the flap (arrow)

Fig. **60** The conchal flap is held in place, and the mastoid process is exposed

As in the Shambaugh and Lempert incisions, Farrior's modification is suitable for atticotomies, atticoantrostomies, and canal wall-down mastoidectomies. If the air-cell system is large and extends towards the apex of the mastoid process, then the vertical skin incision superiorly and the conchal incision inferiorly can be enlarged.

For tympanoplasty or other work inferiorly and anteriorly in the tympanic cavity, the Lempert, Shambaugh and Farrior incisions are not particularly suitable, because the large Surdille flap is somewhat in the way during surgery. It can be dissected and pressed forward (Figs. **52, 56, 57**) but often has to be removed. If the circumferential incisions are placed more medially towards the fibrous annulus, then the Surdille flap will be smaller and less disturbing during the tympanoplasty. By further diminishing the Surdille flap to a size similar to that of a Rosen flap, the Lempert and Shambaugh incisions become more and more similar to the Heermann incision, with a small tympanomeatal flap and a large conchal skin flap.

Canal Skin Removal

Ear-canal skin removal techniques were developed after the Lempert and Shambaugh incisions, partly because of the disturbance of a large tympanomeatal flap during tympanoplasty, and partly because the ear-canal skin, as a free graft, is used to reconstruct the outer layer of the new eardrum in the socalled sandwich myringoplasty.

After the completed Shambaugh (Fig. **52**) and Lempert incisions (Fig. **56**), the elevated canal-skin flap can be removed from the annulus with a sickle knife. In principle , there are three major modifications, relating to which part of the canal skin is left in place as a vascular strip: a) inferior vascular strip (Farrior); b) anterior vascular strip (Wolfermann); c) superior vascular strip (Fleury).

Inferior Vascular Strip

The Farrior endaural incision (Fig. **61**) has been widely used for myringoplasty. After the circumferential incision and the radial incisions, and after dissection of the conchal flap and placing of the self-retaining retractor, another circumferential incision is made 2 mm lateral to the annulus, connecting the two previous radial incisions. On the right ear, these incisions extend between the 7-o'clock and 4-o'clock positions (Fig. **61**), and on the left side between the 5-o'clock and 8-o'clock positions. The canal skin is elevated with a fine dissector or an angled incision knife. Elevation is started at the anterior canal wall, and then continues to the superior and posterior wall, down to the annulus. Care is taken to preserve the continuity of the tympanomeatal flap, especially at the notch of Rivinus and Shrapnell's membrane. An accurate plane of cleavage has to be established between the canal skin and the fibrous annulus of the drum (Fig. **62**), allowing the keratinized epithelium to be elevated from the drum remnant in continuity with the canal-skin flap (Fig. **63**).

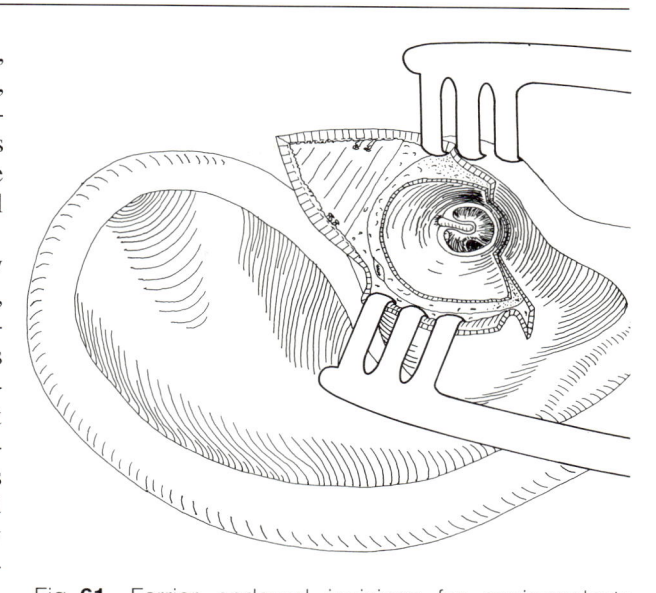

Fig. **61** Farrior endaural incisions for myringoplasty with preservation of an inferior vascular strip. Intercartilaginous, lateral circumferential, and two radial incisions at the 7-o'clock and 5-o'clock positions, and a medial circumferential incision along the inferior fibrous annulus, are performed

3 Endaural Approach

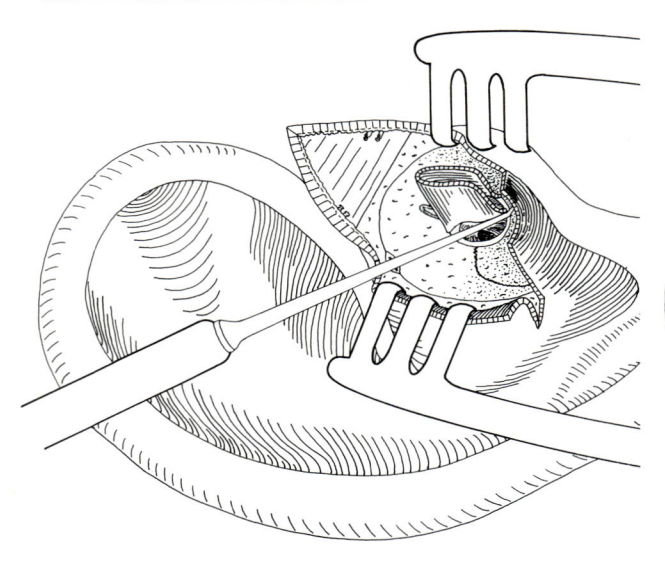

Fig. 62 Dissection of the canal skin from the inferior part of the fibrous annulus

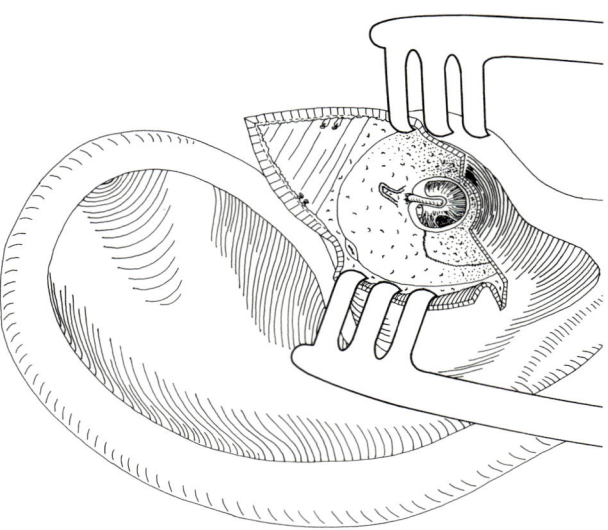

Fig. 63 The canal skin is removed, together with the squamous epithelium of the drum remnant. The inferior canal skin is preserved (Farrior)

Anterior Vascular Strip

Another modification is practised by Wolfermann. The circumferential ear-canal incision starts anteriorly at the 5-o'clock position, goes along the inferior wall, and continues along the posterior and superior walls until the 1-o'clock position (Fig. **64**). The circumferential incision goes along the bone-cartilage junction, like the Farrior incision. On each end of the circumferential incisions, a radial incision is made using straight incision knife perpendicularly to the circumferential incision along the bony canal wall, laterally to the fibrous annulus. The outlined skin flap therefore comprises approximately two-thirds of the skin covering the bony portion of the external auditory canal (Fig. **64**). The skin of the medial part of the ear canal is very thin, and the dissection should be careful, especially at the 12-o'clock position, at the tympanosquamous suture, and at the tympanomastoid suture. The skin is elevated with a small elevator. The fibrous tissue lying in the sutures and around the notch of Rivinus should be cut with a knife or scissors. Wolfermann recommends the use of small cotton balls soaked in topical ephedrine 1/1000, held by a small forceps (Fig. **65**). With these cotton balls, the skin is gently pushed off the bone down to the fibrous annulus. Tearing of the skin can be avoided with this technique. When the annulus is reached, a plane of cleavage between the epithelial and fibrous layer of the drum has to be established. The drum is deepithelialized by pushing the flap toward the edges of the perforation. The skin flap with the epithelial layer of the drum remnant is finally removed in one piece all around the perforation (Fig. **66**). The skin flap is preserved in Ringer's solution to be reused later, either in sandwich myringoplasty or simple replacement on the denuded ear canal bone.

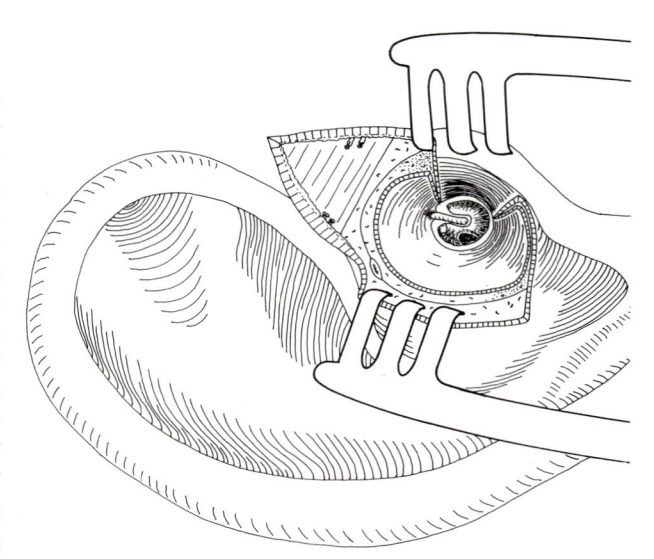

Fig. **64** **Wolfermann's modification of the endaural approach,** with preservation of an anterior vascular strip

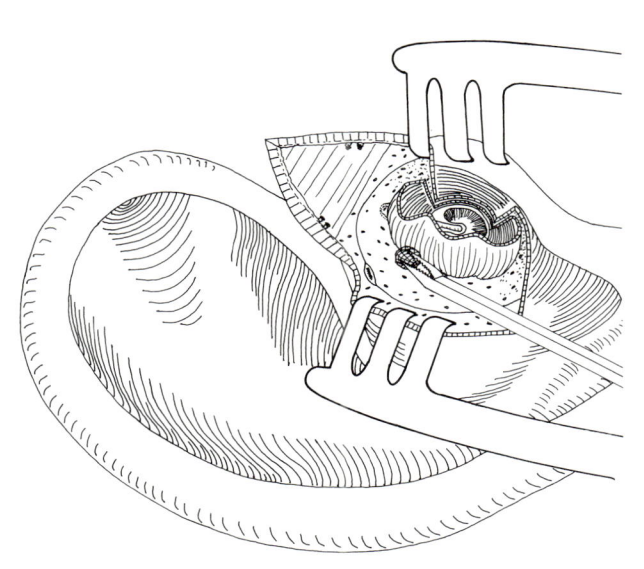

Fig. 65 Elevation of the canal-wall skin from the superior, posterior, and inferior canal walls

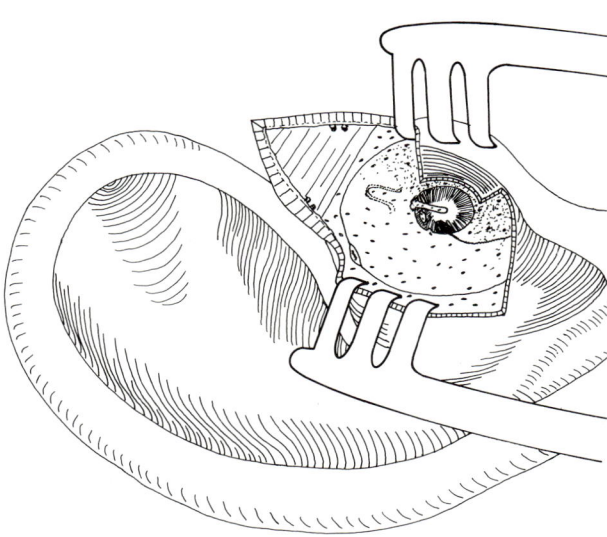

Fig. 66 The canal-wall skin and the drum remnant epithelium are removed, and the anterior annulus is deepithelialized

Superior Vascular Strip

This modification is mainly practised by Fleury and some of the French school. The incision is an interesting modification of the Shambaugh and Lempert incisions. First, the lateral circumferential incision is started anteriorly at the 2-o'clock position at the bone-cartilage junction with a scalpel, and continued inferiorly (Fig. 67). The lateral circumferential incision is then started at the 12-o'clock position and continued posteriorly and inferiorly, joining the anterior part of the incision (Fig. 68). A small intercartilaginous incision is performed laterally in the meatus, allowing a pair of blunt, curved scissors to undermine the skin little by little. The progress of the scissors may be visualized under the skin (Fig. 69). The vertical skin incision is performed using scissors (Fig. 70). After incision through the subcutis and the periosteum along the lower edge of the temporalis muscle, the cortical bone of the mastoid process is exposed by elevating the periosteum. The elevated tissue is held in place by two selfretaining retractors (Fig. 71). Elevation of the canal skin starts posteriorly, and continues down to the annulus. The annulus is elevated, together with the canal skin and the drum remnant, in its total circumference (Fig. 72). Elevation then continues towards the anterior and inferior canal skin (Fig. 73), and finally all the annulus, together with the canal skin and the drum remnant epithelium, is pushed superiorly (Fig. 74). The fascia can now be placed as the underlay graft either on the denuded malleus handle or medial to it. This technique, which includes several interesting moments, is suitable for total and subtotal perforations, and has been modified by Fleury for other perforations as well.

3 Endaural Approach

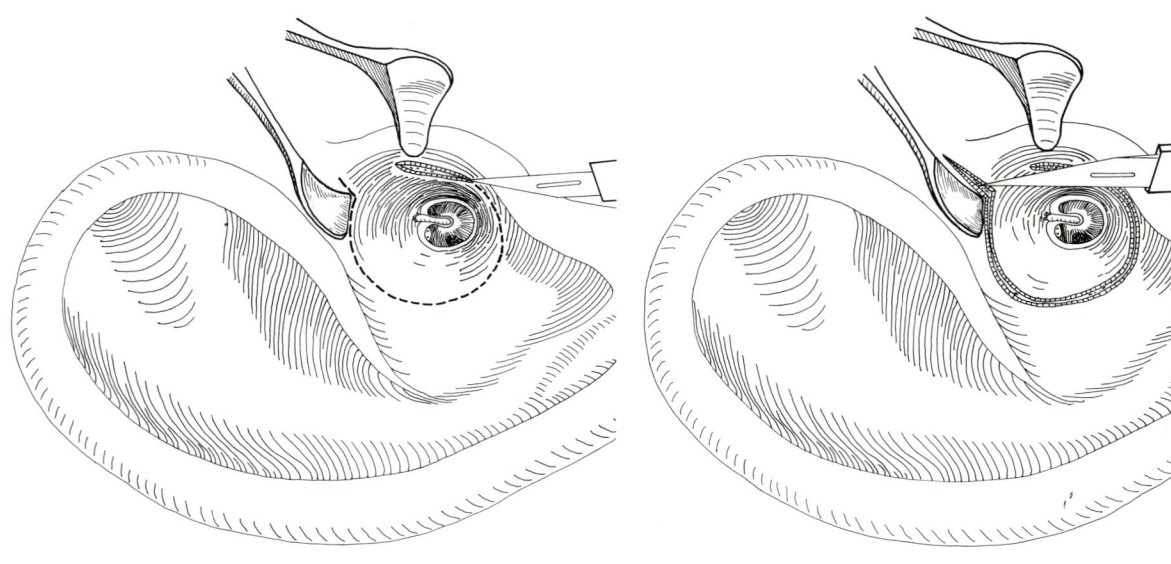

Fig. 67 **The superior vascular strip technique (Fleury)**, with a lateral circumferential incision starting at the 2-o'clock position

Fig. 68 The Lateral circumferential incision is completed, leaving a superior vascular strip. A small intercartilaginous incision is performed

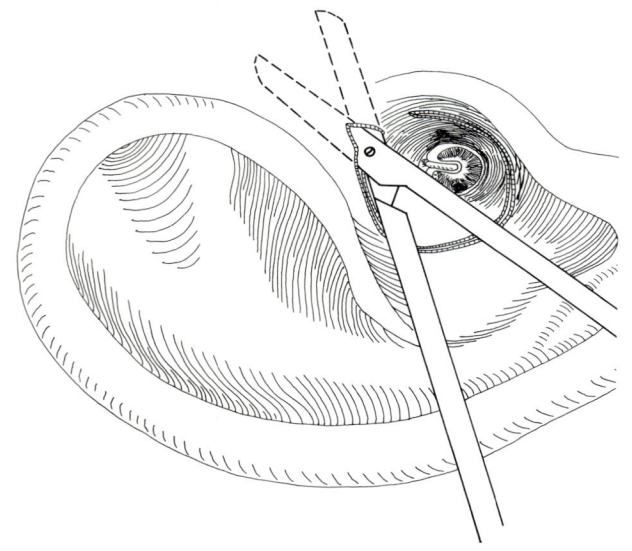

Fig. 69 Through the intercartilaginous incision, the skin superior to the ear canal is undermined

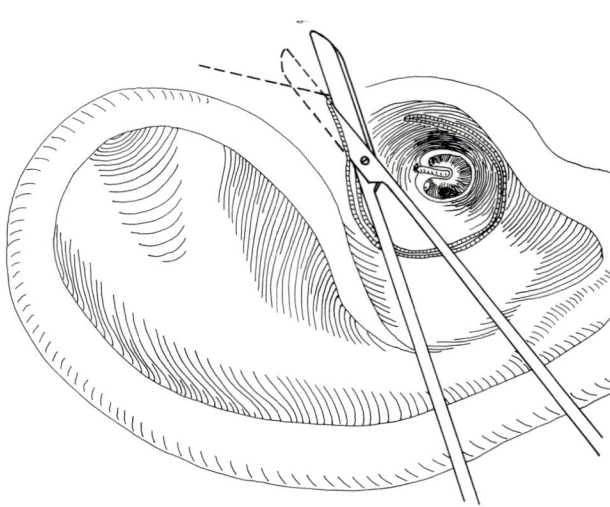

Fig. 70 The vertical skin incision is performed using scissors

Farrior Incision

Fig. 71 The periosteum is elevated, and the mastoid process is exposed

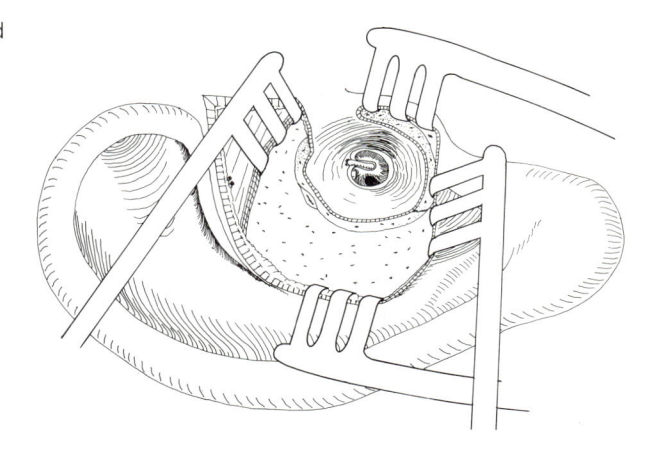

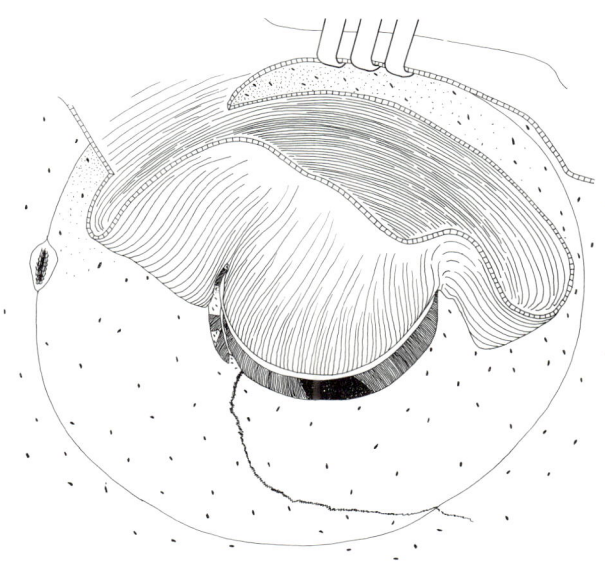

Fig. 72

Fig. 73

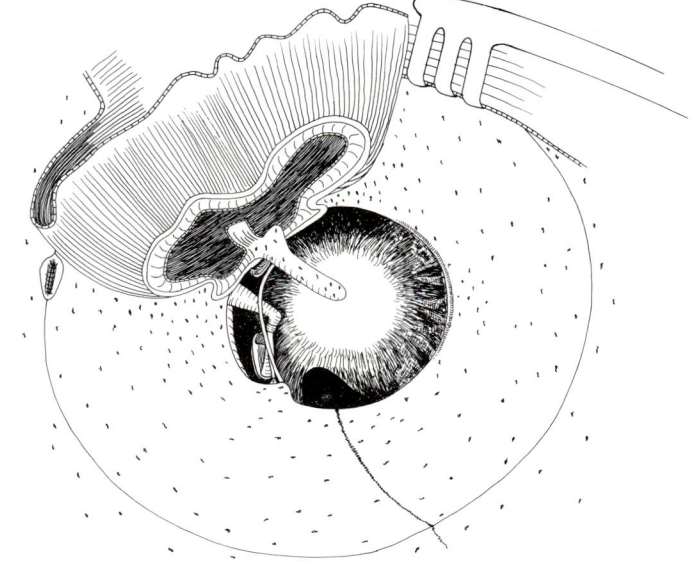

Fig. 72 The posterior canal skin is elevated, together with the annulus

Fig. 73 The anterior canal skin, with the annulus and drum remnant, is elevated

Fig. 74 All canal-wall skin, the annulus, and the drum remnant, are pushed superiorly, completing the superior vascular strip technique

Fig. 74

4 Retroauricular Approach

The incision is made behind the auricle, which is pulled anteriorly. In contrast to the endaural approach, in which the auricle is pushed posteriorly and the surgery takes place through the enlarged meatus, in the retroauricular approach the auricle is pushed anteriorly and the surgery takes place initially behind the auricle and behind the auditory meatus. The exposure is generally wider than in the endaural approach, and it can easily be further widened in ears with large air-cell systems, or in ears with complications requiring extensive surgery. In fact, today all inner ear surgery, facial nerve surgery, and translabyrinthine acoustic neuroma surgery procedures are performed by retroauricular incision at various distances behind the retroauricular fold (Fig. 75). In addition, all intact canal wall mastoidectomies, and the majority of cavity obliteration techniques, as well as ear-canal reconstructions, require the retroauricular approach, mainly because the various musculoperiosteal flaps are dissected through this approach. The retroauricular skin incision can be made in the retroauricular fold or elsewhere posterior to it, depending on the purpose of the surgery, the pathology to be operated on, and the surgical methods or obliteration methods to be used (Figs. 75, 76). These incisions are called retroauricular flap incisions.

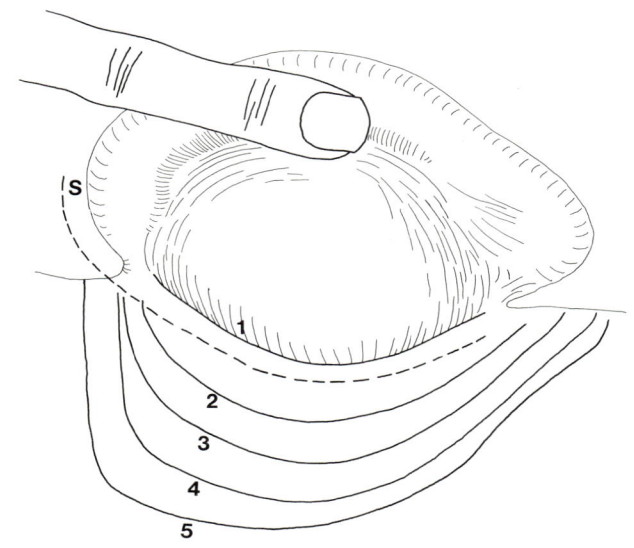

Fig. 75 A retroauricular fold incision in the retroauricular fold (1), and retroauricular flap incisions at various distances behind the fold (2–5). Posterosuperior incision (S)

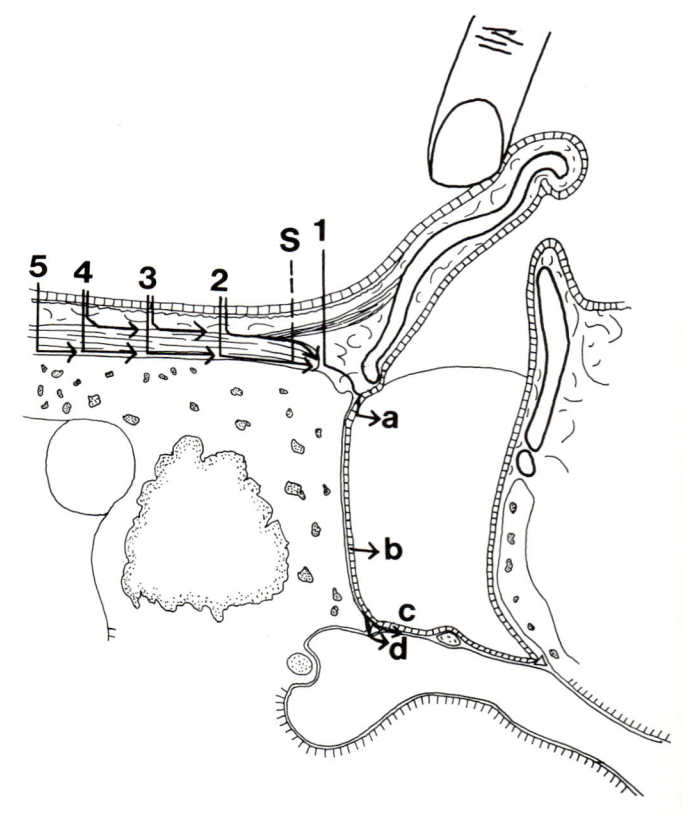

Fig. 76 The retroauricular incision seen from the side. The incision in the retroauricular fold, or the posterosuperior incision, goes through the posterior auricular muscle, fibrous tissue, and periosteum on the mastoid cortex, and just behind the suprameatal spine, making a small (or no) musculoperiosteal flap. In incisions 2–5, the musculoperiosteal flaps are larger. Dissection towards the concha can either continue subcutaneously, leaving the musculoperiosteal flap in place, or between the periosteum and the cortex of the mastoid process, elevating the musculoperiosteal flap. The levels of the lateral (a) and medial (b) circumferential incisions are indicated. Elevation of the entire canal skin together with the drum remnant epithelium (c), and the drum with the annulus (d)

Retroauricular Fold Incision

An incision in the retroauricular fold is performed in myringoplasty and in tympanoplasty cases with no need for extensive mastoidectomy. By pressing in the auricle anteriorly with the fingers, the skin of the retroauricular fold is stretched. The incision goes from a point 1 cm lower than the upper attachment of the auricle to 1 cm above its lower attachment. Through the superior part of the skin incision, the superior auricular muscle and the oblique muscle of the auricle are seen, and sometimes cut. The posterior auricular muscle, extending from the conchal prominence towards the mastoid process, is always cut (Fig. 77), and the dissection continues through the deeper subcutaneous tissue towards the mastoid bone. By firm traction of the auricle in an anterior direction, the edge of the junction of the mastoid process surface with the bony meatus can be palpated with the finger, and a curved incision through the fibrous tissue and periosteum about 5 mm behind the bony edge is made (Fig. 77). Using a strong raspatory, the periosteum is elevated from the mastoid process and around the bony auditory meatus. The roof of the bony meatus, the root of the zygoma, the suprameatal spine, and the posterior and inferior walls of the bony meatus are all delineated. After further elevation of the ear-canal skin a few millimeters medial to the suprameatal spine, the ear-canal skin can be visualized.

Several modifications of the postauricular fold approach are used (Fig. 76). These are based on the level of the circumferential incision, and can be classified as follows:

1. Lateral circumferential skin incision, located between the level of the suprameatal spine and approximately 7 mm medial to it.
2. Medial circumferential incision, located between the drum level and approximately 7 mm lateral to it.
3. No circumferential incision in the canal skin, but elevation of the canal skin over its entire length, with or without elevation of the annulus.

Lateral Circumferential Incision

With a lateral circumferential skin incision through the posterior meatal skin, further surgery becomes transcanal, and this approach is also termed the retroauricular–transcanal approach. There are several modifications of the lateral circumferential skin incision method. These relate to:

1. The extension of the circumferential incision around the ear-canal skin.

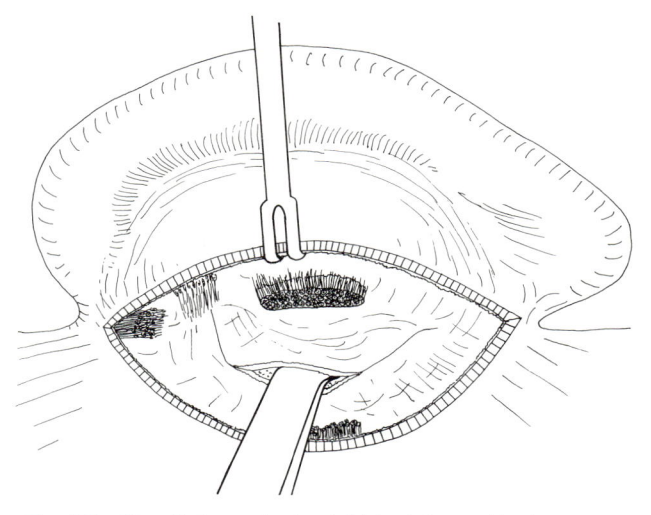

Fig. 77 The Retroauricular fold incision, with the superior, oblique, and posterior auricular muscles. After an oval subcutaneous-periosteal incision on the mastoid process, elevation of the periosteal flap is performed

2. The localization of the incisions and the size of the tympanomeatal flap.
3. The level of the lateral circumferential incision, either at the level of the suprameatal spine or further medially to it, up to 7 mm medially.
4. Removal of the tympanomeatal flap.

Plester Technique

The canal-wall skin between the 12-o'clock and 6-o'clock positions is further elevated with a raspatory (Fig. 78). In ears with a narrow ear canal,

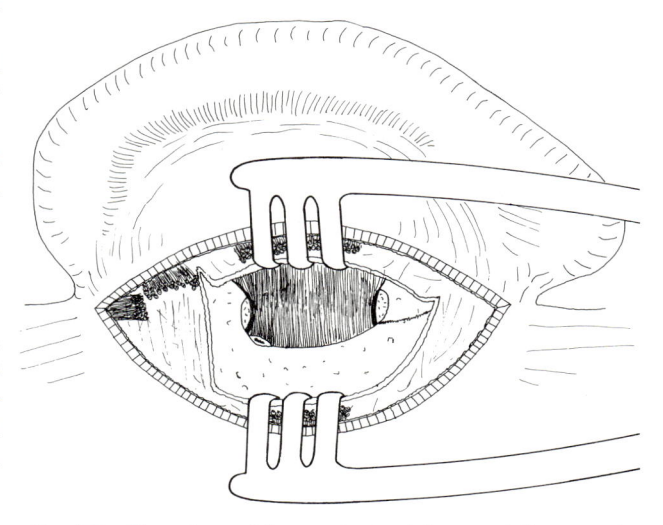

Fig. 78 Elevation of the periosteal flap and the canal-wall skin between the 12-o'clock and 6-o'clock positions

4 Retroauricular Approach

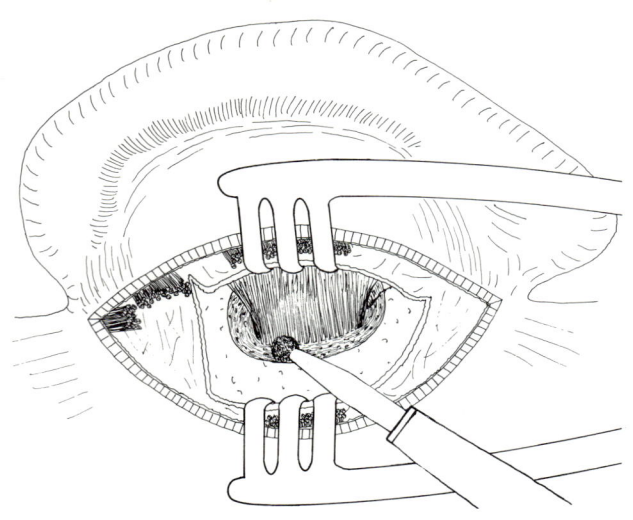

Fig. **79** Drilling of the entrance to the bony ear canal, and further exposure of the ear-canal skin

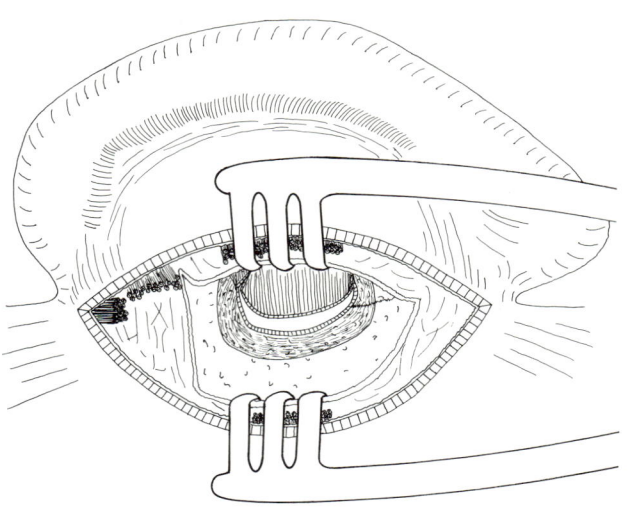

Fig. **80** Circumferential skin incision from the 12-o'clock to 6-o'clock positions, and the radial incision, running outwards from the superior edge of the circumferential incision (Plester technique)

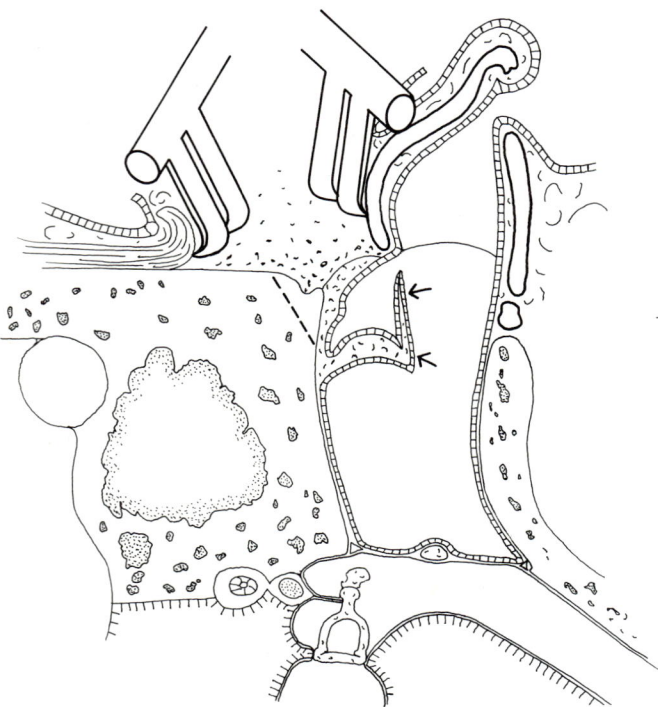

Fig. **81** The circumferential and radial skin incisions in the superior wall of the auditory meatus, seen from the side (arrows)

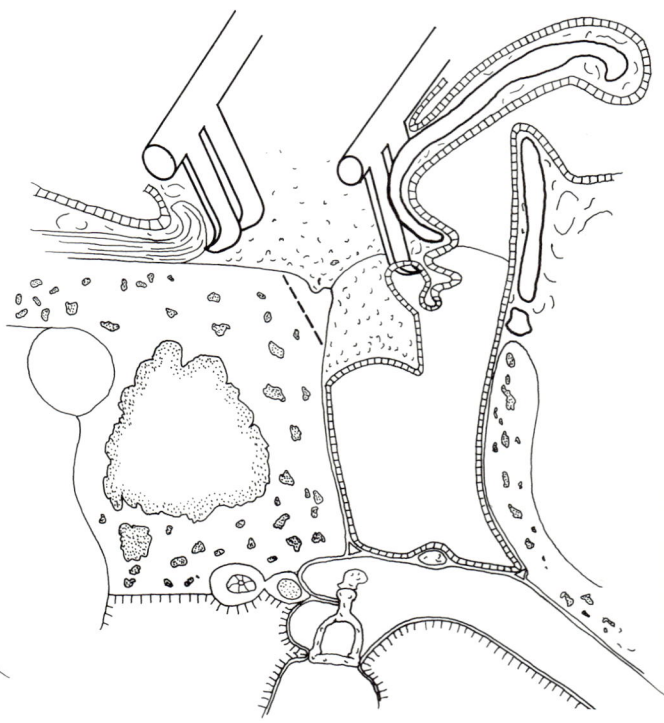

Fig. **82** A long selfretaining retractor is placed on top of the radial incision, pulling the skin and the lateral part of the auditory meatus, with the auricle, outward

the entrance of the bony canal is widened using a 3 mm cutting drill. The drilling starts at the suprameatal spine, and continues inferiorly along the border between the bony canal and the cortex of the mastoid process. Medially, the canal-wall bone is drilled away as much as is needed to facilitate the

view of the proposed canal-wall skin incision (Fig. **79**). The circumferential incision is made by a scalpel from the 12-o'clock to the 6-o'clock positions at a level 4–5 mm medial to the suprameatal spine (Fig. **80**). From the superior edge of the circumferential incision, a 1–1.5 cm-long outward-

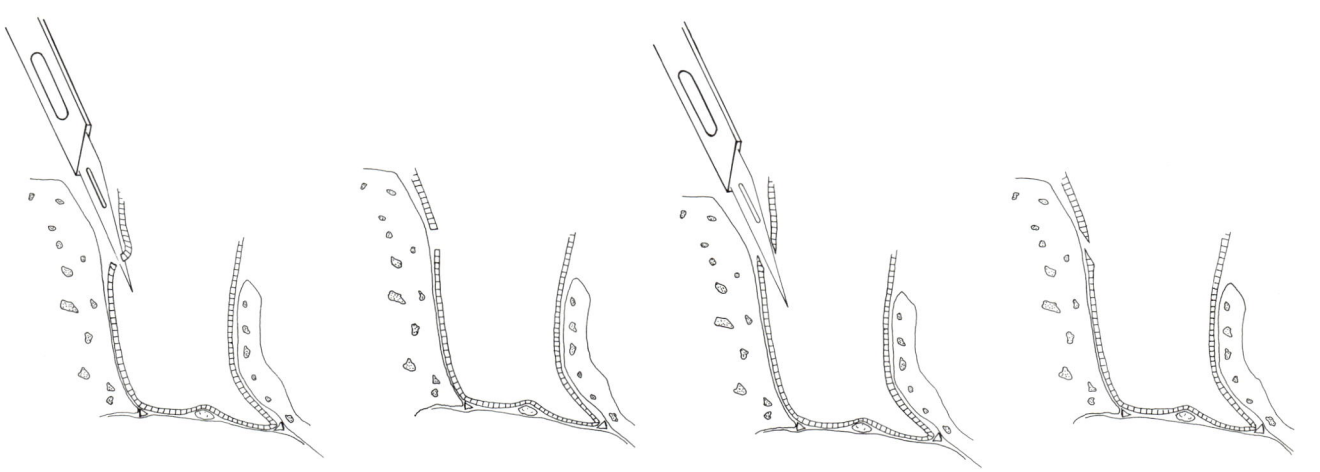

Fig. 83 Perpendicular cutting of the circumferential canal skin incision with a scalpel

Fig. 84 Oblique cutting, illustrating easier adaptation of the skin to the bone

directed radial incision is performed (Fig. 80). This forms a triangular skin flap, based inferiorly and laterally in the ear canal (Fig. 81). Using an especially long selfretaining retractor, this flap is pulled outward, together with the lateral part of the auditory meatus and the auricle, providing a good view of the anterior part of the drum (Fig. 82). Because a strong selfretaining retractor is needed to keep the auricle and the lateral part of the meatus retracted, visualization of the posterior tympanum, and especially the sinus tympani, can be hampered by the anterior arm of the retractor (Fig. 82). By rotating the operating table towards the surgeon, a better view of the sinus tympani can be obtained, and the laterally-positioned retractor can also be rotated to leave only a small cleft with insufficient visualization (Fig. 82).

Several authors believe that the lateral circumferential incision should be performed perpendicularly to the skin and periosteum to make clean perpendicular skin edges for closure of the wound (Fig. 83). Morimitsu (1991) believes that a circular incision through the skin should be oblique, and while this is indeed easier to perform in the auditory canal, it also elongates the skin. The covering of bony defects is easier, and the flap edges are thinner (Fig. 84).

The radial skin incisions are usually made at the 11-o'clock and 7-o'clock positions on the right side (Fig. 85) and between the 1-o'clock and 5-o'clock positions on the left side, depending on the situation and size of the drum perforation. The large tympanomeatal flap is elevated medially towards the annulus, exposing the bone of the entire posterior half of the ear canal. Together with the meatal skin the fibrous annulus is elevated between the 11-o'clock and 6-o'clock positions, and the entire tympanomeatal flap is pushed anteriorly in the auditory canal (Fig. 86). A more extensive elevation of the annulus is necessary in total and subtotal perforation.

This approach is used in myringoplasty with underlay grafting. Visualization of the anterior edge can be hampered by the large tympanomeatal flap lying in the ear canal together with the fibrous annulus (Fig. 86).

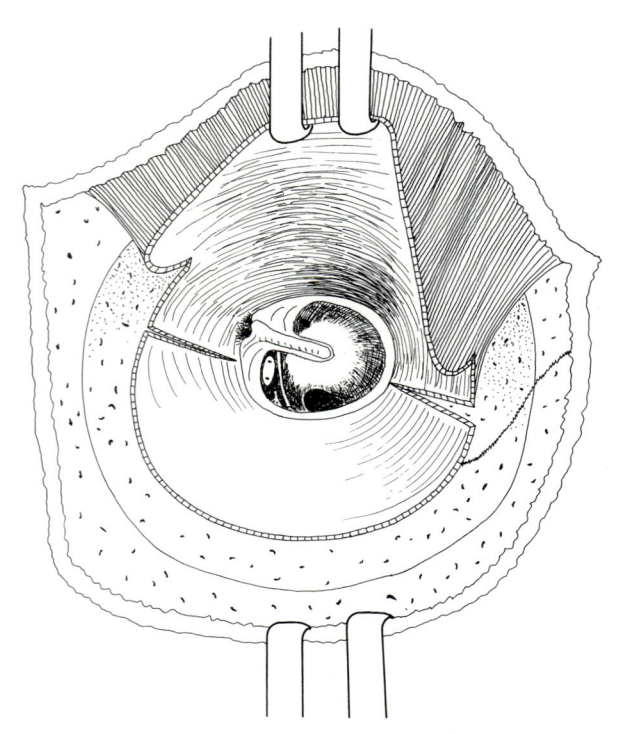

Fig. 85 A retroauricular fold incision. Radial incisions at the 12-o'clock, 7-o'clock positions

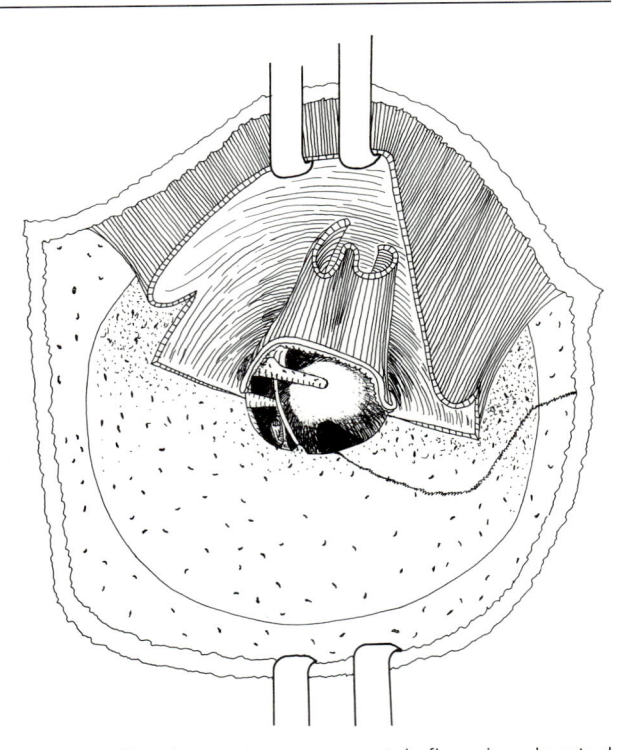

Fig. 86 The large tympanomeatal flap is elevated, together with the fibrous annulus

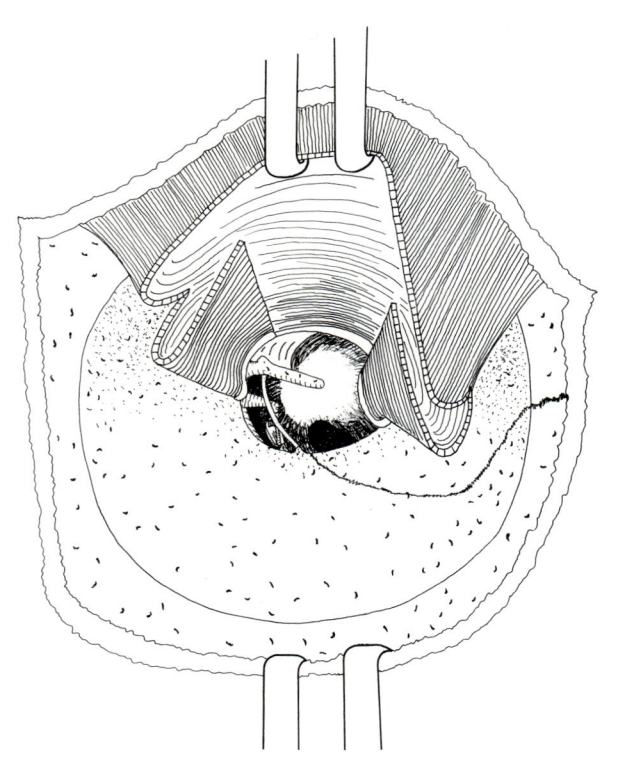

Fig. 87 **The swing-door technique (Palva)**, with a radial skin incision through the tympanomeatal flap at the 9-o'clock position

Palva's Swing-Door Technique

To avoid the drawback of poor anterior visualization by a large tympanomeatal flap, one radial incision at the 9-o'clock position is made, and the tympanomeatal flap is divided into superior and inferior flaps (Fig. 87). The view of the anterior part of the fibrous annulus is not impaired in this swing-door modification (Palva 1963). In fact, it seems that the swing-door modification is a very popular method in the retroauricular fold approach. The radial incision can be made with a straight incision knife or a sickle knife before elevation of the skin, or the skin can be first elevated in total posteriorly, and then cut at the 9-o'clock position from lateral to medial with a pair of scissors, also continuing through the annulus.

Circumferential incisions involving more than the posterior half of the ear-canal circumference, or the majority of the circumference, are used in several modifications. The difference between these modifications lies in the placing of the vascular strip with intact ear-canal skin.

Fisch Technique

From the exposure of the external ear canal as shown in Figure **78**, Fisch starts the postauricular part of the circumferential incision with a scalpel a few millimeters medial to the spine of Henle, continuing along the superior and anterior meatal walls (Fig. **88**).

The purpose of the circumferential incision over the anterior meatal wall is to eliminate the overhang around the anterior wall. The skin over the anterior meatal wall is elevated, and the bony overhang is drilled away with a diamond burr (Fig. **89**). The flap is then replaced, and the myringoplasty can proceed.

The swing-door technique can be used, with a radial incision in the posterior meatal wall skin at the 9-o'clock position down to the annulus and through the annulus (Fig. **89**), elevating the superior and inferior skin flap as shown in Figure **87**, and performing the myringoplasty with underlay fascia grafting.

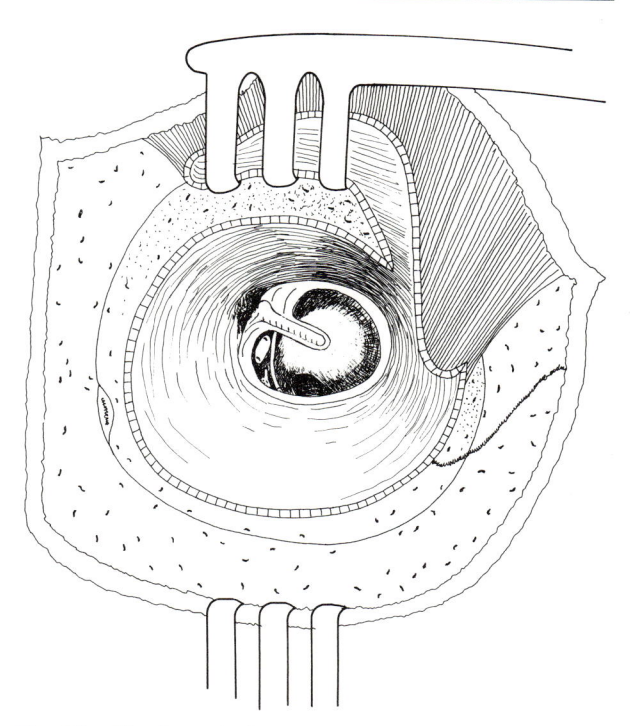

Fig. **88** **Fisch technique**. A large lateral circumferential incision 5 mm medial to the suprameatal spine, leaving only the inferior part of the meatal skin intact. The lateral part of the ear canal is elevated

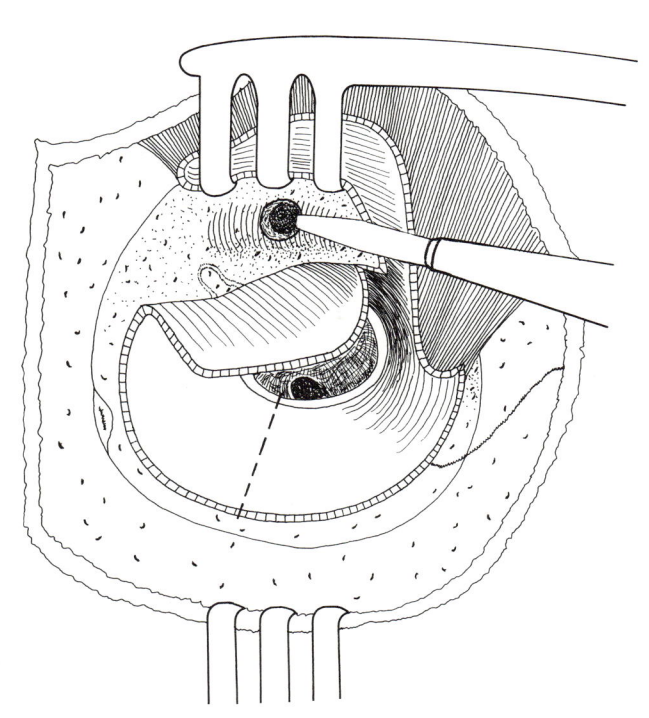

Fig. **89** The anterior skin is elevated, and the bony prominence is drilled away. The dotted line indicates the incision for the swing-door technique

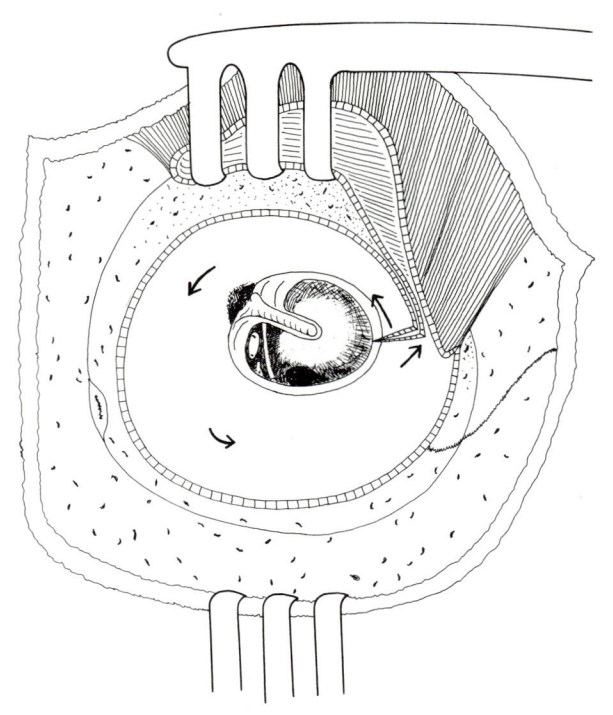

4 Retroauricular Approach

Fig. 90 Further extension of the circumferential incision, and a radial incision at the 6-o'clock position in order to elevate the entire flap (Fisch)

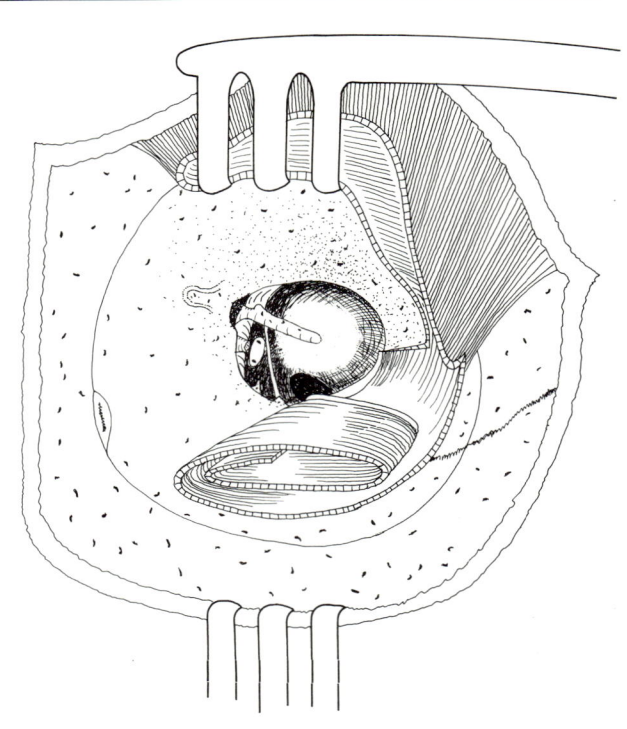

Fig. 91 The tympanomeatal flap, together with the annulus, is partly elevated

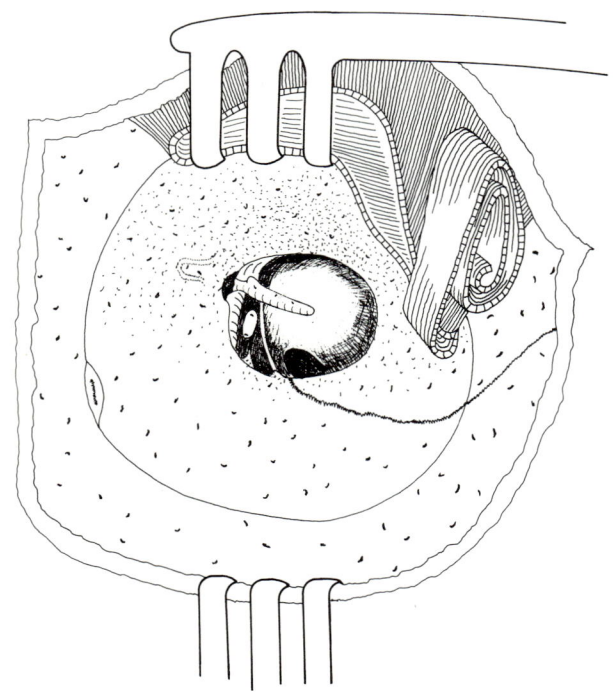

It is sometimes necessary to remove the entire annulus together with the tympanomeatal flap in order to get sufficient exposure of the tympanic cavity. Fisch prolongs the anterior part of the circumferential incision to the 6-o'clock position, and continues with a radial incision through the canal skin and the annulus (Fig. 90). Then the flap is elevated, just as in the counterclockwise direction (Figs. 91, 92).

Fig. 92 The entire tympanomeatal flap, with the annulus, is elevated and folded inferiorly

Farrior Technique

The circumferential incision is extended through four-fifths of the circumference of the canal skin (Fig. **93**). It starts at the level of the spine of Henle, continuing superiorly to the 12-o'clock position. Inferiorly, it continues to the 6-o'clock position and on then to the 3-o'clock position, leaving only the anterosuperior meatal skin intact (Fig. **93**). In this approach the inferior part of the canal skin can be elevated to drill away the bony prominence of the ear canal, the entire large tympanomeatal flap can be elevated together with the annulus, and the skin can be removed (Figs. **94, 95**).

Canal Skin Removal

Several surgeons remove the canal skin of the entire tympanomeatal flap and replace it in a different way in sandwich myringoplasty (Farrior) (Figs. **94, 95**), as a free graft, or cover the bone of the cavity after mastoidectomy. Plester removes canal skin flaps when there is a risk of damage during drilling, or when they disturb surgery in the tympanic cavity.

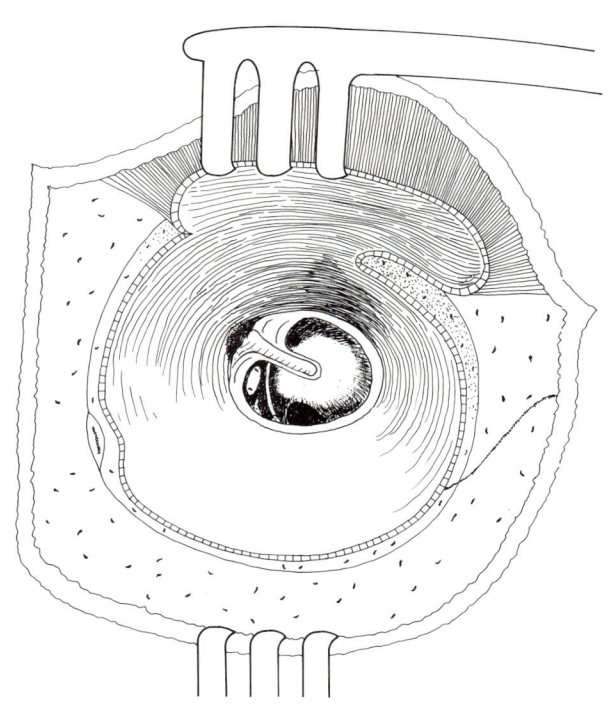

Fig. **93 Farrior technique.** A large lateral circumferential incision at the level of the suprameatal spine, leaving the anterosuperior meatal skin intact. The lateral part of the ear canal is elevated

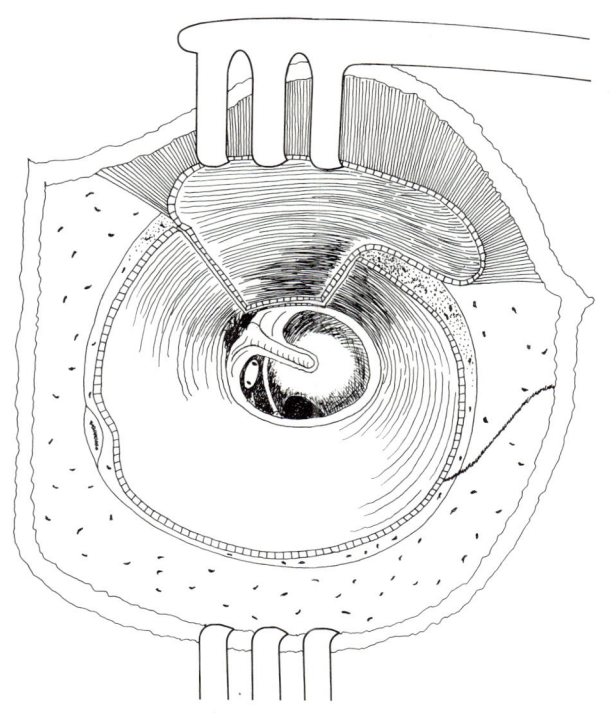

Fig. **94** Radial skin incisions before removal of the entire tympanomeatal flap

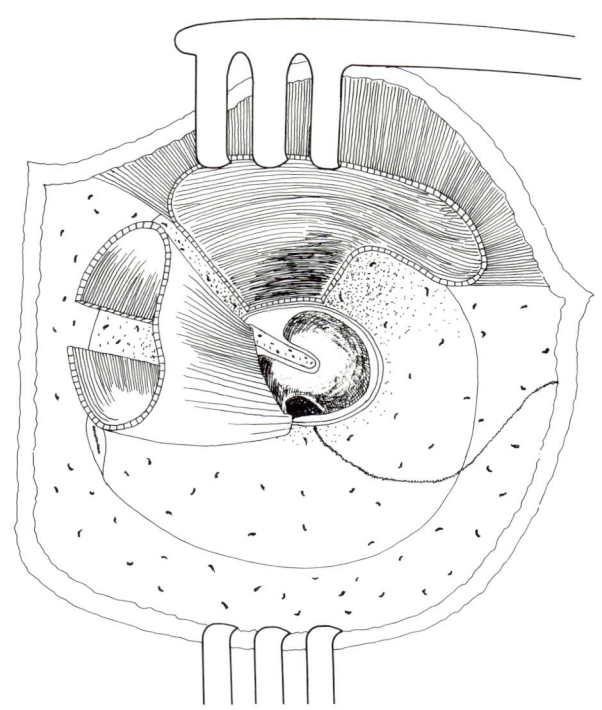

Fig. **95** The entire tympanomeatal skin flap, together with the drum remnant epithelium, is elevated and removed

4 Retroauricular Approach

Medial Circumferential Incision

Medial circumferential incisions are localized at any level between the drum and the middle of the ear canal, approximately 7 mm lateral to the drum.

The circumferential incision is performed with a scalpel between the 12-o'clock and 6-o'clock positions. The tympanomeatal flap is shorter than in the lateral circumferential techniques, but the laterally pedicled ear-canal skin flap is longer. Medial circumferential incision techniques are the most common ones used in tympanoplasty. They are used in all cases with a primary endaural approach through the speculum, when larger access, or an atticotomy or antrotomy, is not required. Compared to the lateral circumferential incision techniques with large tympanomeatal flaps, the medial circumferential incision methods with a small tympanomeatal flap are used much more often today.

There are several modifications in the handling of the lateral skin flap and the tympanomeatal flap.

Lateral skin flaps in medial circumferential incisions are always large. In relation to the size and location of the radial incision, the flap can be:

1. An inferolaterally-based flap, with a superior radial incision.
2. A superolaterally-based flap, with an inferior radial incision.
3. A laterally-based flap, with both the superior and inferior radial incisions.

Wullstein–Kley Technique

The Wullstein–Kley technique, with an inferolaterally-based skin flap, is similar to the Plester technique in some respects. The lateral radial incision is performed superiorly, and the skin flap is thus based inferolaterally. The bony ear canal is further widened for about 2–3 mm by drilling with a sharp drill (Fig. **96**), and the canal skin is elevated further medially towards the drum level. When drilling, care should be taken not to open the mastoid cells in cases with good pneumatization. If the cell system is opened, the meatus should later be completely covered by skin or fascia to prevent infection of the cell system.

A circumferential skin incision at a level about 10 mm medial to the spine of Henle (or 5–6 mm lateral to the drum) is performed with a scalpel. The incision extends from the 12-o'clock to the 6-o'clock positions (Fig. **97**). A small radial incision starts at the 12-o'clock position perpendicular to the circumferential incision, and continues a few

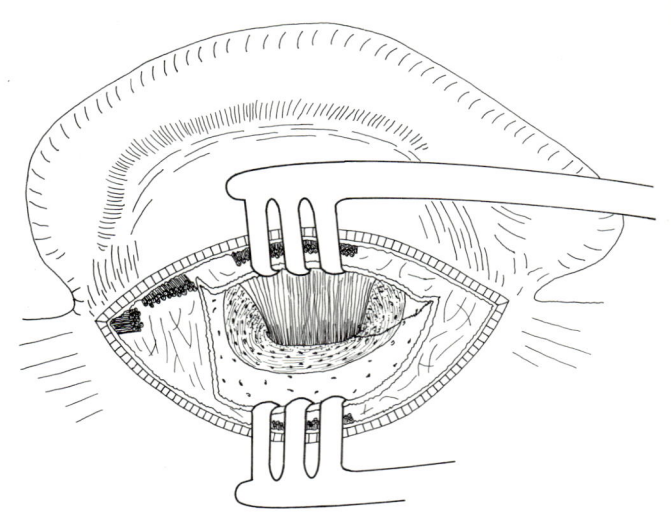

Fig. **96 Wullstein–Kley technique.** The bony ear canal is widened for 2—3 mm, before the medial circumferential incision is performed

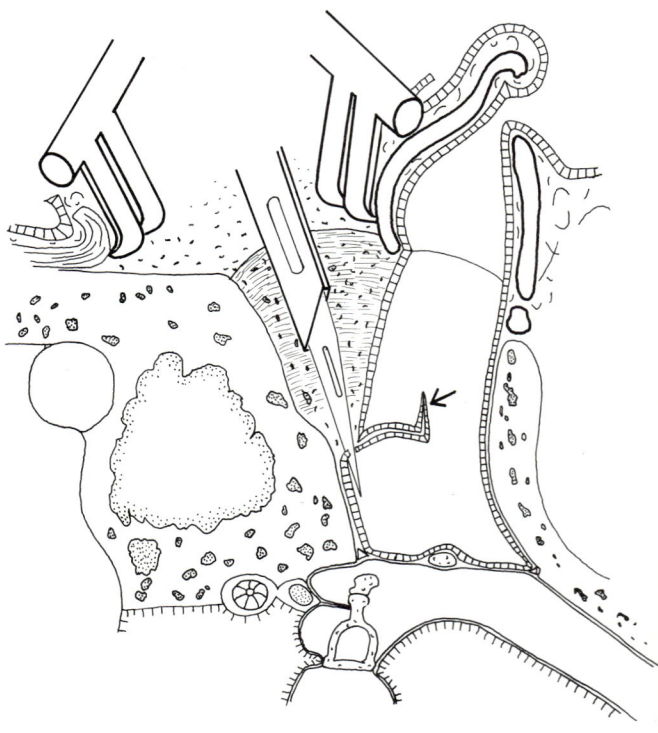

Fig. **97** Side view of the circumferential incision 5–6 mm lateral to the ear drum, and a radial incision at the 12-o'clock position (arrow).

millimeters in a lateral direction along the roof of the ear canal. A similar small radial incision is performed at the 6-o'clock position (Fig. **98**). With a tissue forceps (Fig. **99**), this small flap is pulled posteriorly, and the radial incision at the 12-o'clock position is continued for about 1 cm laterally (Fig. **100**).

The selfretaining retractor is placed in a far lateral position, and the canal-skin flap is turned backward and outward and sutured to the prominence of the conchal cartilage (Figs. **101, 102**). Visualization of the entire drum is possible, especially the anterior tympanomeatal angle (Fig. **102**).

The principle of the Wullstein–Kley technique is to protect the posterior canal skin by turning the inferolaterally-based skin flap posteriorly and pulling it outwards.

An inferolaterally-based skin flap facilitates a good view of the superior half of the drum and the attic, and is most often used when pathology is localized superiorly. In closure, it is usually necessary to support the closure of the attic region with the fascia.

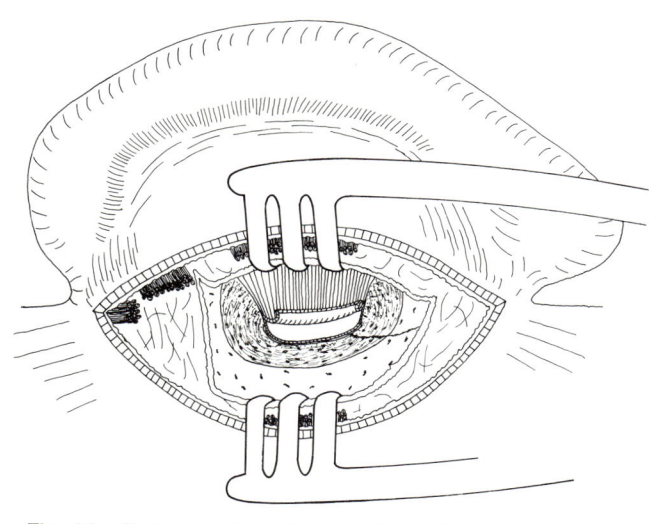

Fig. **98** Both small radial incisions, the superior and the inferior, have beer performed, and a small, laterally-based skin flap is turned posteriorly

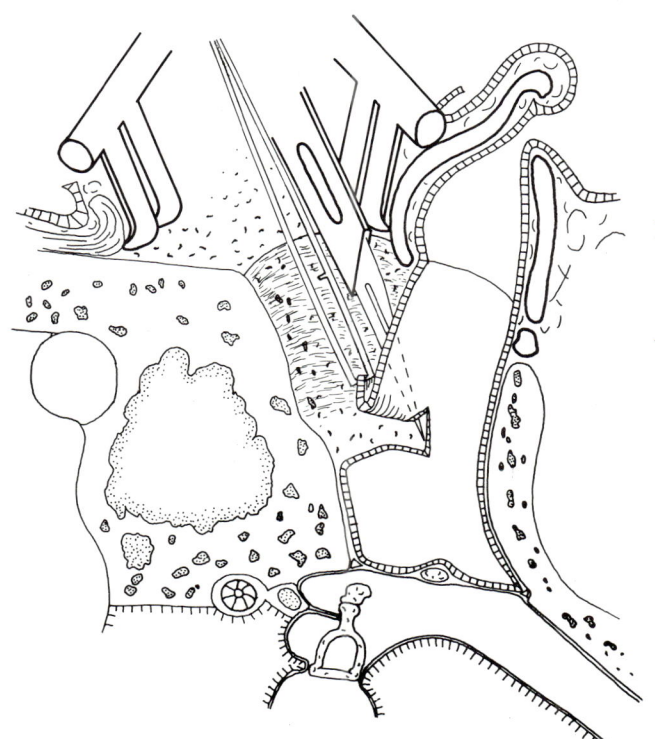

Fig. **99** The superior radial incision is prolonged outwards (dotted line), enlarging the lateral skin flap

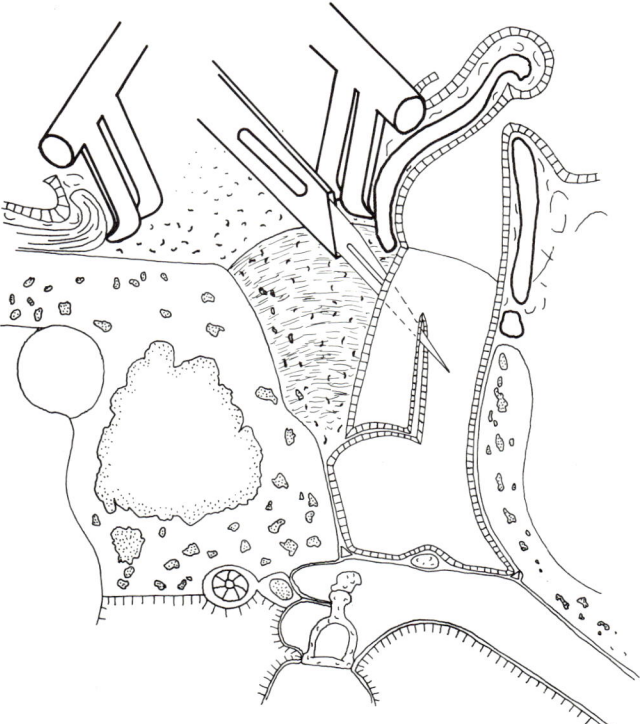

Fig. **100** Side view of the Wullstein–Kley technique, with a completed radial incision

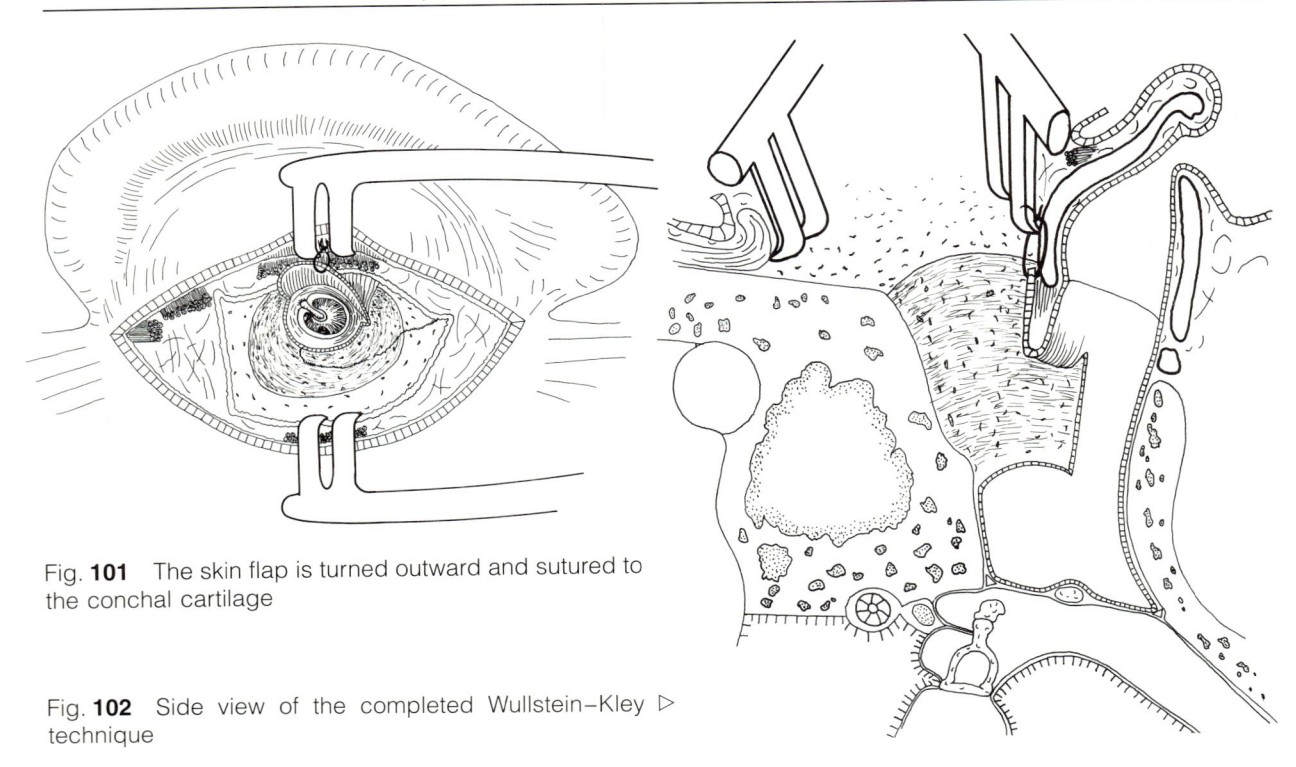

Fig. 101 The skin flap is turned outward and sutured to the conchal cartilage

Fig. 102 Side view of the completed Wullstein–Kley technique

Superolaterally-Based Flap

After the medial circumferential incision between the 12-o'clock and 6-o'clock positions, a small radial incision is made as shown in Figures **98** and **99**. The inferior radial incision is extended 1–1.5 cm laterally with a scalpel (Fig. **103**), forming a superolaterally-based skin flap which is pressed anteriorly by a large protecting speculum (House–Sheehy) (Fig. **104**).

The superolaterally-based skin flap is suitable for inferior and posterior drum pathology. Inspection of the attic is hampered by the canal-skin flap, but closure of the attic region is easier.

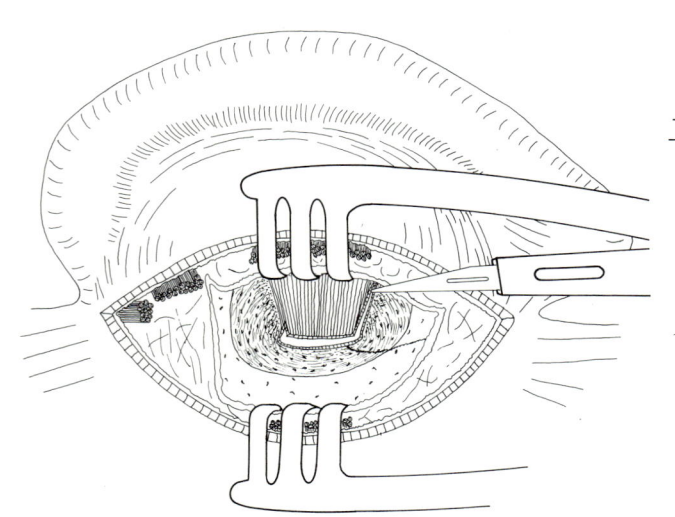

Fig. 103 **Technique for a superiorly-based skin flap.** After the circumferential incision, a large lateral, radial incision is performed inferiorly in the ear canal

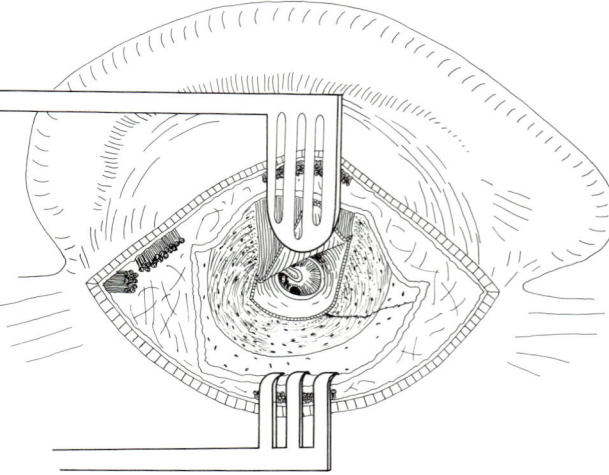

Fig. 104 A superolaterally-based flap is pushed anteriorly, and protected by a speculum

Laterally-Based Flap

After the medial circumferential incision between the 12-o'clock and 6-o'clock positions, the lateral radial incisions are performed superiorly and inferiorly at the 12-o'clock and 6-o'clock positions, respectively. Both incisions are made by a scalpel and are 1–1.5 cm long (Fig. 105), resulting in a large, laterally-based skin flap, which is pushed anteriorly and protected by a large speculum (Fig. 106). The broad protecting blade of the speculum (House–Sheehy) is long enough to push the flap far anteriorly, nearly touching the anterior canal wall (Fig. 107).

Management of the Tympanomeatal Flap

As mentioned above, the medial circumferential incision can be placed at any level between the drum and the middle of the ear canal. The tympanomeatal skin flap can therefore have various sizes, depending on the pathology and the myringoplasty technique employed. Several technique are used to manage the tympanomeatal flap:

1. No tympanomeatal flap. After careful elevation of the posterior half of the canal skin down to the annulus, the medial circumferential incision

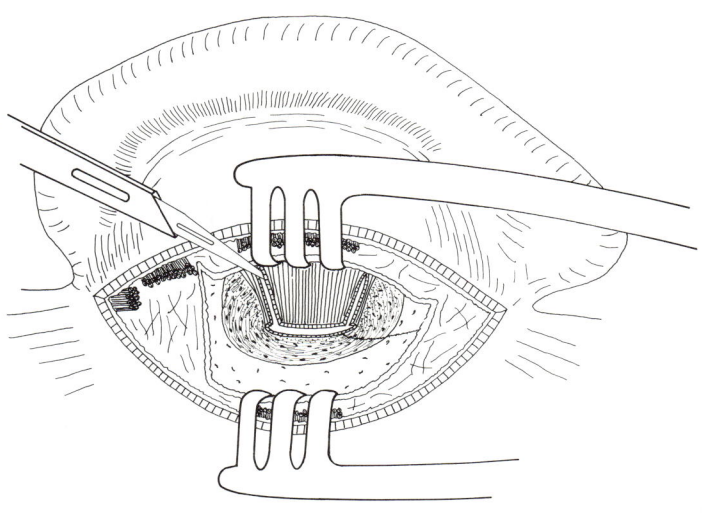

Fig. 105 Modification, with a laterally-based flap and two long lateral radial incisions performed at the 12-o'clock and 6-o'clock positions

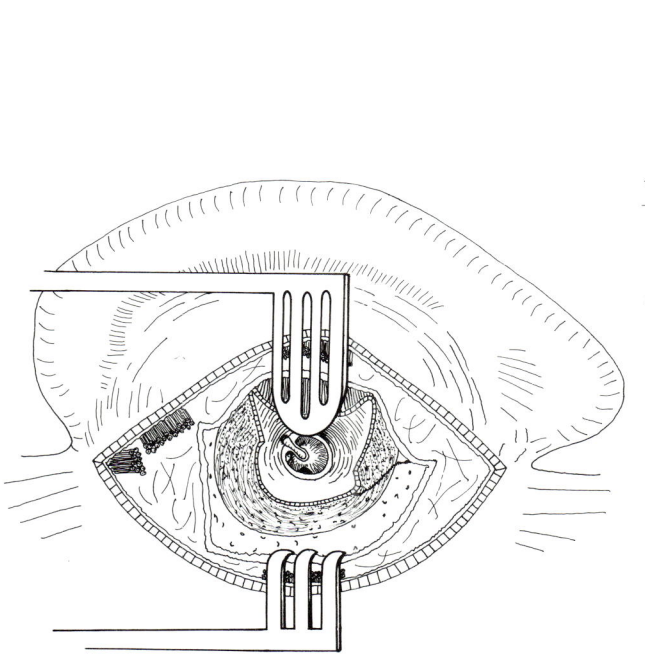

Fig. 106 The laterally-based flap is protected by a large retractor

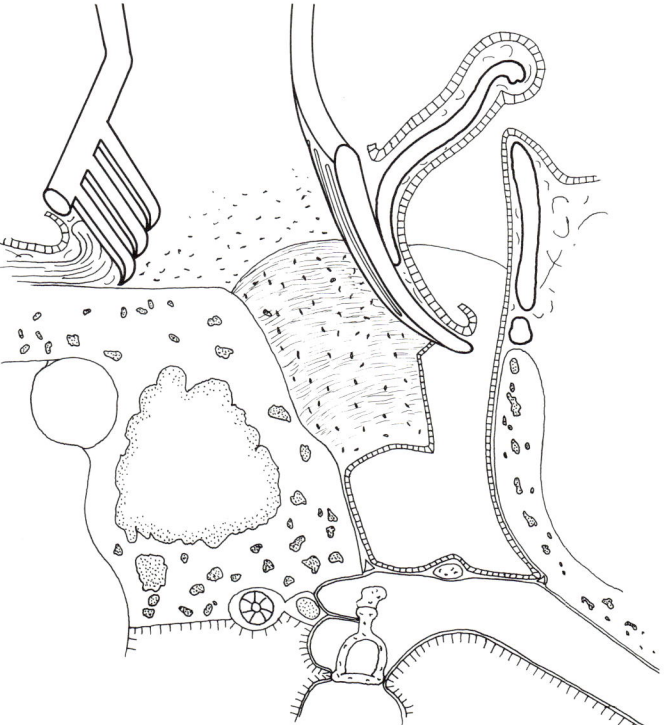

Fig. 107 A long, protective retractor blade pushes the flap anteriorly, providing an excellent view of the anterior tympanomeatal angle

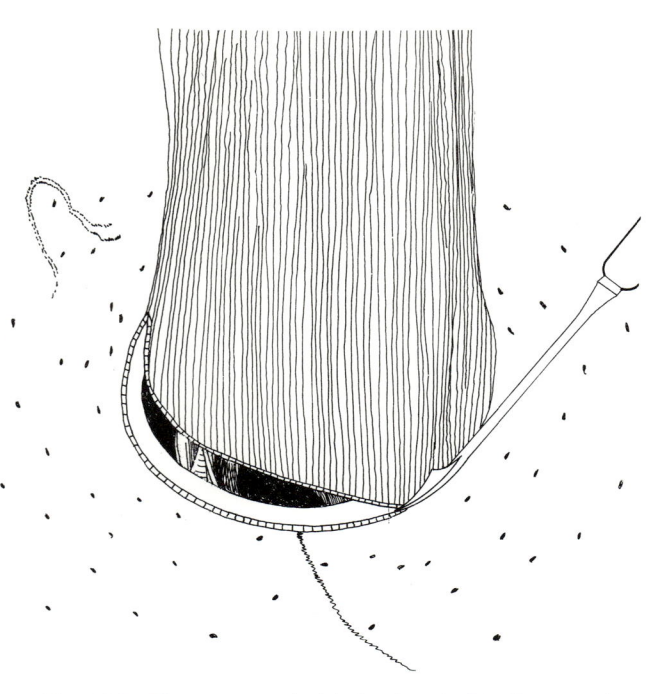

Fig. 108 The ear-canal skin is elevated to the annulus, and incised with a sickle knife at the annulus level, between the 12-o'clock and 6-o'clock positions

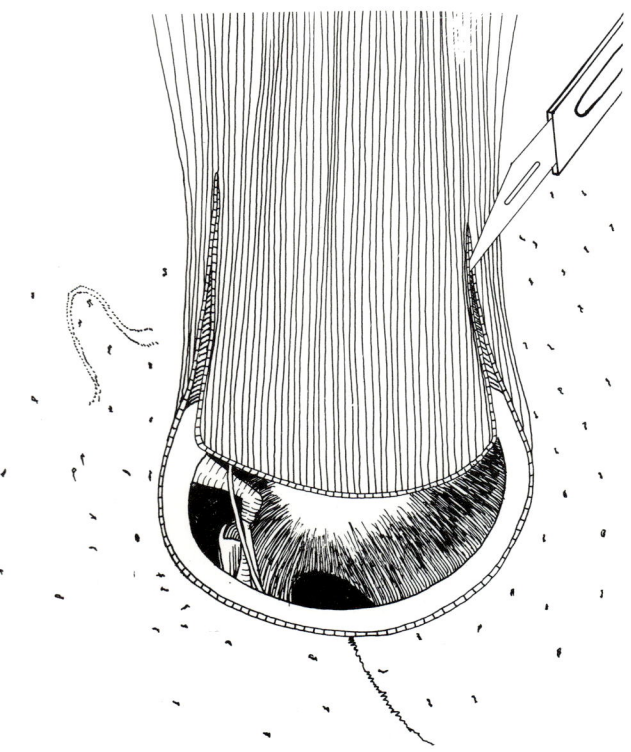

Fig. 109 Two long radial incisions at the 12-o'clock and 6-o'clock positions are performed with a scalpel, forming a very long, laterally-based skin flap

is performed with a sickle knife, either a) close to the annulus (Fig. 108), or b) at the annulus itself, or c) not at all, in cases with peripheral posterior or total perforation. In the latter cases, elevation of the canal skin is continued with a round knife or a small elevator over the annulus, and the instrument enters the tympanic cavity between the epithelium of the drum remnant and the lamina propria. Mobilization of the canal skin can be performed either by placing a long lateral radial incision superiorly and a small incision inferiorly; or a long radial incision inferiorly and a small incision superiorly; or two long radial incisions at the 12-o'clock and 6-o'clock positions, respectively (Figs. 109–111).

2. The tympanomeatal flap can be elevated and managed, as in exploratory tympanotomy, by two radial incisions at the 11-o'clock and 5-o'clock positions, and elevation of the skin and annulus, entering into the tympanic cavity. This technique is suitable for myringoplasty with an underlay fascia graft (Fig. 112).

3. The tympano-meatal flap can be elevated down to the fibrous annulus. The epithelial covering of the drum remnant can then be elevated all around the drum remnant (Fig. 113). The fascia graft is placed on the annulus as an intermediate graft.

4. The tympanomeatal flap can be elevated together with the annulus along its entire circumference (Fig. 114), in order to place the underlay fascia graft.

5. Palva's swing-door technique starts with elevation of the tympanomeatal flap, cutting off the flap and annulus at the 9-o'clock position, and further elevation of the superior and inferior flaps. This method is suitable for an underlay fascia graft (Fig. 115).

6. With a circumferential incision 1 mm lateral to the annulus starting at the 11-o'clock position, continuing inferiorly and anteriorly up to the 1-o'clock position (Fig. 116). The squamous epithelium from the annulus and the drum remnant is removed together with a small strip of the canal skin (Tos 1980). The fascia is placed mainly as an onlay graft. Posterosuperior and anterosuperior skin flaps and, in the middle, a malleus flap, are formed (Fig. 117). The fascia will here be placed as an intermediate flap, and the flaps turned back.

Posterosuperior skin flaps can involve the entire tympanomeatal flap with the annulus (Fig. 118), which is cut at the 9-o'clock position. The fascia will be partly an intermediate graft and partly an underlay graft. The present author has used these techniques since 1960, both in the endaural approach and the postauricular approach.

7. The tympanomeatal flap can be cut by a radial incision at the 11-o'clock position, elevated, and cut with a sickle knife along the annulus, forming an inferiorly-based skin flap (Fig. **119**).
8. Finally, the inferiorly-based tympano-meatal flap can be removed by another radial incision at the 6-o'clock position and later reimplanted at the same place, or elsewhere.

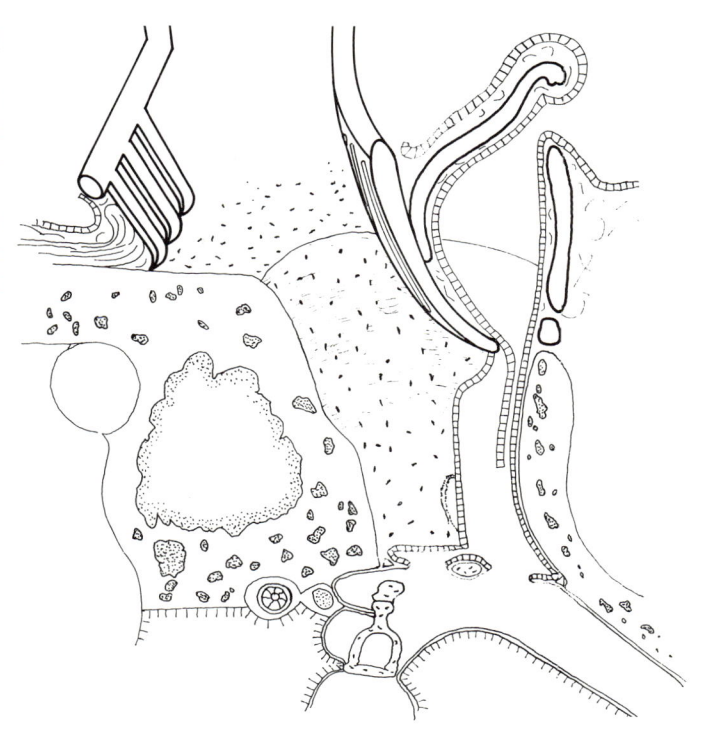

Fig. **110** The long skin flap is pushed anteriorly with a protecting retractor blade

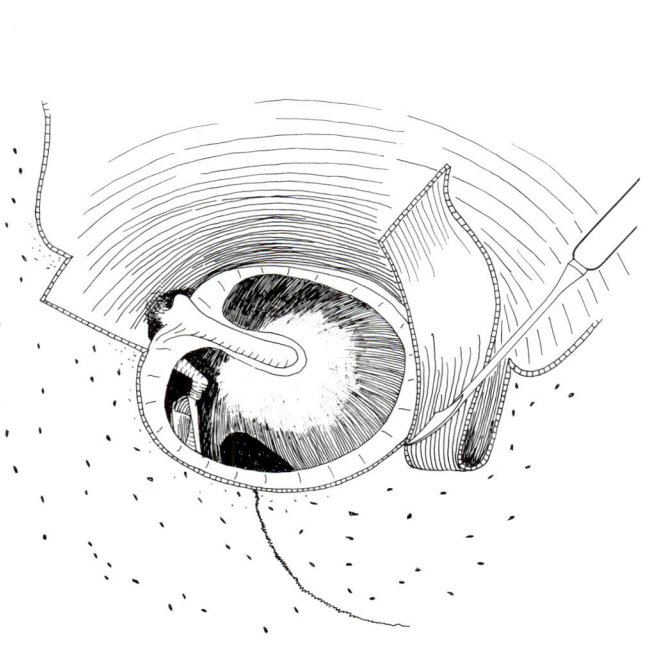

Fig. **111** The long skin flap is turned backward and sutured to the lateral part of the canal skin

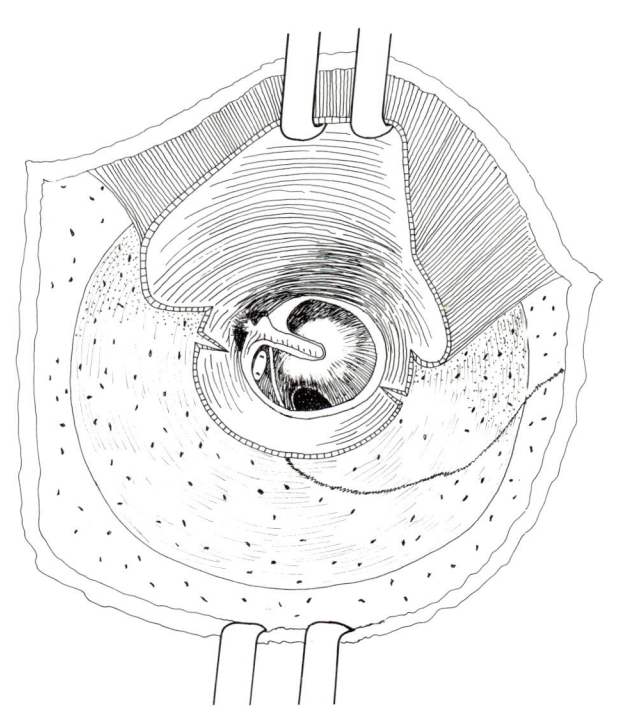

Fig. **112** A medial circumferential incision, with superior and inferior radial incisions facilitating elevation of the tympanomeatal flap together with the annulus, as in exploratory tympanotomy

4 Retroauricular Approach

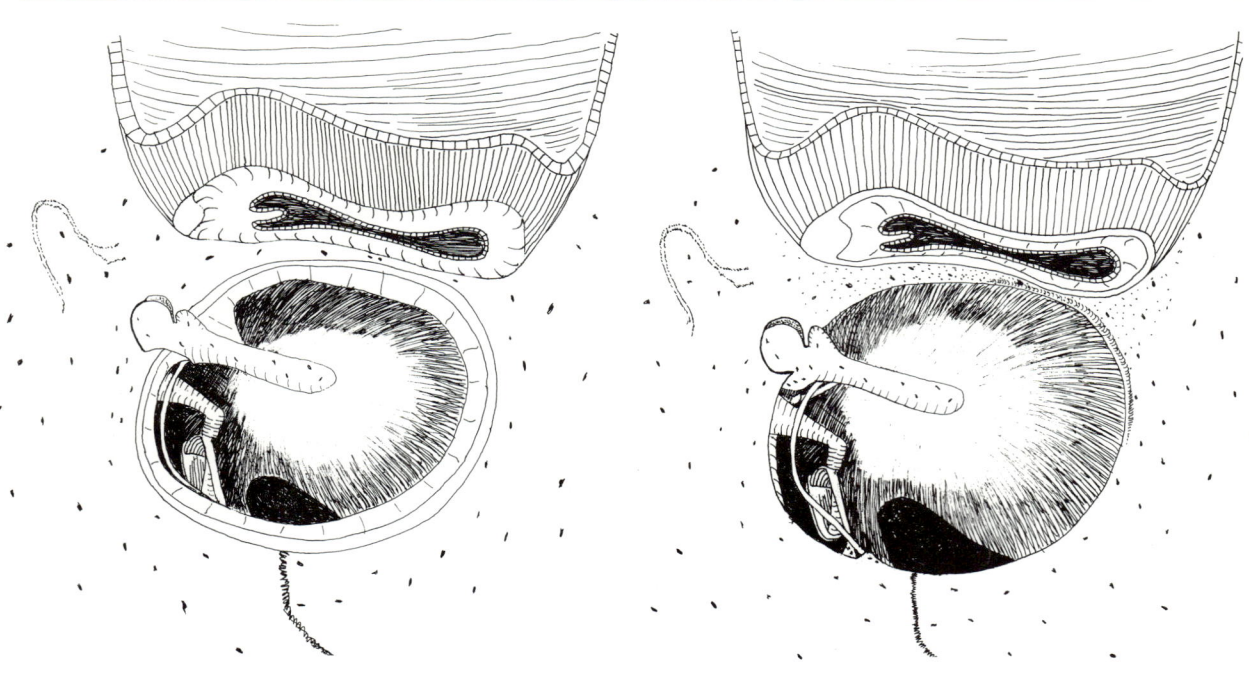

Fig. **113** The tympanomeatal flap and the epithelium of the drum remnant are elevated. The annulus is left in place

Fig. **114** The tympanomeatal flap, together with the drum remnant and the annulus, is elevated along the entire circumference

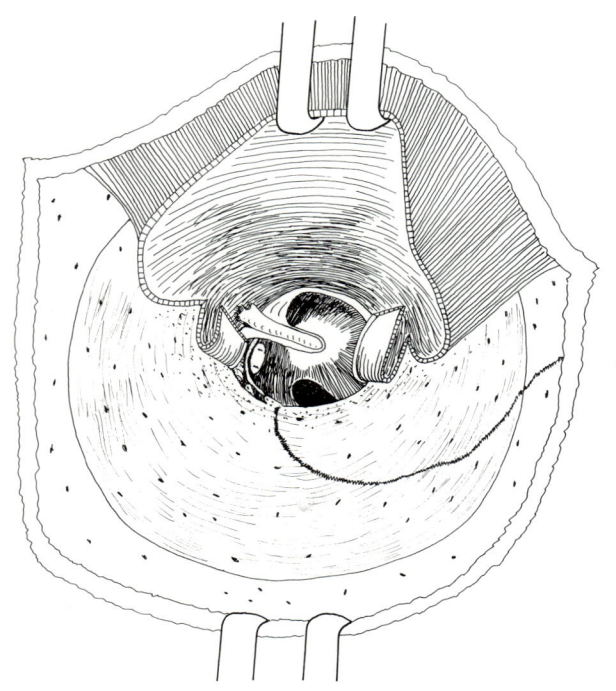

Fig. **115** The swing-door technique (Palva), with an elevated tympanomeatal flap and the annulus cut at the 9-o'clock position

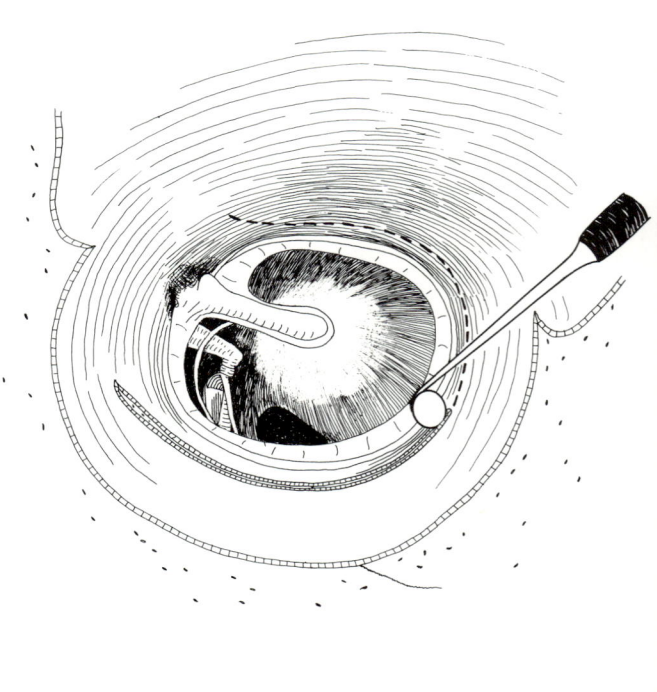

Fig. **116** A circumferential incision close to the annulus from the 11-o'clock to the 1-o'clock positions, all the way round (Tos)

Wullstein–Kley Technique

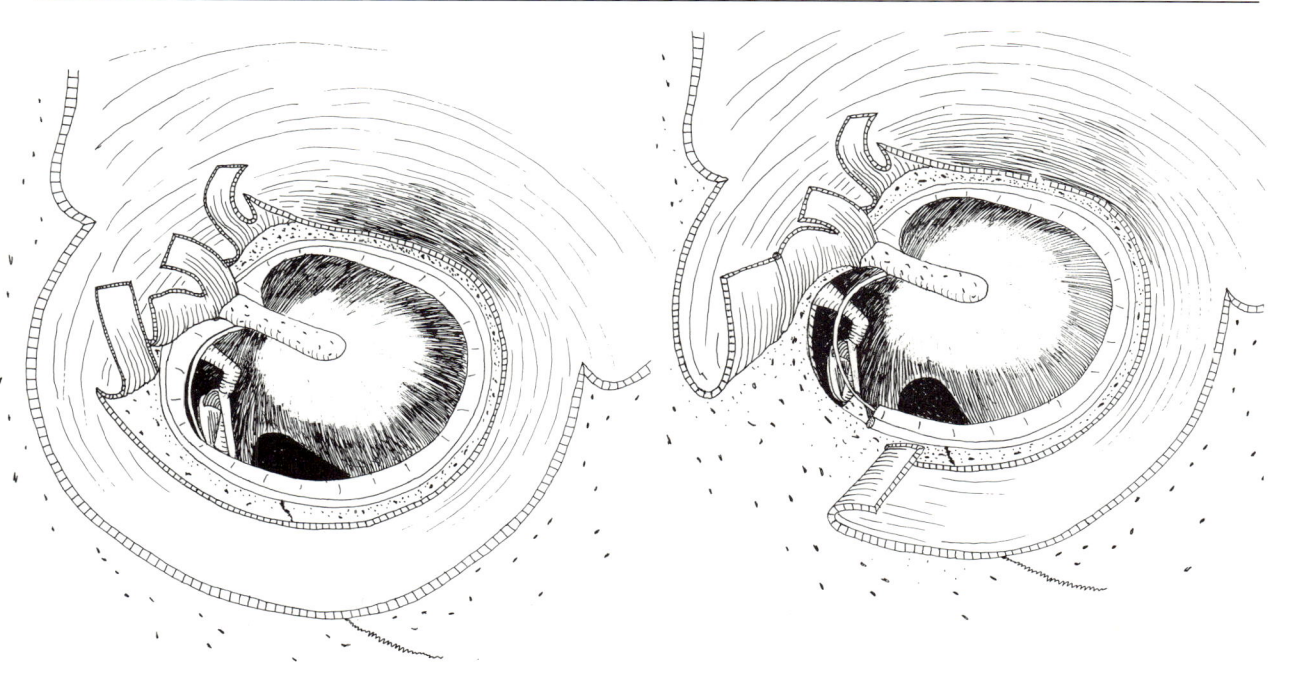

Fig. **117** The skin is removed from the bony annulus, and the drum remnant and three small flaps are formed superiorly

Fig. **118** The posterosuperior flap can involve the entire tympanomeatal flap and the annulus

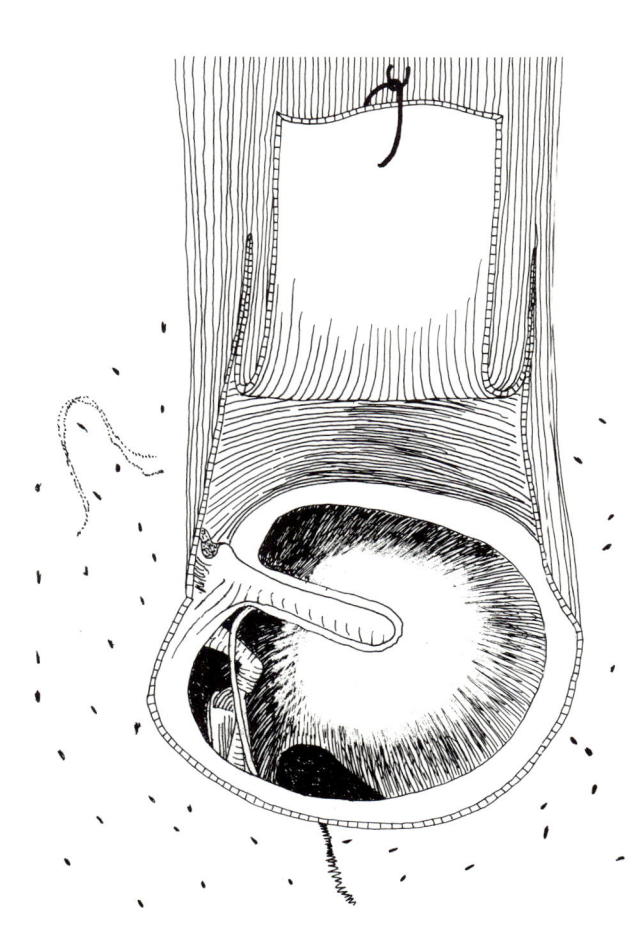

Fig. **119** The tympanomeatal flap has been elevated, and cut superiorly and along the annulus to be preserved as an inferiorly based flap (or removed)

No Circumferential Incision

The canal skin is not cut by a circumferential or radial incision, and the canal skin is elevated in one piece down to the annulus.

After the same retroauricular fold incision and some widening of the bony canal as described in Wullstein–Kley technique (Fig. 96), the canal skin can be further elevated medially, as far as the annulus (Morimitsu 1991, Schobel 1965). In patients with a narrow bony ear canal, some more drilling of the canal may be necessary to widen it. Elevation should be performed carefully with a sharp elevator, to avoid tearing of the skin. At the notch of Rivinus, fibrous tissue should be cut using scissors or a knife. There are two methods.

1. Elevation of the canal skin together with the epithelium of the drum remnant.
2. Elevation of the canal skin together with the entire drum remnant with the fibrous annulus.

Drum Remnant Epithelium Elevation (Morimitsu)

This method was perfected by Morimitsu. With a curved, golf club-like dissector, Morimitsu dissects all the epithelium from the annulus and drum remnant in one piece (Fig. 120). Shrapnell's membrane, together with the epithelium covering the short process and the malleus handle, are included in the elevated skin. Anteriorly, the epithelium is elevated from the annulus by circumferential movements with the elevator from the 6-o'clock towards the 3-o'clock position and from the 12-o'clock towards the 3-o'clock position. Anteriorly, the canal skin is elevated up to 2 mm lateral to the annulus, exposing the bone (Fig. 121). The fascia is placed as the intermediate graft on the annulus and surrounding bone. This method is delicate, and there can be problems with removing the keratinized epithelium from the retracted Shrapnell's membrane.

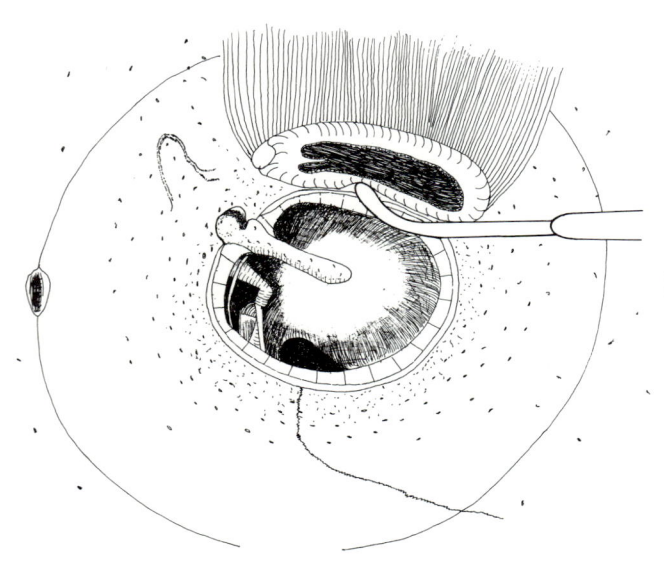

Fig. 120 **Morimitsu technique**. The canal wall and epithelium from the annulus and the drum remnant is elevated along its entire circumference

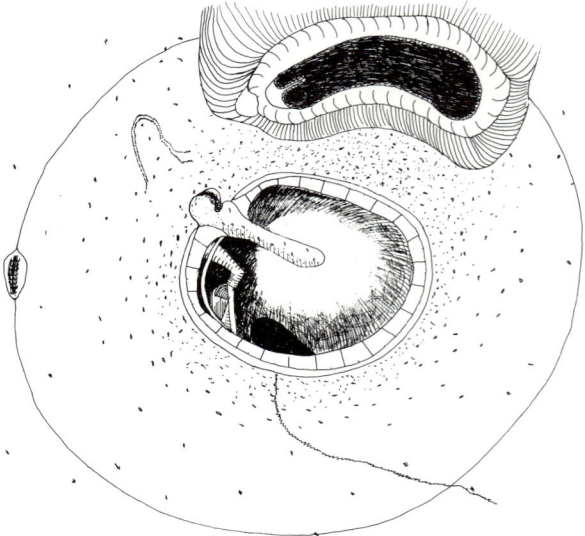

Fig. 121 Completed elevation of the skin in the Morimitsu technique

Annulus and Drum Remnant Elevation

This method was used by Bennet (1971). Elevation of the entire drum remnant together with the annulus is used in methods in which the drum is removed and replaced by homograft drum. After elevation of the canal skin as far as the fibrous annulus posteriorly, inferiorly, and superiorly, the annulus is elevated at the 8-o'clock position by a round knife or sickle knife, and the tympanic cavity is entered. The annulus is then elevated in a superior direction, passing the tympanic chorda prominence and localizing the chorda, cutting the posterior ligament, and elevating Shrapnell's membrane (Fig. **122**). Shrapnell's membrane is elevated in toto. Any possible adhesion to the neck of the malleus and the short process is dissected off. The epithelium from the malleus handle is elevated along the length of the malleus. Inferiorly and anteriorly, the annulus is elevated all the way around, and phushed about 1 mm laterally. The perforation is closed by underlay fascia.

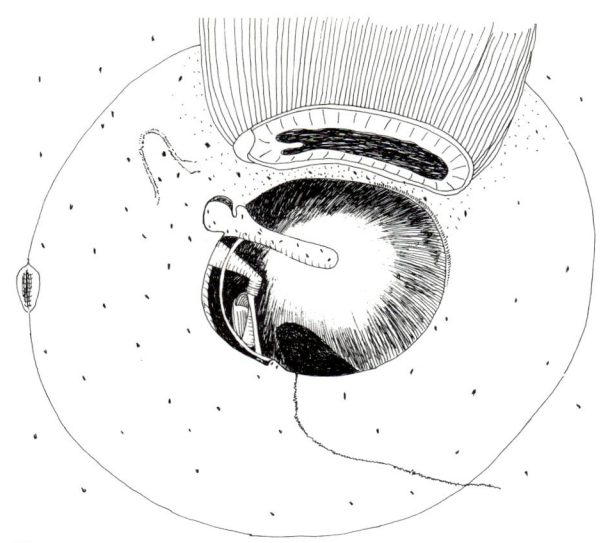

Fig. **122** Elevation of the canal skin together with the entire fibrous annulus and the drum remnant

Posterosuperior Incision (Portmann)

This incision is not only popular among French otologists (Portmann 1979, Charachon 1990, Magnan 1972), but also with others (Morimitsu 1991). The skin incision is localized in the supra-auricular and retroauricular fold. The upper part of the auricle is pulled inferiorly, and the incision is started just above the attachment of the auricle and 2 mm posterior to the attachment of the helix (Fig. **123**). The first 2 cm of the incision run anteroposteriorly, and then it curves inferiorly and around the postauricular fold. Inferiorly, it ends about 1 cm higher than the postauricular fold incision. Superiorly, the scalpel cuts through the superior auricular muscle. The posterior auricular muscle is cut (Fig. **124**) with a knife or a pair of scissors. The auricle is detached and freed, especially superiorly, exposing a relatively large area of the temporalis muscle fascia. It is important to detach the auricle as far anteriorly as the anterior wall of the meatus. A circular periosteal incision is performed by a scalpel perpendicular to the bone and close to the meatal wall, not leaving any periosteal flap attached to the ear-canal skin (Fig. **125**). During the periosteal incision, the auricle is pulled outward to hold the meatus rigid and straight, and the index finger is pressed into the meatus (Fig. **124**). In this way, the fibrous tissue attached to the ear canal is separated from the canal skin while avoiding an incision of the skin and open-

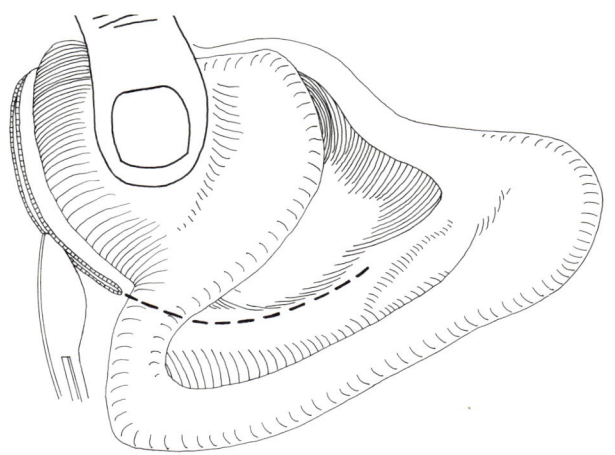

Fig. **123 Portmann incision.** A posterosuperior incision, starting superiorly to the attachment of the auricle

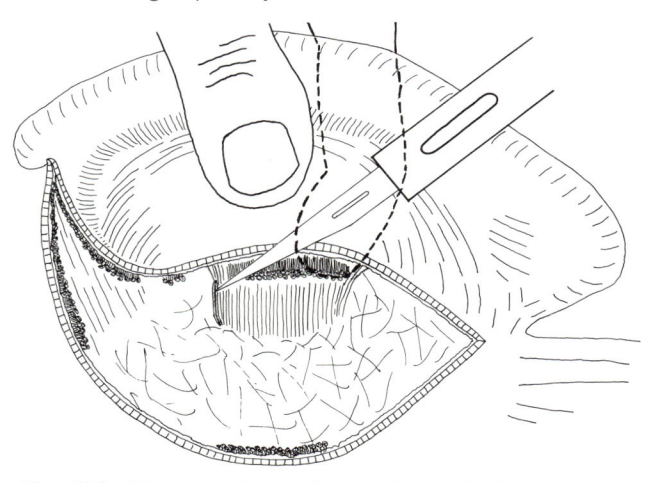

Fig. **124** The superior and posterior auricular muscles are cut. The circular periosteal incision is started anterosuperior to the ear canal

4 Retroauricular Approach

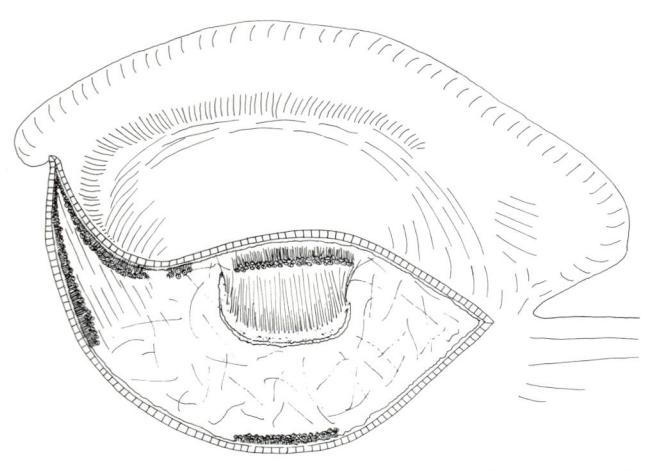

Fig. 125 The periosteal incision close to the ear-canal skin is completed, exposing the entrance to the bony ear canal

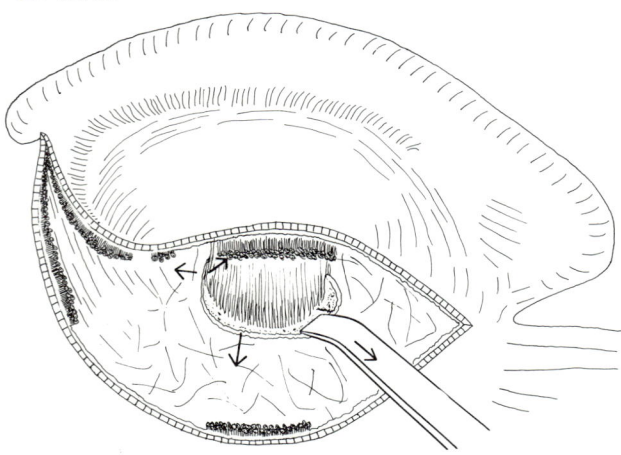

Fig. 126 Periosteal elevation using four strokes, as recommended by Portmann

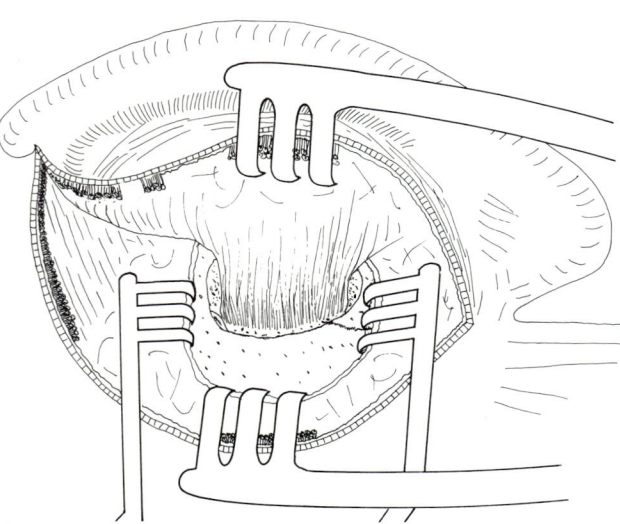

Fig. 127 Elevated ear-canal skin and the periosteum from the mastoid process

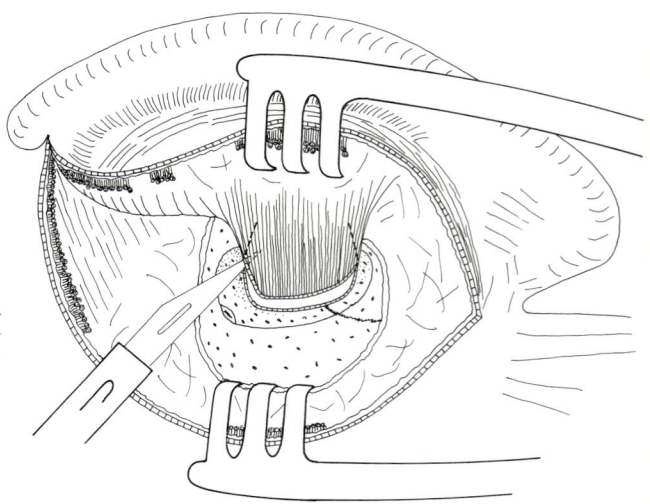

Fig. 128 The circumferential incision is completed, and the superior radial incision at the 12-o'clock position is started

ing the meatal wall (Fig. 125). Portmann recommends periosteal elevation with a large periosteal elevator using four strokes (Fig. 126): the first in a posteroinferior direction, the second in a posterior, the third in a superior, and the fourth in an anterior direction, along the superior edge of the bony ear canal, elevating the canal skin from the bone. The tympanosquamous suture and the notch of Rivinus are exposed. After removal of the conchal perichondrium or temporalis muscle fascia, or both, for graft material, two selfretaining retractors keep the auricle and the elevated periosteum retracted, exposing the mastoid process (Fig. 127).

After further elevation of the skin towards the drum, a lateral circumferential incision of the posterior canal skin from the 12-o'clock to the 6-o'clock position is performed with a scalpel (Fig. 128). The incision is localized approximately 8 mm laterally to the ear drum. Then a lateral radial incision at 12 o'clock along the roof of the meatus and one along the bottom at 6-o'clock are performed. The radial incisions are 1 cm long. By these incisions, a laterally based skin flap is formed (Fig. 129). The flap is similar to the flap described in the posterior fold incision (Fig. 127), but somewhat shorter.

Posterosuperior Incision (Portmann)

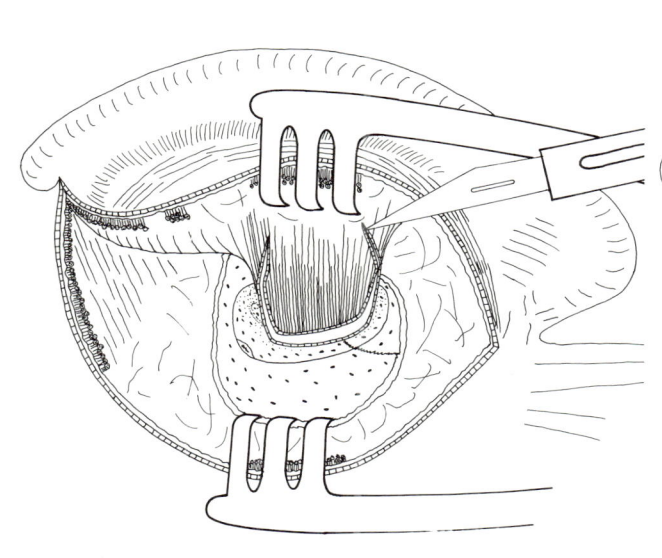

Fig. **129** The radial incision the at 6-o'clock position is completed

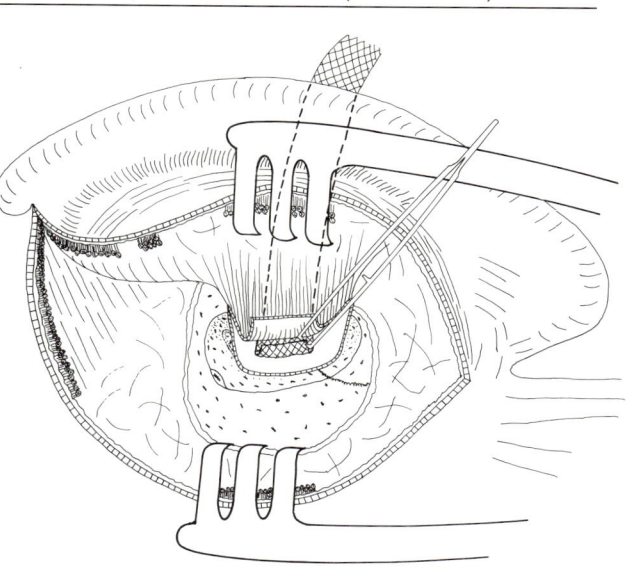

Fig. **130** The strip of gauze is elevating the mobile, laterally-based skin flap

The laterally based skin flap is held in place by a strip of gauze placed in the ear canal, before placement of the selfretaining retractor (Fig. 130). With a tissue, forceps or a clamp, the gauze can be pulled out of the ear canal and the skin flap held in place by the gauze (Fig. 131).

The tympanomeatal flap can be managed in different ways in relation to the pathology of the tympanic membrane:

1. Elevated together with the annulus, as in tympanotomy and underlay fascia grafting.
2. Leaving the posterior skin flap in place, but elevating an anterior flap for underlay fascia grafting of an anterior perforation.
3. Dissecting the skin flaps outwards, in inferior or total perforations (Portmann).

There are several important differences between the posterosuperior incision and the retroauricular fold incision. In Portmann's posterosuperior incision:

1. The skin incision goes more anteriorly, as far as the anterior edge of the helix, but the incision is 1 cm shorter in its inferior course.
2. In the posterosuperior incision, there is more bleeding superiorly, because of the cutting of the superior auricular muscle and the anterior auricular artery and vein.
3. Mobilization of the auricle is larger.
4. Exposure of the temporalis muscle fascia is larger.
5. The periosteal circular incision runs closer to the ear canal.

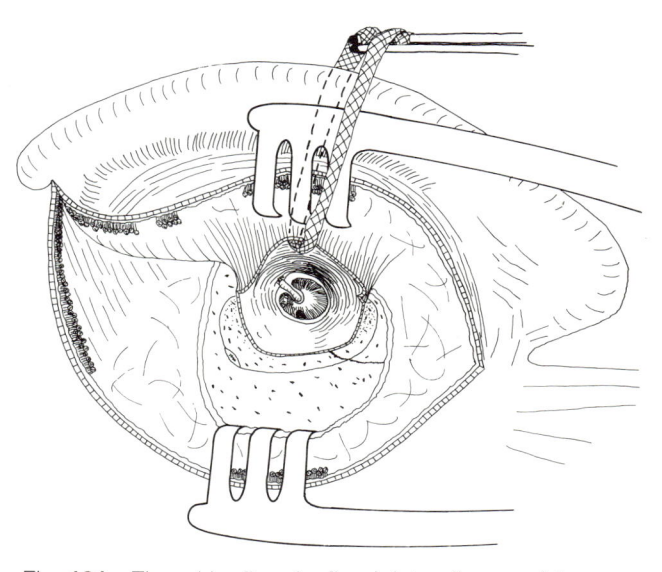

Fig. **131** The skin flap is fixed laterally, providing a good view of the tympanic membrane

6. The periosteal circular incision goes more anteriorly, exposing the bony wall anterior to the tympanosquamous suture.
7. There is no musculoperiosteal flap attached to the ear canal, and obliteration of a possible cavity with an anteriorly-based Palva flap is not possible.
8. Elevation of the periosteum to achieve larger exposure of the mastoid process exposure is difficult without additional incisions, although additional incisions are relatively easy.
9. There is a good opportunity to make some thin skin flaps from the ear-canal skin, free of attached fibrous tissue.

In cases requiring mastoidectomy and large exposure of the mastoid process, Portmann recommends two backward-directed incisions of the periosteum, one superiorly, one inferiorly, allowing further elevation of the periosteum posteriorly (Fig. 132). This type of posteriorly-based musculoperiosteal flap is held in place by two selfretaining retractors, allowing larger exposure of the cortical bone of the mastoid process (Fig. 133). Morimitsu, using the posterosuperior incision, recommends two incisions of the periosteum running convergently from the superior and inferior edges of the ear canal towards the plane of mastoideum. This creates an anteriorly-based musculoperiosteal flap, allowing traction of the canal skin backward and easier closure (Fig. 134).

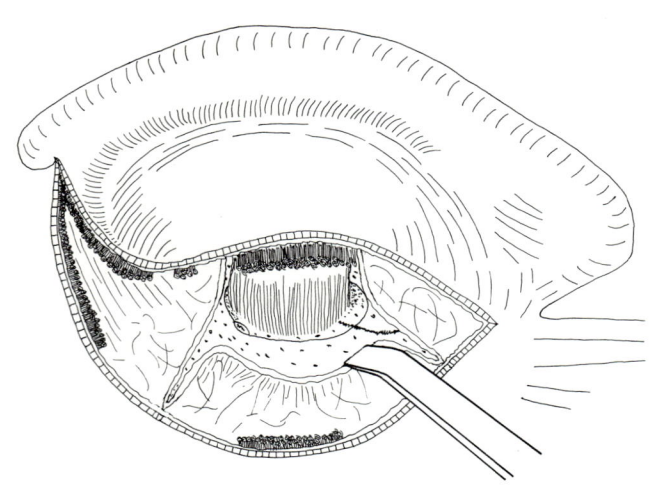

Fig. 132 Two subcutaneous-periosteal incisions, allowing more extensive bone exposure

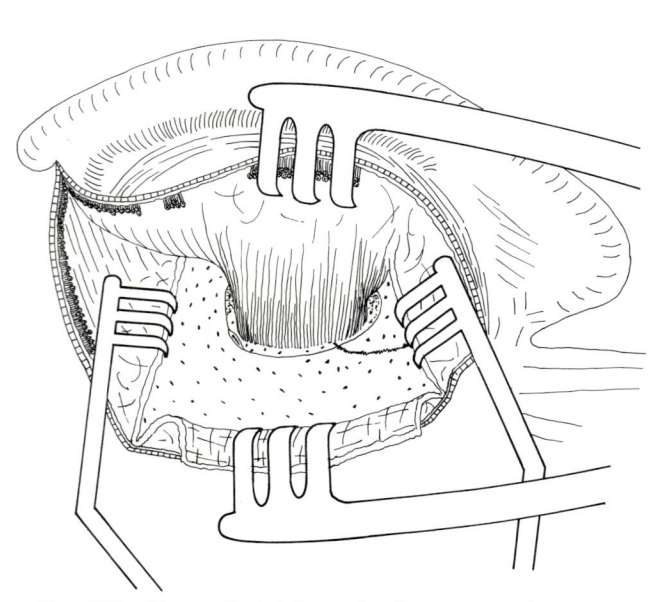

Fig. 133 Two selfretaining retractors are in place

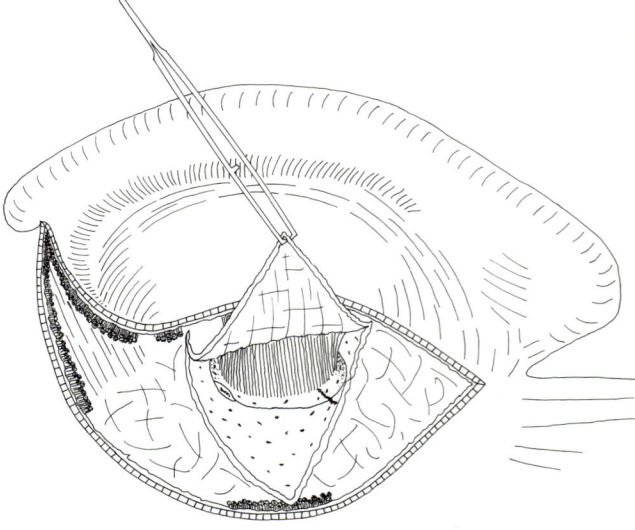

Fig. 134 The Morimitsu modification of the periosteal incisions

Retroauricular Flap Incisions

In contrast to retroauricular fold incisions and Portmann's posterosuperior incision with no, or very little, subcutaneous musculoperiosteal flap attached to the posterior ear-canal skin (Fig. 125), retroauricular flap incisions allow substantial subcutaneous musculoperiosteal flaps. These flaps are based anteriorly, and can be used in reconstruction of the ear canal, or obliteration of the cavity, or both, as Palva flaps. The retroauricular fold incision and the posterosuperior incision are mainly used for tympanoplasty without mastoidectomy, retroauricular flap incisions are used for intact canal-wall mastoidectomy or other canal wall–up or canal wall–down mastoidectomies, as well radical operations requiring major exposure of the mastoid process. If the flap is not used for obliteration or ear canal reconstruction, i.e. in canal wall–up techniques with re-aeration, it is helpful for tight closure of the wound, preventing retraction of the skin into the mastoid cavity or a postauricular fistula.

For all inner ear surgery, facial nerve surgery, translabyrinthine acoustic neuroma and glomus tumor surgery requiring mastoidectomy, the retroauricular flap incision will be used. In these cases, the subcutaneous musculoperiosteal flap provides tight closure of the mastoidectomy cavity, which is of major importance for successful obliteration with fatty tissue and prevention of CSF leakage.

The skin incision for mastoidectomy and chronic ear surgery is usually placed 1–2 cm posterior to the retroauricular fold (Fig. 75). The incision through the subcutis and periosteum goes behind the insertion of the postauricular muscle, which is included in the subcutaneous-musculoperiosteal flap (Fig. 135). The postauricular skin can be elevated separately up to the posterior surface of the conchal prominence, allowing exposure of the perichondrium and conchal cartilage for grafting materials in myringoplasty and obliteration (Fig. 136). The incision through the periosteum and subcutis goes approximately 1–2 cm behind the ear canal. The periosteum is elevated around the ear canal, and the suprameatal spine can be located (Figs. 137, 138). The bone around the introitus of the bony ear canal is exposed as far anteriorly as possible in order mobilize the flap (Fig. 139). If the incision is made directly to the periosteum without previous separation of the skin, the subcutaneous periosteal flap also includes skin (Fig. 138). The elevation of the ear-canal skin is in principle the same as in retroauricular fold incisions. The difference is only that the musculoperiosteal flap obstructs the view of the ear canal. The flap should

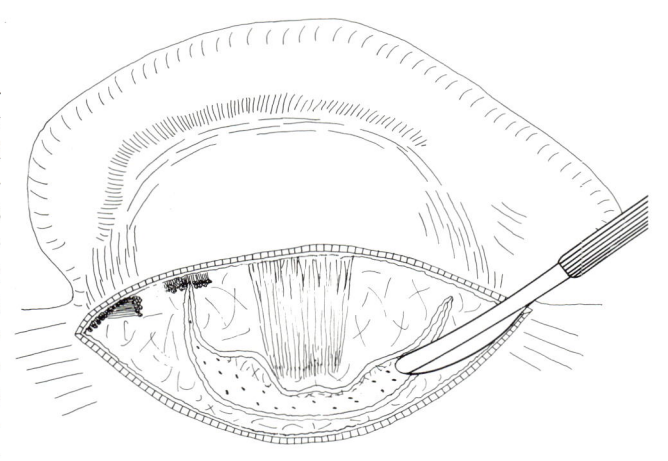

Fig. 135 A retroauricular flap incision, 1–2 cm behind the retroauricular fold, and a curved incision through the subcutis and the periosteum

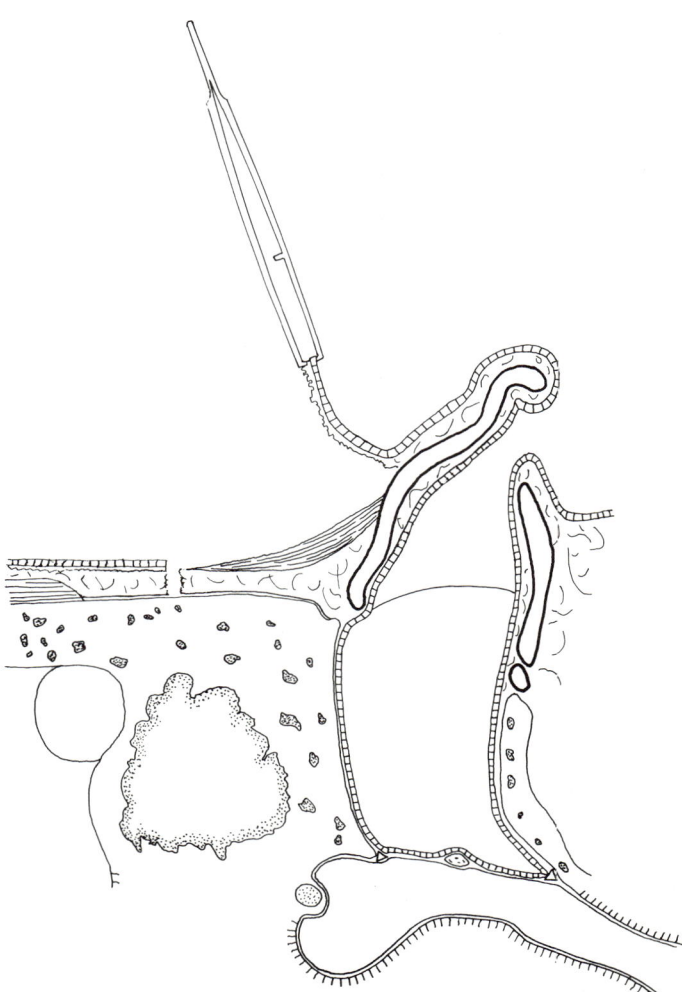

Fig. 136 The skin is elevated separately up to the eminence of the concha

56   4 Retroauricular Approach

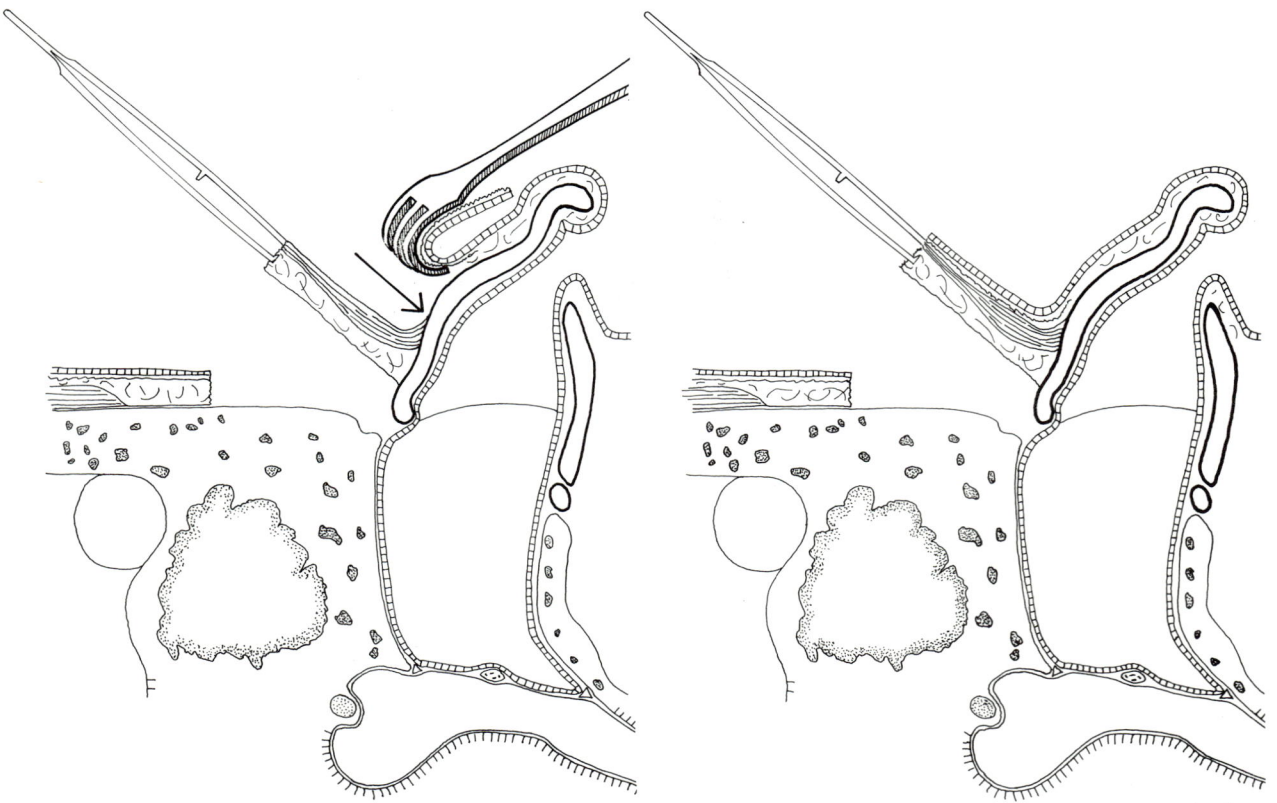

Fig. **137** Access to the perichondrium and conchal cartilage (arrow)

Fig. **138** The subcutaneous-musculoperiosteal flap, with the skin, is elevated

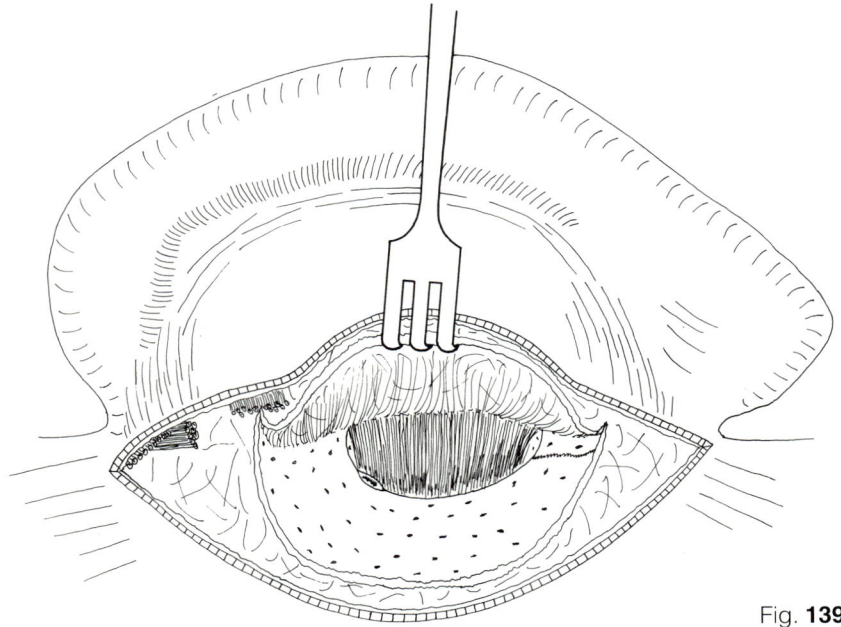

Fig. **139** The ear-canal skin is elevated

toto. Care is taken not to elevate the annulus and the lamina propria of the tympanic membrane. The dissection is superficial to the fibrous annulus. In this way, the canal skin can be elevated in continuity with the drum-remnant skin. Elevation of the epithelium from the malleus handle, the posterior and anterior malleus folds, and from the short process of the malleus, can be performed together with elevation of Shrapnell's membrane (Fig. 153). Finally, elevation of the skin from the superior wall along the notch of Rivinus and tympanosquamous suture is performed without tearing the epithelium (Fig. 153).

The skin is removed and kept moist in a physiological irrigation solution until reinsertion, usually in sandwich myringoplasty.

A curved retroauricular skin incision 1–3 cm behind the postauricular fold, going through the subcutaneous tissue and the periosteum, is performed (Fig. 135). The subcutaneous musculoperiosteal flap is elevated towards the suprameatal spine and the cortical bone of the mastoid process, as well as the entrance of the bony ear canal. With a periosteal elevator, the most lateral part of the posterior canal skin is elevated, making all of the posterior vascular strip mobile. Additional lateral radial incisions are performed superiorly at the 12-o'clock (Fig. 154) and inferiorly at the 5-o'clock position. The canal skin of the posterior vascular strip is turned posteriorly, pulled outwards, and fixed with a surgical stay (Fig. 155). With a protecting ear speculum, the auricle and the canal are pushed anteriorly and held in place. Sufficient bone exposure for intact canal-wall mastoidectomy is thus achieved.

Instead of transcanal removal of the canal skin, it can be removed after the retroauricular incision and after the vascular strip has been completely elevated and fixed with a selfretaining retractor (Fig. 156). Removal of the canal skin through the retroauricular approach is faster. In cases where the primary goal is to perform intact canal-wall mastoidectomy, this modification is usually used, but the end results of the approach are the same whether the canal skin is performed through the ear canal or from behind (Fig. 157).

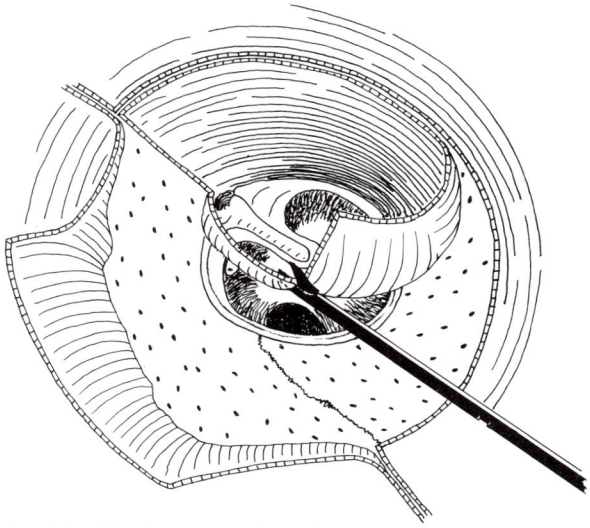

Fig. 152 Further elevation of the ear-canal skin inferiorly. The small skin bridge between the two sutures is cut by scissors

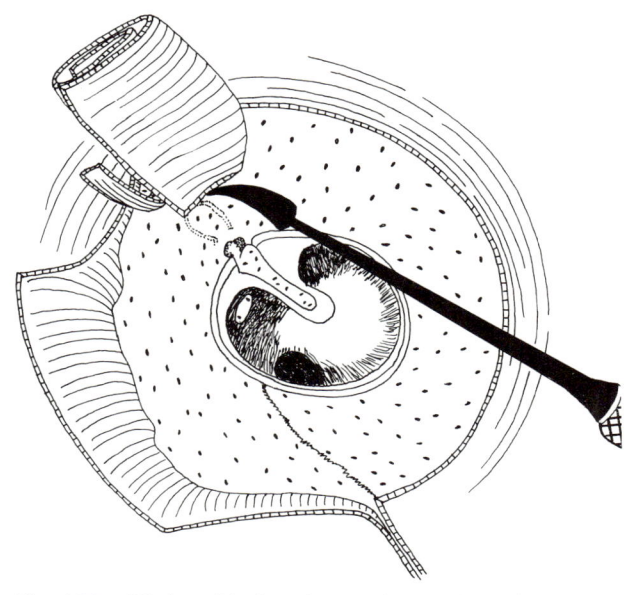

Fig. 153 All the skin has been elevated, and the last part of the section is taking place around the tympanosqaumous suture and the notch of Rivinus

4 Retroauricular Approach

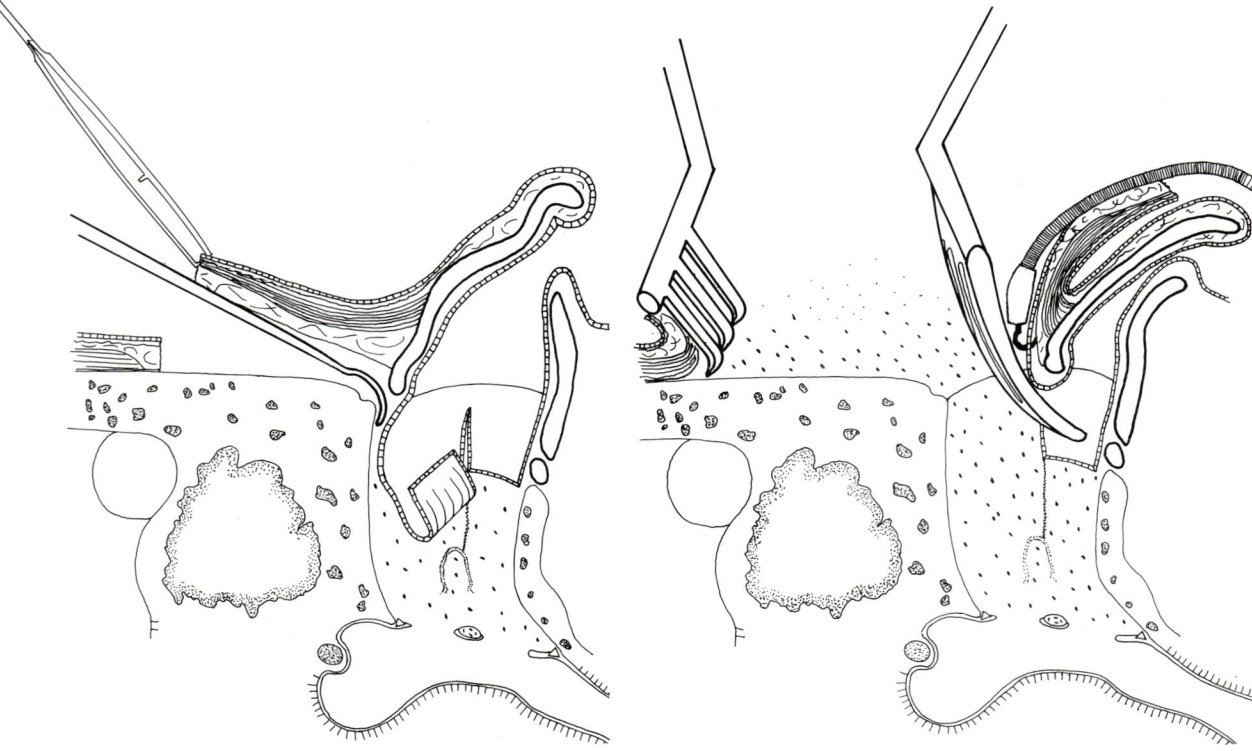

Fig. **154** Side view of the elevated posterior vascular strip. The musculoperiosteal flap is elevated, and the ear canal is entered from behind

Fig. **155** The posterior canal skin is turned posteriorly around the posterior surface of the auricle and fixed with a surgical stay. The auricle, with the ear-canal skin, is pushed anteriorly, and protected with a selfretaining retractor, providing a good view of the ear canal without canal skin

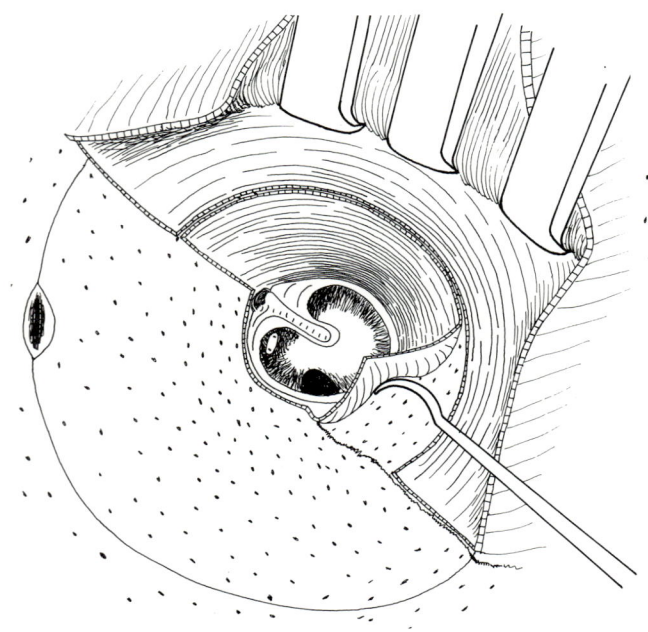

Fig. **156** Dissection of the canal skin through the posterior flap incision. First, the posterior flap is elevated and protected; then the circumferential incision is made; and finally, the skin from the ear canal and ear-drum remnant is removed

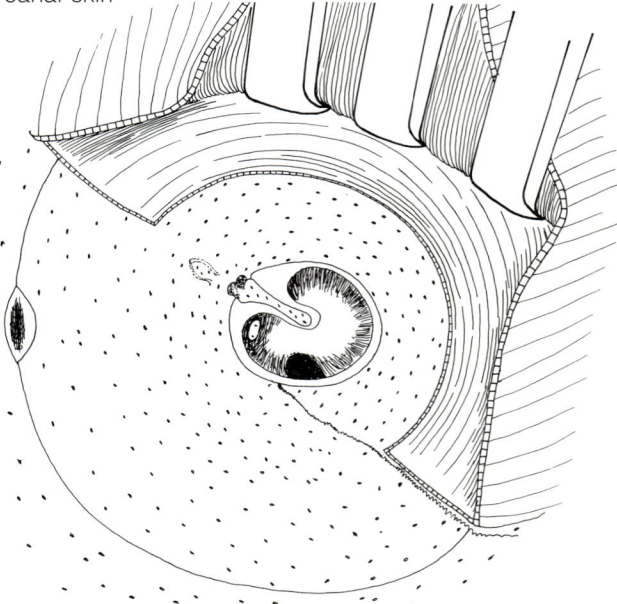

Fig. **157** The final situation after the posterior vascular strip technique. There is no skin in the medial half of the ear canal, and complete elevation of the posterior vascular strip

5 Superior Approach

Sabina Wullstein (Wullstein 1974) developed the superior approach for osteoplastic epitympanotomy. The principle in this approach is wide exposure of the superior wall of the ear canal and widening of the ear canal. This is achieved by drilling the superior meatal wall (temporal squama) up to the middle fossa bony plate, and continuing drilling so medially that the entire lateral attic wall can be exposed and removed in toto as a bony lid. This is done in such a way that the attic can be covered again using the same bony lid.

The philosophy of osteoplastic epitympanotomy is:
1. Rapid exposure of the entire pneumatic system of the middle ear, from the tympanic tubal orifice and mesotympanum to the attic and aditus.
2. The opportunity to extend the dissection anteroinferiorly to the hypotympanum, and posteroinferiorly to the apex of the mastoid process.
3. Preservation of the intact posterior bony ear canal wall.
4. Preservation of the skin of the auditory meatus and canal widely intact, as a skin sleeve.
5. Preservation of all the aeration pathways from the tympanic cavity to the attic and aditus.

The surgeon's position differs from the classic posterior position. The surgeon is seated superior to the patient's head, and the position is similar to that in the middle cranial fossa (or transtemporal) approach to the inner ear canal or the facial nerve (Fig. **158**). The surgeon should also have the option of changing to the retroauricular position if this is required.

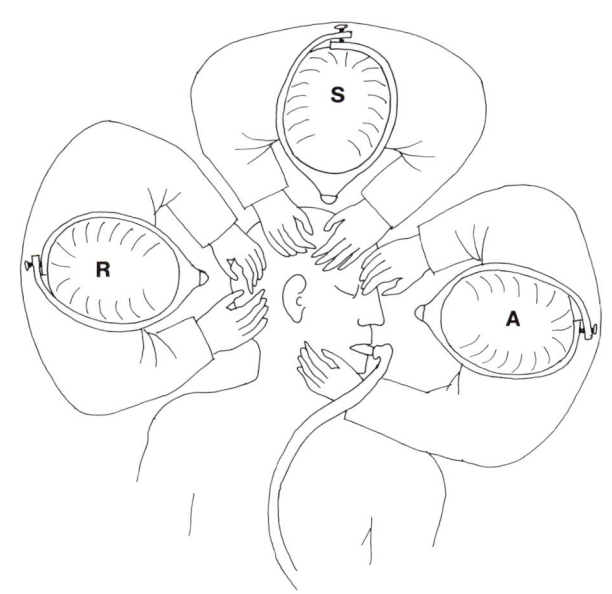

Fig. **158** The three positions for the surgeon in middle-ear surgery
R The most common retroauricular position
S The superior position for the superior approach (S. Wullstein)
A The seldom-used anterior position (A), recommended by Goodhill

Osteoplastic Epitympanotomy (S. Wullstein)

The standard skin incision starts just anterior to the helix, and the level of the supratragal notch. It continues superiorly parallel to the helix, turns posteriorly just under the superior edge of the helix, and runs as a slightly convex curve posteriorly and inferiorly, ending at a somewhat lower level than the anterior origin of the incision (Fig. **159**). The standard incision is used for limited processes in the tympanic cavity and attic, as well as for cases with small or absent pneumatization. In cases with a wide antrum and extensive pneumatization, two additional small incisions are performed, one anteriorly above the zygomatic root, and one posteriorly behind the auricle (Fig. **158**).

For a wide mastoid exposure, the posterior part of the incision is extended around the posterior border of the helix (Fig. **159**). For surgery of a focus above the attic, the incision is extended further superiorly, similar to the incision for middle cranial fossa surgery (Wullstein and Wullstein 1990).

The standard superior incision differs from the Heermann C incision in several ways:
1. Its vertical part is shorter, and there is no intercartilaginous incision.
2. The ear canal skin is elevated in toto superiorly and posteriorly, and pushed as a sleeve inferiorly.
3. The superior incision runs far more superiorly than the Heermann C incision (Figs. **27, 159**).

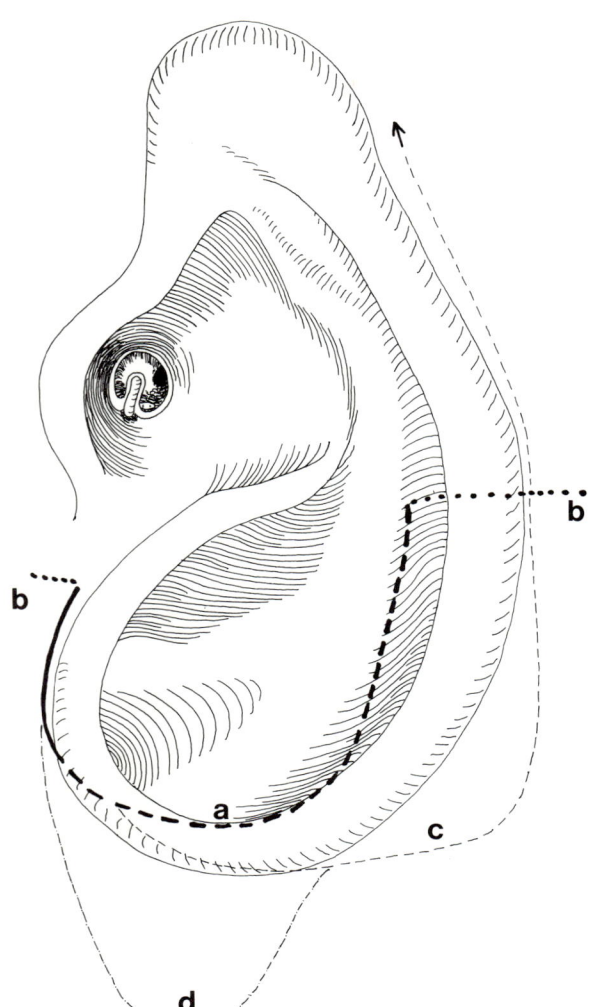

5 Superior Approach

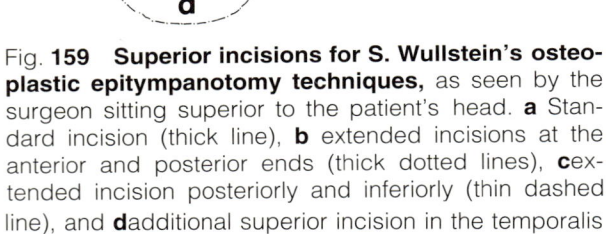

Fig. 159 **Superior incisions for S. Wullstein's osteoplastic epitympanotomy techniques,** as seen by the surgeon sitting superior to the patient's head. **a** Standard incision (thick line), **b** extended incisions at the anterior and posterior ends (thick dotted lines), **c** extended incision posteriorly and inferiorly (thin dashed line), and **d** additional superior incision in the temporalis squama region (thin dotted and dashed line)

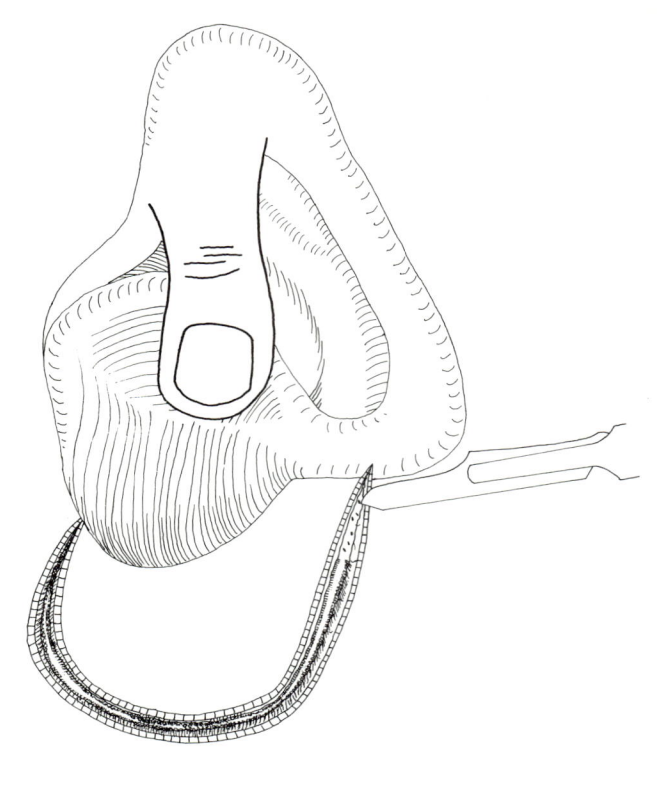

Fig. 160 The standard superior skin incision, cutting through the superior auricular muscle down to the temporalis muscle fascia. The lower posterior part of the skin incision goes through the periosteum

After the skin incision, the entire superior auricular muscle lying superficial to the temporal muscle fascia is cut (Fig. 160), but the incision does not involve the anterior auricular muscle, the anterior ligament, or the posterior auricular muscle, since the lower edges of the incision are situated cranially to these structures. After meticulous coagulation of the small parietal branches of the superficial temporal artery, the auricle with the superior auricular muscle is elevated from the temporalis muscle fascia, and turned inferiorly over the entrance of the ear canal. The auricle is held in place by surgical stays (Fig. 161) or a large selfretaining retractor. The dissection of the auricle should go close to the meatal skin, but without damaging it. It should remain as an intact sleeve during further elevation from the bony ear canal. The temporalis muscle is elevated along the linea temporalis, and the muscle with the periosteum is pushed superiorly. The temporal squama, part of the zygomatic root, the bony ear canal from the tympanosquamous suture to the tympanomastoid suture, as well as the posterosuperior part of the mastoid process, are exposed (Fig. 162).

The initial drilling of the superior edge of the bony ear canal is performed, facilitating further elevation of the canal skin around the notch of Rivinus (Fig. 162). Further drilling down to the lateral wall of the attic is done by thinning the roof of the bony meatus, close to the middle fossa dura, leaving only a thin bony plate of the internal cortex, which is recognized by slightly discoloured reddish bone with small blood vessels and bleeding points.

Osteoplastic Epitympanotomy (S. Wullstein) 65

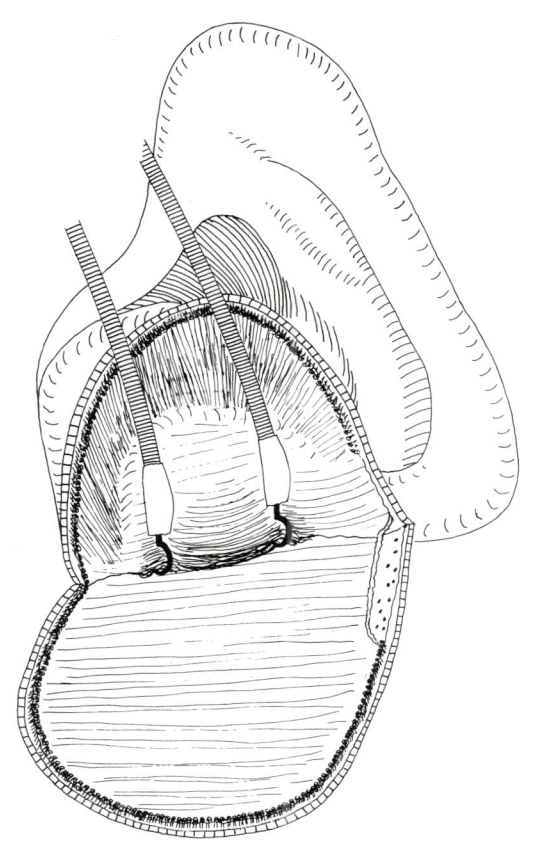

Fig. 161 The auricle is turned inferiorly, and the meatal skin is exposed

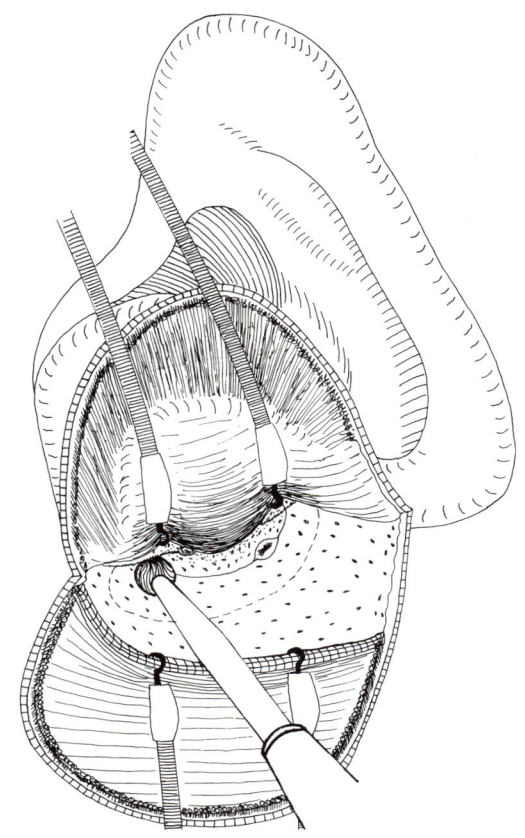

Fig. 162 The temporalis muscle is elevated superiorly, and held in place by surgical stays. The ear-canal skin is elevated from the tympanosquamous suture to the tympanomastoid suture, and bone drilling is started. The dotted line indicates the superior border for bone removal

Development and thinning of the bony lid requires quite extensive drilling. The lateral wall of the epitympanum lies further medially and anteriorly at the zygomatic root than posteriorly at the aditus ad antrum. The drilling of the bony lid starts anteriorly at the bony annulus, and continues along the anterior wall of the attic upwards to the tegmen tympani. There it bends at a right angle posteriorly, and follows the middle cranial fossa bony plate along the tegmen tympani to the aditus and the beginning of the tegmen antri (Fig. **163**).

Before dislocating the bony lid outward, the entire Shrapnell's membrane and the upper part of the annulus of the pars tensa are elevated in order to inspect the incudostapedial joint (Fig. **164**). The posterior groove of the bony lid starts at the bony annulus posterior to the long process of the incus, and then continues posterosuperiorly towards the incudal fossa, which is the most posterior limit at the facial-nerve region. The incudal fossa can be palpated with a long hook. At the incudal fossa, the

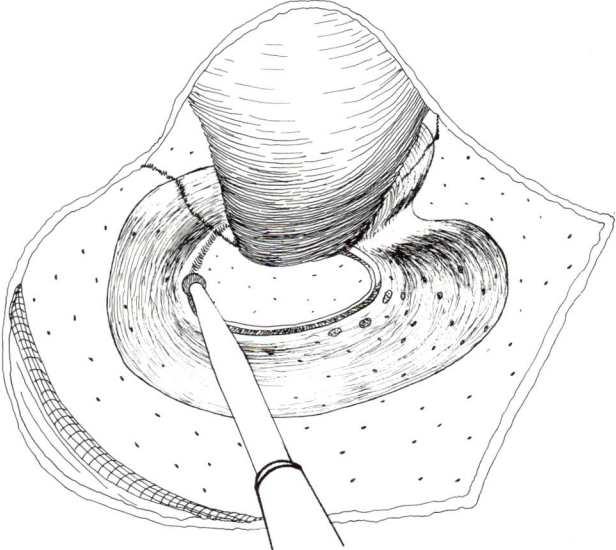

Fig. **163** The canal skin is elevated medially towards the annulus at the 10-o'clock position, and drilling with a diamond burr of a groove in the lateral attic wall is initiated

5 Superior Approach

drilling is carefully performed with a diamond burr to form the fulcrum, where the bone lid will later be fractured, rather than cut through. This precaution is taken to protect the facial nerve, which is situated underneath. An incorrectly-placed bone groove represents the only danger of injury to the facial nerve. Finally, the epitympanic bony lid is cut out along the already prepared bony groove with a 0.3–0.4 mm-thick diamond burr, beginning at the anterior tmypanic spine (Fig. 165). An elevator is inserted under the lid from the tegmen tympani to break it off. After elevation of the bony lid, an excellent view of the attic walls, and the malleus and incus, both with the ligaments and mucosal folds intact, is achieved. To inspect the hypotympanum, the annulus is elevated to about the 9-o'clock position posteriorly and the 3-o'clock position anteriorly, and if necessary, the drum is dissected off the malleus handle as far as the umbo (Fig. 166).

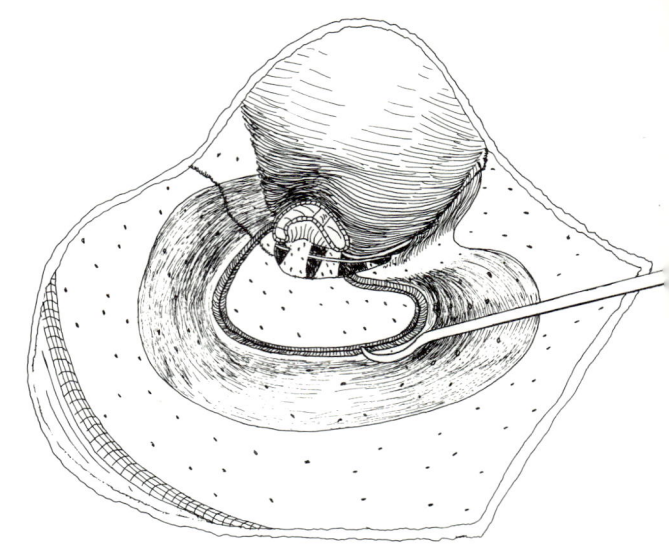

Fig. **164** The ear-canal skin, with the superior part of the drum, is elevated. The small epithelial flaps around the short process of the malleus are elevated. The posterosuperior part of the pars tensa, with its annulus, is elevated. The bony lid is drilled thin, and a groove is drilled out for luxation of the lid outward with a strong elevator, completing the osteoplasty epitympanotomy

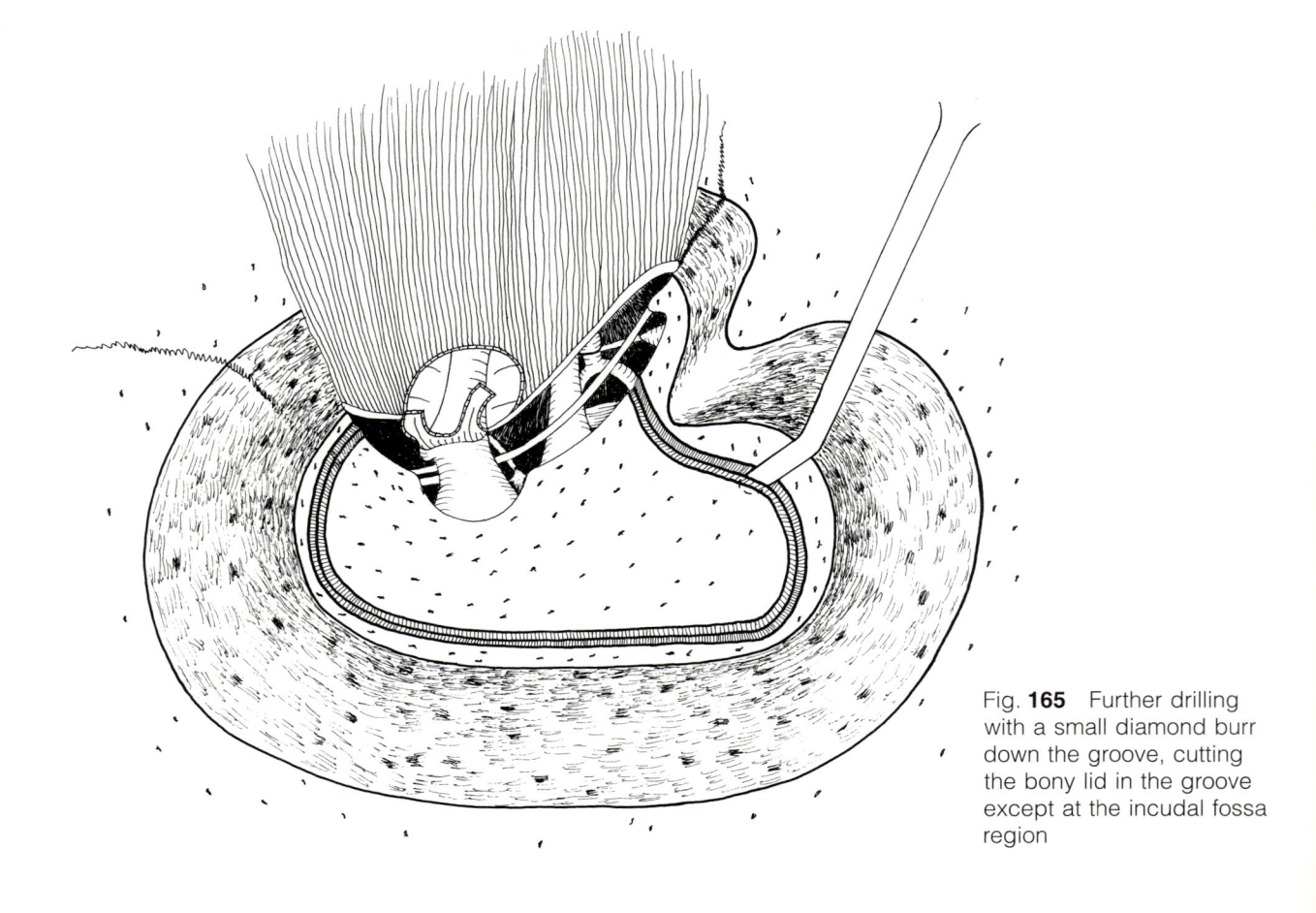

Fig. **165** Further drilling with a small diamond burr down the groove, cutting the bony lid in the groove except at the incudal fossa region

Osteoplastic Epitympanotomy (S. Wullstein)

Fig. **166** The situation after removal of the bony lid, with wide exposure of the attic structures, and the tympanic cavity after elevation of the ear drum from the malleus handle

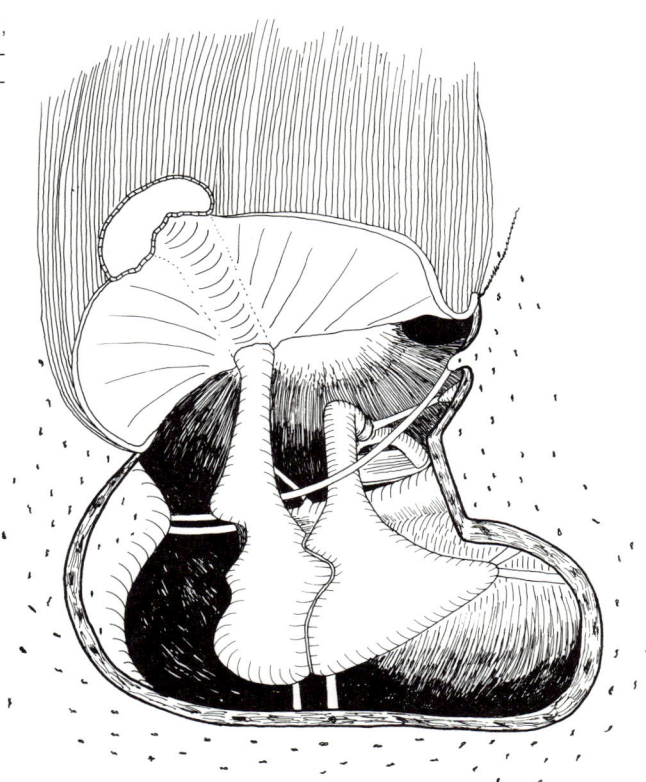

6 Anterior Approach

In the anterior approach, the surgeon is seated in front of the patient's face (Fig. 158), looking into the ear canal in a posterior direction, mainly exploring the posterior tympanum and sinus tympani (Popper technique).

Popper Technique

The anterior approach was introduced by Popper (1935) for the fenestration operation. He used a 3-cm long vertical incision just anterior to the tragus (Fig. 167), pushed the tragus and the ear-canal skin posteriorly, and performed a lateral circumferential incision anteriorly at the bone–cartilage junction (Fig. 168). With a selfretaining retractor, the anterior wall of the auditory meatus, together with the tragus, is retracted in a posterior direction, providing a good view of the posterior part of the drum, posterior tympanum, and the entire superior ear canal (Figs. 169, 170). This approach has only been used in tympanoplasty extremely rarely.

Goodhill Technique

Goodhill introduced the anterior approach using an ear speculum. With the surgeon sitting in front of the patient's face, a speculum is introduced into the meatus, pushing the tragal cartilage anteriorly (Fig. 171).

The anterior approach is seldom used, either with the Popper technique or the Goodhill technique, but it can be the only possible approach for removing cholesteatoma located deep in the tympanic sinus and hidden by the prominent facial nerve. This region cannot be reached by posterior tympanotomy (Fig. 172) or any of the other posterior approaches. Cholesteatoma located in the posterior tympanum, posterior to the round window niche and under the pyramidal process, is also diffi-

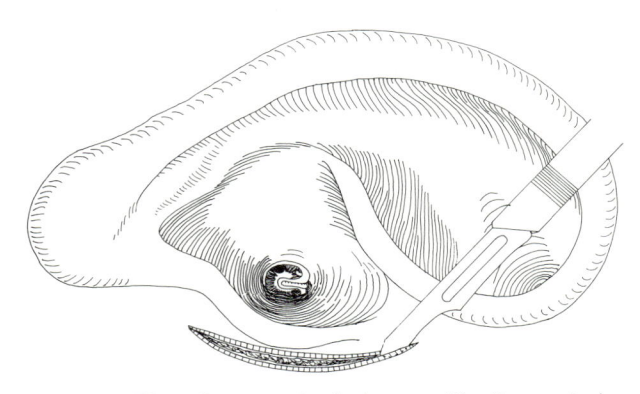

Fig. 167 **The Popper technique** with the anterior approach, with a 3 cm long incision anterior to the tragus

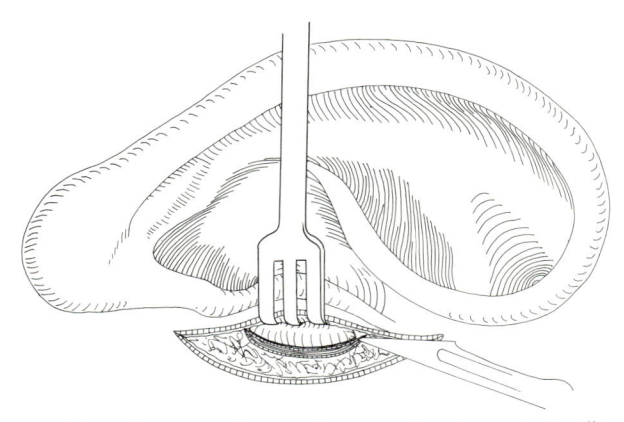

Fig. 168 The anterior surface of the tragus is dissected, and the tragus pulled posteriorly with a retractor. A lateral circumferential incision is carried out using a no. 11 scalpel blade

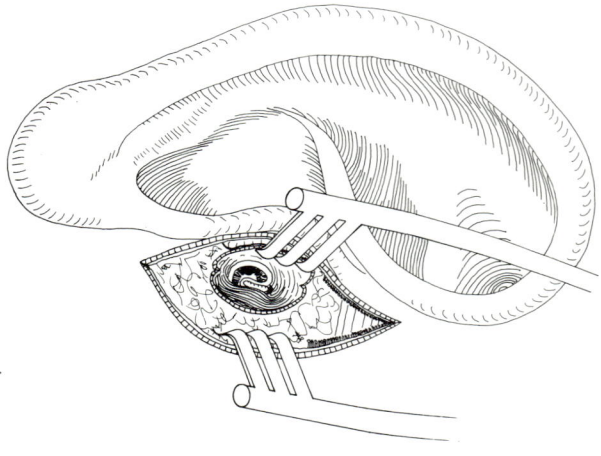

Fig. 169 The tragus and the anterior meatal skin are ▷ elevated and held in place with a selfretaining retractor, and the posterior surface of the ear drum is visible

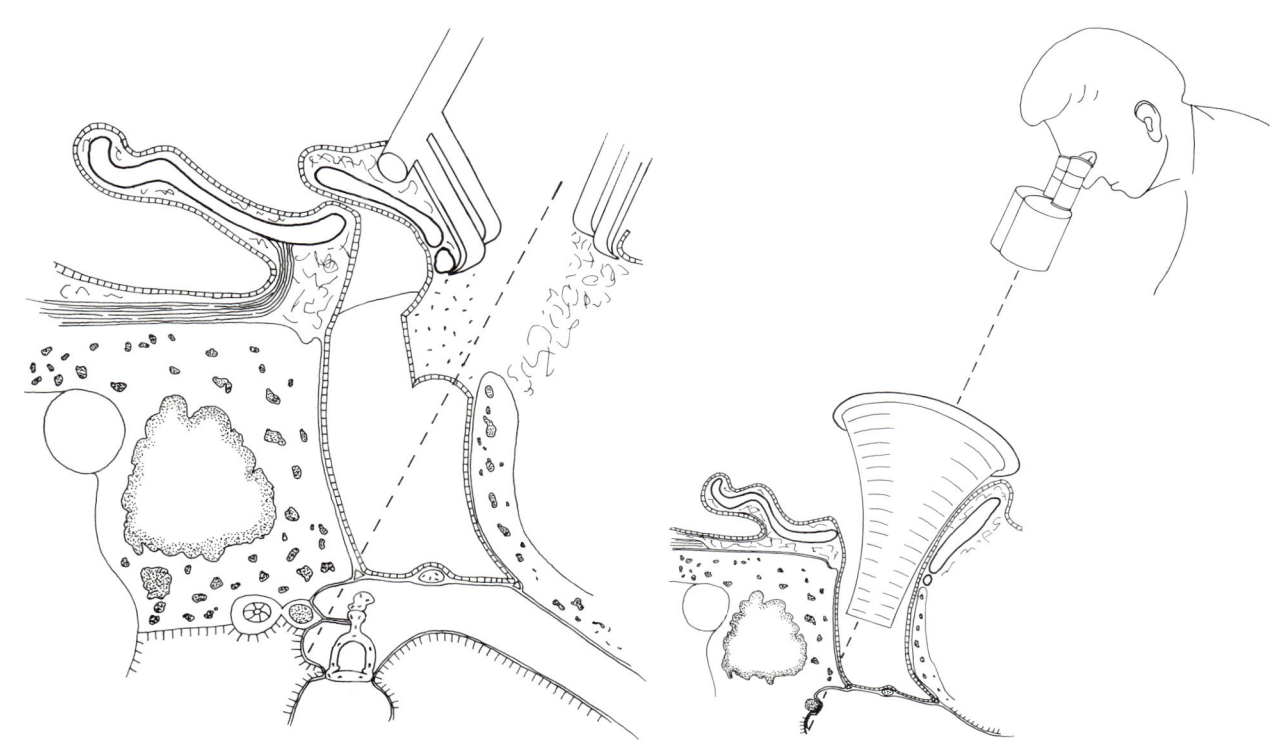

Fig. 170 Side view of the Popper incision, illustrating the good view of the sinus tympani

Fig. 171 **Goodhill's proposal** for the anterior approach with an ear speculum, and the surgeon sitting anterior to the patient's face

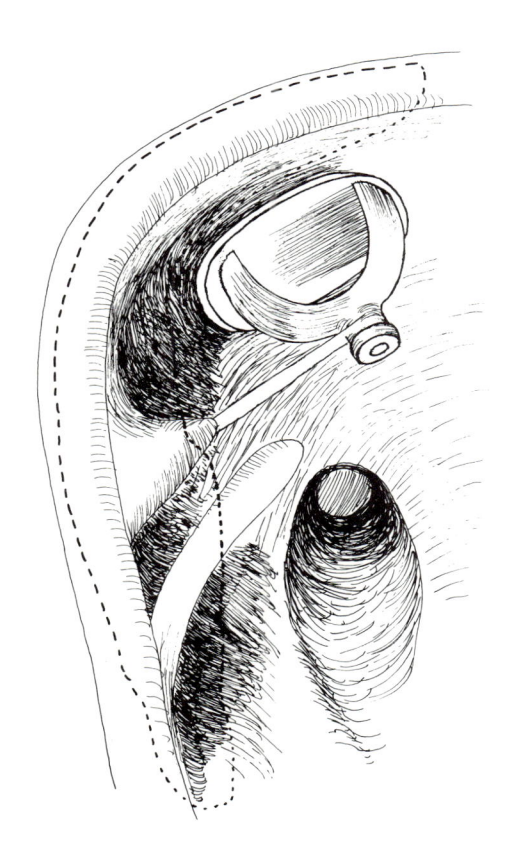

cult to reach by posterior or endaural approaches. In these cases, the anterior approach can also be applied.

When a tympanoplasty is being carried out by the endaural approach with a speculum, and difficulties arise in removing the squamous epithelial membrane of the posterior tympanum, it is not difficult to shift from the posterior position to the anterior position. This circumferential access to the middle ear, from a posterior to a superior or anterior position, allows rotation of the surgeon over 270° from a posteroinferior position to an anteroinferior position (Goodhill 1978) (Fig. **158**).

◁ Fig. **172** The region of the horizontal part of the facial nerve canal, the stapes, and the tympanic sinus. The dotted line illustrates the borders of the area, which is difficult to visualize using any approach except the anterior one

7 Tympanotomies

Tympanotomy means opening the tympanic cavity by elevating a tympanomeatal flap together with the fibrous annulus. As a diagnostic surgical procedure, exploratory tympanotomy is used in many unclear cases of conductive hearing loss, or to diagnose a hidden cholesteatoma in the tympanic cavity. Depending on the location of the elevation of the tympanomeatal flap, tympanotomies can be divided into:

1 Posterior tympanotomy
2 Inferior tympanotomy
3 Anterior tympanotomy
4 Superior tympanotomy

In fact, Wullstein (1952) described control windows on the middle ear: an upper control window (*obere Paukenkontrolle*), with elevation of Shrapnell's membrane after a skin incision just above it; an upper middle control window by elevating the posterosuperior fibrous annulus between the 12-o'clock and 9-o'clock positions after a small skin incision 1–2 mm lateral to the annulus, including drilling of the bony annulus; and a lower control window (*untere Paukenkontrolle*) with elevation of the annulus below the round window.

Since the introduction of intact canal-wall mastoidectomy, drilling from the posterior attic through the facial recess to the tympanic cavity has also been termed "posterior tympanotomy" by Jansen (1972). This procedure was originally called "middle ear inspection" by Wullstein (1952, 1968). Although the term "posterior tympanotomy" has become very popular, it is not a correct term, in the present author's view. The term "posterior atticotympanotomy," proposed by Farrior, is preferable, as it indicates that the procedure starts in the posterior attic and ends in the tympanic cavity. The term "anterior tympanotomy" has also been introduced in intact canal-wall mastoidectomy by Morimitsu (1991), denoting the removal of the bony plate between the anterior attic and the supratubal recess. A better term for this procedure would be "anterior atticotympanotomy."

Posterior Tympanotomy

Posterior tympanotomy is the most common procedure in middle-ear surgery. Exploratory tympanotomy mostly involves posterior tympanotomy, searching for pathology in the posterior tympanum. It is also the opening maneuver in stapes surgery, in nearly all ossiculoplasties with an intact drum, and in many myringoplasty methods with underlay placement of the graft.

The skin incision can be curved, starting at the 12-o'clock position close to Shrapnell's membrane, and ending at the 6-o'clock position at the annulus. The other commonly-used incision is a medial circumferential incision placed about 6 mm lateral to the annulus, running from the 11-o'clock to the 5-o'clock position, and two medial radial incisions running towards the annulus (Fig. **173**).

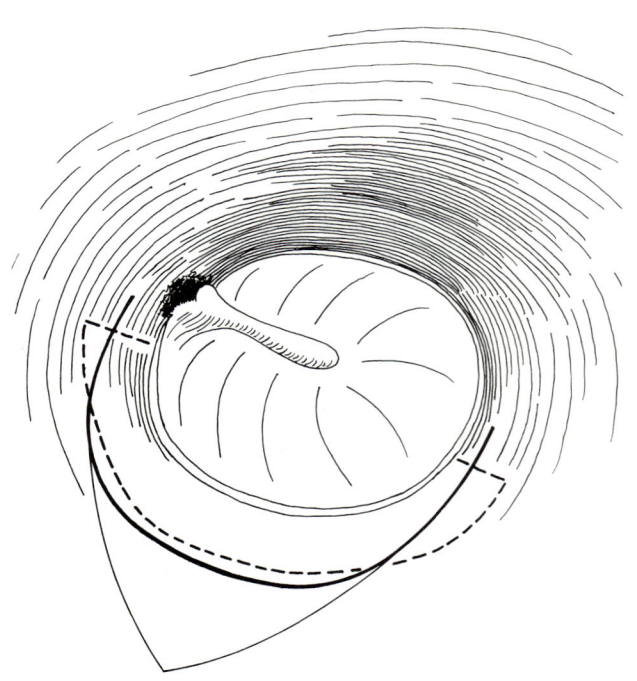

Fig. **173 The most common incisions for posterior tympanotomy:** a curved Rosen incision (thick solid line) from the 12-o'clock to 6-o'clock positions; a circumferential incision with radial incisions at the 12-o'clock and 6-o'clock positions (dotted line); and a laterally-placed conic incision (thin solid line)

Posterior Tympanotomy

The level of the skin incision, and thus the size of the canal skin flap, depends on the purpose of the procedure. For stapedectomy and ossiculoplasty, a classic Rosen incision with a 6-mm long skin flap is sufficient (Fig. **174**). In cases requiring more extensive drilling of the bony annulus, for instance in removal of a sinus cholesteatoma, a more laterally-placed skin incision is needed to cover the bony defect after drilling of the posterosuperior bony annulus.

The Rosen incision can start with a round or oval knife at the 12-o'clock position and continue to the 9-o'clock one (Fig. **174**). The inferior part of the incision starts at the 6-o'clock position at the annulus, and continues laterally, reaching the superior part of the incision at the 9-o'clock position (Fig. **175**). With the same round knife, the skin flap together with the periosteum is elevated down to the fibrous annulus (Fig. **176**). The tympanic cavity is usually entered inferiorly, at the 7-o'clock or 8-o'clock position. The fibrous annulus is carefully dislocated out of its bony sulcus, and the middle ear is entered by incision of the mucosa with the incudostapedial knife (Fig. **177**).

With the same instrument, the annulus is dislocated further down to the 6-o'clock position and up to the eminence of the chorda, which is at the 10-o'clock position. Care is taken not to damage the chorda tympani, which runs from the eminence of the chorda anterosuperiorly towards the long process of the incus and malleus handle (Fig. **178**).

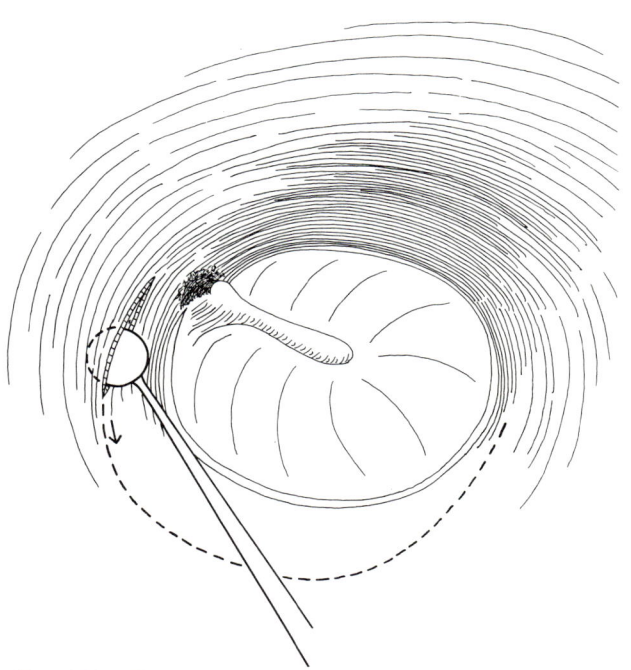

Fig. **174** The Rosen incision is started superiorly

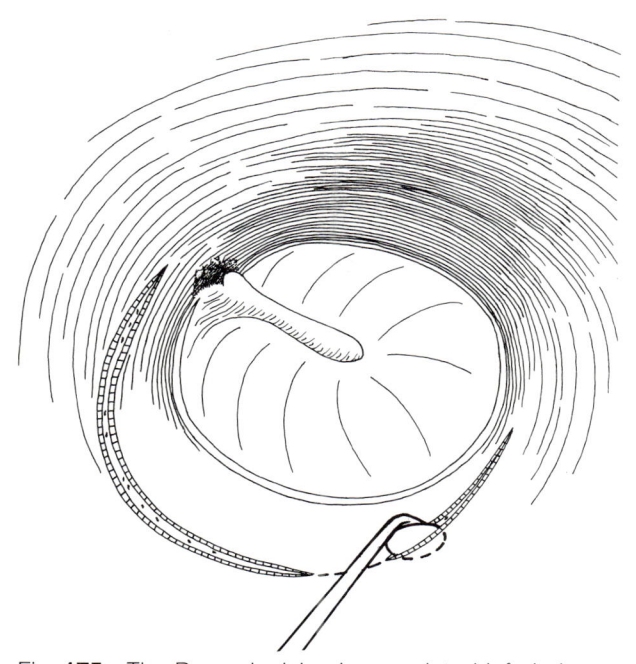

Fig. **175** The Rosen incision is completed inferiorly

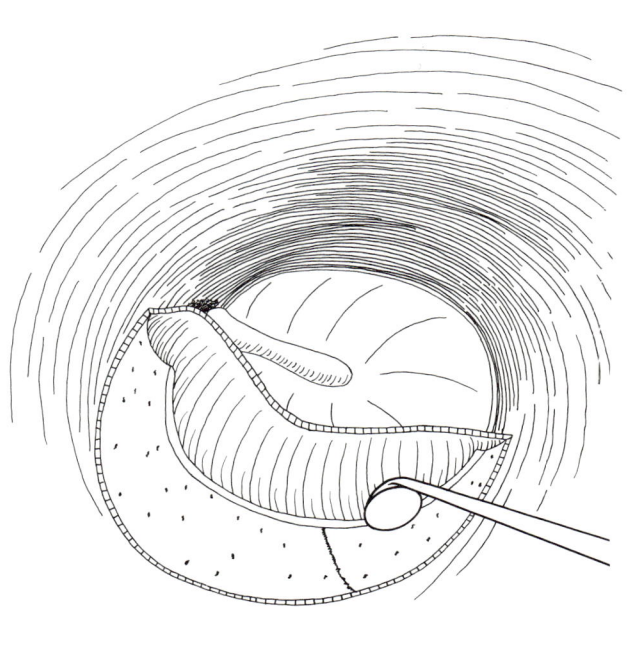

Fig. **176** The skin flap is elevated down to the fibrous annulus

7 Tympanotomies

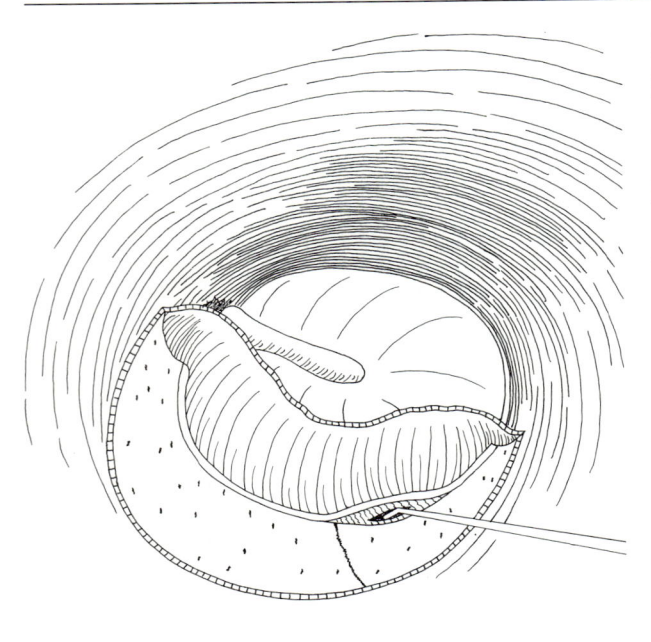

Fig. 177 The annulus is luxated at the 5-o'clock position, and the mucosa is incised with an incudostapedial knife

In fact, the chorda is the best guide for locating the incudostapedial joint and the handle of the malleus. Following the chorda, it crosses the long process of the incus somewhat superior to the lenticular process, and runs under the neck of the malleus, just superior to the attachment of the medial ligament of the malleus. The upper part of the malleus handle can be safely located.

Superior to the eminence of the chorda, the posterior malleolar ligament is attached to the bony annulus (Fig. **178**). When the exact location of the chorda tympani is known, the thin fibrous annulus superior to the chorda is dislocated for further exposure of the incudostapedial joint (Fig. **179**). Some of the bony annulus can be removed, either using a House curette or a small diamond drill, and the attachment of the posterior malleolar ligament to the bony annulus is torn using a hook (Fig. **180**). Further bone removal facilitates the view to the stapes region and the sinus tympani (Figs. **181, 182**). The removal of the posterosuperior bony annulus, termed "otosclerosis drilling," is an important part of stapedectomy, tympanoplasty, and several mastoidectomy methods, providing an ade-

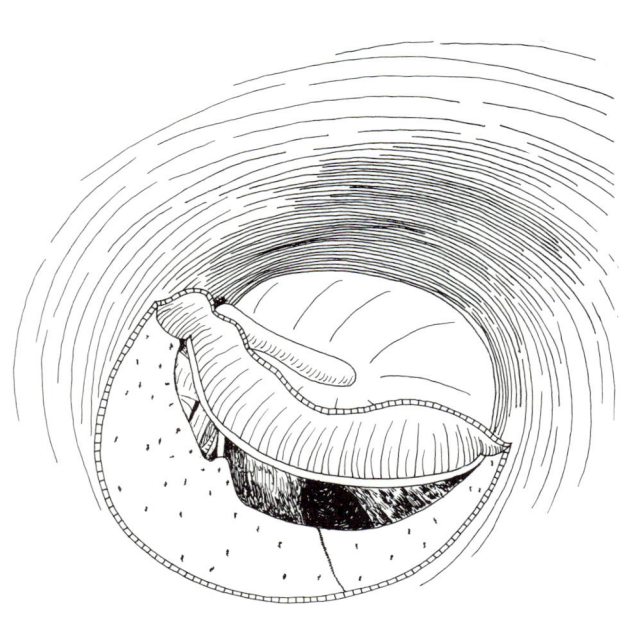

Fig. 178 Further luxation of the fibrous annulus, exposing the posterior part of the tympanic cavity

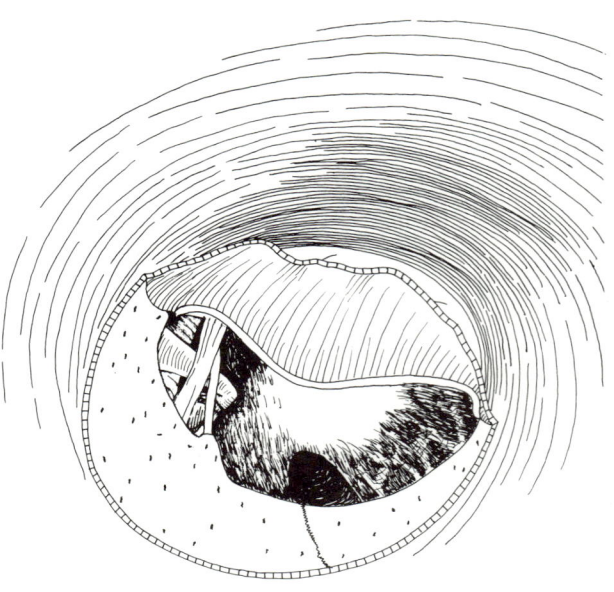

Fig. 179 The annulus is luxated from the 6-o'clock to the 12-o'clock positions, and the posterior half of the tympanic cavity is completely exposed

quate view of the sinus tympani, stapes, and horizontal segment of the facial nerve. Otosclerosis drilling is necessary in stapes surgery, for removal of the incus remnant from the attic in ossiculoplasty, in all cases with posterosuperior retraction, and in the presence of epithelial membranes extending down to the tympanic sinus. The bone removal makes it possible to place the instruments behind the retracted membrane, and to elevate the retracted membrane.

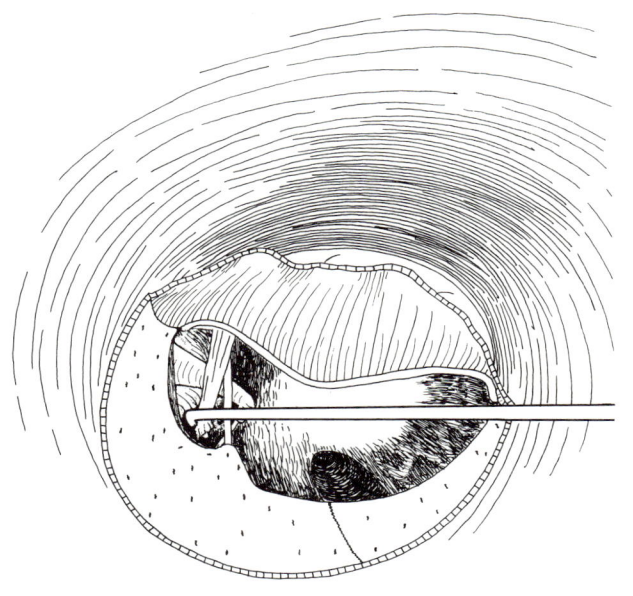

Fig. **180** Some drilling of the bony annulus has taken place, and the posterior malleus ligament is torn with a hook

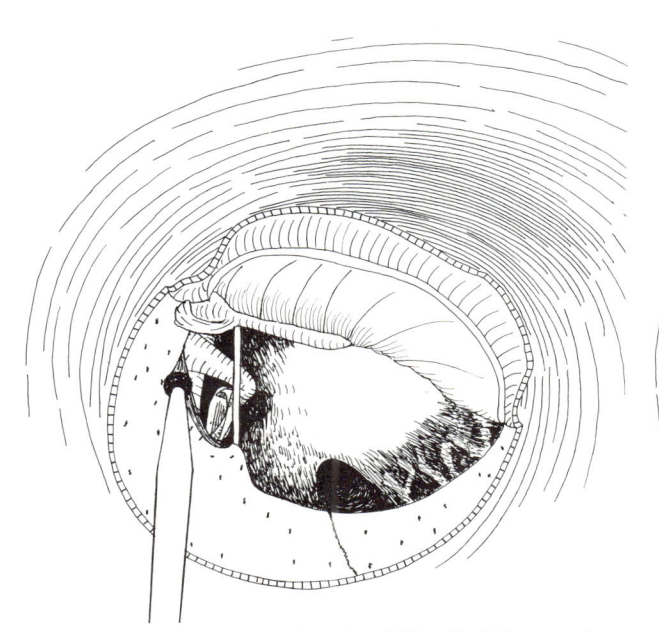

Fig. **181** Further "otosclerosis drilling" of the posterosuperior bony annulus, using a diamond drill

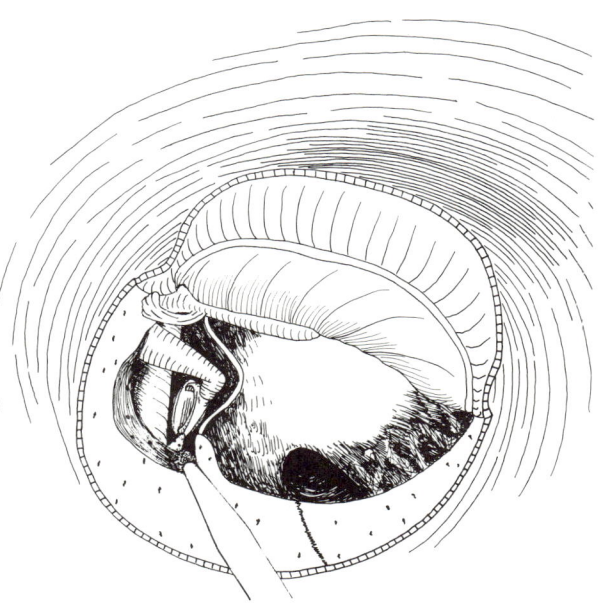

Fig. **182** The bone posterior to the chorda tympani is drilled away

7 Tympanotomies

The chorda tympani can and should be spared during drilling in posterior tympanotomy. This can safely be done by drilling posterior to the chorda, leaving a small piece of bone around the chorda (Fig. **183**). With a curette, the posterior covering of the chorda can be fractured away and removed (Fig. **184a**). After liberation of the chorda posteriorly and laterally, the bone is removed by a curette anterior and medial to the chorda (Fig. **184b**). The chorda is now liberated, and can be pushed away without stretching (Fig. **184c**). As can be seen in Fig. **184**, the entire stapes region, tympanic sinus, pyramidal process, and ponticulus region are all visible, and the cholesteatoma matrix or a retraction membrane can safely be removed from the sinus.

Posterior tympanotomy can be performed either with endaural, retroauricular, superior, or anterior approaches, and it is included in most modifications of these basic approaches.

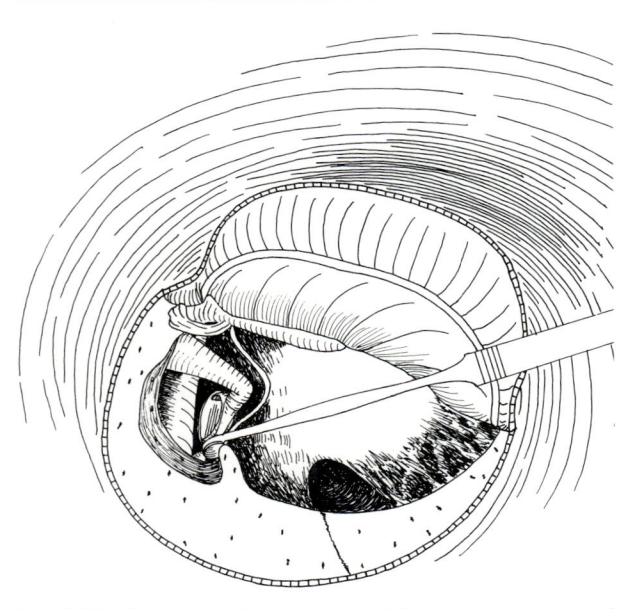

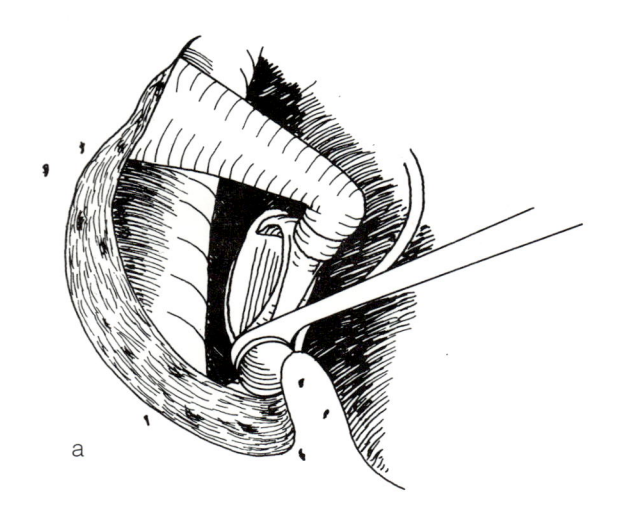

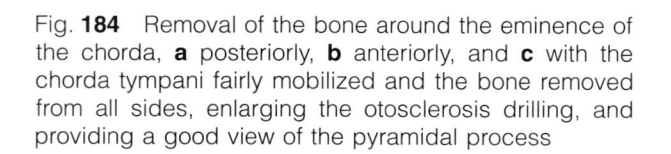

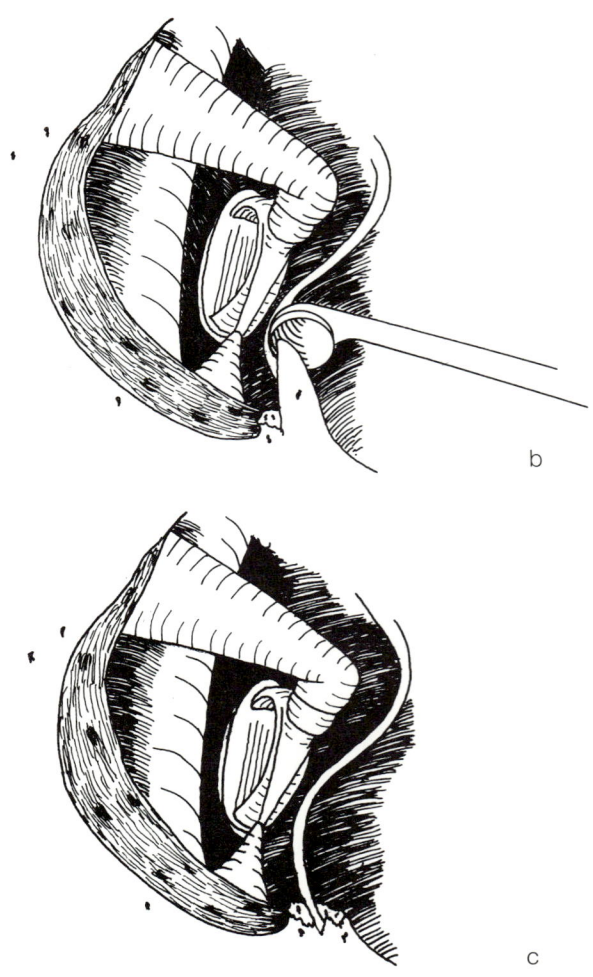

Fig. **183** The posterior remnant of the bony covering of the chorda tympani is removed with a curette

Fig. **184** Removal of the bone around the eminence of the chorda, **a** posteriorly, **b** anteriorly, and **c** with the chorda tympani fairly mobilized and the bone removed from all sides, enlarging the otosclerosis drilling, and providing a good view of the pyramidal process

Inferior Tympanotomy

Inferior tympanotomy is characterized by an inferiorly-placed curved skin incision running from the 9-o'clock to the 3-o'clock position (Figs. **185, 186**). This tympanotomy is an extension of posterior tympanotomy. Inferior tympanotomy as a sole procedure is used on a few occasions, for instance in the extra-annular placement of a ventilating tube, or as an exploratory hypotympanotomy in hidden cholesteatoma cases and small glomus tympanicum cases.

In connection with posterior tympanotomy, inferior tympanotomy is used to remove cholesteatoma located in the hypotympanic air cells. After skin incision with the round knife between the 9-o'clock and 3-o'clock positions (Fig. **186**), the meatal skin is elevated down to the fibrous annulus. The tympanic cavity is entered at the 5-o'clock position by dislocating the fibrous annulus from the bony sulcus and perforating the middle-ear mucosa with a small elevator (Fig. **187**). Dislocation of the fibrous annulus is continued all the way around to the 3-o'clock position. The tympanomeatal flap, with the annulus and drum, is turned superiorly as far as the lower edge of the umbo. The lower half of the tympanic cavity is now exposed and clearly visible (Fig. **188**). To place a ventilating tube, a groove is drilled in the bony annulus (Fig. **189**), the tube is placed in the hypotympanum (Fig. **190**), and the tympanomeatal flap is then turned back to its original position (Fig. **191**).

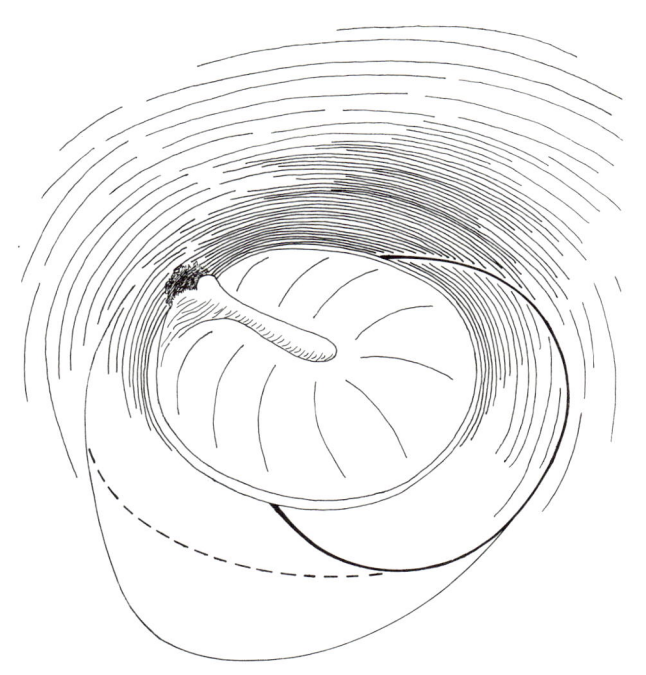

Fig. **185** **Incision for inferior tympanotomy** (solid line), together with an incision in combination with posterior tympanotomy (dotted line), and an extended incision far lateral to the annulus, including posterior tympanotomy and inferior tympanotomy (thin solid line)

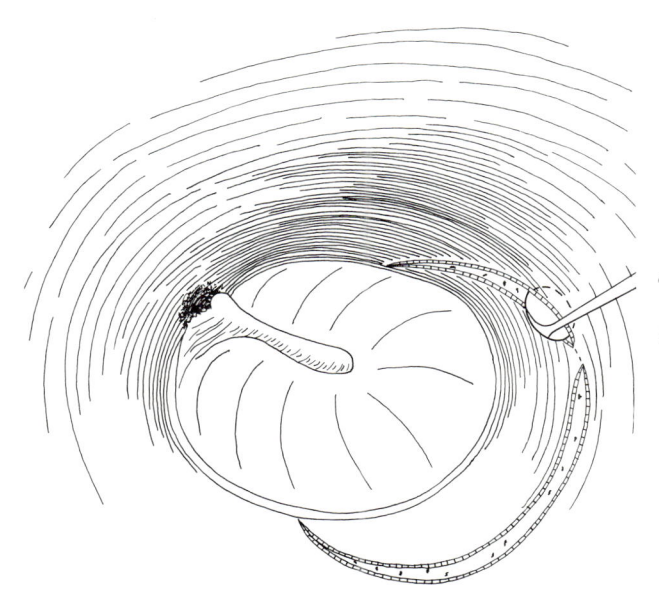

Fig. **186** A curved incision of the skin

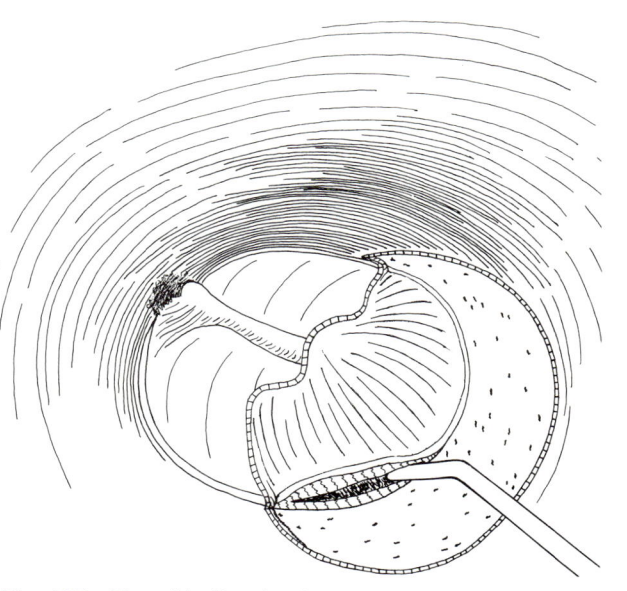

Fig. **187** The skin flap is elevated, the fibrous annulus luxated at the 5-o'clock position, and the tympanic cavity entered

7 Tympanotomies

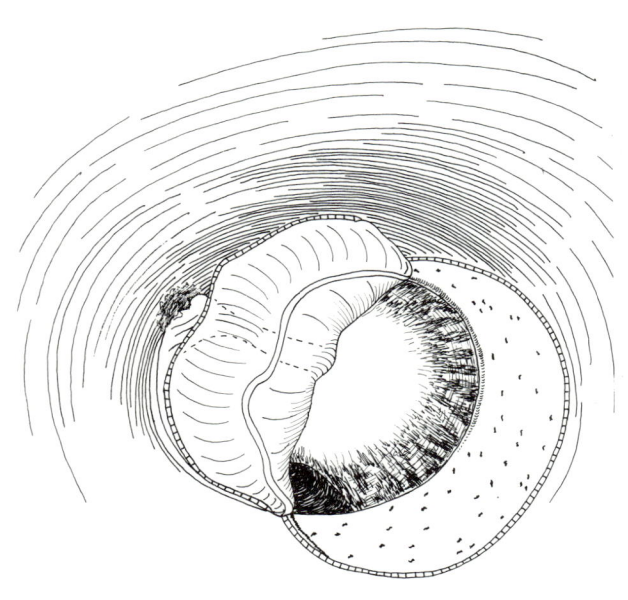

Fig. **188** Total exposure of the inferior half of the tympanic cavity, up to the umbo

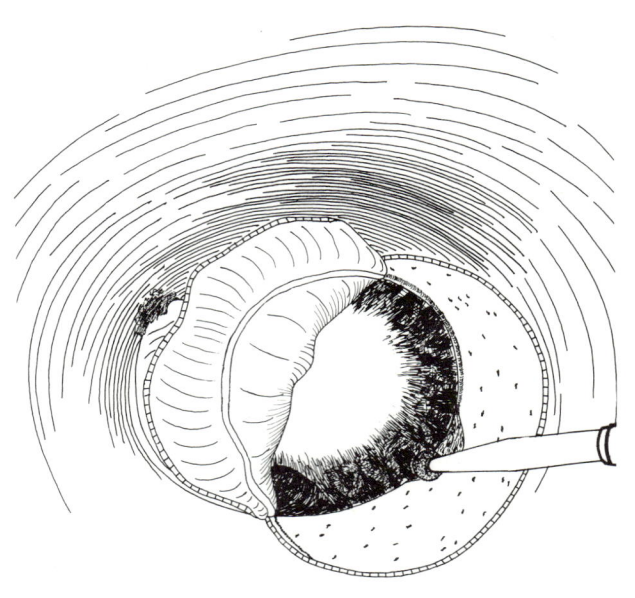

Fig. **189** Drilling of the bony annulus for placement of the extra-auricular ventilating tube

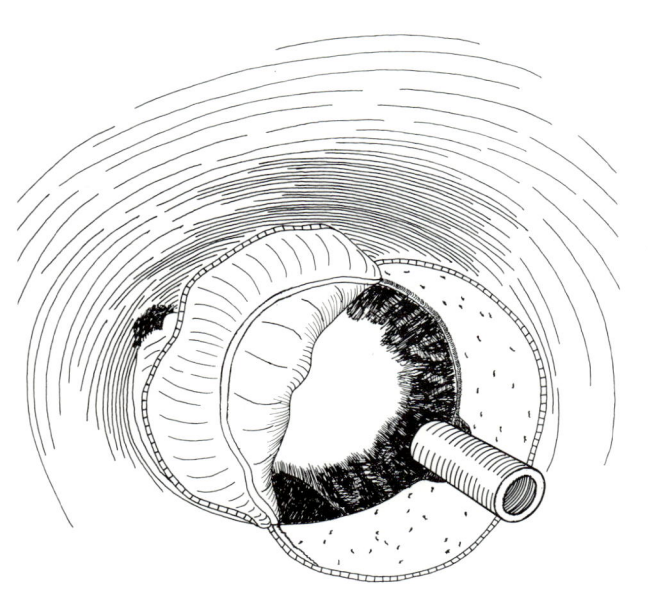

Fig. **190** The ventilating tube has been placed

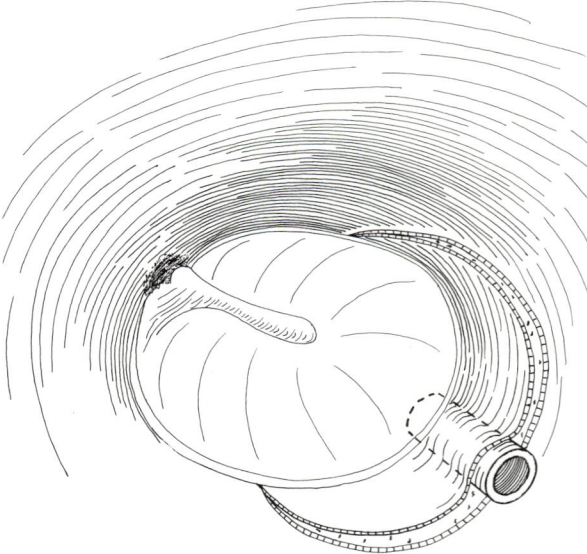

Fig. **191** The tympanomeatal flap is returned to its original position

Hypotympanotomy

Hypotympanotomy means removing the bone from the inferior annulus and opening the hypotympanum. Hypotympanotomy is an extension of inferior tympanotomy, and can be performed with all aproaches, both endaural ones (including the speculum) and postauricular ones. It is sometimes necessary to remove the inferior bony annulus in order to get better access to the hypotympanum and widen it (Fig. 192). This can be the case in tensa-retraction cholesteatoma, glomus jugulare tumors (Farrior), and in pericochlear drainage of cholesterol granulomas of the petrous apex.

After drilling of the bony annulus from the 3-o'clock to the 9-o'clock position, much of the hypotympanum can be visualized (Fig. 192), and the exposed bone can easily be covered by a sufficiently large tympanomeatal flap (Fig. 193).

For more extensive pathology, e.g., larger glomus tumors, the hypotympanotomy has to be extended. The approach can be endaural or postauricular, and the canal-skin incision involves an extended encision of the posterior and inferior tympanotomies, starting superiorly at the 12-o'clock position and ending at the 3-o'clock one (Fig. 194). The tympanomeatal flap is large, and the circumferential incision is placed at least 8 mm lateral to the annulus. The canal skin is elevated, the annulus is dislocated from the bony sulcus from the 12-o'clock to 3-o'clock positions, and the posterior

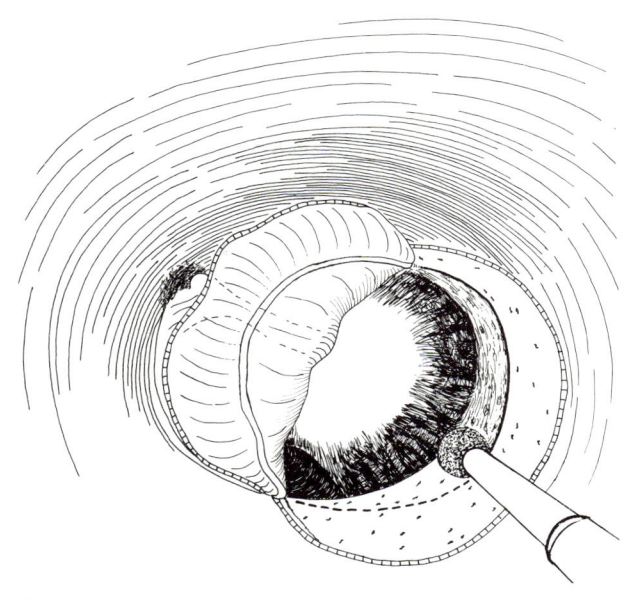

Fig. 192 **Hypotympanotomy.** The inferior bony annulus is drilled away, enlarging the hypotympanum and providing better exposure of the hypotympanic cells

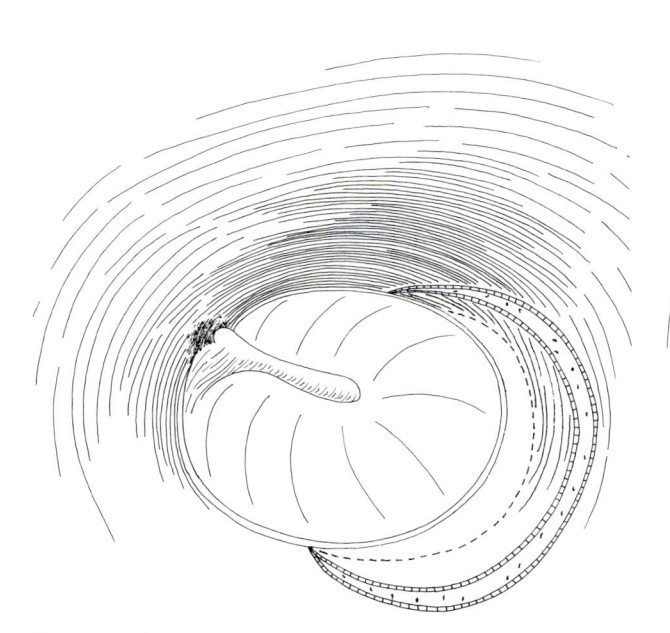

Fig. 193 The tympanomeatal flap is replaced. The dotted line indicates the extent of the bone drilling

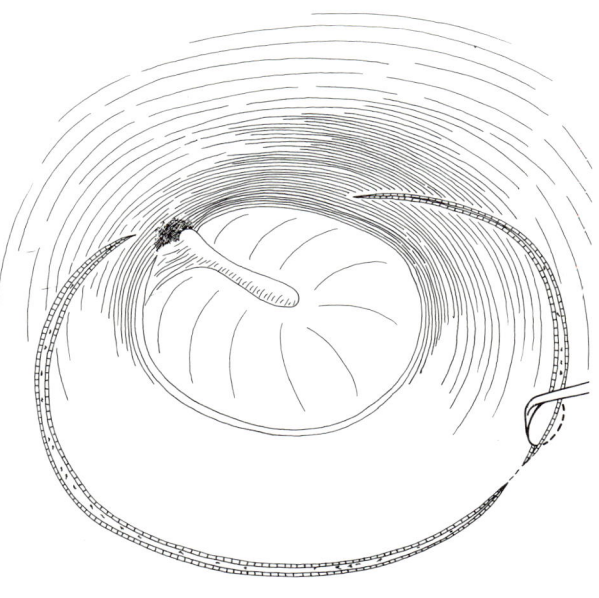

Fig. 194 Extension of the incision, including posterior and inferior tympanotomy

7 Tympanotomies

Fig. **195** The annulus is luxated all the way around from the 12-o'clock to the 3-o'clock position, and the posterior and inferior parts of the tympanic cavity are exposed. The bone is drilled inferior to the bony annulus, preserving the bony annulus

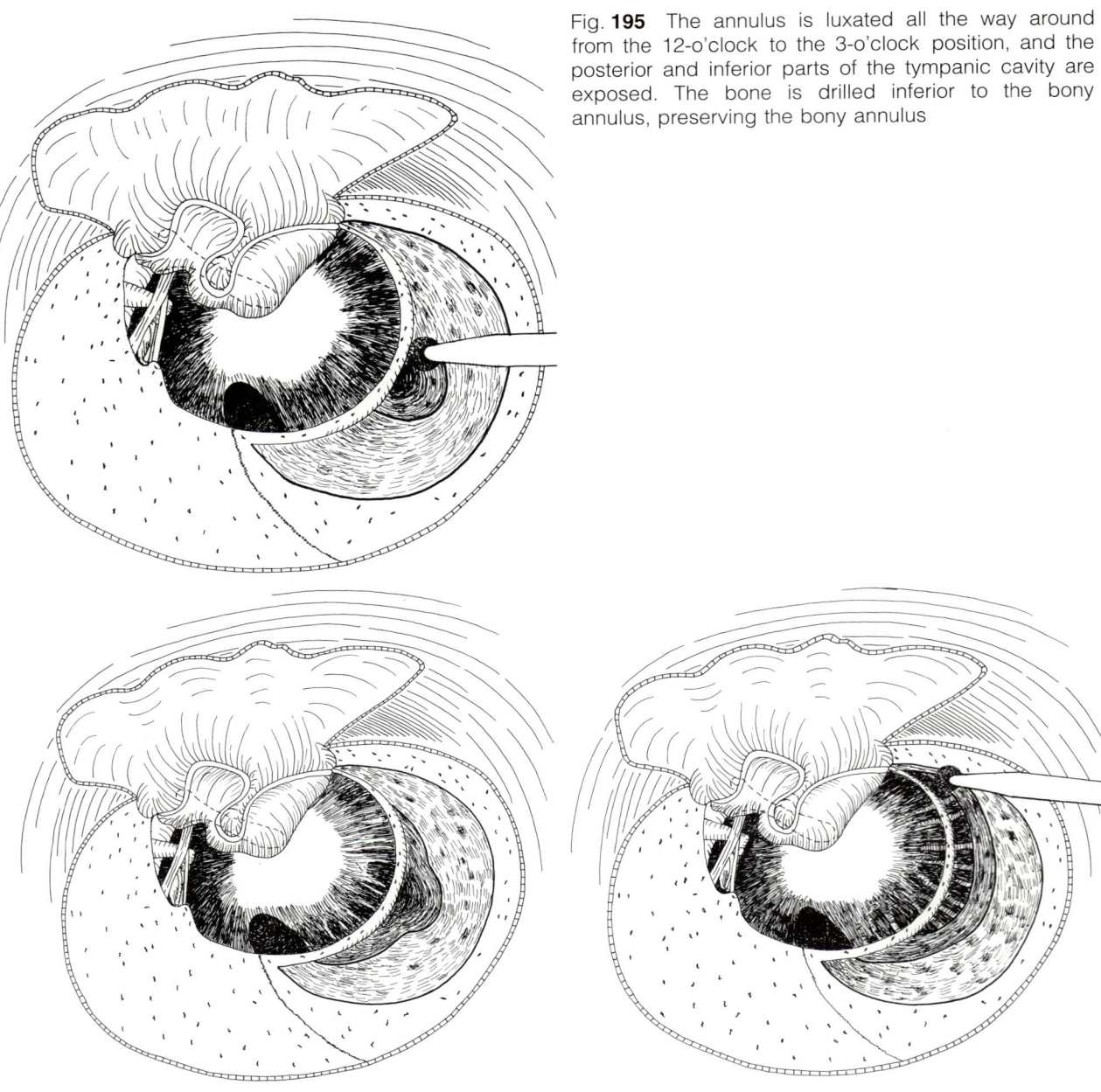

Fig. **196** Further drilling of the bone, enlarging the hypotympanum

Fig. **197** Further enlarging of the hypotympanum anteriorly

and inferior parts of the drum, together with the skin flap, are pushed anterosuperiorly (Fig. **195**). The posterior and inferior parts of the tympanic cavity are exposed. After extensive drilling inferiorly on the tympanic bone, the ear canal is enlarged inferiorly, preserving a small bony bridge for drum support (Fig. **195**). Further drilling under the bridge is started at the 6-o'clock position, proceeding down to the floor of the hypotympanum (Fig. **196**). The enlargement of the entrance to the hypotympanum is widened by further drilling posteriorly and anteriorly (Fig. **196**), still trying to preserve the bony bridge. Further removal of bone from the anterior part of the hypotympanum is possible without damage to important structures (Fig. **197**). If much of the bone is removed, a piece of fascia can be placed on the preserved bony bridge and the bony defect inferior to it. The replaced tympanomeatal flap will cover the fascia. The fibrous annulus is replaced exactly on the bony bridge (Fig. **198**).

Inferior Tympanotomy

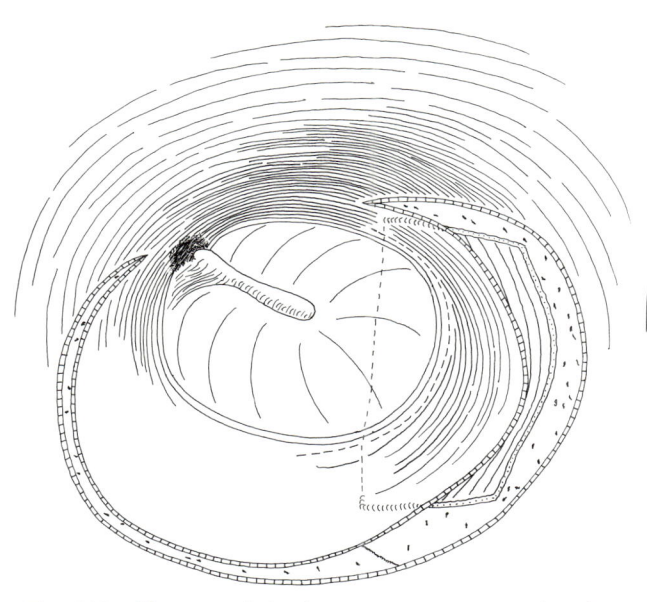

Fig. **198** Closure of the hypotympanotomy using fascia placed on the bony annulus, and on the drilled bone. The tympanomeatal flap is replaced

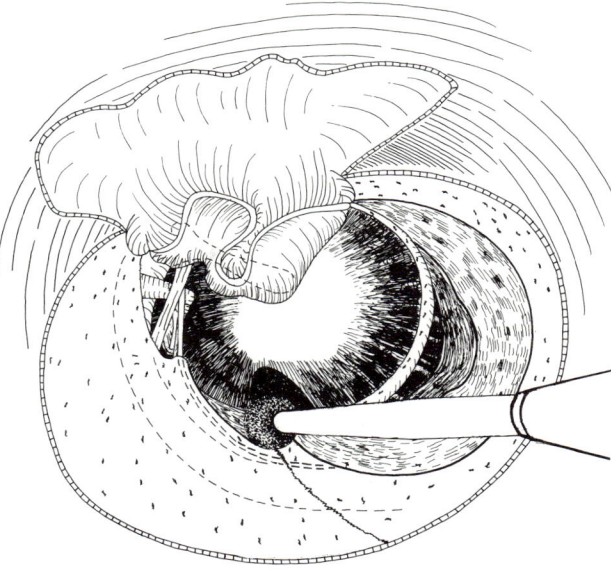

Fig. **199** Extension of the hypotympanotomy by drilling of the posterior bony annulus along the chorda

For further exposure of the hypotympanum, the course of the chorda tympani and the vertical part of the facial nerve should be taken into consideration. It is best to start drilling with a diamond burr at the 9-o'clock position, gradually exposing the chorda tympani at the eminence of the chorda. With gentle drilling of the bony annulus in an inferior direction and along the course of the chorda (Fig. **199**), much of the posterior tympanum inferiorly and around the round window niche can be exposed (Fig. **199**). The bony bridge has to be disrupted at this point (Fig. **200**). The small pieces of bone around the chorda have to be removed with a curette (Fig. **200**) and the bone gradually drilled away (Fig. **201**) until the entire chorda and its entrance into the facial nerve are exposed (Fig. **202**). Further exposure of the vertical segment of the facial nerve depends on the pathology, but once a small area of the perineurium of the facial nerve is visible, further exposure and decompression of the whole facial nerve down to the stylomastoid foramen can be performed.

The bony bridge can be removed, providing wide exposure of all the hypotympanic air cells, facilitating entrance into the pericochlear air cells and into the perimeatal and apical air cells (Fig. **203**). With continuous drilling inferior to the cochlea, the jugular bulb will be exposed posteriorly and the carotid artery anteriorly. The space between these two structures and the cochlea varies in size (Giddings et al. 1991). Closure of the

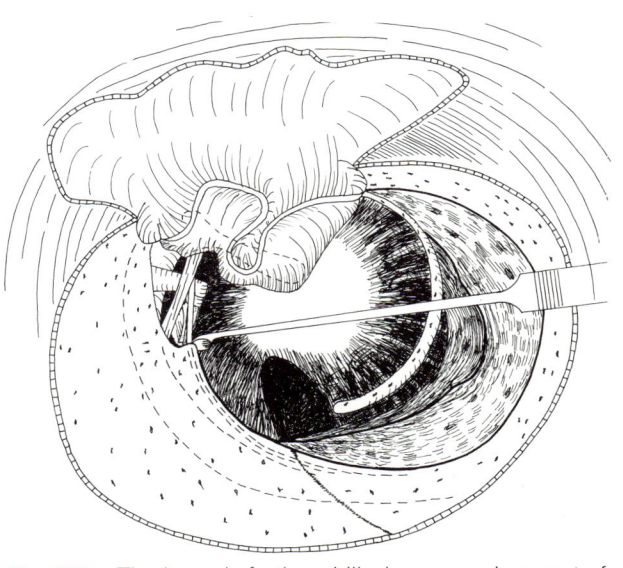

Fig. **200** The bone is further drilled away, as is a part of the bony bridge

hypotympanotomy can be performed by placing the tympanomeatal flap back on the preserved annulus without the fascia (Fig. **204**), or with the fascia placed on the bony bridge, as described above (Fig. **202**).

If the bony bridge is removed, the tympanomeatal flap can be fortified by fascia, or just placed on the bone (Fig. **205**). In any case, there will be a large area of the bone not covered by the meatal skin, which has to be epithelialized.

7 Tympanotomies

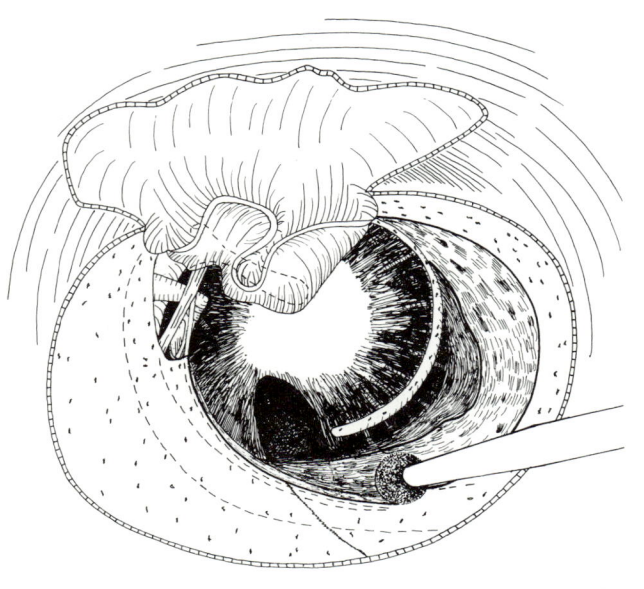

Fig. 201 The chorda tympani is exposed along its course to the vertical segment of the facial nerve

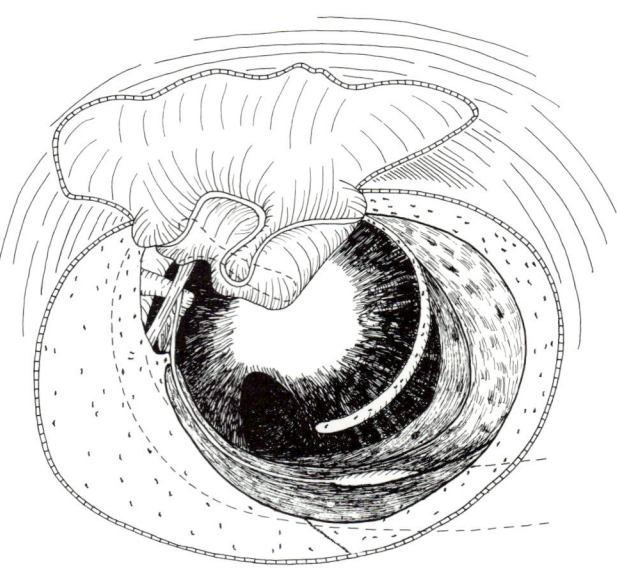

Fig. 202 Total exposure of the chorda tympani and a small part of the facial nerve after extensive drilling of the bone. The bony bridge is partly preserved

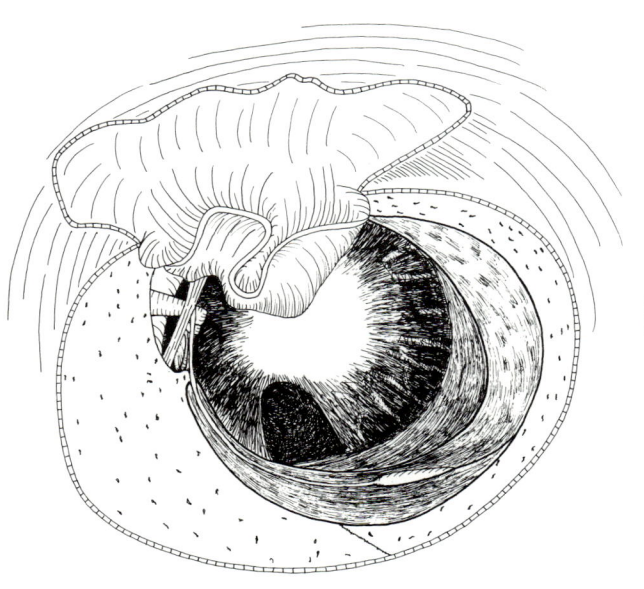

Fig. 203 Hypotympanotomy with the bony bridge removed, and extensive exposure of the hypotympanum, with a small area of the facial nerve

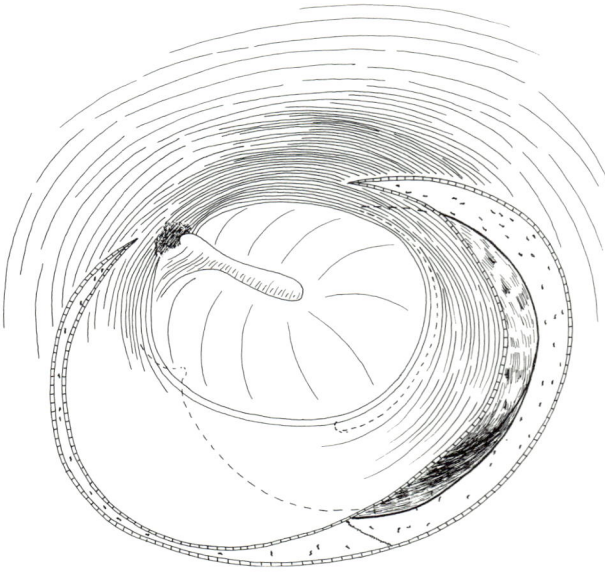

Fig. 204 The tympanomeatal flap is replaced on the preserved bony bridge, covering the most of the drilled area in the hypotympanum

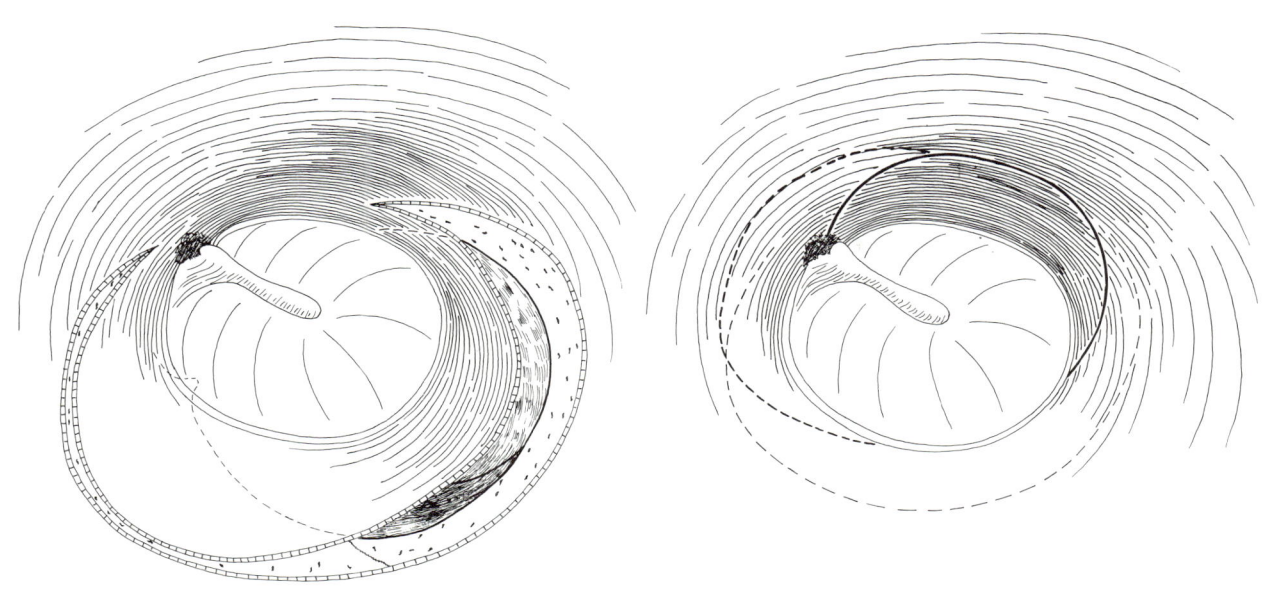

Fig. **205** The tympanomeatal flap is replaced, covering the bony defect

Fig. **206** **Anterior tympanotomy** with an curved incision from the 12-o'clock to the 6-o'clock position (solid line) which may be combined with a superior tympanotomy (dotted line) or inferior or posterior tympanotomies.

Anterior Tympanotomy

Anterior tympanotomy means entering the anterior part of the tympanic cavity from the ear canal by elevating of the anterior ear-canal skin flap together with the fibrous annulus. Generally, this type of tympanotomy is seldom used as a sole procedure, although it is sometimes used as an exploratory tympanotomy for cholesteatoma in posterior perforations, and occasionally for exploration of the tympanic orifice of the Eustachian tube. More often, it is used in special myringoplasties with underlay graft techniques.

In combination with posterior tympanotomy and inferior tympanotomy, an anterior tympanotomy will follow the extension of tensaretraction cholesteatoma into the Eustachian tube (Fig. **206**). In combination with superior tympanotomy, the anterior tympanotomy may be used to follow an extension of an attic cholesteatoma towards the tympanic orifice of the Eustachian tube.

The incision for the anterior tympanotomy goes as a curved line from the 12-o'clock to the 6-o'clock position about 5 mm lateral to the annulus. The skin flap is elevated, the anterior annulus is dislocated out of its bony sulcus, the mucosa is disrupted, and the tympanic cavity is entered (Fig. **207**). For further exposure of the tympanic orifice of the Eustachian tube, the anterior bony annulus is drilled away using a diamond burr (Fig. **208**), and the lateral lamina of the Eustachian tube mucosa is exposed. The mucosa can be elevated from the bone (Fig. **209**), and excised with a sickle knife (Fig. **210**). Exposure down to the isthmus of the Eustachian tube is possible (Fig. **211**). Membranes with keratinized squamous epithelium can be dissected away from the mucosa of the medial and lateral walls of the Eustachian tube, preserving the mucous membrane intact. Further exposure of the Eustachian tube is possible with further drilling of the bone of the tube's lateral wall.

Closure of the tympanotomy does not cause problems, as the skin flaps can easily cover the bone defect (Fig. **212**).

7 Tympanotomies

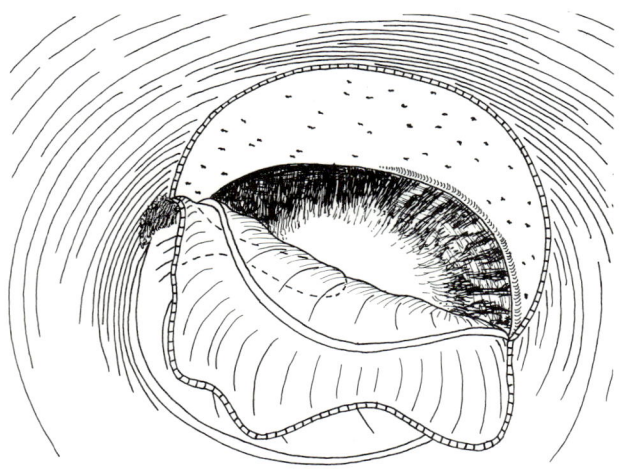

Fig. 207 The tympanomeatal flap is elevated. The annulus is elevated from its sulcus, and the anterior half of the tympanic cavity is exposed

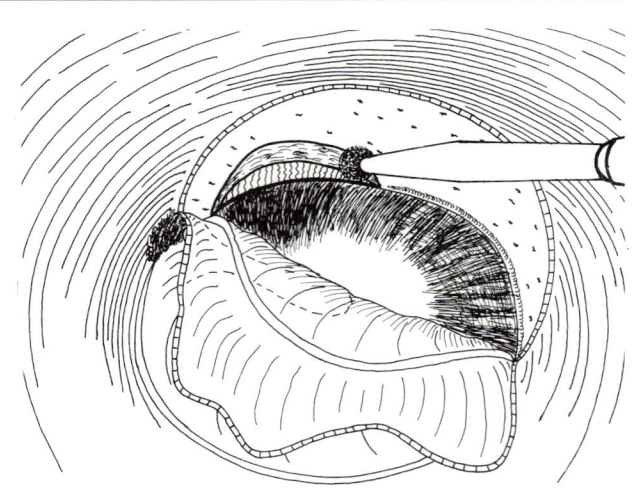

Fig. 208 The bony annulus is drilled away

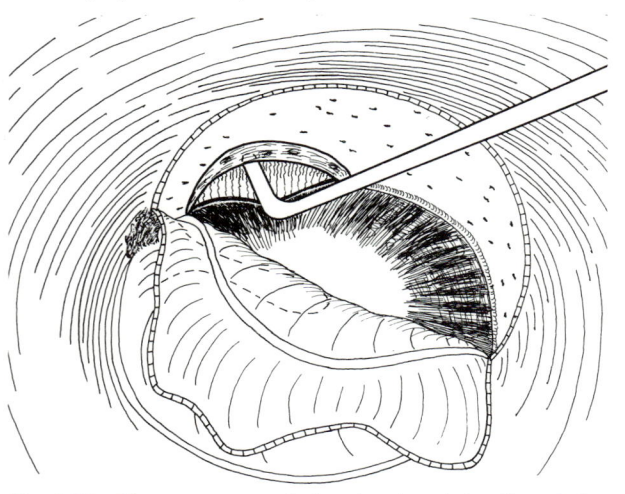

Fig. 209 The mucosa of the lamina lateralis of the Eustachian tube is further elevated

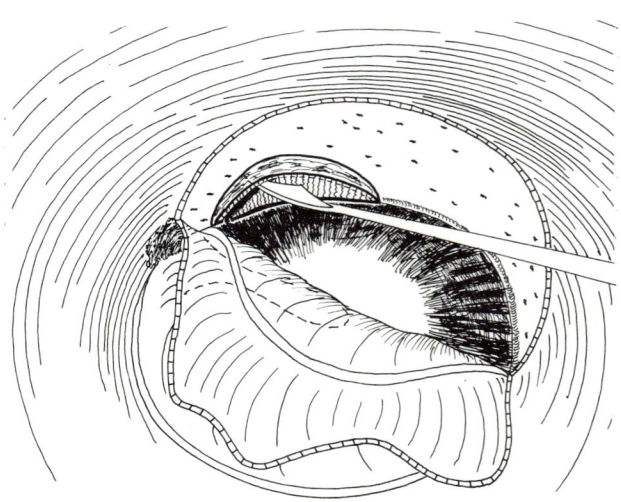

Fig. 210 The mucosa of the lamina lateralis is excised

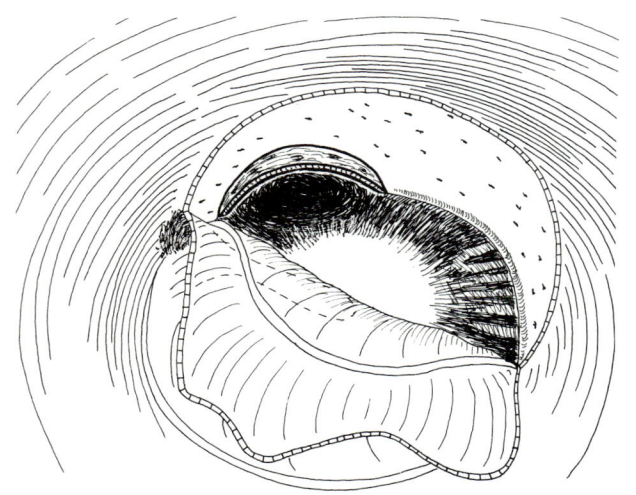

Fig. 211 After excision, a good view of the isthmus tuba is possible

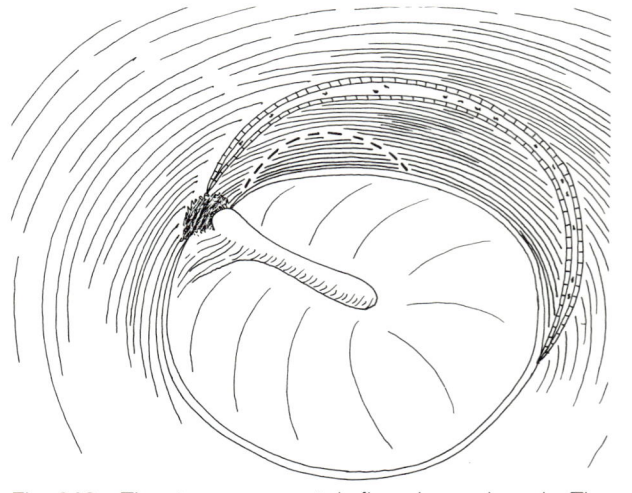

Fig. 212 The tympanomeatal flap is replaced. The dotted line indicates the extension of bone drilling

Superior Tympanotomy

The superior tympanotomy provides an opportunity to explore the attic. The curved skin incision goes from the 9-o'clock to the 3-o'clock position about 5 mm lateral to Shrapnell's membrane (Fig. **213**). The skin is firmly attached to the notch of Rivinus (Fig. **214**), and the fibrous connections usually have to be cut with a sickle knife (Fig. **214**). The tympanomeatal flap is elevated together with Shrapnell's membrane (Fig. **215**). Posteriorly, the fibrous annulus is also elevated, exposing the long process of the incus and the Shrapnell's membrane region (Fig. **216**). Inspection of the part of the attic anterior to the neck of the malleus is possible. Posterior tympanotomy is completed, and the tympanomeatal flap is replaced and eventually fortified by a small plate of perichondrial fascia or cartilage placed under Shrapnell's membrane.

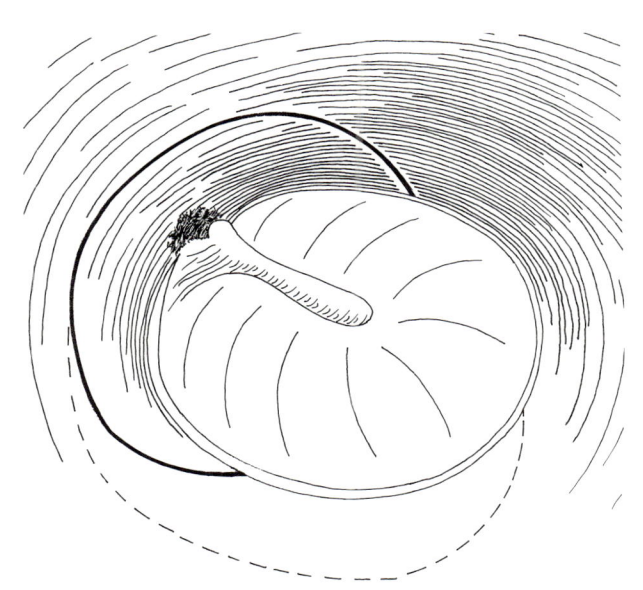

Fig. **213** **The superior tympanotomy line of incision** (solid line) in combination with posterior tympanotomy (dotted line)

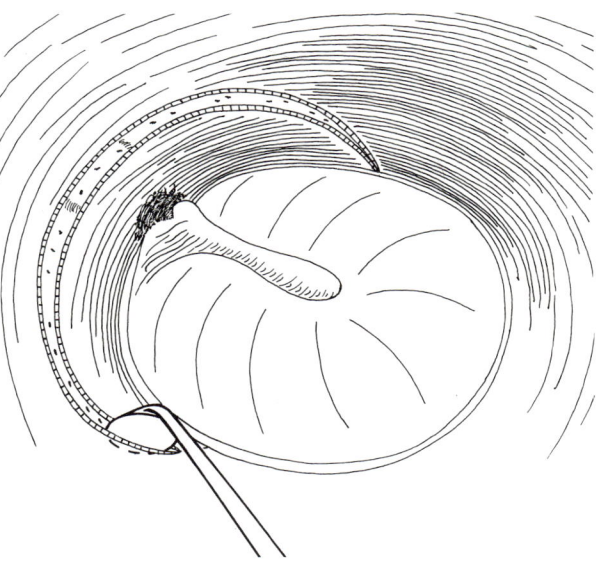

Fig. **214** The skin is incised with a round knife

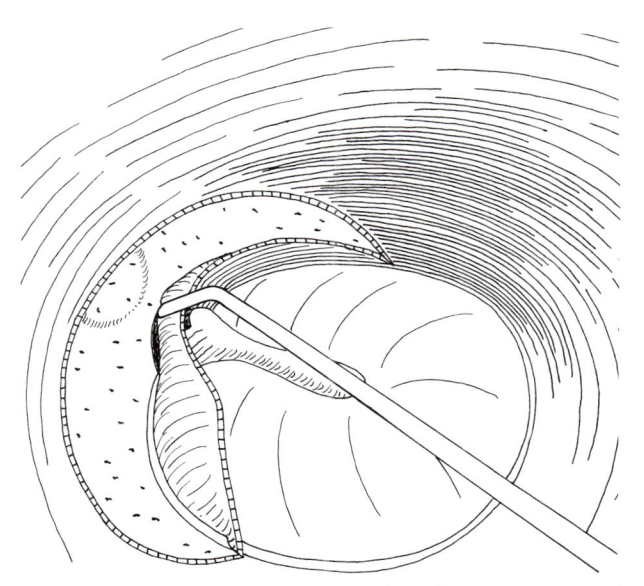

Fig. **215** The tympanomeatal skin flap is elevated, together with Shrapnell's membrane

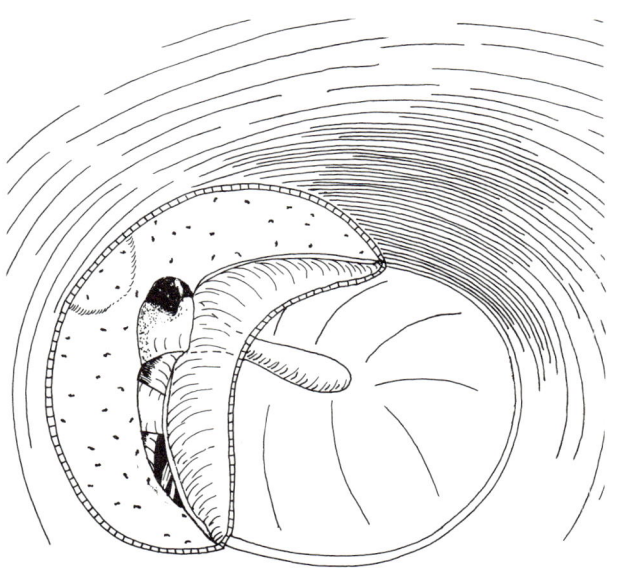

Fig. **216** Posteriorly, the fibrous annulus is elevated. The superior tympanotomy is completed, and inspection in the anterior attic is possible

Atticotomy

In the Heermann B incision or retroauricular incision, a large posterior and superior tympanomeatal flap is elevated (Fig. 217). After elevation of the tympanic chorda from the bony annulus, the mucosa is incised, and the tympanic cavity entered posterosuperiorly. After the otosclerosis drilling and inspection of the stapes region, the drilling of the superior ear-canal wall is started (Fig. 218). The atticotomy drilling is extended to the entire attic region, with careful preservation of the bony bridge separating the Shrapnell's membrane region (Fig. 219). Further enlargement of the atticotomy opening takes place, and the bone of the lateral attic wall has become thin, but is still intact (Fig. 220). The anterosuperior bony annulus is visualized by luxating the fibrous annulus. Drilling is extended further towards the anterior attic, with careful preservation of the bony bridge. The mucosa between the anterosuperior bony annulus and the fibrous annulus is incised, and the anterosuperior tympanum is inspected. The thin bone from the lateral attic wall is drilled away, exposing the mucosa of the attic at the level of the malleus head (Fig. 221).

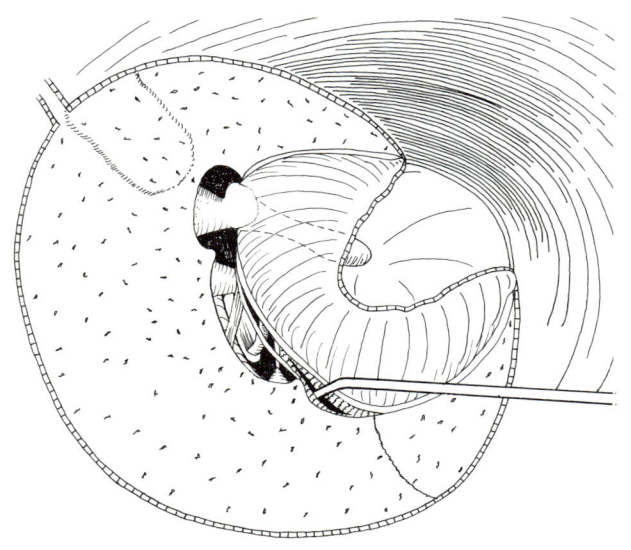

Fig. 217 **Atticotomy.** Large superior and posterior tympanomeatal flaps are elevated, the annulus is luxated, and the tympanic cavity is entered

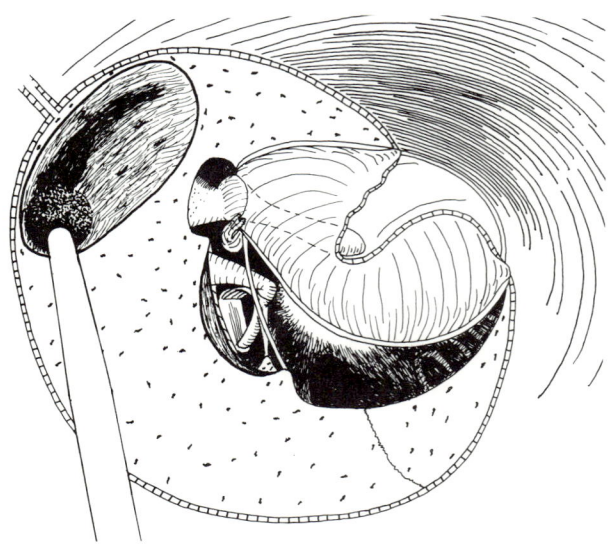

Fig. 218 Drilling of the superior ear-canal wall is started

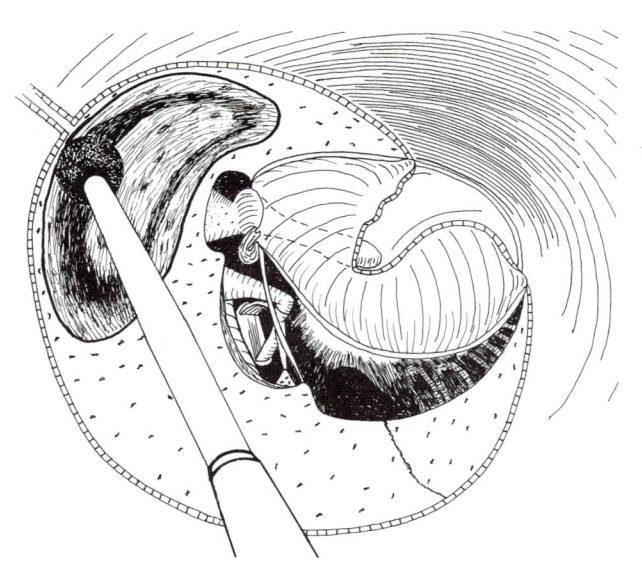

Fig. 219 The atticotomy opening is widened by further drilling, with preservation of the bridge

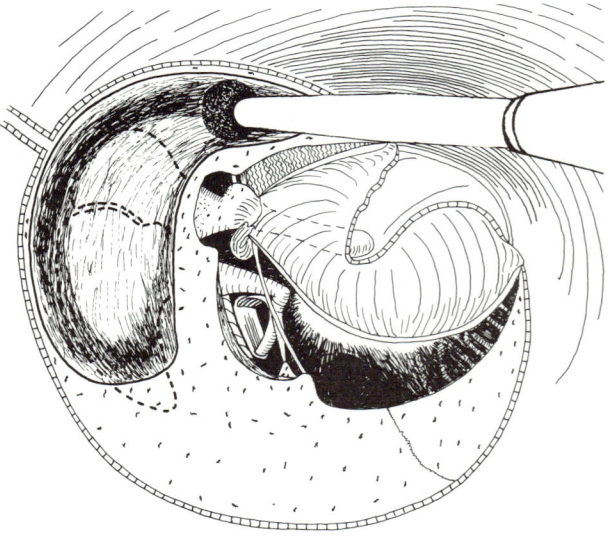

Fig. 220 Drilling is extended anteriorly, with careful preservation of the bridge

The attic mucosa is opened, exposing the malleus head, a part of the incus body, and a part of the anterior attic (Fig. 222). After further drilling, the anterior attic and Prussak's space are exposed, with the bridge still being preserved intact (Fig. 223).

Atticotomy with preservation of the bony bridge is the cornerstone of the author's modification of the intact canal-wall technique (Tos 1984). It provides a safe surgical procedure in the anterior attic, where much more bone can be removed if necessary, still preserving the bridge intact. In fact, the superior part of the Eustachian tube can be reached through the anterior atticotomy.

Aditotomy

By opening the posterior attic around the incus body and the short process of the incus, a good view of the aditus ad antrum can be achieved (Fig. 224). The aditotomy can be part of a large atticotomy if required, but if there is no suspicion for pathology in the anterior attic, bone removal can be carried out in the posterior attic region and in the aditus alone. The aditotomy will mainly be indicated in sinus cholesteatoma, starting as a posterosuperior retraction of the pars tensa, continuing into the tympanic sinus, and from there through the facial recess into the aditus ad antrum. After removal of a cholesteatoma membrane from the tympanic

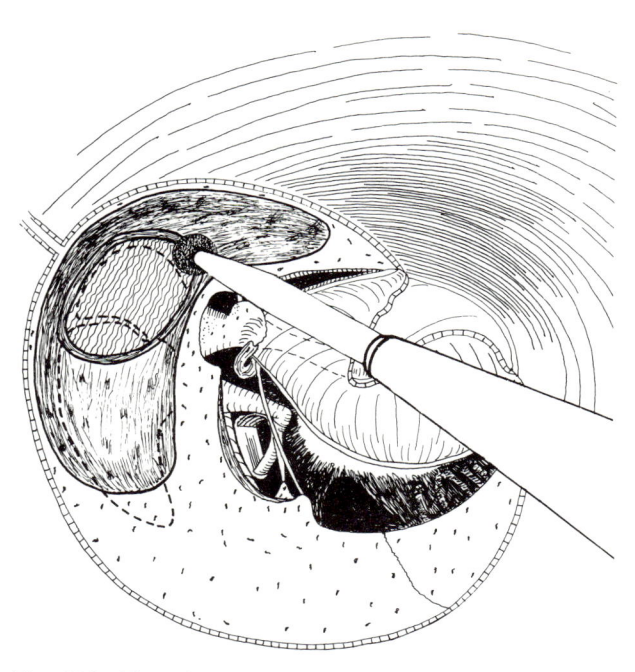

Fig. **221** The bone from the lateral attic wall is removed, exposing the mucosa of the attic

cavity an aditotomy will show whether any cholesteatoma membrane is left around the incudal fossa. With further removal of the bone posterior to the incudal fossa, the entire prominence of the lateral semicircular canal can be exposed. With

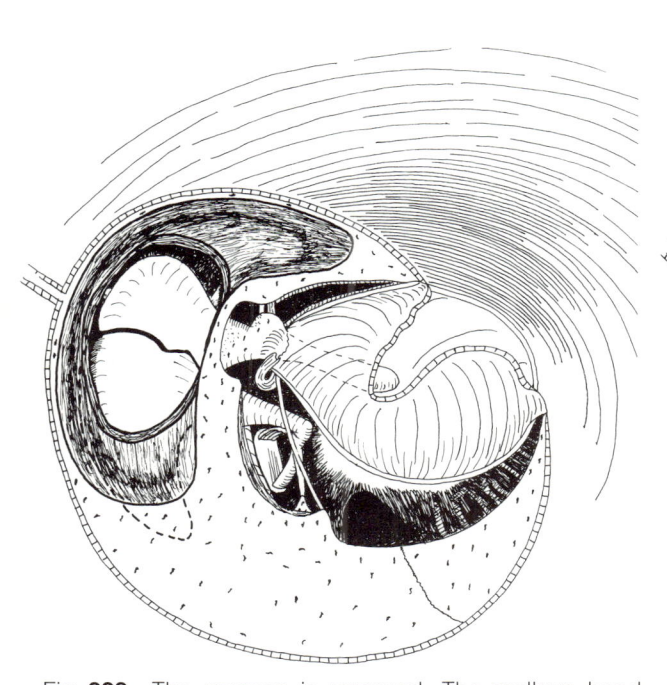

Fig. **222** The mucosa is removed. The malleus head and part of the incus body, as well as part of the anterior attic, are visualized

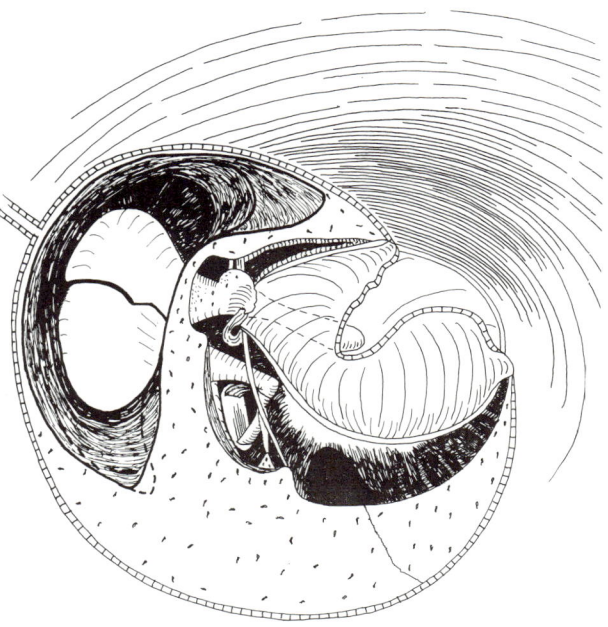

Fig. **223** Further removal of the bone from the anterior attic wall, with preservation of the bridge

further drilling of the bridge, pathology in the facial recess can be removed.

Closure of an atticotomy or an aditotomy can be achieved with a shaped piece of cortical bone or cartilage. The present author prefers to close it with fascia only (Fig. 225), followed by replacement of the tympanomeatal skin flap (Fig. 226). Retraction will not occur because of the bone has been removed superior to the bridge, and is even less likely if the incus body and malleus head are still in place. Any eventual retraction will usually occur inferior to the bridge at the Shrapnell's membrane region or in the posterosuperior part of the pars tensa.

Superior tympanotomy can be performed to inspect or remove a deep and suspicious attic retraction, or to control an attic precholesteatoma. The retraction is elevated from the head of the malleus, fortified with a slice of cartilage, and the tympanomeatal flap replaced.

The author very often uses atticotomy in cases with a bony fixation of the head of the malleus in the attic. Instead of removing the incus, and resecting and extracting the malleus head, ending with a type II tympanoplasty with interposition of the incus, the author prefers an atticotomy, drilling away the bone fixing the malleus with a diamond drill, and preserving the ossicular chain intact. Atticotomy is also performed in tympanosclerosis of the attic.

Most often, atticotomy has to be performed through Heermann B or other endaural incisions, or through a retroauricular incision. Even a small atticotomy can be performed using an endaural approach with an ear speculum (Figs. 213–216); drilling in the lateral attic wall requires good access to the superior ear-canal bony wall (Figs. 217–222).

In this chapter, only atticotomy and aditotomy *with preservation* of the bridge are described. Surgical procedures involving the attic with removal of the bridge are described in Volume 2.

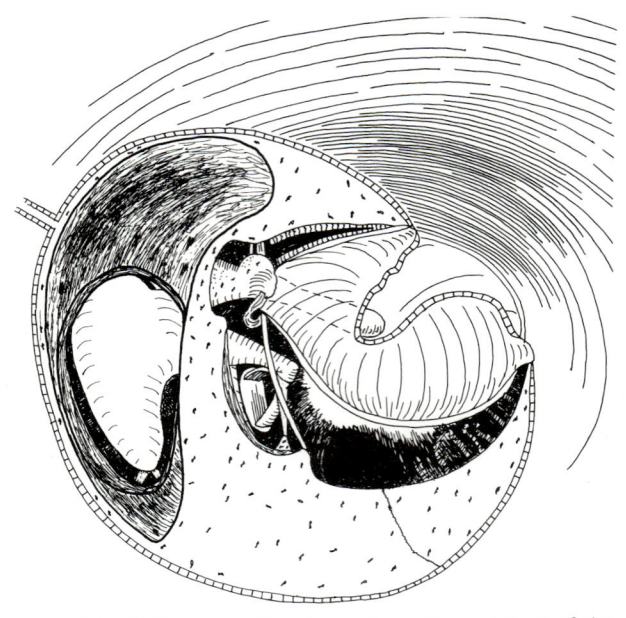

Fig. 224 **Aditotomy.** The bone from the regions of the incus body and the short process of the incus, as well as the incudal fossa, is removed, providing a good view of the aditus ad antrum

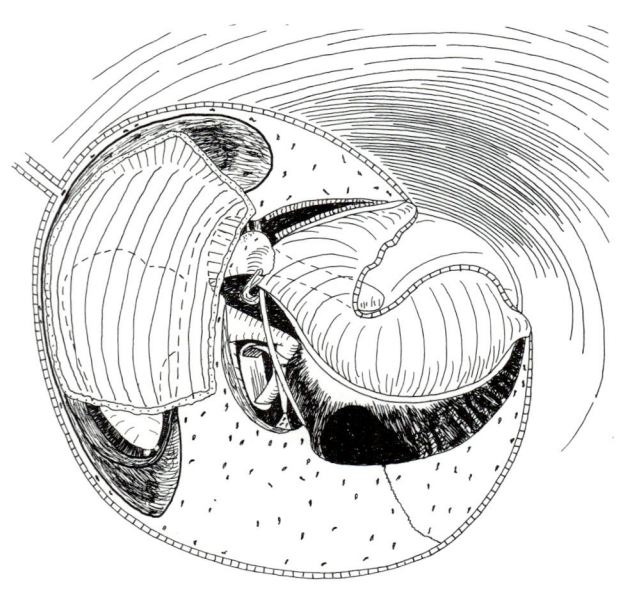

Fig. 225 The atticotomy and aditotomy are covered with fascia

Fig. 226 The tympanomeatal flap is replaced

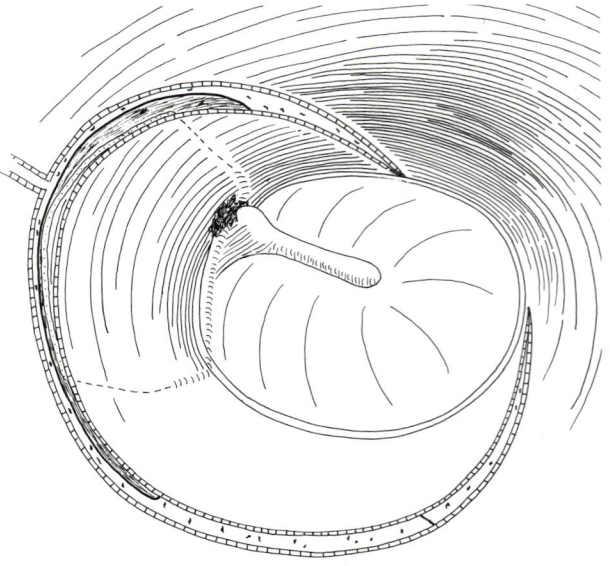

Part II
Myringoplasty

8 Graft Materials

Many autogenous, several allogenous (homogenous), and a few xenogenous (heterogenous) graft materials have been used for closure of the eardrum perforation and reconstruction of the middle ear and ear canal. The majority are still used today as routine procedures for special conditions and in specific techniques.

Terminology of Grafts

The terminology of graft implants and transplants in tympanoplasty has changed during the last few year (Frootko 1985). The term "autograft" (autogenous graft), denoting a graft from the same person, remains unchanged. The term "homograft" (homogenous graft), denoting a graft from another person, has been changed to allograft (allogenous graft). The term "heterograft" (heterologous graft), denoting a graft from animals, has been changed to xenograft (xenogenous graft). Isograft denotes a transplant from a genetically identical person; it is not appropriate in tympanoplasty, but is used in organ transplantation. In contrast to transplants, the ear-drum implant consists of nonbiological material.

Autogenous Grafts

Autogenous grafts are the most popular grafts. They are usually easily available, do not involve any immunological problems, are inexpensive, and, most important of all, there is no risk of HIV infection. These grafts include:

Temporalis muscle fascia
Tragal perichondrium
Conchal perichondrium
Tragal or conchal cartilage
Periosteum
Vein
Fatty tissue
Subcutaneous tissue
Fascia lata
Ear-canal skin
Heterotopic skin

Temporalis Muscle Fascia

Temporalis muscle fascia was first used in myringoplasty by Ørtegren (1958–59), Heermann (1961), and Storrs (1961). It is the most commonly used autogenous material. It is very popular for several reasons: 1) It is easy to harvest. 2) It can be used as an onlay, intermediate, or underlay graft. 3) For primary operations, there are no size limitations. 4) It can be used in more than one piece, each piece overlapping the other. 5) For reconstruction of the tympanic cavity and ear canal, fascia is the only suitable autogenous material, because of its size. 6) It can be used in the sandwich technique as one of the double grafts with ear-canal skin on the fascia.

The temporalis muscle fascia is an extension of the deep fascia of the neck. It covers the temporalis muscle, which arises from the deep layer of the temporalis muscle fascia itself, and from the periosteum of several cranial bones: the parietal, sphenoidal, frontal, and temporal bones (Fig. **227**). The attachment of the upper part of the temporalis muscle is the temporal plane, and that of the lower part is the temporal fossa. Muscle fibers run toward the temporalis fossa under the zygomatic arch, inserting into the coronoid process of the mandible.

The temporalis muscle fascia consists of two layers: the superficial layer, situated just under the superior auricular and anterior auricular muscles, consisting of loose areolar fibrous tissue. When cutting through the superior auricular muscle, this tissue can easily be elevated with Freer's rugine and dissected away. The superficial fascia layer is not strong enough for reconstruction of the drum. In the inferior part of the temporalis muscle, along the attachment of the fascia to the linea temporalis and the zygomatic root, the superficial layer becomes thicker, and here it cannot be separated from the deeper layer.

The deeper layer of the temporalis fascia (the lamina profunda) is aponeurotic and strong, with a clear arrangement of the fibers (Fig. **228**). On the posteroinferior, posterior, superior, and anterior borders of the temporalis muscle, the deep fascia runs together with the superficial layer, and both are firmly attached to the pericranium (Fig. **229**).

Temporalis Muscle Fascia

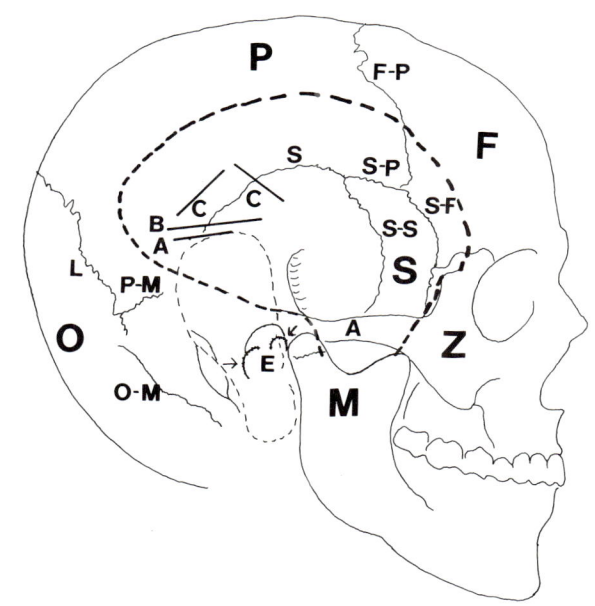

Fig. 227 The borders of the temporalis muscle fascia (thick dotted line); incision lines A, B and C, for removal of the temporalis muscle fascia graft related to the borders of the auricle (thin dotted line); and the entire area of the right side of the skull, with the following sutures: squamous suture (S), sphenosquamous suture (S–S), frontoparietal suture (F–P), sphenoparietal suture (S–P), sphenofrontal suture (S–F), lambdoid suture (L), parietomastoid suture (P–M), and occipitomastoid suture (O–M). The neighboring cranial bones involved with the temporalis muscle fascia are the parietal bone (P), frontal bone (F), sphenoidal bone (S) zygomatic bone (Z) with the zygomatic arch (A), mandible (M), and temporal bone in the middle

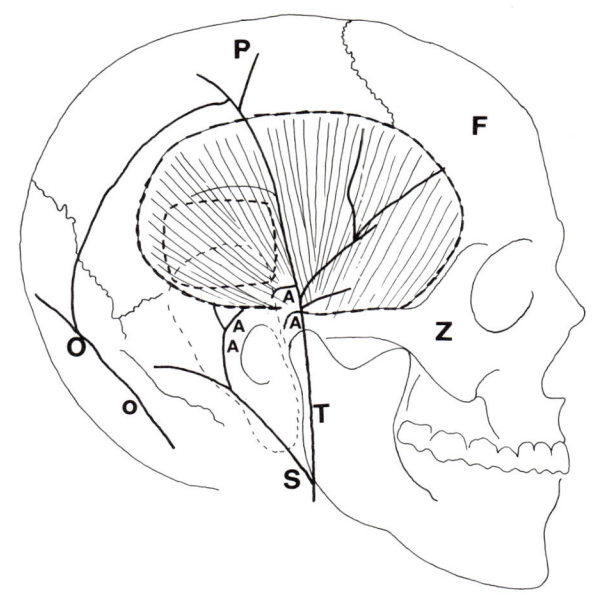

Fig. 228 The direction of the fibers in the temporalis muscle fascia projected onto the cranium (thick dotted line). Projection of the auricle (thin dotted line), and of the arteries (solid line) related to the temporalis muscle fascia. The superficial temporal artery (T) with auricular branches (A), dividing into a frontal and a parietal branch. The stylomastoid artery (S), giving off some auricular branches (A) and the occipital artery (O). The dotted line indicates the large posterior area of the temporalis muscle fascia without major vessels. Parietal bone (P), frontal bone (F), zygomatic bone (Z) and occipital bone (O)

On the anteroinferior border, the fascia attaches to the zygomatic arch—the superficial layer attaches mainly to the lateral surface of the arch, and the deep layer to the medial edge of the arch. Between the two layers lies fatty tissue.

The following practical tips may be useful in harvesting temporalis muscle fascia:

1. For reconstruction of the ear drum, the most suitable region for fascial harvesting is the area superior to the helix.
2. The inferior half-centimeter of the temporalis muscle fascia is too thick for immediate ear-drum reconstruction, and the inferior incision through the fascia should therefore be made about 0.5 cm superior to the lower attachment of the muscle, leaving the thick strip of fascia in place. If the fascia is to be used as a large piece for ear-drum and ear-canal reconstruction, the thick strip is excellent for reconstruction of the

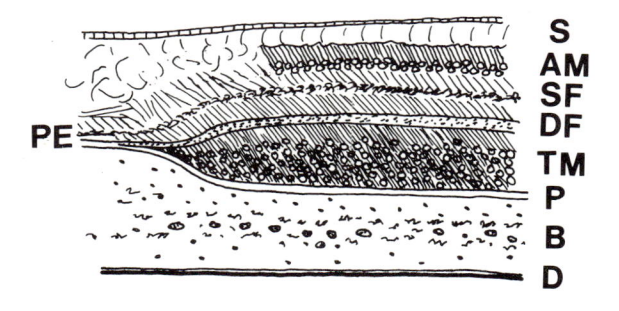

Fig. 229 A cross-section of the temporalis muscle area posterosuperior to the auricle, with the posterior connection of the deep and superficial fascia layers to the pericranium (PE). The dura (D) with the bone of the squama (B), and the periosteum (P). The temporalis muscle (TM), the deep layer of the temporalis fascia (DF), the superficial layer of the temporalis fascia (SF), the superior auricular muscle (AM), and skin with subcutaneous tissue (S)

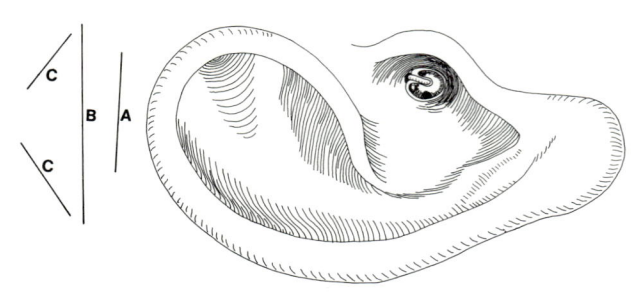

Fig. 230 Separate incisions superior to the auricle (A) for small fascia, (B) for large fascia, and (C) in reoperations where fascia has been previously removed (see also Fig. 227)

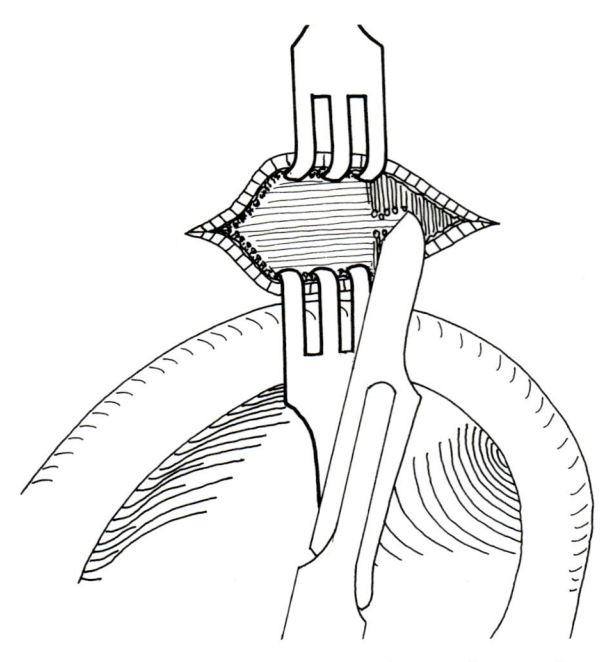

Fig. 231 Incision A for removal of a small area of temporalis muscle fascia. The remaining fibers of the superior auricular muscle are cut with a no. 15 scalpel

ear canal. On the other hand, the inferior, thick strip of the fascia is a good support for the temporalis muscle when used as a superiorly-based muscle flap in cavity obliteration. For this reason, the inferior strip should stay connected to the muscle.

3. The fascia is stretched over the muscle and will contract after excision; the area of the fascia will therefore be smaller after excision than before. The borders of the remaining fascia will also retract, making additional removal of fascia from the same incision difficult.
4. If a very large fascia graft is needed, or if some fascia has already been removed in a previous operation, a large, separate incision about 2 cm superior to the helix is necessary (Fig. 230).

Fascia in the Endaural Approach

In myringoplasty or tympanoplasty with an endaural approach *using the speculum*, the fascia will be taken at the beginning of the operation through a separate incision 1 cm above the helix (Fig. 230). The length of the incision is 2–3 cm, depending on the size of the fascia required. Immediately after the skin incision and incision through the superior auricular muscle (Fig. 231), the wound is maximally divided by two strong retractors held by a scrub nurse, to separate the subcutaneous tissue, and elevate the skin borders. Additional incisions through fibers of the superior auricular muscle that may have been cut (Fig. 231) provide a sufficient view of the loose areolar tissue of the superficial layer of the temporalis muscle fascia, lying directly under the superior auricular muscle. With a Freer rugine, this loose tissue is dissected away from the clearly visible deep layer, exposing a sufficient area of the fascia. The lateral surface of the uncut and stretched fascia will be carefully cleaned from the remaining fibrous tissue of the superficial layer (Fig. 232). With scalpel blade no. 15, an incision through only the fascia is performed, exposing the muscle fibers underneath (Fig. 233). By elevating the fascia graft and placing a Freer's rugine under the fascia, its undersurface can be cleaned from muscle fibers (Fig. 234). After further cutting of the fascia with a scalpel or a pair of scissors, and simultaneous elevation of the graft with a forceps (Fig. 235), the fascia is placed on a plastic plate, spread out, and separated from the remaining muscle fibers with the back of scalpel blade no. 23 (Fig. 236). Finally, all edges are cut using the same knife (Fig. 237). The fascia is then covered with a wet piece of gauze. It will be cut again to the necessary size before use.

Temporalis Muscle Fascia

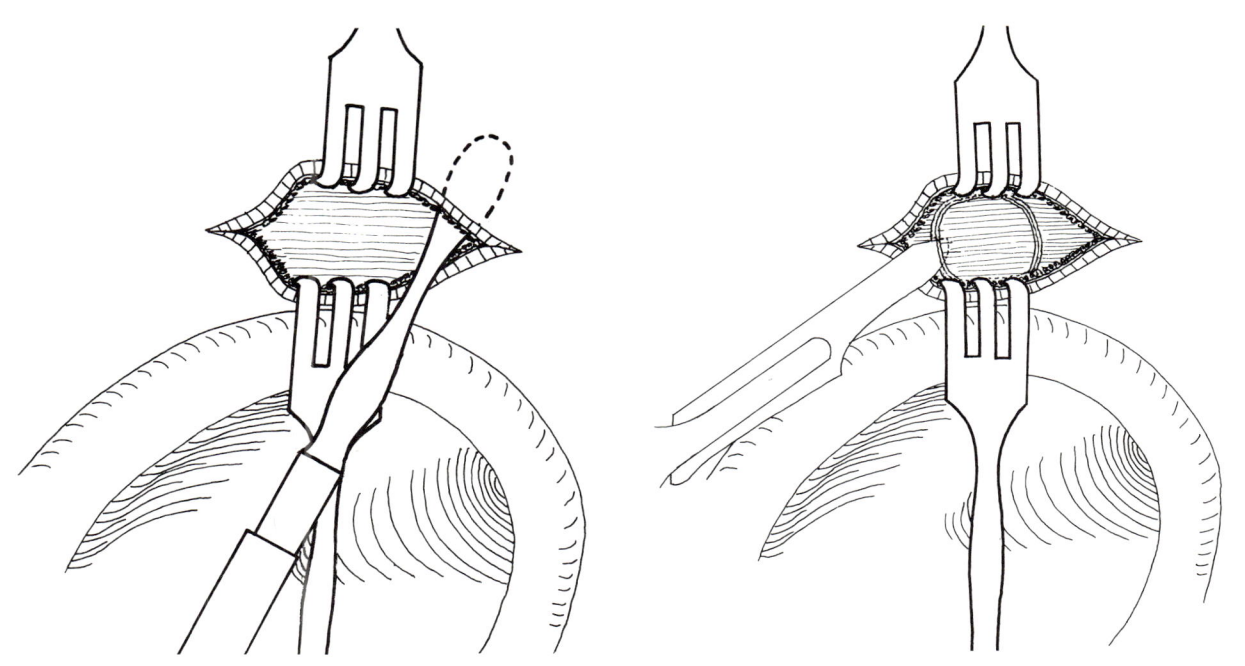

Fig. 232 The deeper layer of the fascia is cleaned using a Freer's rugine for the fibers belonging to the superficial layer

Fig. 233 Incision through the deep fascia layer

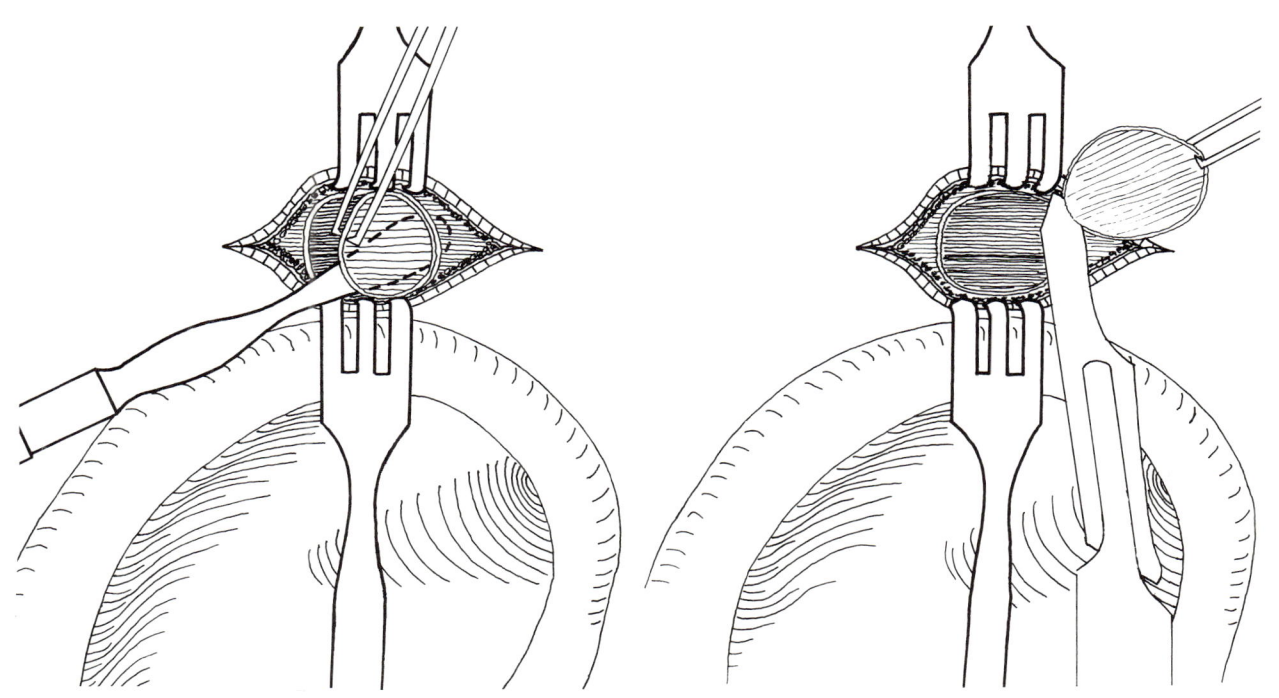

Fig. 234 The undersurface of the fascia is cleaned using a Freer's rugine

Fig. 235 The fascia is removed

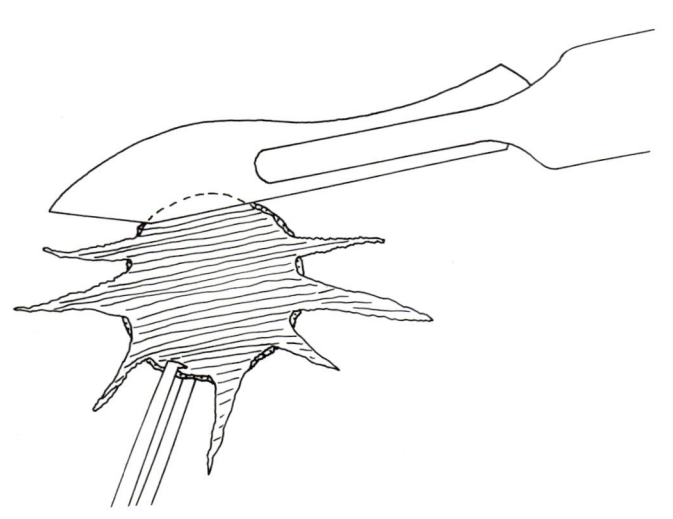

Fig. 236 The fascia is placed on a plastic plate, and cleaned with the back of a no. 23 scalpel blade

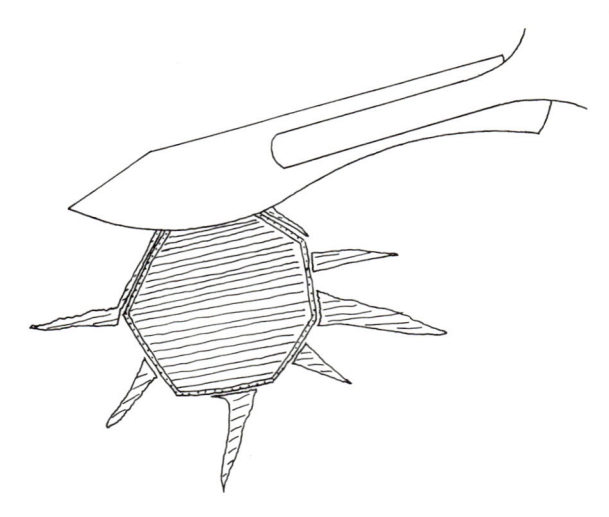

Fig. 237 Further cutting of the edges of the fascia with a no. 23 scalpel blade

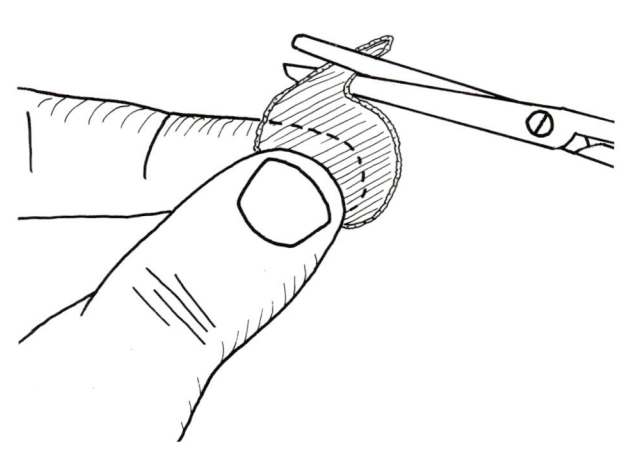

Fig. 238 Cutting a dry fascia with scissors

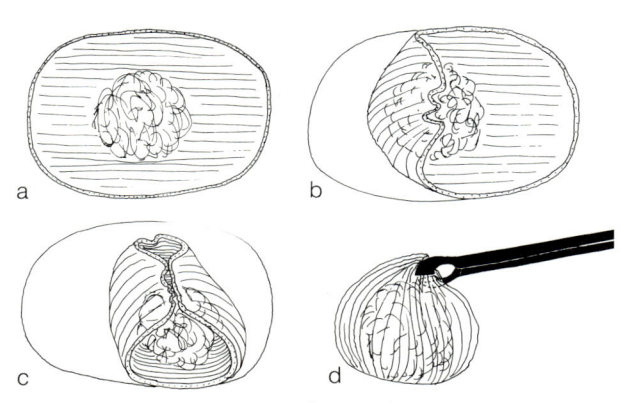

Fig. 239 Preparing a bag for wet fascia to bring it onto the drum remnant as an onlay graft. **a** Gelfoam is placed on the fascia, **b, c** fascia is elevated around the Gelfoam, **d** the bag is lifted with forceps

Many surgeons use dried fascia and cut it with scissors while holding it with the fingers (Fig. **238**). Immediately before insertion, this dried fascia will be made wet or semiwet by placing drops of water on it, or simply by immersing it in water or in a solution with antibiotics.

The present author uses both types. Wet fascia is used in the endaural approach with an ear speculum, or with the Heermann incision for onlay closure of total, subtotal, or large inferior perforations. The fascia is brought through the ear speculum onto the drum remnant as a bag, containing a semiwet, small Gelfoam ball (Fig. **239**). On the drum remnant, the bag is opened with a forceps, and the fascia is rolled out onto the annulus. In posterior perforations, a dry or semidry fascia is used as the underlay graft (Fig. **240**). In small anterior or inferior perforations, a semiwet fascia is used as an onlay graft (Fig. **240**). In the retroauricular approach, especially in cases with mastoidectomies or ear-canal reconstructions, a large piece of fascia is needed, and a semidry fascia is used both in onlay or underlay techniques (Fig. **240**).

In the endaural approach with *Heermann* incisions, a small piece of temporalis muscle fascia can be obtained by the Heermann A incision, but usually the Heermann B incision is used (Fig. **27**). With the Heermann B incision, there will be enough space to obtain an even larger piece of fascia. By further elevating the skin around the superior part of the vertical incision, and by removing the superficial layer of the fascia with a Freer's rugine, the posterosuperior area of the deeper temporalis

Temporalis Muscle Fascia

muscle fascia layer can be exposed (Fig. **241**). The fascia is incised anteriorly with scalpel blade no. 15, elevated with a pair of forceps, and cleaned of muscle fibers on the undersurface with a Freer's rugine (Fig. **242**). After exposure of enough fascia, and after cleaning of both sides, the fascia graft is excised using a pair of blunt scissors (Fig. **243**).

After larger exposure of the mastoid process in the Heermann B incision, a very large piece of fascia can be obtained (Fig. **38**). This is also the case with the Heermann C incision (Fig. **48**).

In *Shambaugh's* incision (Fig. **52**), *Lempert's* incision (Fig. **55**), *Farrior's* incision (Fig. **60**), and *Fleury's* incision (Fig. **71**), a large piece of temporalis muscle fascia can be obtained in a way similar to that described for the Heermann incision.

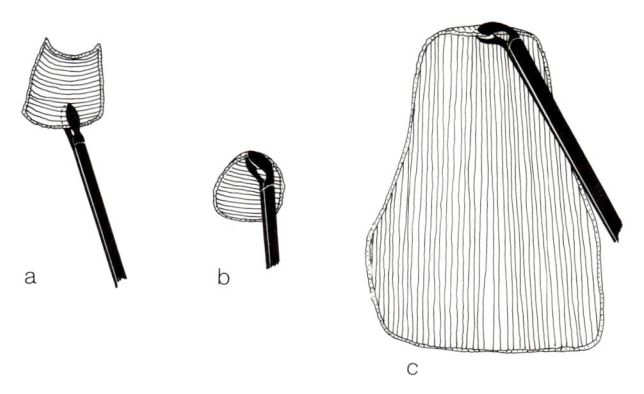

Fig. **240** Bringing the dry fascia **a** as an underlay graft, or **b** a small, dry fascia as an onlay graft, or **c** a large dry fascia as an underlay or onlay graft

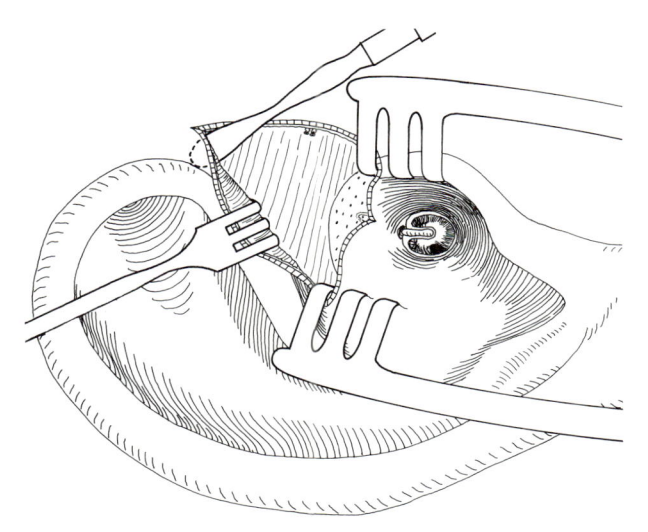

Fig. **241** Exposure of the fascia in a Heermann B incision, with elevation of the auricle and dissection of the superficial layer with a Freer's rugine

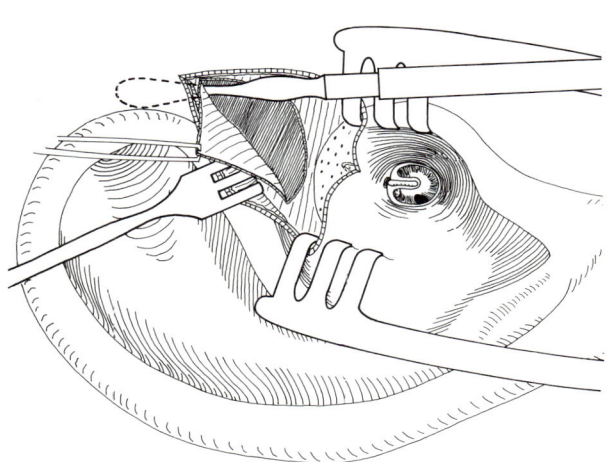

Fig. **242** Cleansing of the undersurface of the fascia with a rugine

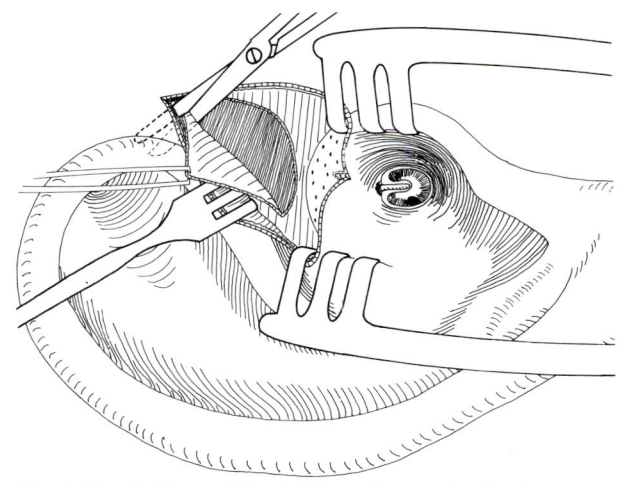

Fig. **243** Cutting of the fascia with a pair of scissors

94   8   Graft Materials

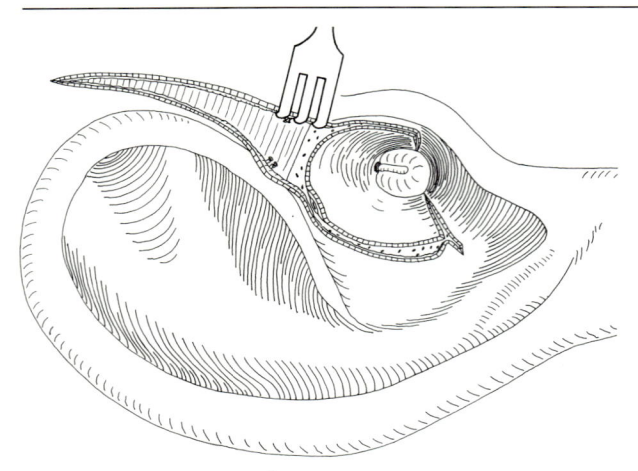

Fig. 244 Extension of the vertical incision in an endaural approach, with Heermann B, Lempert, of Shambaugh incisions, about 2 cm superiorly, to obtain wider access to the fascia

If a large piece of fascia is needed, or if the inferior part of the fascia has already been removed during a previous operation, the vertical incision can be extended for about 2 cm superiorly (Fig. 244). The skin, anterior and superior auricular muscles, and superficial temporalis fascia are elevated, and a large area of the deep temporalis muscle fascia is exposed and cleaned (Fig. 245). With scalpel blade no. 15, fascia is incised about 5 mm superior to the lower border of the muscle, and the undersurface of the fascia is then cleaned with a pair of scissors (Fig. 245). The fascia is gradually cut along the anterior border of the incision, as far superior as possible (Fig. 246). Care is taken to avoid the superficial temporal artery and vein. Finally, the fascia is cut posteriorly after further elevation of the auricle (Fig. 247).

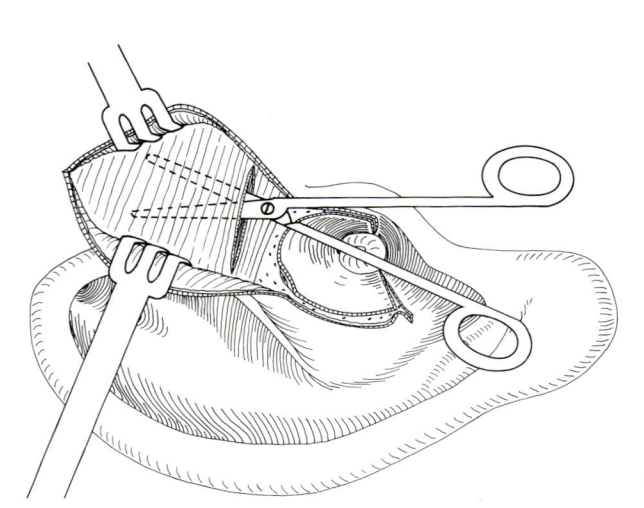

Fig. 245 The fascia is exposed, incised inferiorly, and cleaned on its undersurface with a pair of scissors

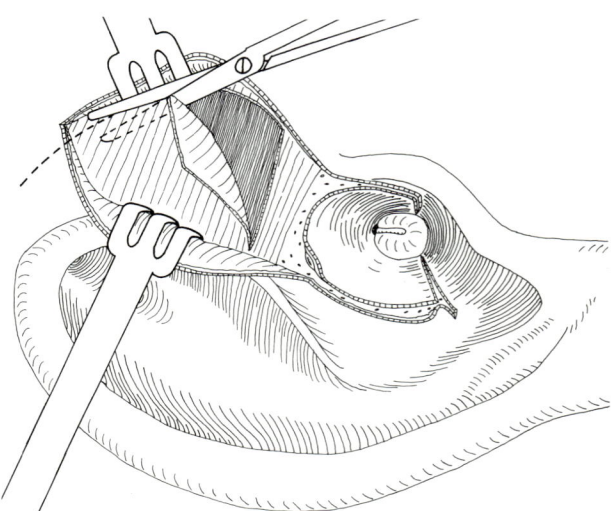

Fig. 246 The anterior incision of the fascia with a pair of blunt scissors

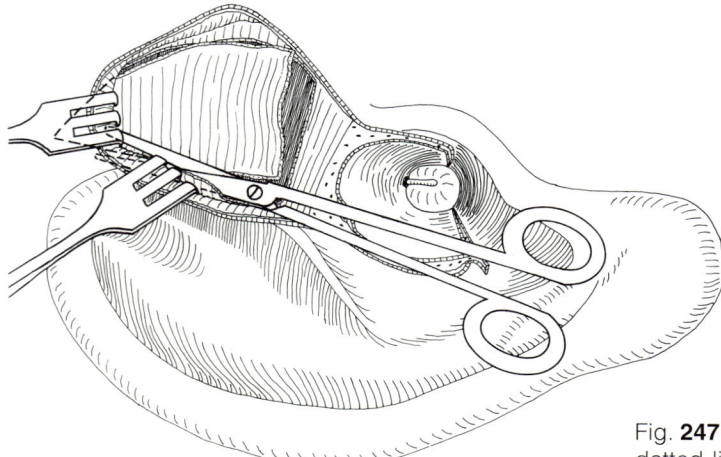

Fig. 247 The posterior cutting of the fascia, along the dotted line

Fascia in the Retroauricular Approach

A small piece of temporalis muscle fascia, for closure of a total perforation, can easily be obtained in the retroauricular approach by elevating the skin at the superior borders of the postauricular incision, exposing the fascia. This can be performed immediately after the postauricular skin incision, or after elevating the skin from the entrance of the ear canal (Fig. **78**). The lateral surface of the deep fascial layer is cleaned using Freer's rugine. A round incision in the temporalis fascia is performed with scalpel blade no. 15 (Fig. **248**). The fascia elevated with forceps, and its undersurface is again cleaned of remaining muscle fibers (Fig. **249**).

If a large piece of fascia is required, e.g., for reconstruction of the drum and the ear canal, the fascia can be incised 0.5 cm superior to and parallel to the linea temporalis, avoiding the thick lower strip of the fascia. With a Freer's rugine, or a pair of blunt scissors, the surface is cleaned of the loose fibers belonging to the superior layer of the fascia. This is performed far superiorly. The undersurface is then cleaned in the same way (Fig. **250**). After liberating a large area of the fascia superiorly to the skin-incision borders, a pair of blunt scissors is inserted to make the anterior cutting far superiorly under the skin (Fig. **251**). No vessels lie on or under the fascia in this posterosuperior region (Fig. **228**). The posterior incision is then made in a similar way (Fig. **252**), connecting the anterior incision. With forceps, the fascia is pulled out, and further cleaned with a rugine. The fascia is spread out on a plastic plate, further cleaned, and covered with moist gauze of, if dry fascia is desired, simply spread out.

In posterosuperior (Fig. **123**, **127**) or superior (Figs. **159**, **161**) approaches, there are no problems in obtaining sufficiently large pieces of fascia.

In retroauricular flap techniques with canal wall–down mastoidectomies, or total reconstruction of the middle ear, a large piece of fascia is usually required. It can be obtained in the same way as described in Figures **250**, **251**, and **252**. At the same time the temporalis muscle and other muscles may be required for possible obliteration of the cavity.

A very large retroauricular fold incision, as described in Fig. **146**, makes it possible to remove all the posterosuperior part of the temporalis fascia and still use the muscle with the inferior part of the fascia for obliteration. The skin is maximally elevated, and a large area of fascia is exposed (Fig. **253**). Its surface is cleaned of fibrous tissue from the superficial fascia. The fascia is also cleaned on its undersurface. With a pair of curved blunt scissors, the fascia is cut far superiorly, nearly at the attachment of the muscle (Fig. **254**), and the cutting is then continued far anteriorly, and the fascia pulled out.

In cases with several reoperations, there will be no fascia to take at the area around the auricle. In such cases, a separate incision is necessary (Fig. **230**). Sometimes it is necessary to take the fascia from the temporalis muscle of the opposite side, or to use fascia lata.

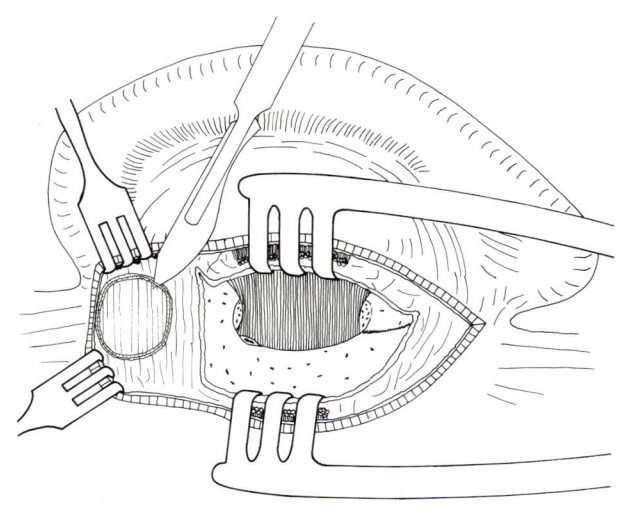

Fig. **248** Removal of a small piece of the temporalis muscle fascia in a retroauricular incision. The superior edge of the incision is spread. The fascia is exposed and incised with a scalpel

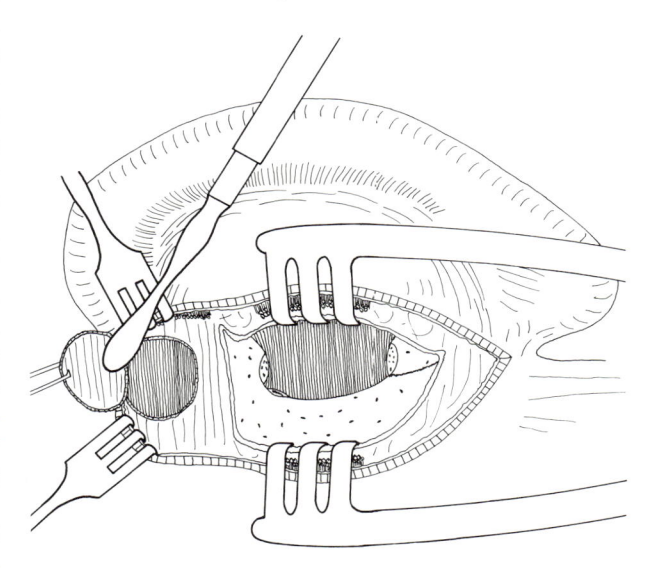

Fig. **249** The fascia is removed and cleaned

8 Graft Materials

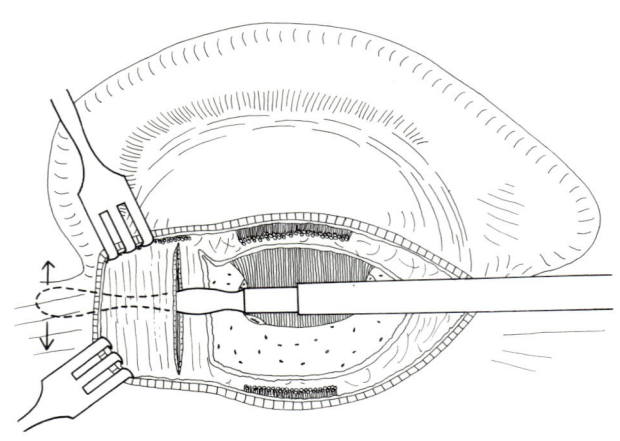

Fig. 250 Removal of a large piece of temporalis muscle fascia in a retroauricular approach. After exposing the fascia, the incision is performed 5 mm superior to the inferior border, and the fascia is cleaned on both sides with a Freer's rugine

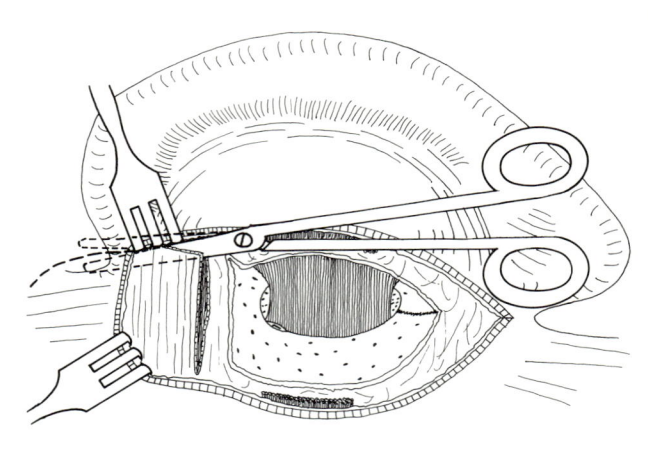

Fig. 251 With a pair of curved blunt scissors, the fascia is cut anteriorly and far superiorly under the elevated skin

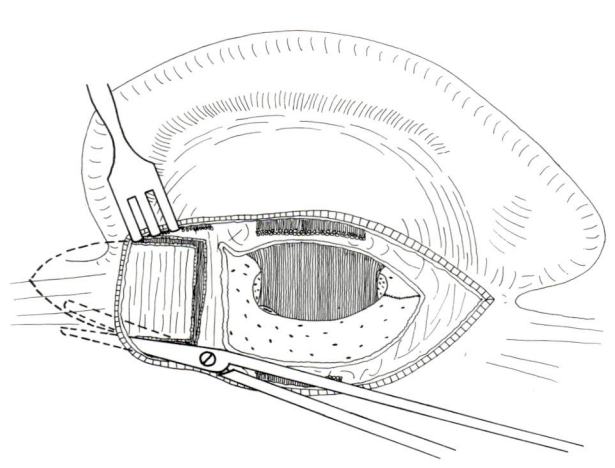

Fig. 252 The fascia is cut posteriorly and connected with the previous anterior incision

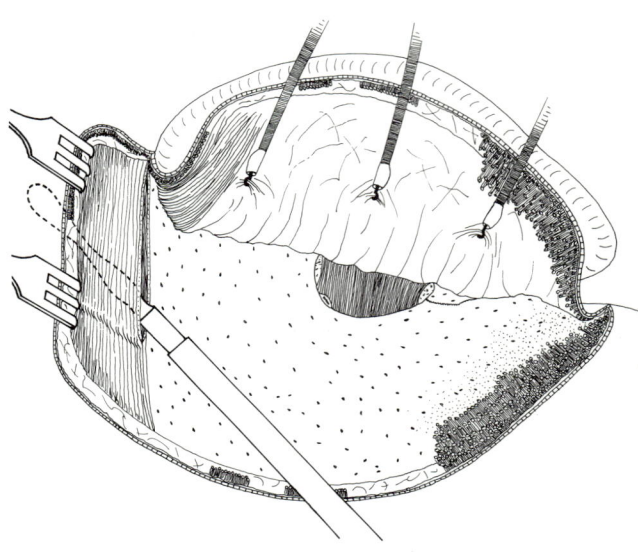

Fig. 253 Removal of the fascia in a large retroauricular flap incision. The skin of the superior edge of the incision is maximally elevated with two strong retractors. The surface of the fascia is cleaned with a Freer's rugine on the upper and lower surfaces

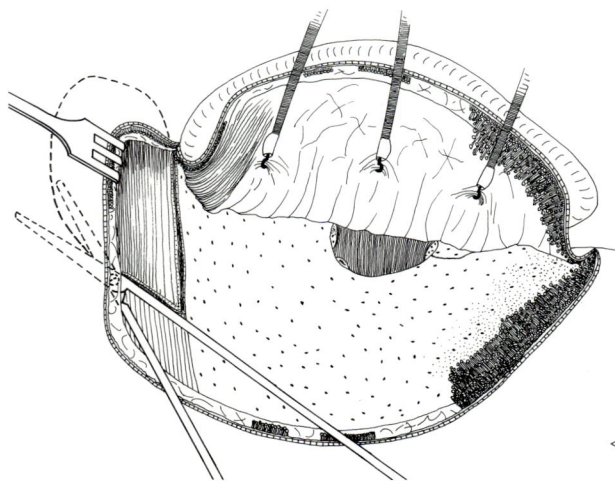

◁ **Fig. 254** The fascia is cut off with a pair of blunt curved scissors far superior to the skin incision

Tragal Perichondrium

Tragal perichondrium was introduced into myringoplasty by Goodhill et al (1964), after being used in stapedectomy as an oval window graft for some years before that. Like temporalis muscle fascia, tragal perichondrium has several advantages:

1. It is easily accessible.
2. It is a mesodermal graft.
3. It has a good chance of postoperative survival.
4. It has a conical contour.
5. It is sufficiently large for myringoplasty of a total perforation, but not for larger reconstructions of the ear canal. In these conditions, tragal cartilage is inferior to temporalis muscle fascia.

Tragal perichondrium can be obtained as a partial graft, a) *hemigraft*, either a from the posterior (canal) tragal surface, or b) from the anterior (facial) tragal surface, or c) the entire tragal cartilage may be removed, and both perichondrial surfaces used in continuity as a *total graft*.

The size of the drum perforation to be covered decides whether a hemigraft or a total graft should be used. The Goodhill technique of harvesting of the tragal cartilage was described as an anterior approach, i.e., with the surgeon sitting in front of the face (Fig. 158). The technique described here differs very little from Goodhill's original but the surgeon is sitting behind the head.

A 1.5 cm long incision on the dome of the tragal cartilage is performed with scalpel blade no. 15 (Figs. **255**, **256**). The tragal cartilage can immediately be seen under the skin. Using a pair of small blunt curved scissors the subcutaneous tissue from the *posterior surface* of the tragus is dissected away, and the entire posterior surface of the tragal cartilage is exposed (Fig. **256**). The perichondrium is incised along the entire dome (Fig. **257**), and the posterior plate of the perichondrium is elevated from the cartilage with a Freer elevator. When the entire posterior perichondrium is maximally elevated and cleaned on both sides, it can be cut out by scalpel blade no. 11, first at the inferior margin, then by a cut as medially as possible without damaging the canal skin, and finally with an outward-directed cut along the superior margin (Fig. **258**). The perichondrium is gently held by a tissue forceps during the cutting.

About 1.5 cm^2 of the already cleaned perichondrium can be obtained. The perichondrium is covered with wet gauze during the operation, and is generally not used as a dry graft, because its consistency is somewhat more solid than the consistency of the fascia. The wet graft of the perichondrium is stiff enough to be placed as an underlay or onlay graft.

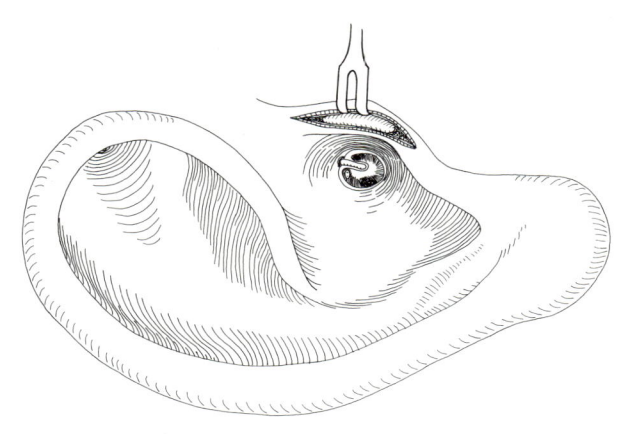

Fig. **255** Incision for removal of tragal cartilage

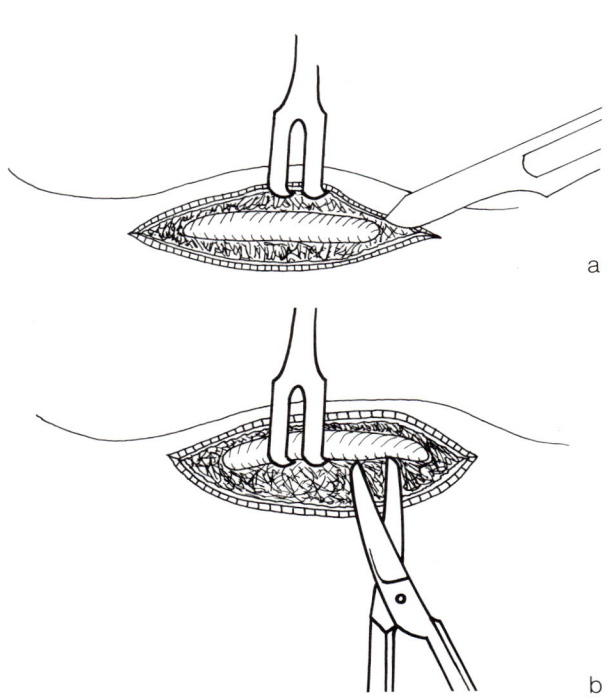

Fig. **256a** Skin incision over the dome of the cartilage. **b** The posterior surface of the cartilage is cleaned

The anterior surface of the tragal cartilage can be removed at the same stage if desired (Fig. **259**), e.g., in a major reconstruction. In fact, it is easier to acquire a larger area of the perichondrium from the anterior part after the posterior perichondrium has been removed. Because of the fibers from the parotideomastoid fascia attached to the anterior perichondrium plate, it has to be cleaned more than the posterior plate.

98 8 Graft Materials

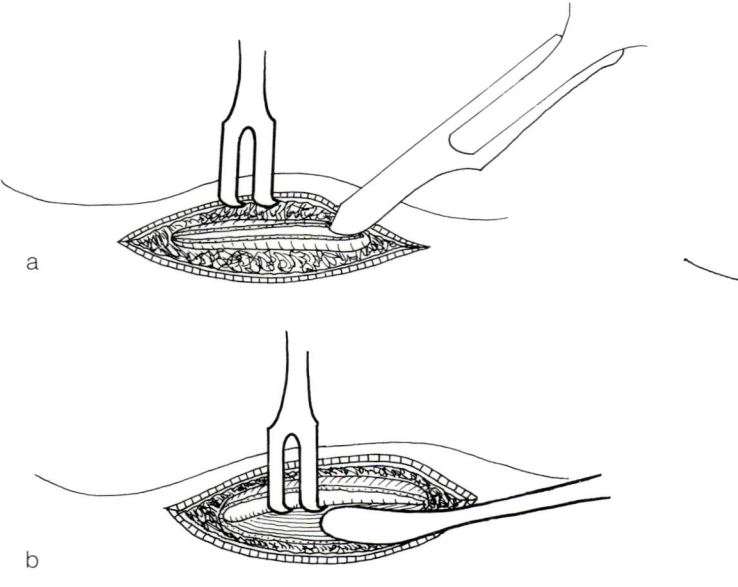

Fig. **257a** The perichondrium is incised. **b** The posterior blade of the perichondrium is elevated from the cartilage

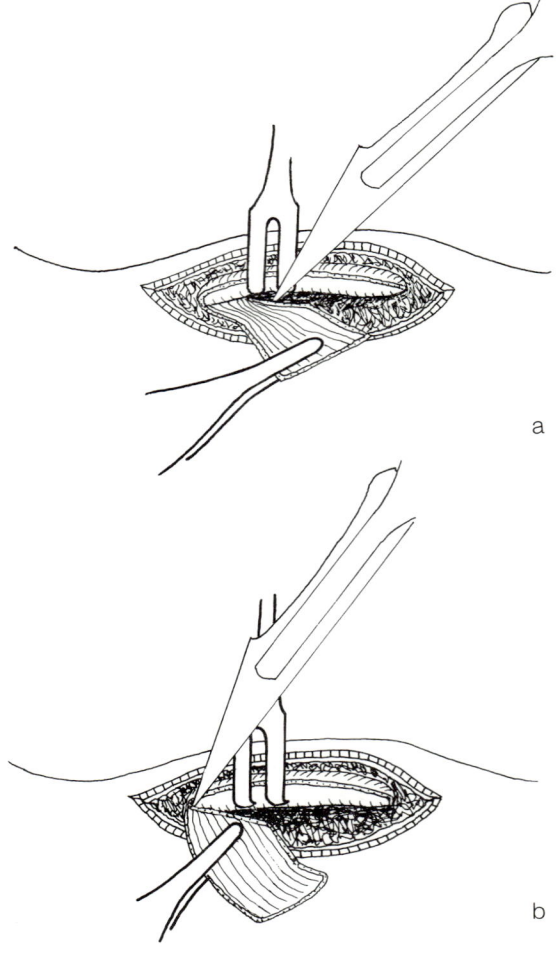

Fig. **258a** The posterior blade of the cartilage is excised inferiorly and medially. **b** The excision is continued along the superior border

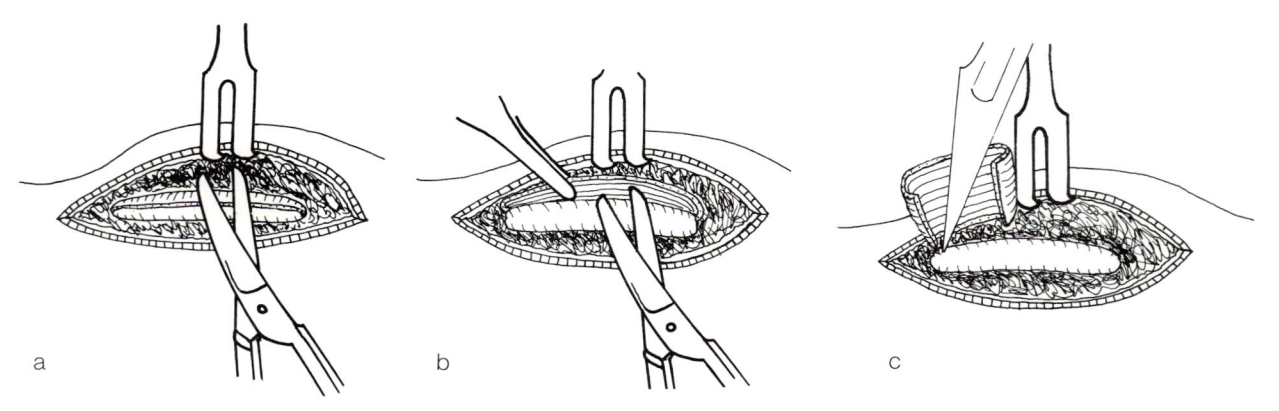

Fig. **259a** The anterior perichondrial hemigraft is cleaned. **b** The perichondrium has been excised, and is elevated from the cartilage. **c** The anterior hemigraft is excised

Tragal Perichondrium

The perichondrium can be removed as a *total graft*, from the entire tragus. Using the same skin incision, the subcutaneous tissue from the tragal cartilage is dissected away on both sides of the cartilage and the free superior and inferior edges. This dissection is performed thoroughly with a pair of blunt scissors. It is easier to clean the perichondrium if it is still attached to the cartilage and the tragus is still fixed in place. With a forceps, without damaging the perichondrium, the tragus is gently pulled outwards, and superiorly (Fig. **260**), and the cutting of the inferior edge of the tragus, as far medially as possible, is started. This is continued superiorly, leading to total removal of the tragus (Fig. **260**).

By fixing the tragus with the finger, the perichondrium is gradually elevated from one side of the cartilage (Fig. **261**). It is turned around, and again fixed with the finger to dissect the other side. Finally, both sheets of the perichondrium are folded together, pressed down on the plate with the finger, and the final attachment of the cartilage is gently dissected away with a Freer rugine (Fig. **261**).

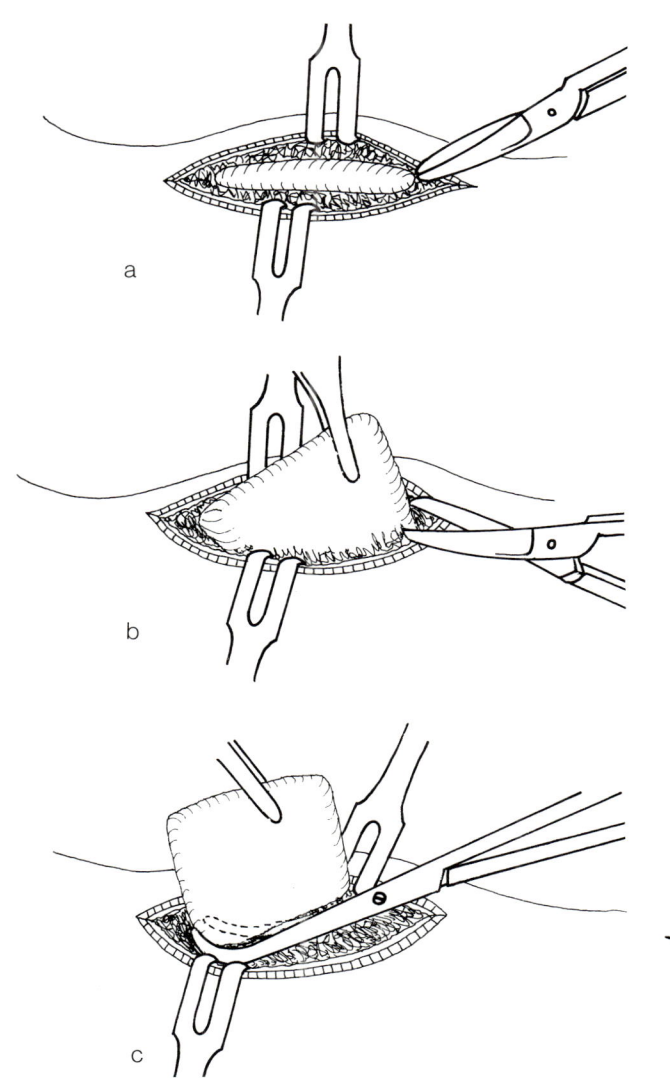

Fig. **260** Removal of the entire tragal cartilage with the perichondrium. **a** After the skin incision, the tragal cartilage is cleaned on both sides. **b** The cartilge is pulled in a superior direction, and **c** cut as medially as possible

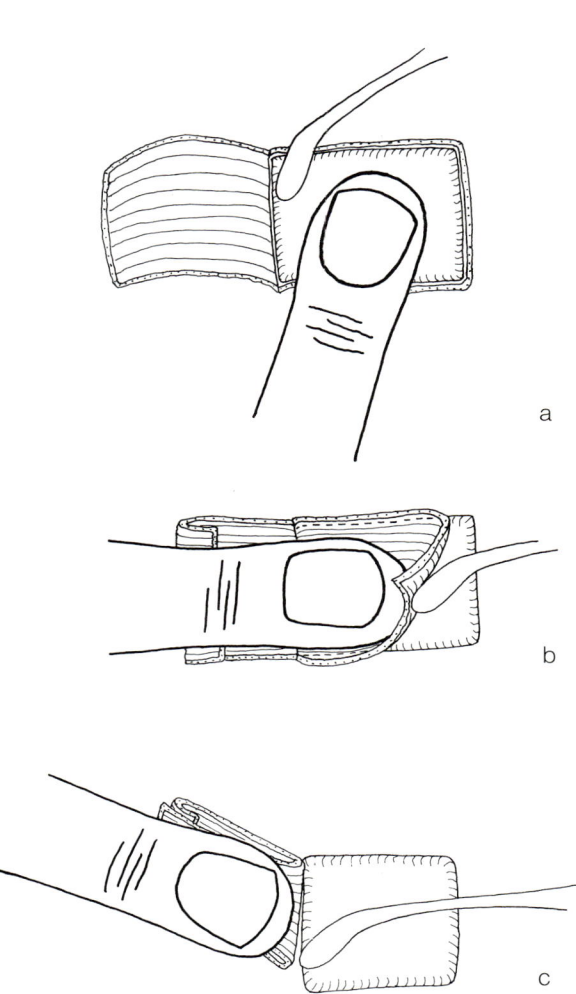

Fig. **261** The elevation of the perichondrium from the cartilage **a** on one side, **b** on the opposite side, **c** on the last edge

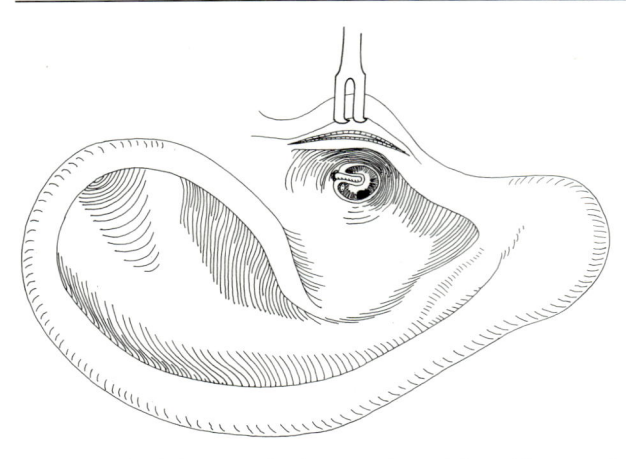

Fig. 262 Incision to obtain tragal perichondrium and cartilage 2 mm medially in the ear canal

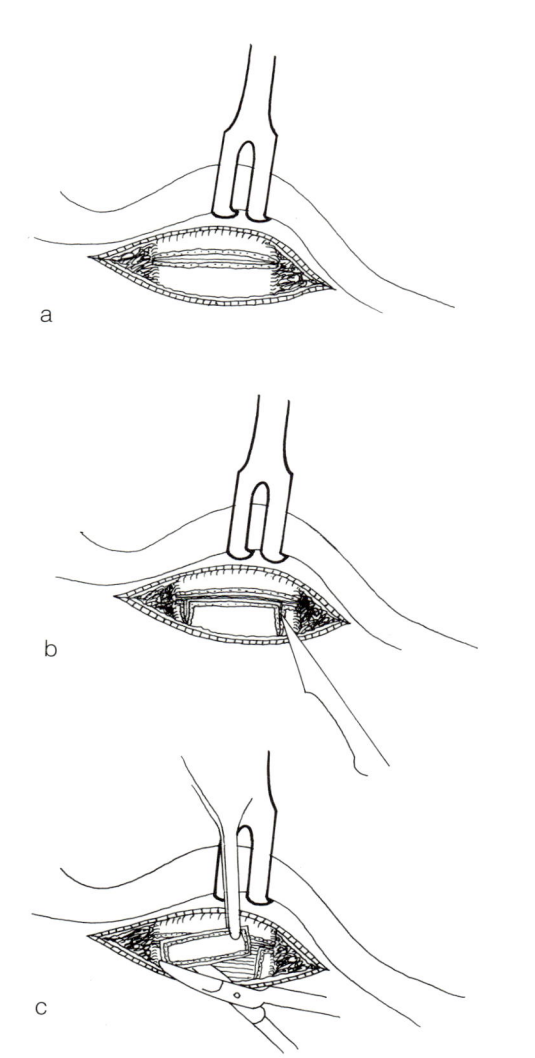

Fig. 263 Removal of a piece of cartilage with perichondrium. **a** The perichondrium is incised. **b** The cartilage is incised. **c** A piece of cartilage with perichondrium is cut out with a pair of scissors

Tragal Cartilage

The cartilage is reinserted in the same place, and in the same position, as before. Even if some pieces of the cartilage may be removed for purposes of ossiculoplasty, or if it is otherwise damaged, the remnant should be reinserted. Reinsertion will to some extent prevent retraction of the tragus skin, which is the only complication of tragal cartilage removal.

The present author prefers to use perichondrium in small perforations, and especially in cases previously operated on using fascia. In addition, total perichondrial graft with the entire tragal cartilage is routinely used in reconstructing old radical cavities. In ossiculoplasty, the cartilage is widely used as interposition material in type II and III tympanoplasty, and especially as thin cartilage slices placed on top of the head of total or partial ossicular replacement prostheses. Heermann uses palisades of tragal (or conchal) cartilage for myringoplasty, without other graft material. Several methods of myringoplasty using cartilage–perichondrium grafts, or cartilage alone, to prevent posterior retraction, are described below (pp. 210–216).

To avoid retraction of the tragal skin and a visible scar, the skin incision can be made 2 mm inside the ear canal (Fig. **262**). If perichondrium alone is desired as a posterior hemigraft, it can be removed in the way shown above (Fig. **258**). If both perichondrium and a minor piece of tragal cartilage is required for ossiculoplasty, a quadrangular piece is cut with scalpel blade no. 11, and cartilage with the perichondrium is detached with a rugine (Fig. **263**).

Tragal Perichondrium

Tragal cartilage with perichondrium can be removed through a Heermann incision or other endaural incisions. With a pair of blunt, small, curved scissors pushed through the intercartilaginous skin incision (Fig. 264) towards the posterior and anterior surfaces of the tragal cartilage, the subcutaneous tissue is elevated from the tragus, which is gradually exposed on all sides (Fig. 265). Using a tissue forceps, tragal cartilage is pulled out through the intercartilaginous incision, and cut as far medially as possible with a pair of scissors (Fig. 266).

A separate skin incision 2–3 mm medial to outer edge of the tragus top can be performed, and this incision should not extend to the intercartilaginous incision. Further dissection of perichondrium and tragus is carried out as described above.

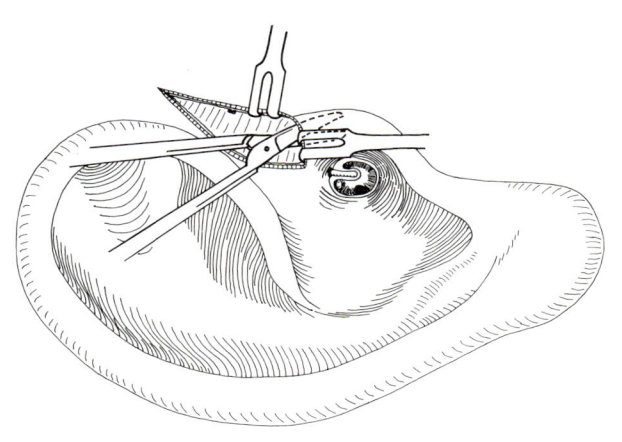

Fig. 264 Removal of tragal cartilage through the intercartilaginous incision

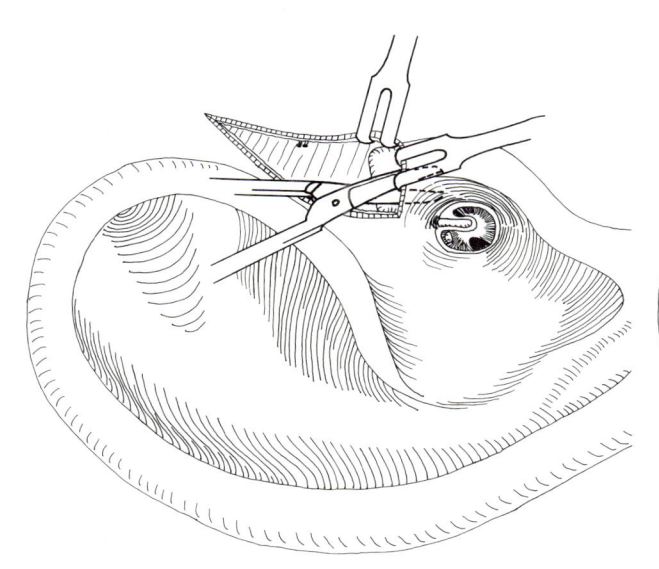

Fig. 265 The posterior aspect of the tragal cartilage is dissected from the subcutaneous tissue with a pair of scissors

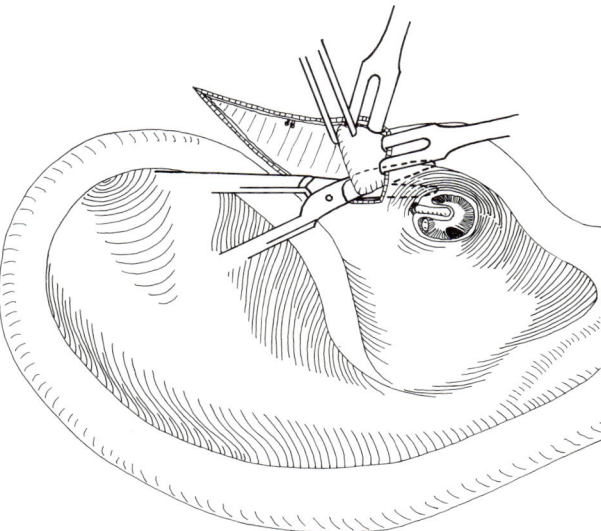

Fig. 266 The anterior surface is dissected, as well as the inferior edge. The cartilage is pulled out with an anatomical forceps, and subsequently cut medially with a pair of scissors

Conchal Perichondrium and Cartilage

A major piece of conchal perichondrium or conchal cartilage, or both, can be harvested a) by a separate posterior incision; b) in a retroauricular incision, c) in an endaural incision. The conchal perichondrium and cartilage is used for the same purposes as the tragal cartilage in myringoplasty and tympanoplasty and in various reconstructions of the ear canal. Because of its concave shape, conchal cartilage is especially suitable for ear-canal reconstruction. Some authors claim that all cartilage from the cavum conchae can be removed without any sequelae (Fig. **267**). In ears with canal wall–down mastoidectomy, where enlargement of the introitus of the external auditory meatus is required because of the large cavity, the medial edge of the conchal cartilage should be resected to enlarge the canal (Fig. **268**). Because of the postoperative retraction, the auricle will be retracted down to the mastoid process and the conchal cartilage will become prominent, gradually diminishing the entrance of the ear canal, and thus causing problems with selfcleansing of the cavity.

Cartilage Via a Separate Posterior Incision

Some surgeons prefer to use a separate incision to acquire the conchal perichondrium before starting with an endaural incision.

After the auricle has been retracted anteriorly with the fingers, a 3-cm long skin incision is performed over the conchal eminence 1 cm anterior to the retroauricular fold (Fig. **267**). A possible infiltration of the region with local anesthetic containing adrenaline can be used prior to the incision. The skin and the subcutis are elevated with a pair of blunt scissors. The attachment of the posterior auricular muscle to the auricle is freed, and the muscle is pushed posteriorly. A major part of the conchal eminence, as well as the anterior edge of the concha, can be exposed by further dissection of the loose tissue from the concha (Fig. **267**).

A curved incision through the perichondrium is performed with scalpel blade no. 15 (Fig. **269**). The perichondrium is elevated from the cartilage using a Freer rugine (Fig. **270**), and a large piece is resected with a pair of scissors. If both conchal cartilage and perichondrium are desired, the incision is made through the posterior layer of the perichondrium and the cartilage (Fig. **271**), but the anterior layer of the periochondrium is not incised and is left in place. With a Freer's rugine, the cartilage is elevated from the anterior layer of the perichondrium (Fig. **271**), and gradually luxated posteriorly. The cartilage with the perichondrium can easily be excised by a pair of scissors.

If the perichondrium is desired separately, it is worthwhile elevating it from the cartilage with a Freer's rugine before removing the cartilage, since this type of elevation is easier. The cartilage and the perichondrium can be removed separately (Fig. **272**).

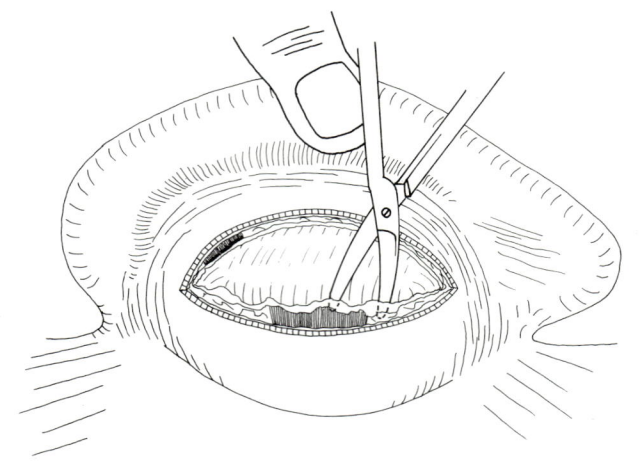

Fig. **267** Removal of conchal perichondrium through a separate retroauricular incision. The subcutaneous tissue and posterior auricular muscle are elevated from the perichondrium

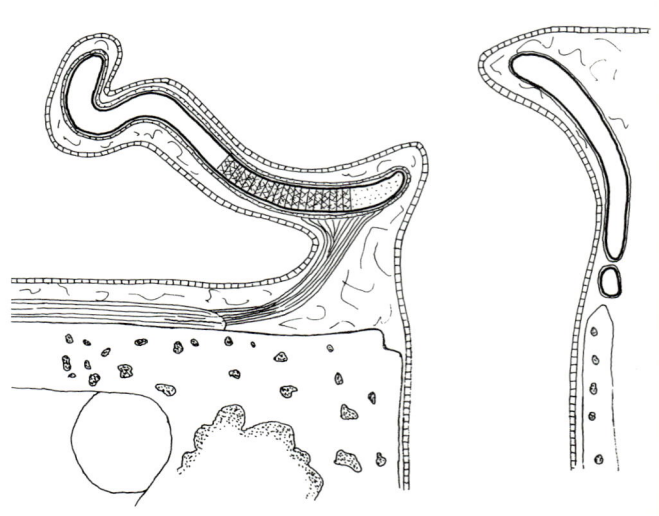

Fig. **268** Auricle in side view. Part of the conchal cartilage, which can be removed (shaded area), and the conchal cartilage with its edge (dotted area), which ought to be removed, to enlarge the ear canal

Conchal Perichondrium and Cartilage

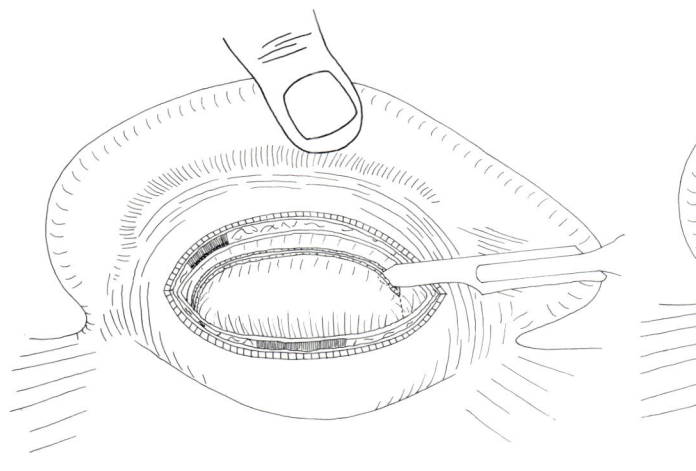

Fig. 269 Incision in the perichondrium

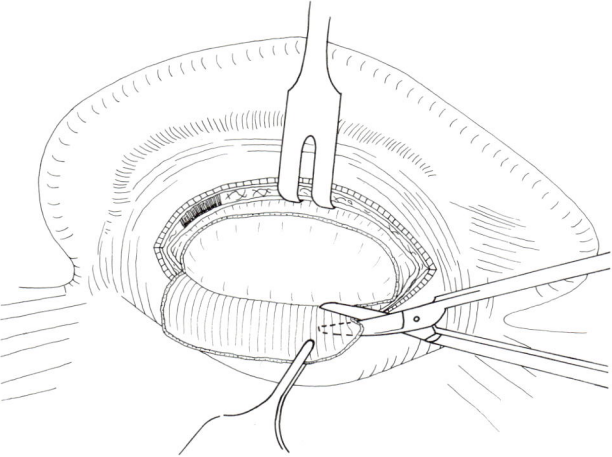

Fig. 270 The perichondrium is elevated and cut

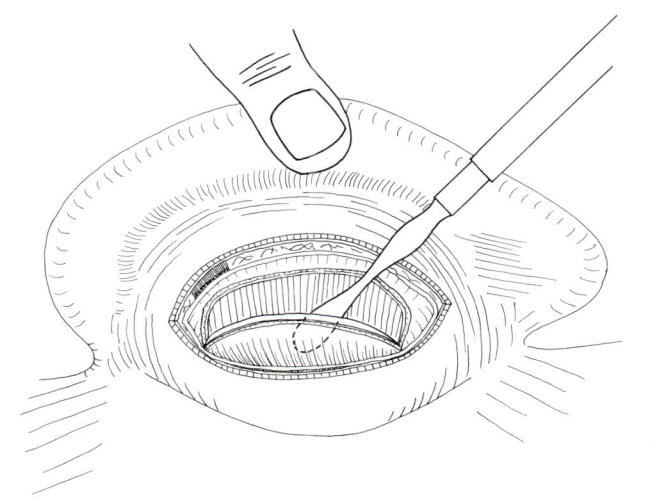

Fig. 271 The perichondrium and conchal cartilage are incised, and the cartilage is luxated posteriorly with a Freer's rugine and elevated from the anterior blade of the perichondrium

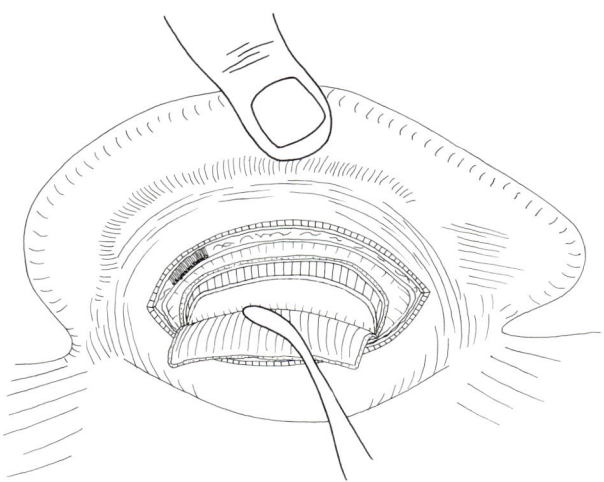

Fig. 272 The perichondrium ist elevated from the cartilage with a rugine. The perichondrium and cartilage will be cut off separately

Cartilage Via Retroauricular Incisions

In the retroauricular fold incision and posterosuperior incision running close to the auricle (Figs. **75, 77, 123**), a large area of the conchal eminence can easily be exposed by elevating the subcutaneous tissue and the postauricular muscle from the conchal perichondrium. Removal of the conchal perichondrium or conchal cartilage, or both, takes place in the same way as described above in a separate posterior incision (Figs. **268–272**).

In retroauricular flap incisions running far posterior to the conchal prominence (Fig. **75**), the postauricular skin can be elevated separately up to the conchal eminence (Figs. **136, 137**). From here, the subcutaneous tissue and the insertion of the postauricular muscle is elevated from the perichondrium of the conchal eminence (Fig. **273**), exposing the entire conchal eminence. By further dissection along the perichondrium, the anterior edge of the conchal cartilage can be reached and exposed (Fig. **274**).

A sufficiently large piece of perichondrium can be acquired through a curved incision and elevation of the perichondrium, which can be cut off (Fig. **275**).

If a large piece of cartilage and perichondrium is desired, an additional curved incision in the cartilage is performed at the same place as the incision of the perichondrium (Fig. 275). With a Freer's rugine, the cartilage is gently elevated from the anterior plate of the perichondrium, and pushed posteriorly. The elevation proceeds until the anterior edge of the concha is reached (Fig. 276). After further dislocation, along the entire anterior edge of the cartilage, from the anterior perichondrial layer, further elevation of the posterior layer of the perichondrium from the conchal cartilage can be performed (Fig. 277). The entire anterior edge of the conchal cartilage is now dissected free from the perichondrium, and can, after cutting of the inferior part, gradually be elevated with a Freer's rugine and removed in one piece (Fig. 278).

The posterior layer of the conchal perichondrium, which has been elevated from both sides, can be resected using a pair of scissors, and used as a graft (Fig. 279).

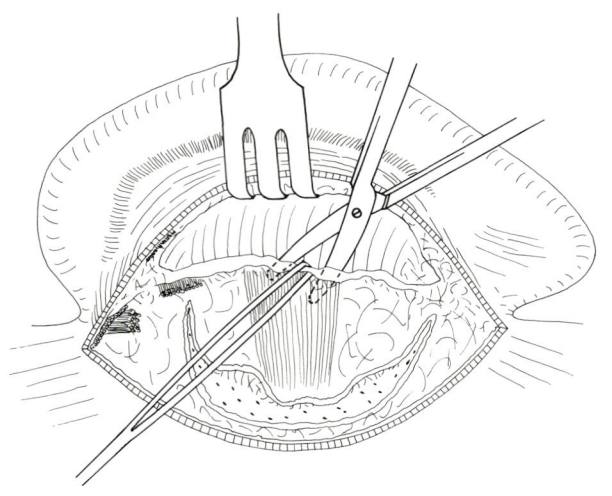

Fig. 273 Obtaining perichondrium and conchal cartilage in a retroauricular flap incision. After a curved incision of the periosteum, the dissection of the retroauricular flap is indicated. The skin is elevated far anteriorly, exposing the conchal eminence. From here, the subcutis is elevated

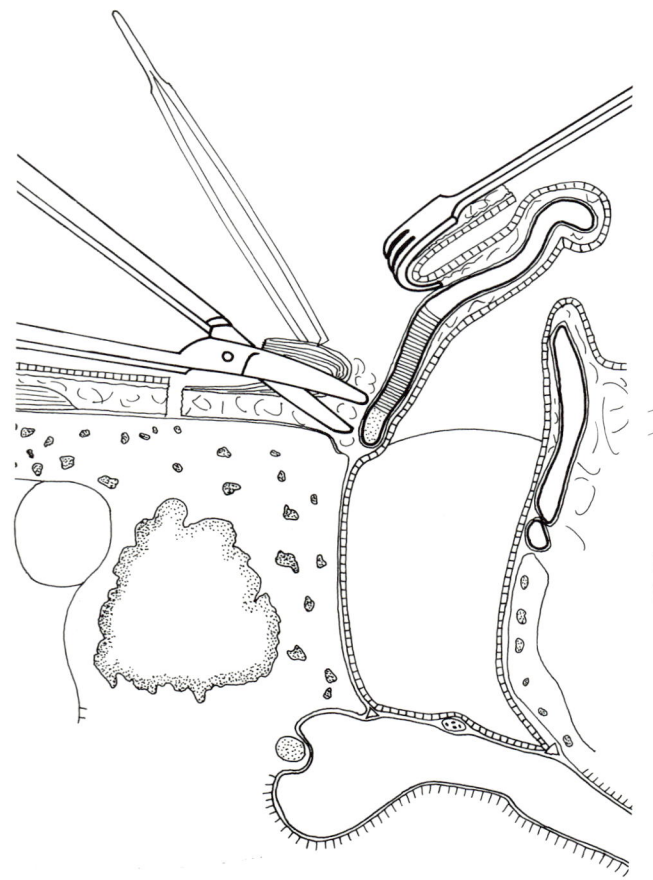

Fig. 274 Exposure of the conchal eminence and entire anterior edge of the conchal cartilage, in a side view

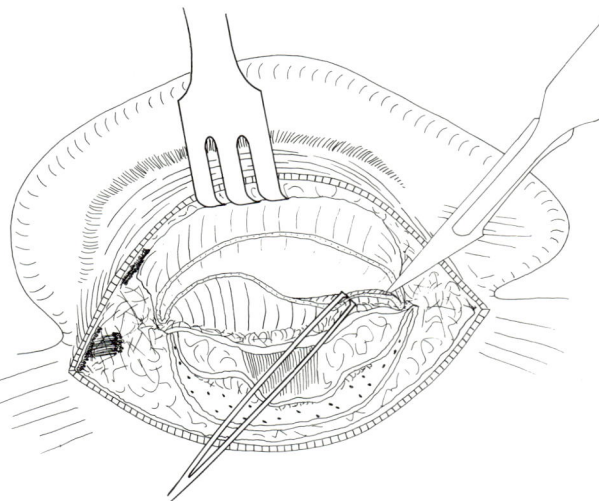

Fig. 275 Excision of the posterior blade of the conchal perichondrium after its elevation from the cartilage

Conchal Perichondrium and Cartilage

Fig. 276 Elevation of the conchal cartilage with the Freer rugine around the anterior blade of the conchal perichondrium. The posterior blade of the perichondrium has already been elevated. The rugine reaches the anterior edge of the cartilage

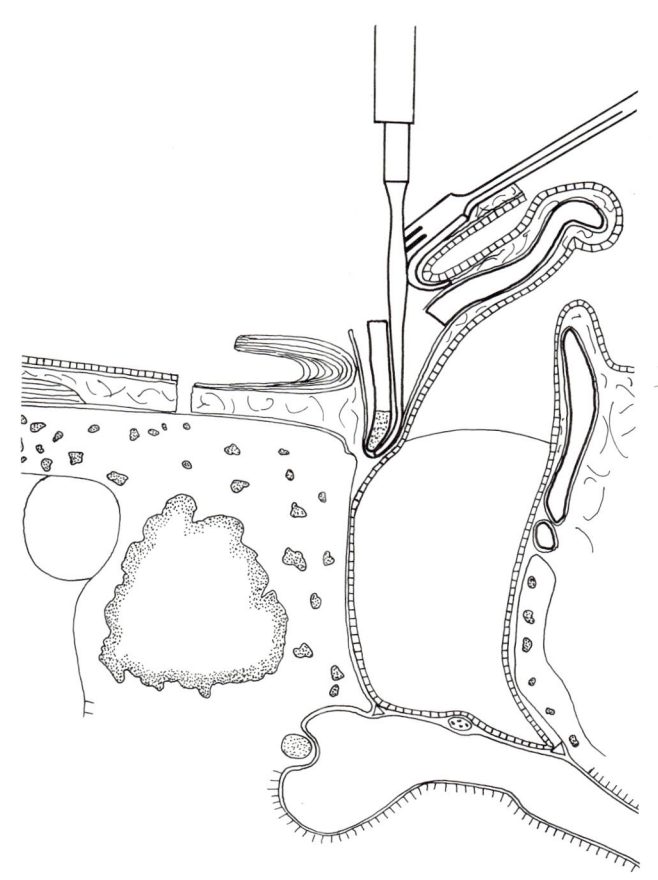

Fig. 277 Elevation of the posterior plate of the perichondrium around the conchal cartilage

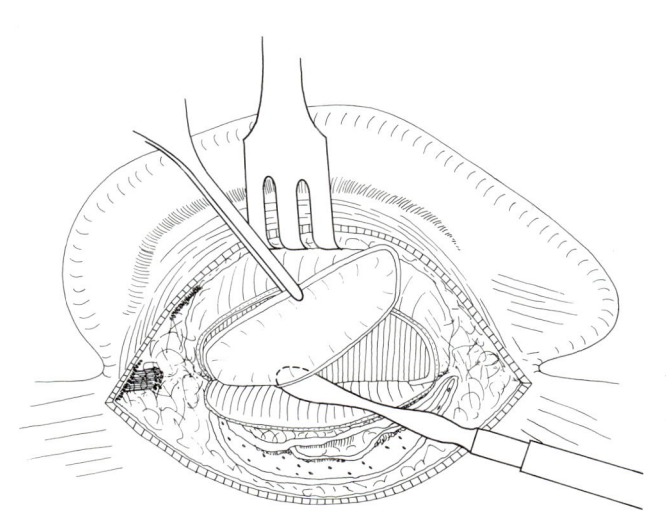

Fig. 278 The conchal cartilage has been cut inferiorly, and can be elevated in one piece from the perichondrium with a Freer rugine

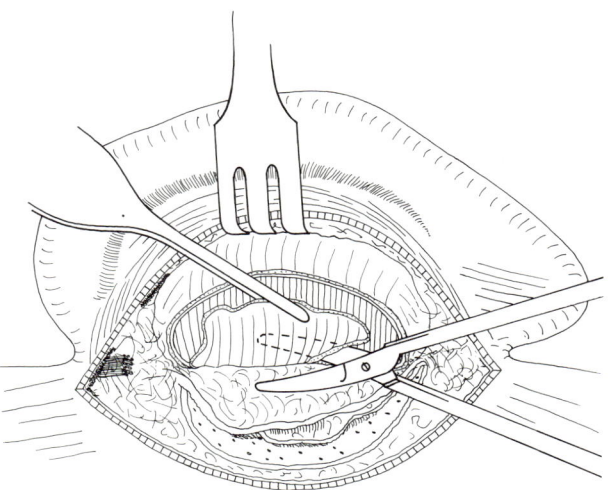

Fig. 279 Removal of the posterior blade of the conchal perichondrium after the cartilage has been removed

8 Graft Materials

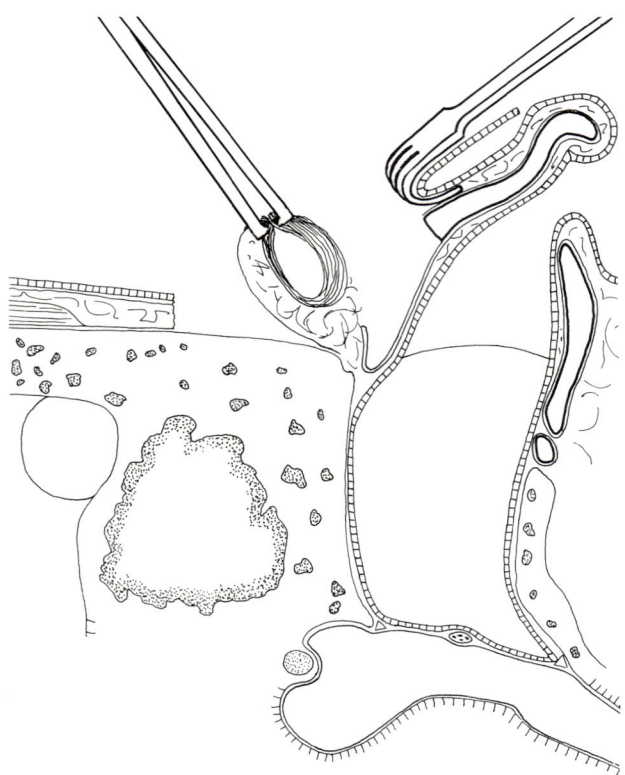

Fig. **280** The situation after removal of the conchal cartilage and posterior blade of the perichondrium. The subcutaneous periosteal flap from the mastoid process has a poor connection with the ear canal, since the subcutaneous tissue from the concha is elevated

The situation after removal of the conchal cartilage and the perichondrium is very poor attachment of the subcutis–periosteal flap. The flap is only attached to the canal skin and the perichondrium with a few fibers (Fig. **280**). Vascularization of this type of anterior-pedicled flap will be poor, but the flap can still be used in reconstruction of the ear canal and in obliteration of the cavity.

In cases where only small pieces of the perichondrium are desired, e.g., in closure of a total or subtotal perforation, a spherical piece of the conchal perichondrium can easily be removed from the conchal eminence (Fig. **281**). The same applies in removal of small pieces of conchal cartilage (Fig. **282**) for ossiculoplasty, or for slices of cartilage placed on top of a total or partial ossicular replacement prosthesis. To prevent retraction into the posterior tympanum or into the attic, small pieces of conchal cartilage, together with the perichondrium, are used to cover an attic bony defect or a bony defect in the posterior bony annulus. They can be obtained in the same way, either via the retroauricular approach (Fig. **273**) or in small, separate posterior incisions. The concave shape of the conchal cartilage is especially suitable for closure of various bony defects, e.g., in atticotomies or antrostomies.

To avoid problems with insufficient attachment of the subcutaneous–periosteal flaps to the concha, the conchal cartilage can be approached far anteriorly. This will also apply in cases in which only minor pieces of cartilage or perichondrium are needed, and in cases in which resection of the anterior edge of the conchal cartilage is desirable.

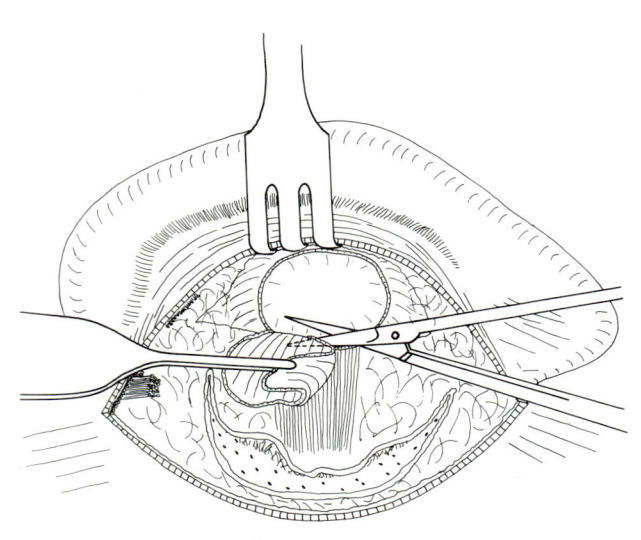

Fig. **281** Removal of the small round piece of perichondrium from the conchal eminence in a retroauricular flap incision

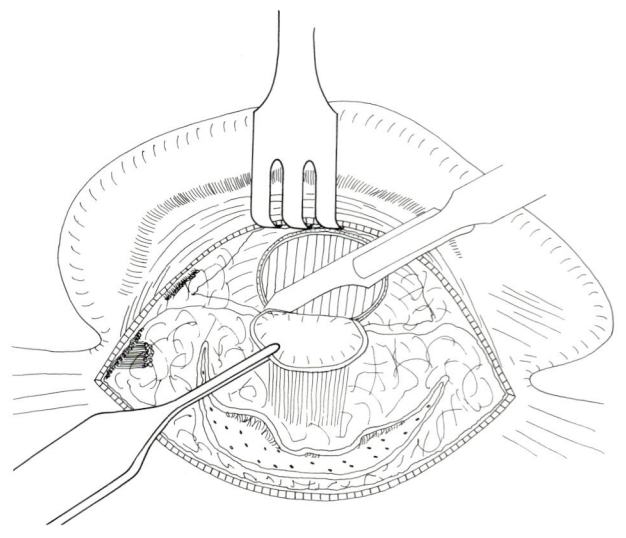

Fig. **282** Removal of conchal cartilage with the perichondrium in a retroauricular incision

Conchal Perichondrium and Cartilage

After the retroauricular incision, the subcutaneous–periosteal flap can be elevated far anteriorly towards and under the conchal eminence. The perichondrium will be exposed after the incision through the subcutis, and the subcutaneous muscle flap is elevated far anteriorly to the perichondrium of the conchal cartilage (Fig. 283). The perichondrium is excised, and elevated from the cartilage far anteriorly and to the edge of the cartilage. The cartilage is then incised with a curved incision running superoinferiorly, and elevated from the anterior layer of the perichondrium. The cartilage to be resected is gently pushed posteriorly with a Freer rugine (Fig. 284), liberating the entire anterior edge of the conchal cartilage (Fig. 285). After cutting its relatively thick inferior connection at the 6-o'clock position close to the antitragal cartilage, the resected conchal cartilage can be pulled out with a forceps and cut at its superior attachment to the crus of the helix (Fig. 286).

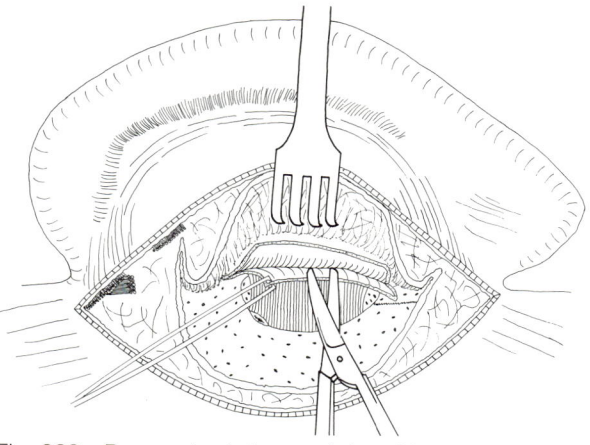

Fig. 283 Removal of the perichondrium or cartilage from the anterior edge of the concha in retroauricular flap incisions. The musculoperiosteal flap is elevated far anteriorly to the lower part of the conchal eminence, which is exposed by pushing the subcutaneous periosteal flap further anteriorly. The posterior blade of the perichondrium is incised and elevated

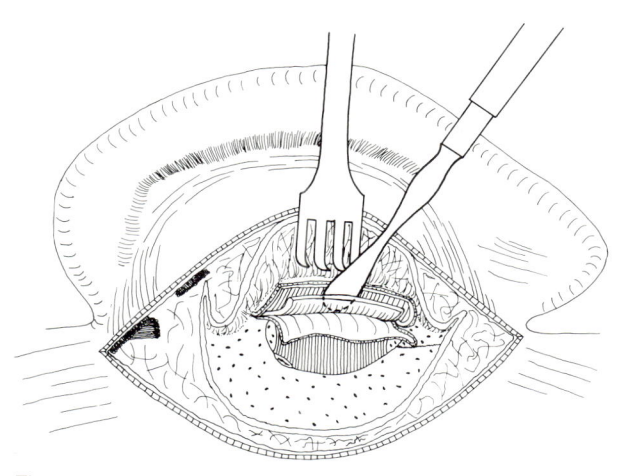

Fig. 284 The cartilage of the anterior part of the conchal eminence is incised by a curved incision, and elevated from the anterior perichondrial blade

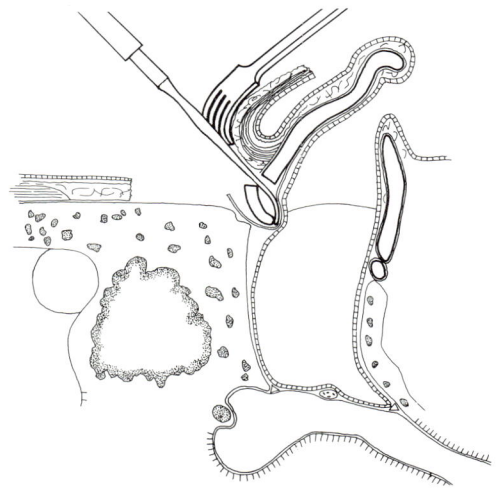

Fig. 285 Side view of the elevation of the anterior edge of the conchal cartilage from the perichondrium by a Freer's rugine

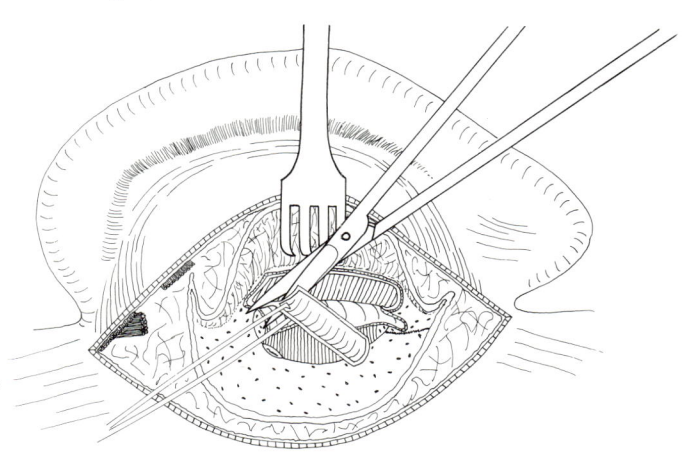

Fig. 286 The anterior edge of the conchal cartilage is resected inferiorly, pulled posteriorly, and resected superiorly at the crus of the helix

108   8 Graft Materials

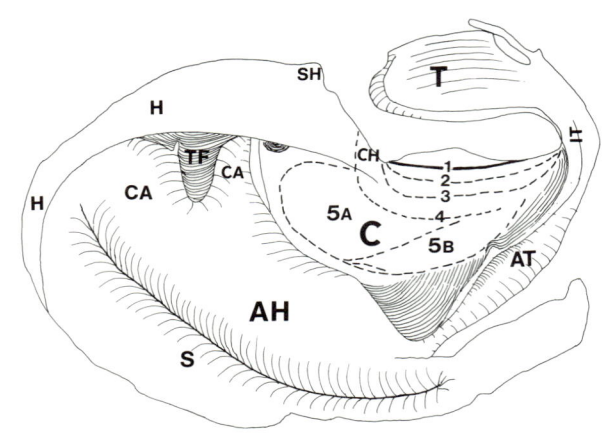

Fig. 287 The front side of the cartilage of the auricle, showing the lines of resection and corresponding areas of resection of the conchal cartilage related to the anatomy of the auricular cartilage. Resection lines 1 and 2 are used to prevent stenosis of the ear canal; lines 3 and 4, running through the crux of the helix and involving inferiorly the antitragus cartilage, are used in stenosis of the ear canal. Lines 5a and 5b mainly delineate areas for obtaining graft materials through retroauricular incisions
AH Antihelix
AT Antitragus
C Concha
CA Crux of the antihelix
CH Crux of the helix
H Helix
IT Intertragal notch
S Scapha
SH Spine of the helix
T Tragus
TF Triangular fossa

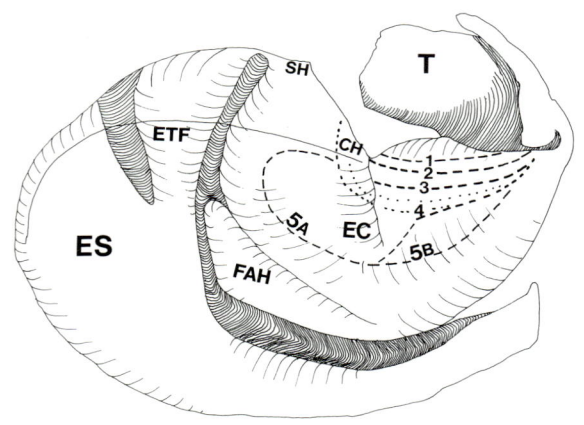

Fig. 288 The reverse of the cartilage of the same auricle as in Figure 287, with the same lines of incision
CH Crux of the helix
EC Eminence of the concha
ES Eminence of the scapha
ETF Eminence of the triangular fossa
FAH Fossa of the anthelix
SH Spine of the helix
T Tragus

Resection Lines of the Conchal Cartilage

To prevent stenosis of the ear canal in cases with canal wall–down mastoidectomy and a large cavity, the anterior edge of the conchal cartilage should be removed during the primary operation. Larger removal is also required in reoperation for ear-canal stenosis caused by prominent conchal cartilage.

The varying curvature and thickness of the cartilage of the auricle make the effect of the resection difficult to predict, and the resection lines are difficult to place, especially when approaching the conchal cartilage from a retroauricular incision. This type of concha can be quite fixed, and may have retracted into the cavity of the mastoid process. The lines of resection of the concha look logical when illustrated in Figure **287** on the front side of the concha. From the posterior side, where the resection usually takes, place it is much more difficult to find the exact position of the resection lines. One of the reasons for this is that retracting the concha with the retractor changes the anatomy of the posterior surface (Fig. **288**). Lines 1 and 2 in Figure **288** indicate the resection of the most anterior 3–4 mm and 4–5 mm, of the concha, respectively, without involving the crux of the helix. They are used in canal wall–down mastoidectomy, to avoid later stenosis. Lines 3 and 4 are applied when treating stenosis of the external meatus caused by conchal prominence after previous canal wall–down mastoidectomy. Considerable areas of the cartilage are removed. Line 5 indicates the large superior area of the concha (Figs. **287, 288**), involving the majority of the actual conchal eminence. This cartilage is exclusively taken as graft material, either as perichondrium, cartilage, or both. Looking at the posterior aspect of the auricle, the conchal eminence is in fact located quite superiorly on the auricle. This part is easy to expose in the retrocochlear approach. The inferior area of the conchal prominence (area 5 b in Fig. **287**) is usually more difficult to expose, but the cartilage is thicker in this region.

Incision of the conchal cartilage and the meatal skin in order to widen the ear canal after canal wall–down mastoidectomy involves formation of the Körner skin flap, which is a laterally-based skin flap in the retroauricular incision. Incision through the canal-wall meatal skin and the concha takes place superiorly at the 10-o'clock position and inferiorly at the 5-o'clock position (Fig. **289**).

Preparation of the Stacke flap, also used in canal wall–down mastoidectomy, with the base of the flap inferior in the ear canal, also requires resecting the conchal cartilage both superiorly and parallel to its anterior edge (Fig. **289**), approximately at resection line 3 (Fig. **288**). The incised conchal cartilage is either left in place, attached to the skin of the flap, or, more usually, it is removed from the skin flap in order to enlarge the introitus of the meatus and improve the mobility of the flaps.

In Portmann's meatoplasty after radical mastoidectomy, a Y-shaped incision is made to enlarge the external meatus. The conchal cartilage is excised in a special way (Fig. **290**).

Cartilage Via an Endaural Approach

Both the anterior edge and the anterior area of the conchal cartilage (Figs. **287, 288**) can easily be harvested via the endaural approach. If necessary, e.g., for closure of a large attic defect, a larger piece of conchal cartilage can be acquired through the endaural approach. In *Hermann B incisions* using the lateral flap technique (Fig. **36**), where the canal skin is elevated laterally out of the ear canal, the conchal cartilage can be exposed. By elevating the skin off the crus of the helix and from the anterior edge of the cartilage, a considerable area, corresponding to resection lines 1–3, can be exposed (Fig. **291**). The resection lines correspond to resection line 3 (Figs. **287, 288**). The exposed cartilage is cut by a scalpel at the same time, enlarging the ear canal (Fig. **292**).

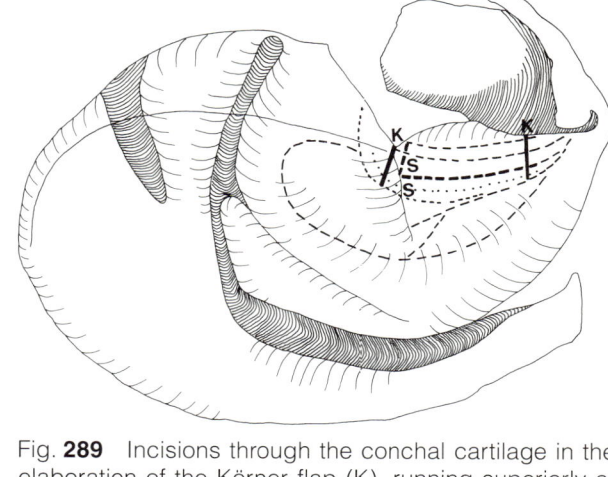

Fig. **289** Incisions through the conchal cartilage in the elaboration of the Körner flap (K), running superiorly at the 10-o'clock position, inferiorly at the 5-o'clock position, and the Stacke flap (S) running superiorly between the 9-o'clock and 10-o'clock positions and along resection line 3 (dotted line).

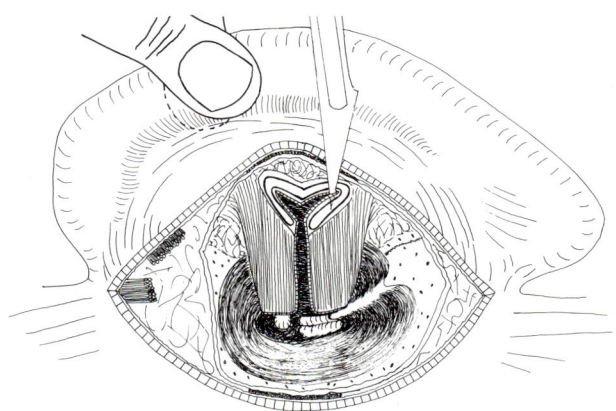

Fig. **290** Y-shaped incision of the conchal cartilage in Portmann's meatoplasty

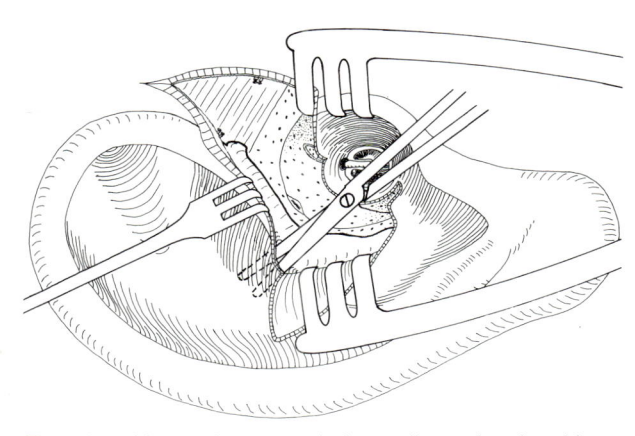

Fig. **291** Harvesting conchal cartilage in the Heermann B incision. The skin from the ear canal is elevated outward and dissected from the conchal cartilage. The skin from the intercartilaginous incision is elevated from the crux of the helix, and further elevated from the conchal cartilage with a pair of scissors

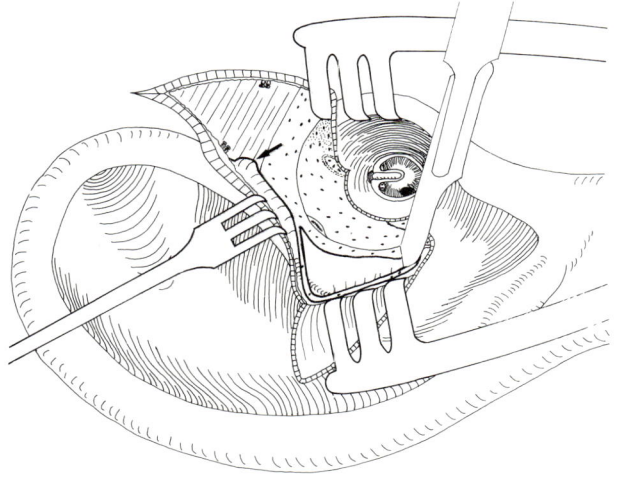

Fig. **292** The conchal cartilage is resected with a knife. The spine of the helix (arrow) can also be resected for use as a graft in ossiculoplasty

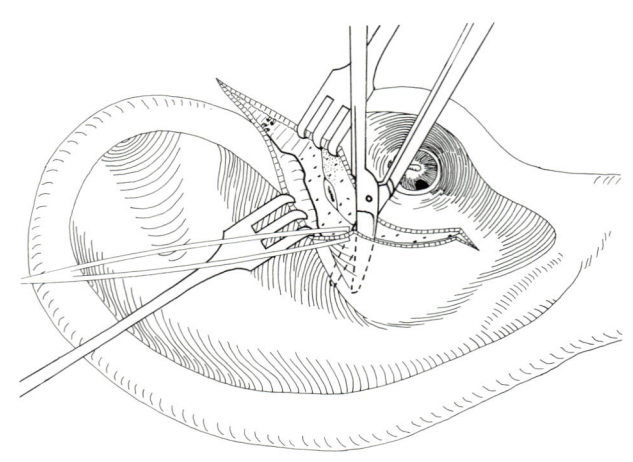

Fig. 293 Harvesting conchal cartilage in the Shambaugh and Lempert incisions. The skin from the crux of the helix and the anterior edge of the conchal cartilage is elevated

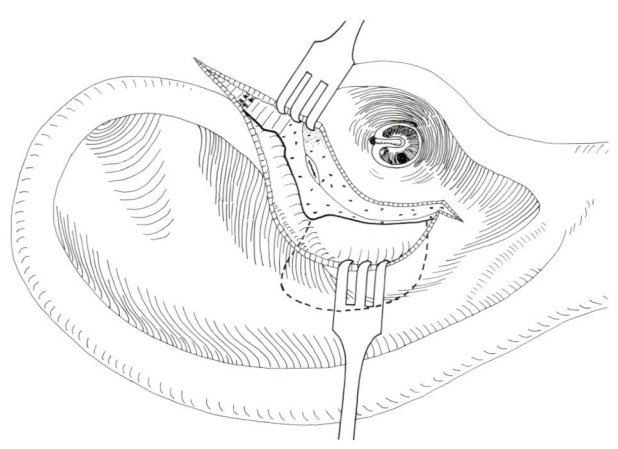

Fig. 294 The anterior edge of the conchal cartilage is exposed. Further skin elevation is indicated by the dotted line

Fig. 295 A major part of the conchal cartilage is to be excised

In *Shambaugh* and *Lempert incisions*, harvesting of the conchal cartilage is relatively easy. After the vertical and lateral circumferential incisions, the skin is elevated from the crus of the helix (Fig. **293**). Along the helix, the skin is further elevated towards the anterior edge of the conchal cartilage, which is exposed. After further careful elevation of the skin with a pair of blunt scissors, more and more of the conchal cartilage can be exposed (Fig. **294**). The anterior edge of the conchal cartilage, back to resection lines 1 or 2 (Fig. **287**), can be resected, or a major part of area 5a can be resected after further elevation of the conchal skin posteriorly, and after mobilization of the undersurface of the conchal cartilage from its attachment to the mastoid process. The conchal cartilage with the perichondrium is excised with a pair of blunt, curved scissors (Fig. **295**). Superiorly, the excision goes below the origin of the helix.

In the *Farrior incision*, a radial conchal skin incision running from the 7-o'clock position outwards from the lateral circumferential incision to the concha allows elaboration of the conchal skin flap (Fig. **61**). By further elevation of the conchal skin flap, the anterior edge of the conchal cartilage is exposed and excised, in order to widen the ear canal (Fig. **296**). Further elevation of the skin allows exposure of a major area of the conchal cartilage (Fig. **297**), which can be elevated from its attachment to the mastoid process, and resected (Fig. **60**).

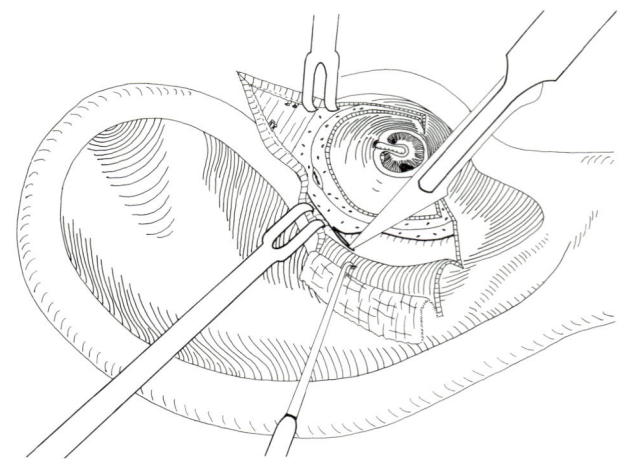

Fig. 296 Exposure and resection of the anterior edge of the conchal cartilage in the Farrior incision, after elevation of the conchal flap

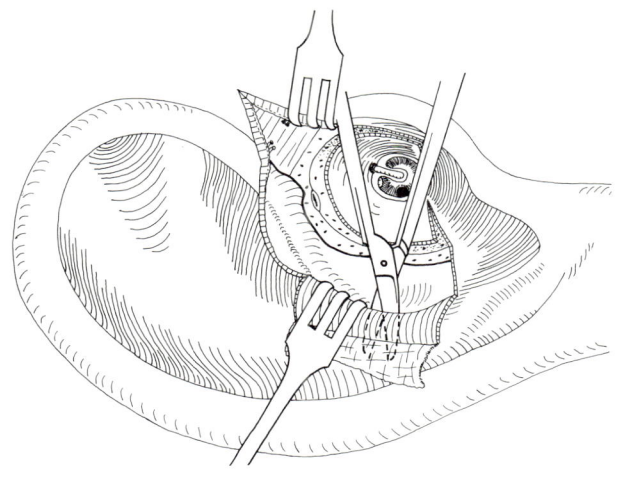

Fig. 297 Exposure of a major area of the conchal cartilage in the Farrior incision. The conchal skin is further elevated

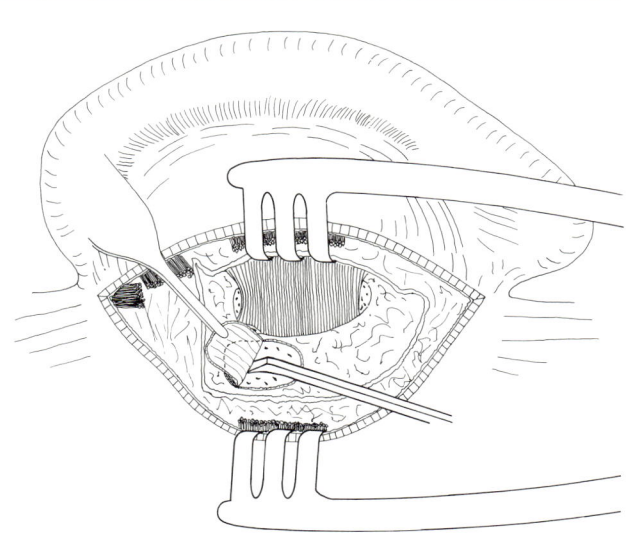

Fig. 298 Harvesting round periosteal graft from the mastoid process in the retroauricular incision. After removal of the fibrous tissue, the periosteum is excised and elevated with a sharp periosteal elevator

Periosteum

Periosteum was the first mesothelial graft ever used in tympanoplasty. Bocca repaired a tympanic membrane defect in 1958 with periosteum taken from the temporal squama (Bocca et al. 1959). Even though it has been shown that periosteum has the same qualities in myringoplasties as temporalis muscle fascia, it is seldom used as a graft of choice. At the beginning of the tympanoplasty era, periosteum was harvested from the tibia (Claros-Domenech 1959).

Mastoid-Process Periosteum

Periosteum can be acquired in sufficient quantities from the surface of the mastoid process behind the ear canal, and below the linea temporalis (Fig. 298). Subcutaneous and fibrous tissue is removed from the surface of the mastoid process, and its surface is cleaned of fibers under the operating microscope. With a scalpel, a round or oval piece of the periosteum is incised and carefully elevated from the underlying cortical bone with a sharp periosteal elevator, avoiding perforation of the periosteum.

The periosteum is usually used as a semiwet graft; it is placed on a plastic plate, covered with wet gauze. The bone side is placed in contact with the plate, so that it can later be placed with a forceps directly onto the ear drum remnant, and used as onlay or underlay graft. In both situations, the bone side of the periosteum should face the tympanic cavity. In double grafts together with fascia, the bone side of the periosteum is directed into the meatus (Krumpholz 1969). The reasons why periosteum is not a popular mesenchymal graft material, compared to temporalis muscle fascia of perichondrium, are the following:

1. In an endaural incision with a speculum, a separate incision is needed to harvest the graft. It is much easier to obtain the fascia by a separate superior incision.
2. It is easier to clean the superior layer of the temporalis muscle fascia from the deeper layers, than the fibrous tissue from the outer surface of the periosteum at the mastoid-process region, especially from its lower region, due to the attachment of the sternocleidomastoid muscle.
3. In endaural approaches (Heermann, Shambaugh, Lempert, Farrior, Fleury) the fascia is easy to obtain through the same vertical incision, and there is no need for a separate incision.
4. If the periosteum has been excised from the mastoid process in a retroauricular incision, it becomes impossible to harvest a useful retroauricular subcutaneous periosteal flap, which is a disadvantage for obliteration of the cavity. Even if only a myringoplasty is performed, suture of the postauricular periosteum is desirable in order to pull the elevated ear-canal skin back into its previous position. Since the fas-

8 Graft Materials

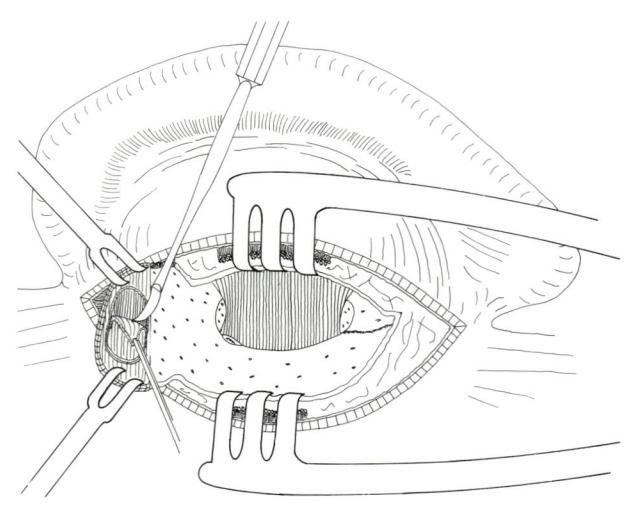

Fig. **299** Harvesting a minor periosteal graft from the temporal squama, above the temporalis line (Wullstein). The lower edge of the temporalis muscle is elevated, and the undersurface exposed. A small, round periosteal graft is excised

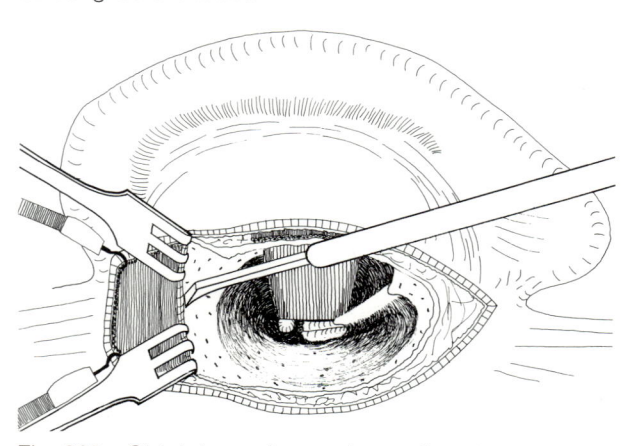

Fig. **300** Obtaining a large piece of periosteum from the temporal squama (Tos), in cases in which fascia and perichondrium are not available. Elevation of the temporalis muscle together with the periosteum

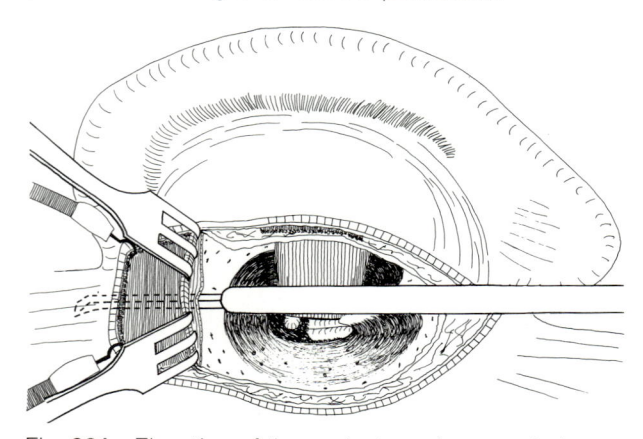

Fig. **301** Elevation of the periosteum far superiorly

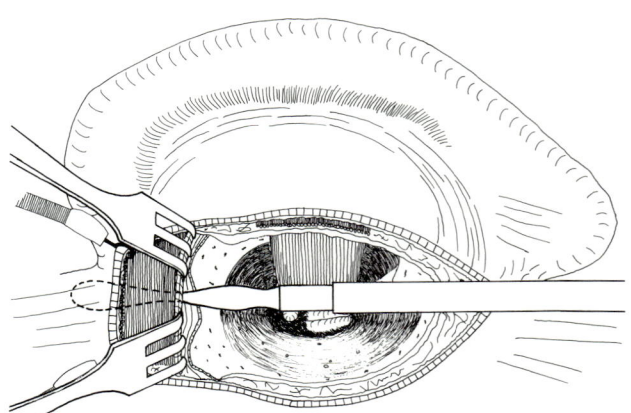

Fig. **302** Separation of the elevated periosteum from the muscle fibers far superiorly and posteriorly

cia is easy to acquire in the retroauricular approach, very few surgeons will use the periosteum in such situations.

Temporal Squama Periosteum

Small pieces of periosteum from the undersurface of the temporalis muscle just above the linea temporalis (Wullstein 1968) can be acquired by elevating the lower edge of the muscle with the periosteum. A small round piece can be excised (Fig. **299**).

A large piece of periosteum can be acquired in revision operations, when all available fascia and perichondrium has already been used, e.g., in reoperation after previous reconstruction of the ear canal. The author has for several years used the following technique to acquire a large piece of periosteum from the temporal squama. As this method has not been published before, it will be described here in detail.

After the end of the bone work, the periosteum is elevated with a periosteal elevator and held in place by two strong retractors (Fig. **300**), facilitating further periosteal elevation from the temporal squama. The instrument elevates the periosteum far superiorly and posteriorly, up to the borders of the muscle attachment (Fig. **301**).

The periosteum is now gently elevated from the muscle fibers by elevating the muscle with blunt retractors, and a plane of cleavage is established between the muscle fibers and the periosteum far superiorly and posteriorly (Fig. **302**). After this, the posterior attachment of the temporal muscle is cut by a pair of scissors about 1 cm superior to the end of the skin incision (Fig. 303). The muscle can now be further elevated and separated from the periosteum (Fig. 304). The border of the periosteum is incised posteriorly by a pair of scissors (Fig. 305). The incision can continue in a superior direction either with a pair of scissors or with a scalpel placed far superiorly under the elevated muscle, cutting the periosteum in a curve (Fig. 306). Finally, the anterior attachment of the periosteum is cut by pulling the periosteum out with a forceps (Fig. 307).

This laborious method is necessary in order to get a sufficiently large piece of periosteum. It has repeatedly been seen that disappointingly small pieces of periosteum are pulled out when the method is not followed exactly.

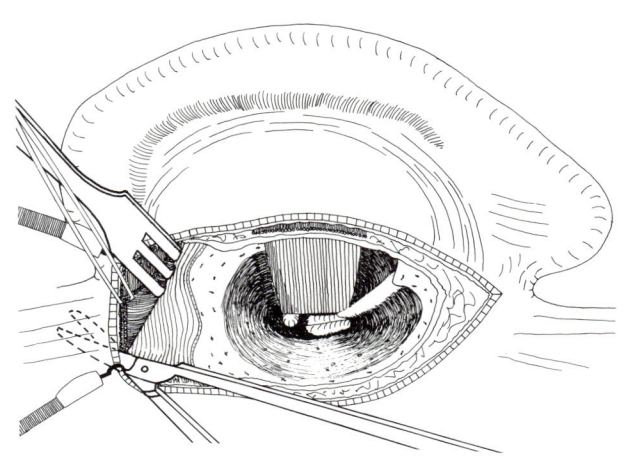

Fig. 303 Incision of the temporalis muscle fibers at the posterior border and elevation of the muscle

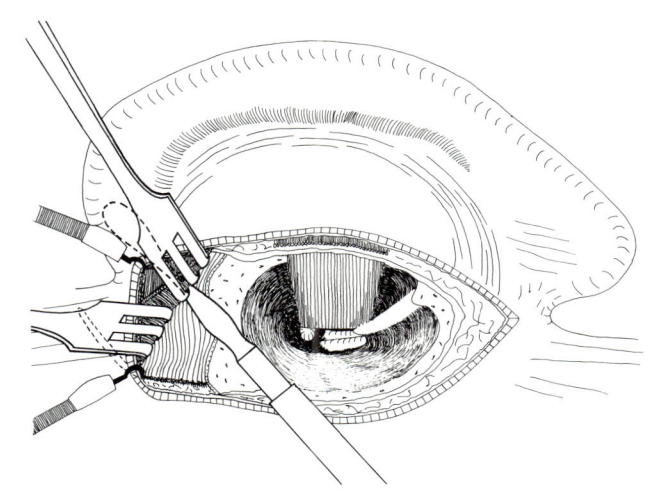

Fig. 304 Further extensive separation of the periosteum from the muscle, which is mobilized posteriorly by incision (dotted line)

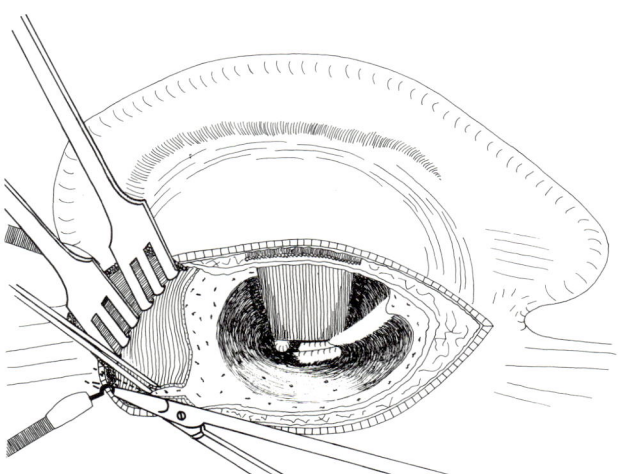

Fig. 305 Elevation of the muscle posteriorly, and cutting of the liberated periosteum with a pair of scissors

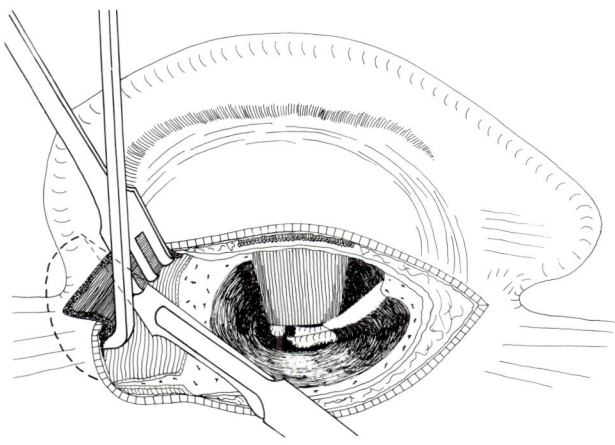

Fig. 306 Incision of the periosteum far superiorly under the muscle

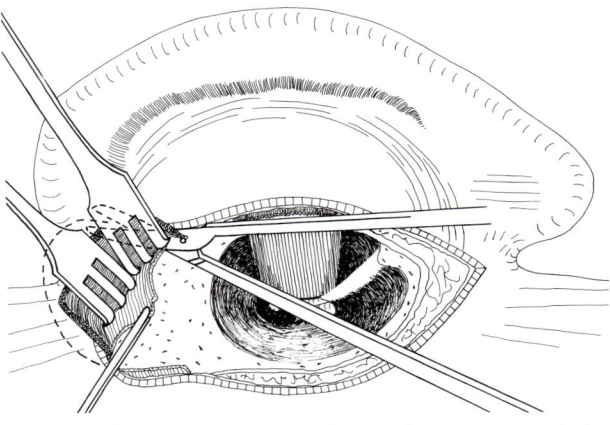

Fig. 307 Final excision of the periosteum anteriorly with a pair of curved scissors

8 Graft Materials

Periosteum Via an Endaural Approach

In the endaural approach with the Heermann, Shambaugh, Lempert, and Farrior incisions, it is generally more difficult to expose a large area of the temporal squama withouth significant cutting of the temporal muscle (Fig. **308**). The periosteum will only be used in an endaural approach in cases where all fascia and all perichondrium has already been used in previous operations.

The temporalis muscle is elevated together with the periosteum, using a small, sharp periosteal elevator, as far superiorly as possible (Fig. **308**). The temporalis muscle is incised on both sides of its exposure and elevated, and the periosteum is then separated from the muscle fibers as far superiorly as possible with a Freer's rugine (Fig. **309**). After further incision of the muscle posteriorly, and after further elevation of the muscle, the periosteum is further separated from the muscle fibers, maximally exposed, and excised with the scalpel or a pair of scissors (Fig. **310**). The muscle will be sutured, and the bleeding points coagulated. In cases with scarring at the lower edge of the temporalis muscle, dissection of the periosteum is difficult or impossible. A blunt separation of the muscle fibers can be performed 1.5–2 cm superior to its lower border. The muscle fibers are separated with blunt retractors, exposing the periosteum (Fig. **311**).

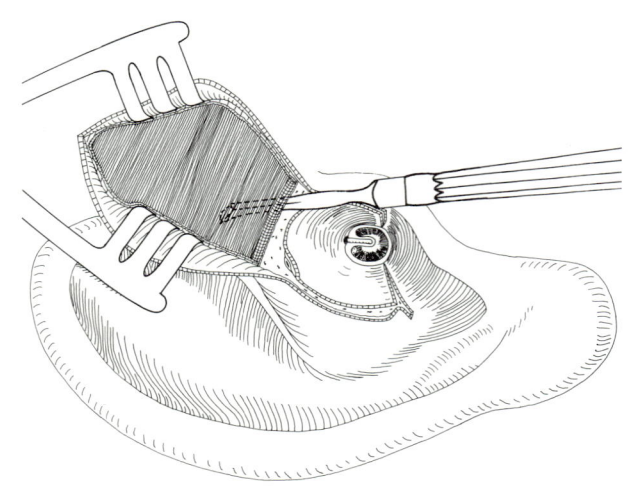

Fig. **308** Harvesting the periosteum in an endaural approach with an extended vertical incision. The temporal muscle fascia has been previously removed. The temporalis fascia with the periosteum is elevated with a sharp periosteal rugine

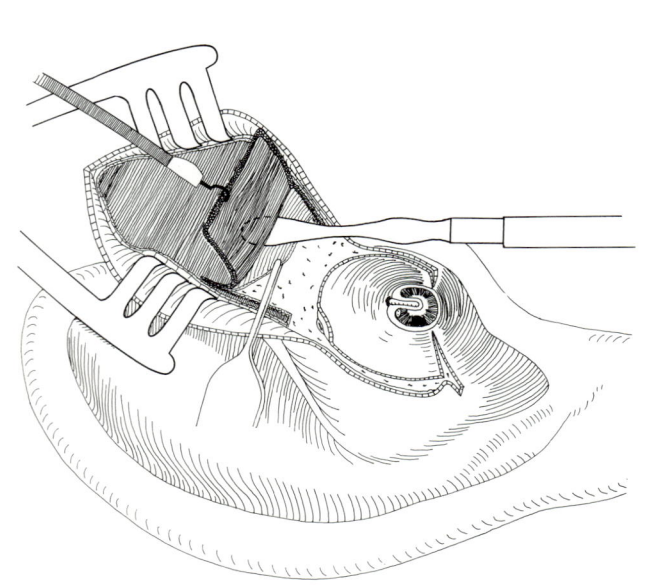

Fig. **309** The temporalis muscle is cut, elevated, and the periosteum is carefully loosened from the muscle fibers

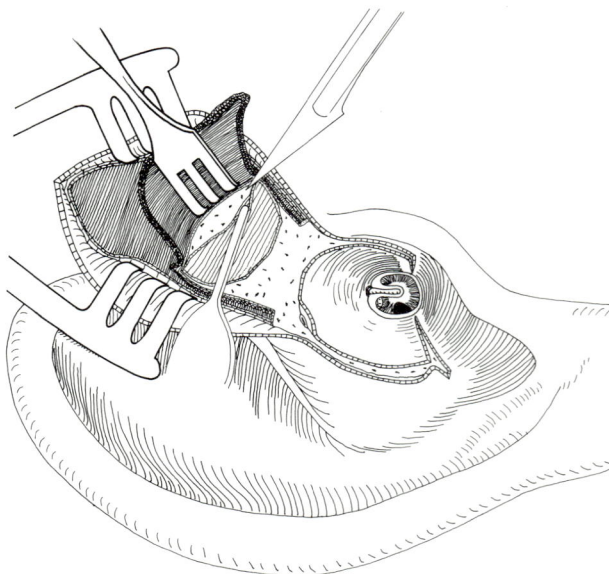

Fig. **310** The elevated temporalis muscle is further elevated and incised, and the periosteum is further exposed. The periosteum is cut with a scalpel as far superiorly as possible

Periosteum

After sufficient exposure of the periosteum, it is incised using an oval incision (Fig. 312), elevated by small sharp elevators, and removed. The muscle fibers are sutured.

In cases in which a large piece of periosteum is needed, in the endaural approach for cavity obliteration, the author has used the following modification. After extending the vertical incision, the temporal muscle is separated 2 cm superiorly to its inferior edge, and the periosteum exposed. With a Freer's rugine, the separation between the muscle and the periosteum is continued downwards to the lower edge of the temporalis muscle (Fig. 313). After total separation between the muscle fibers and the periosteum is established, the temporalis-muscle fibers are cut anteriorly with a pair of scissors, and turned posteriorly (Fig. 314). This part can later be used as a muscle flap or obliteration. The superior part of the temporalis muscle is further elevated from the periosteum, which is now maximally exposed and excised all the way around its borders (Fig. 315). Finally, the cleaned periosteum is carefully elevated from the bone from all sides, and the periosteum is placed on a plastic plate and used as a semiwet graft for reconstruction of the ear canal and the drum. The liberated temporal muscle can either be used as a muscle graft, or can be sutured to its original position (Fig. 316).

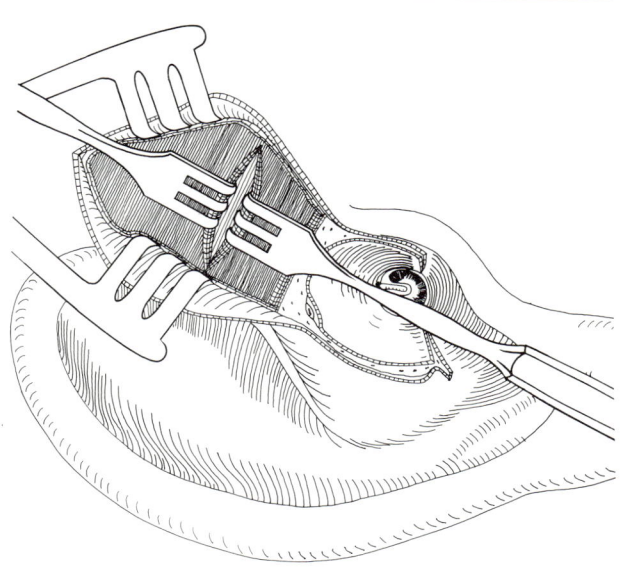

Fig. 311 Harvesting a minor piece of the periosteum in an endaural approach, with scarring at the border of the temporalis muscle. Muscle fibers are separated about 1.5–2.0 cm superior to the inferior border, exposing the periosteum

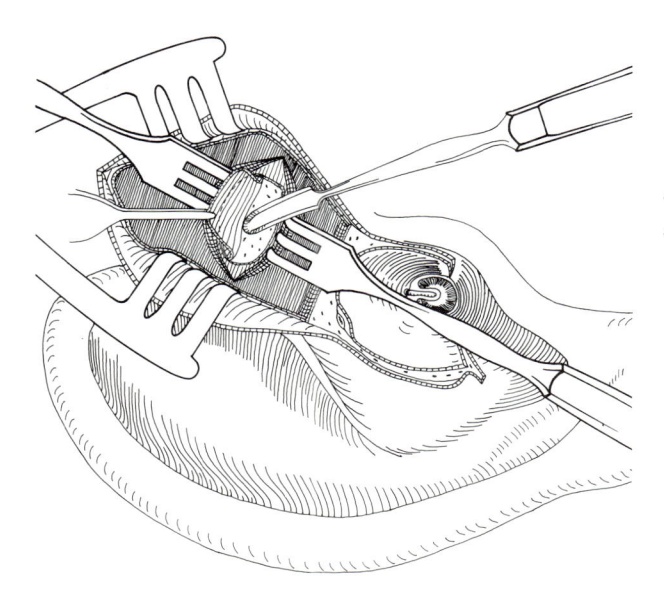

Fig. 312 The periosteum is exposed, incised, and elevated from the bone with a small periosteal elevator

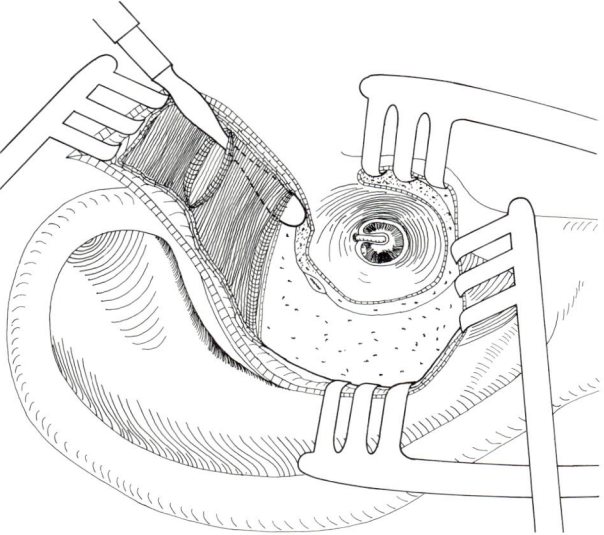

Fig. 313 Harvesting a major piece of the periosteum in an endaural approach, in combination with obliteration of the cavity. Temporalis muscle is separated 2 cm superiorly from the inferior edge, and the periosteum is exposed. Further elevation of the muscle fibers from the periosteum with a Freer elevator

Fig. 314

Fig. 315

Fig. 316

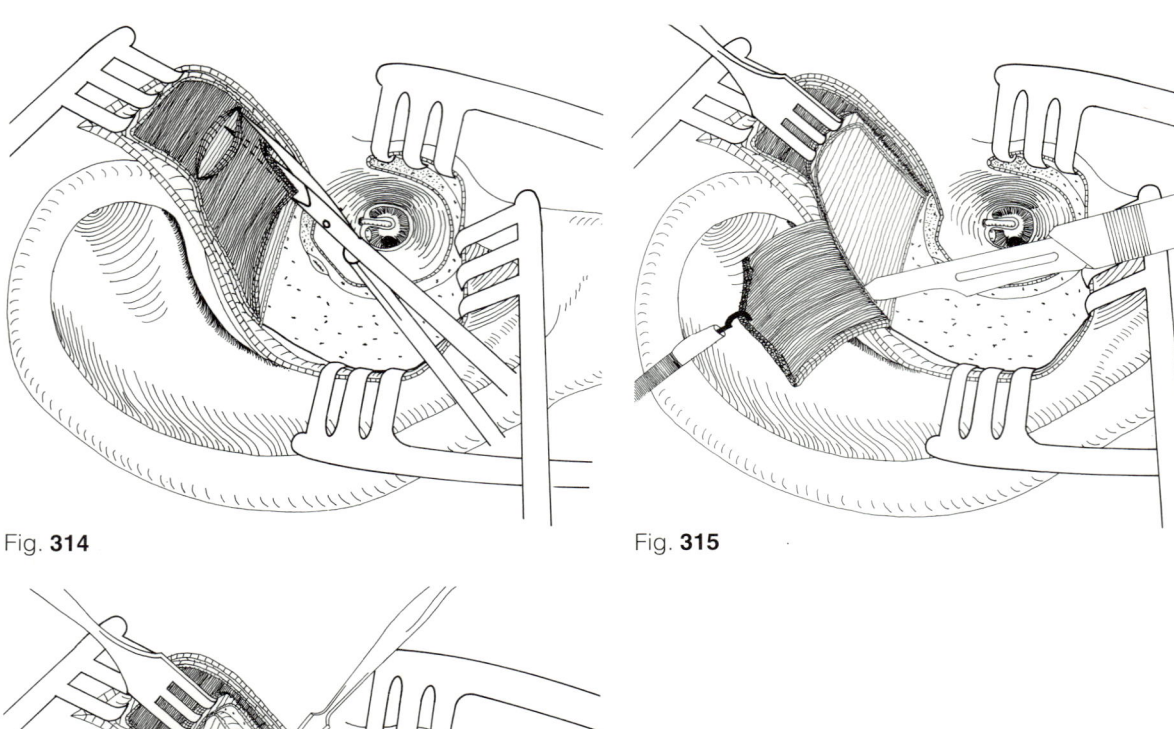

Fig. 314 The temporalis muscle is cut anteriorly with a pair of scissors, leaving the periosteum in place

Fig. 315 The temporalis muscle is elevated, and a larger area of periosteum is exposed and incised all the way round

Fig. 316 The periosteum is carefully elevated from the bone. The posterosuperiorly-based muscle flap can be used as an obliteration graft

Vein Graft

After using vein to cover the oval window in stapedectomy (Shea 1958), Shea introduced the use of vein into myringoplasty as an underlay graft in 1960. In the same year, Tabb published his primary results in closure of perforations with vein graft. Vein for stapedectomy was usually taken from the back of the hand. In myringoplasty for cosmetic reasons, it is usually taken from the greater saphenous vein near the anterior border of the medial malleous, which is larger than the vein from the back of the hand. Another choice is the cubital vein. The vein in front of the malleolus is easy to find, and large enough to cover a major defect of the ear drum.

After ligation of the vein on both sides, approximately 1 cm of the vein is excised (Fig. 317). Perivascular tissue is removed with a fine tissue forceps when the vein is stretched on the blades of a pair of small scissors. The vein is opened, and pressed into Shea's vein-pressing instrument. The vein is mainly used as an underlay graft in smaller perforations. The intima layer of the vein faces into the tympanic cavity.

Because of the insufficient size of the vein in many cases, and because of its tendency to contract back to its original shape, and also because the harvesting is more complicated than with fascia, vein grafting has gradually been totally replaced by the use of fascia and perichondrium, which are easier to acquire.

Fatty Tissue

Fatty tissue is used in myringoplasty in cavity obliteration (Ringenberg 1962). Fatty tissue from the lobule of the ear has been used in small perforations for insertion into the perforation as a cork. This procedure is one of many minor procedures in tympanoplasty, and is always performed under local anesthesia on an outpatient basis.

Harvesting Fatty Tissue

The ear lobule is anesthetized separately, bent upward by an assistant, and held with four fingers to compress the vessels and fix the lobule. With scalpel blade 15, a 1.5-cm to 2-cm long skin incision is made at the margin of the lobule (Fig. 318). A sufficiently large piece of fatty tissue is pulled out with the forceps, and resected (Fig. 319).

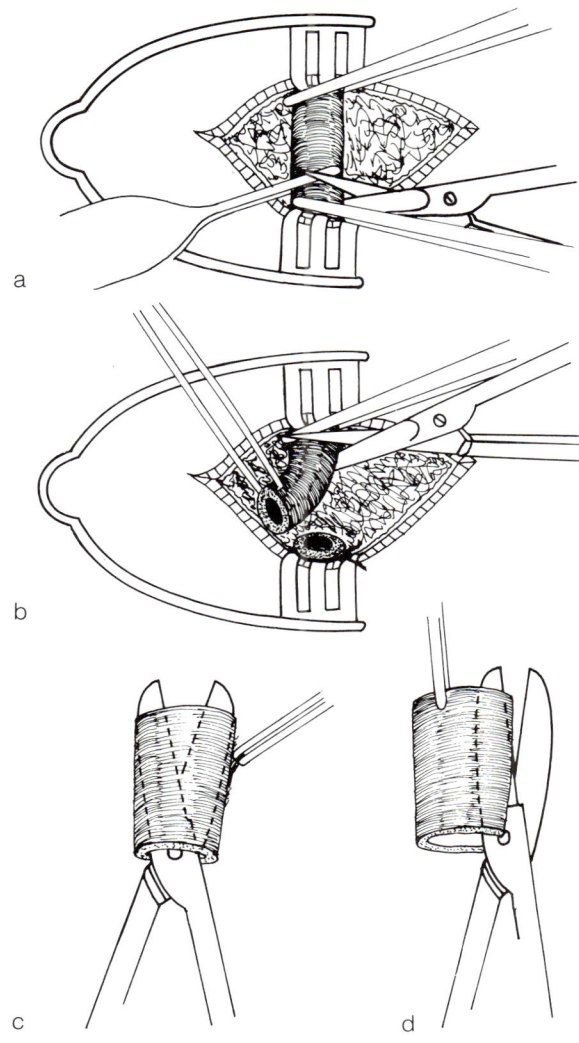

Fig. 317 Harvesting a vein graft. **a, b** Ligation and resection of the vein. **c, d** Cleaning the fibers from the outer layer and opening the vein with a pair of scissors

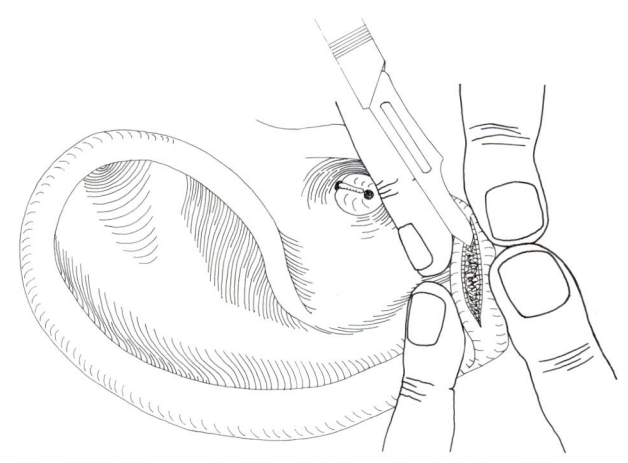

Fig. 318 Removal of the fat from the lobule of the ear. The lobule is bent upward and held by a scrub nurse. The skin incision is made at the lower edge of it

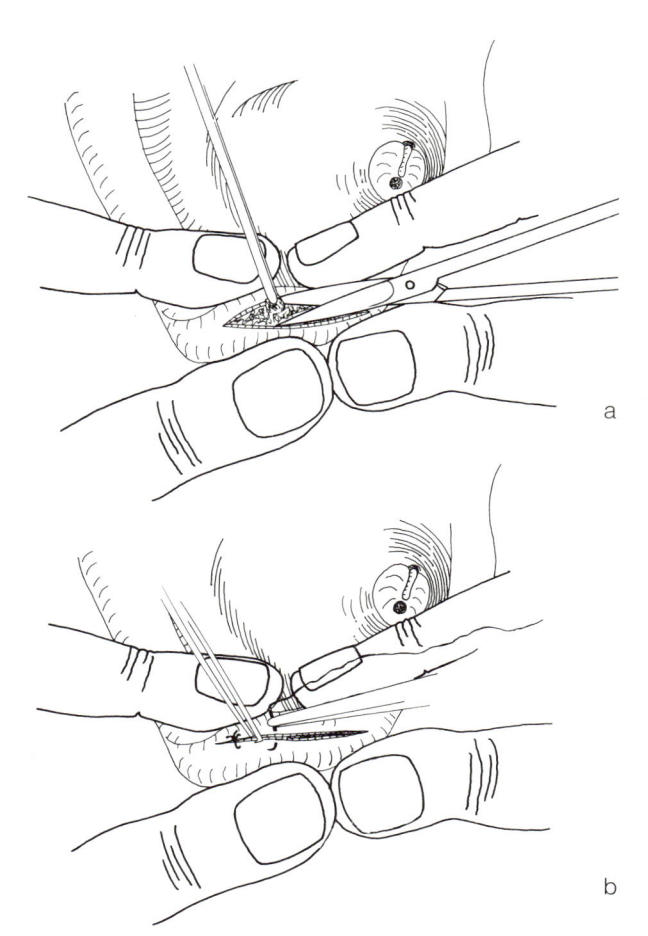

Fig. 319a A sufficiently large piece of fat is pulled out of the lobule and cut. **b** The lobule is fixed during suturing

8 Graft Materials

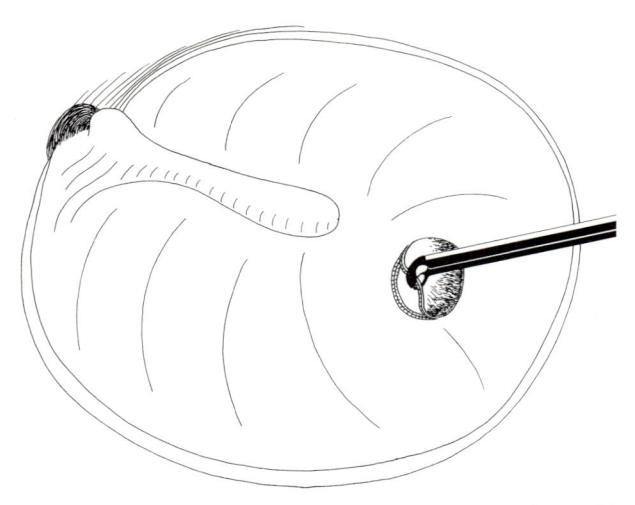

Fig. 320 Closure of a small inferior perforation with fatty tissue. The epithelial edge of the perforation is removed

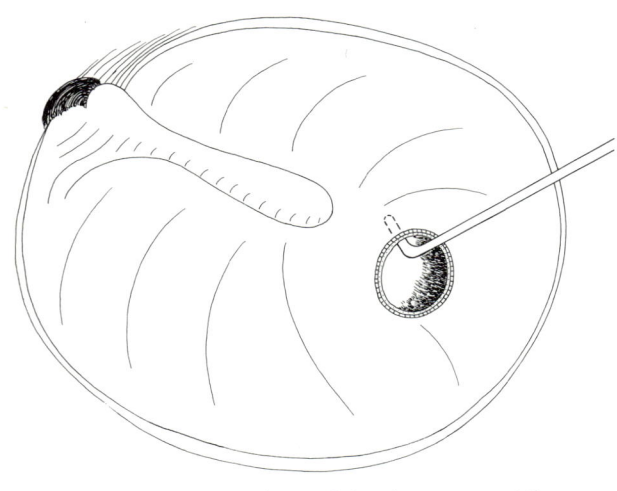

Fig. 321 The undersurface of the drum around the perforation is scarified, and the mucosa is removed

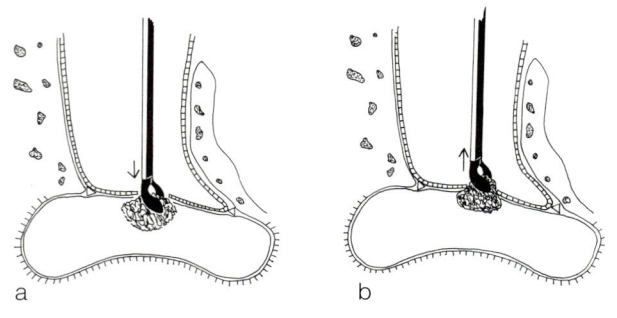

Fig. 322 Placement of the fatty lump. **a** The lump is brought into the cavity, and **b** pulled outward to be fixed inside the edges of the perforation

Fig. 323 The fatty lump is placed in the perforation ▷ and pulled out with a forceps

Myringoplasty with Fatty Tissue

The edge of the drum perforation is carefully removed without significant enlargement of the perforation (Fig. 320), and mucosa from the undersurface of the drum is scarified or removed with a hook or another curved instrument (Fig. 321). The idea behind closure with fatty tissue is to use it to obstruct the hole, like a collar button, with fat protruding into the tympanic cavity and into the ear canal. The lump of fat is placed on the perforation, using forceps to judge its proper size. If the size is appropriate, the fat lump is pushed through the perforation into the cavity (Fig. 322), and again pulled partly back out through the perforation, in order to be securely fixed between the edges of the perforation (Figs. 322, 323). This maneuver can also be performed by suction instead of a forceps. The fat will soon be epithelialized from the sides of the perforation.

It is evident that an attempted closure of a medium-sized, or larger, perforation may easily lead to failure simply because too large a piece of fatty tissue is used. A piece that is too large will protrude into the tympanic cavity, causing partial obliteration, or into the ear canal, causing problems with reepithelialization.

Fat is therefore restricted to use with very small perforations, e.g., those caused by grommets or long-term ventilating tubes. The kind of perforation caused by a long-term ventilating tube may even be too large for fatty-tissue myringoplasty.

Fatty tissue taken from an incision in the abdominal, and specifically the infraumbilical region, is used as the method of choice in obliteration of the cavity after translabyrinthine surgery or glomus tumor surgery; but, strangely enough, it is used extremely rarely in obliteration of the cavity after surgery of chronic ears with canal wall–down methods and obliteration techniques.

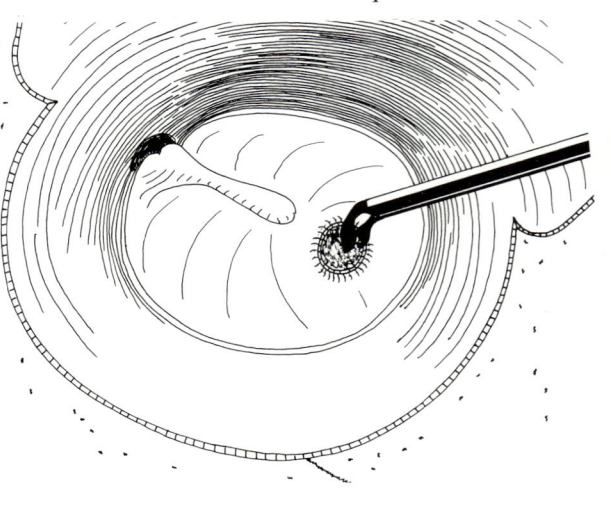

Subcutaneous Tissue

Heermann (1963) used subcutaneous tissue as a tissue graft to the oval window after stapedectomy. Sale (1969) proposed the use of subcutaneous tissue in myringoplasty, taken from the Heermann A incision (Fig. **28**). After undermining the skin on both sides of the Heermann A incision, the skin is held apart by two retractors, and the subcutaneous tissue is exposed (Fig. **324**). With a pair of small, sharp scissors, a graft-sized piece of subcutaneous tissue located superficial to the fascia is excised (Fig. **325**).

Subcutaneous tissue can only be obtained in small pieces. Its surface is not smooth like the surface of the fascia or perichondrium, and is in some places too thick. The subcutaneous flap is usually used as an underlay graft. The present author cannot see any advantages in the use of subcutaneous tissue in cases with small drum perforation that are treated by the retroauricular or endaural approaches. The incision necessary to acquire a subcutaneous graft is the same as that used to acquire temporalis muscle fascia, but the quality of the fascia graft is higher than that of the subcutaneous tissue graft. In the vast majority of cases when a large graft is needed, subcutaneous tissue is definitely not sufficient.

The author sometimes uses subcutaneous tissue from the ear canal in an endaural approach with the ear speculum, in situations in which there is an unexpected tear of the drum, or unexpectedly insufficient length in the tympanomeatal flap due to excessive drilling of the bony annulus. In such cases, fascia has not been taken before the operation, and such minimal closure defects have been supported by a amall piece of subcutaneous tissue, taken at the 12-o'clock position at the superior edge of a Rosen incision, near the notch of Rivinus. At this location, a small piece of subcutaneous tissue is always available.

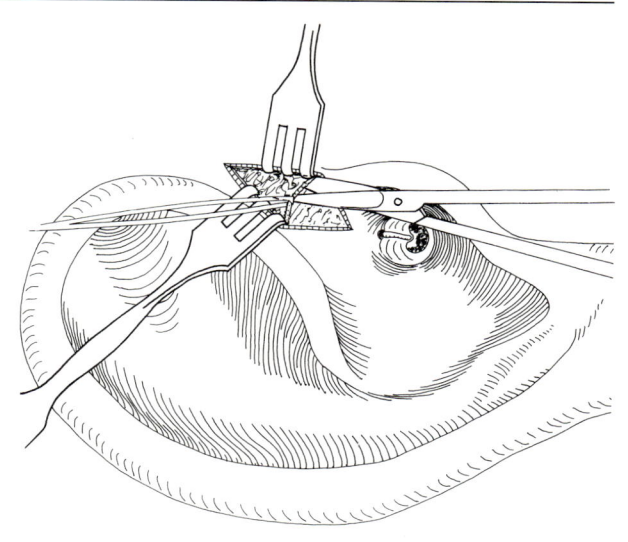

Fig. **324** Harvesting subcutaneous tissue in a Heermann A incision. Superficial to the fascia, a piece of subcutaneous tissue is elevated and dissected

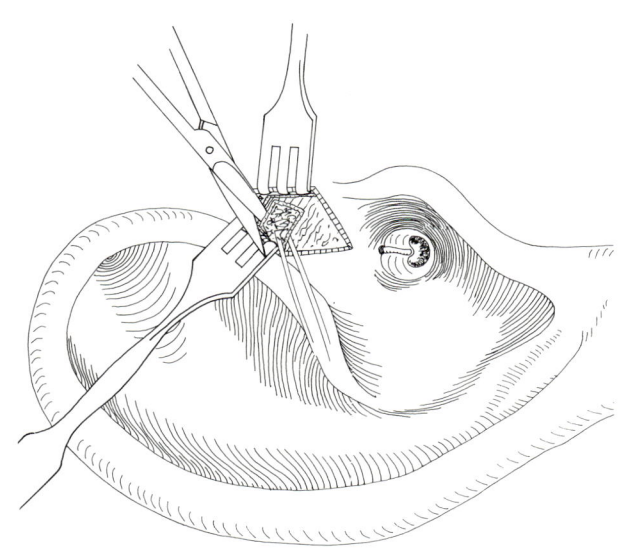

Fig. **325** The subcutaneous tissue is cut out as a small, flat piece

Fascia Lata

Fascia lata is relatively thick—it is too thick to use as an ear-drum graft, but can be used in various ear-canal reconstructions or cavity obliterations. The author only uses it occasionally in cases in which no other autogenous tissue is available around the ear, and the ear-canal reconstruction is a necessity, i.e., in reconstructions of old, wet, and discharging radical cavities. In acoustic neuroma surgery, fascia lata is in our hands the graft of choice in all reoperations for CSF leakage. It is strong, and long enough to be placed in the cavity instead of the dura, and a tight obliteration can take place to prevent repeated CSF leak.

In ear-canal reconstruction with obliteration, a 2.5×3.5 cm large piece of fascia lata is harvested through an 8-cm longitudinal skin incision in the lateral side of the thigh, starting at about 25 cm inferior to the anterior superior iliac spine. The incision continues down through the subcutaneous and fatty tissue, but care should be taken to avoid damage to the nerve branches of the external cutaneous nerve. Fascia is easy to recognize after the subcutaneous and fatty tissue is elevated with a pair of scissors (Fig. **326**). A 3-cm broad and 7-cm long area of the fascia is exposed. At the lower edge of the exposed fascia, it is elevated with forceps and cut with a pair of scissors, exposing the underlying muscle fibers. With continuous cutting along the borders of all exposed fascia and further exposure of the muscle fibers, a sufficiently large piece of fascia is removed. So as to be able to suture the fascia together and avoid muscle prolapse, a long, elliptical piece of fascia should be removed, and the edges sutured.

Fascia is sutured with strong absorbable sutures. The fatty tissue and subcutaneous tissue is also sutured, as is the skin. After closure of the skin, the wound is covered with a strong elastic bandage for one week. The fascia is stored in Ringer's solution, and there is usually no need for major cleaning of the fascia, which is compact and thick.

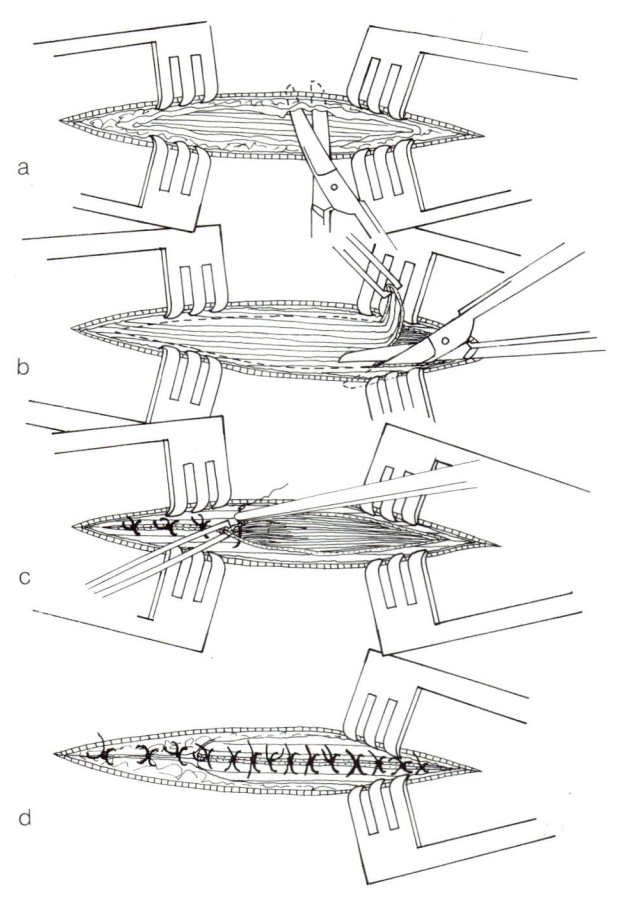

Fig. **326** Harvesting fascia lata. **a** An 8-cm long incision is performed through the skin and the subcutaneous and fatty tissue, down to the fascia, which is exposed. **b** The exposed fascia is held by a forceps at the inferior edge, and cut with a pair of scissors along the dotted line. **c** The edge of the fascia is solidly sutured together with strong absorbable suture. **d** The subcutaneous and fatty tissue are sutured in one layer before closure of the skin

Ear-Canal Skin

Meatal skin flaps of various shapes were used before the tympanoplasty era, and are still used by all surgeons in reconstruction of the ear canal, and in reepithelialization of the mesenchymal drum graft and the bone of the cavity. The Körner, Stacke, Lempert, and Surdille flaps, the Rosen flap, and others, are examples of the use of canal-skin flaps in tympanoplasty. In fact, all the approaches described in the previous chapters are based either on preservation of the canal skin and formation of skin flaps to be placed in particular ways, or on removal of the skin flaps in order to preserve them and reinsert them as free skin grafts, either at the same place or elsewhere.

Pedicled ear-canal skin graft to close the drum perforation was used by Zöllner (1954) and Frenckner (1955). They were used for a period of about two years, and were soon replaced by Wullstein's free skin graft techniques, which used the retroauricular region.

Plester popularized the free canal-skin graft method (1960), and claimed in 1963, after performing 400 myringoplasties with free canal-skin grafts, that this was the ideal material for tympanic membrane closure. It is free of skin appendices, so that graft cholesteatoma cannot form. Because of the absence of elastic fibers, the graft can be cut exactly to the required size. It will not shrink or roll off at the edges, as skin grafts from the skin of the arm or leg, or the postauricular region, do. The canal-skin graft also contains a thin periosteum, providing a smooth undersurface.

Procuring the canal skin in relation to endaural incisions (Heermann, Fig. **44**; Lempert and Shambaugh, Fig. **56**; Farrior, Figs. **62, 63**), and in relation to retroauricular incisions with Farrior (Figs. **94** and **95**) or Sheehy techniques (Fig. **152**), has been described above. In these techniques, the ear-canal skin is used as part of a sandwich graft together with fascia. It is not supposed to be used as a single graft in myringoplasty.

The Plester myringoplasty technique with canal skin in posterior perforations was based on an intercartilaginous Heermann B incision and a lateral circumferential incision starting at the 12-o'clock position and continuing 4–5 mm medially to the suprameatal spine to the 6-o'clock position. The lateral ear-canal skin is retracted posteriorly, exposing the suprameatal spine. After the self-retaining retractors have been placed, radial incisions at the 12-o'clock and 6-o'clock positions are performed down to the annulus, and the canal skin, with the periosteum, is carefully elevated, together with the skin of the posterior part of the drum remnant. After further deepithelialization of the anterior part of the drum, the ear-canal skin is placed on the drum (Fig. **327**). With larger perforations, the lateral circumferential incision continues along the inferior and anterior meatal wall up to the 12-o'clock position, leaving a relatively small superior strip of meatal skin intact. After a further radial incision at the 2-o'clock position, the meatal skin is removed (Fig. **328**), trimmed, and placed on the deepithelialized annulus and drum remnant, and the perforation is closed.

Methods involving closure of the perforation by a canal-skin graft alone are more or less abandoned today, but the methods of skin grafting are still used as sandwich techniques, e.g., by Sheehy and his associates (Fig. **142**).

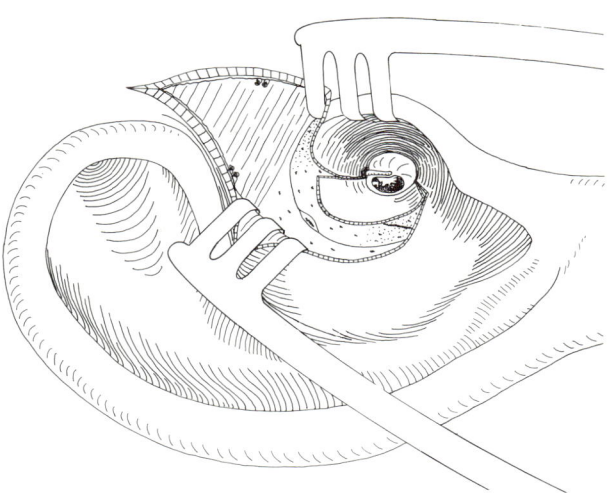

Fig. **327** Harvesting the ear-canal skin from the posterior tympanomeatal flap for closure of minor posterior perforations (Plester). After an endaural incision and a lateral circumferential incision from the 12-o'clock to the 6-o'clock position, the bone of the lateral canal is exposed. After radial incisions are made at the 12-o'clock and 6-o'clock positions, the tympanomeatal flap can be removed together with the drum remnant on the perforation

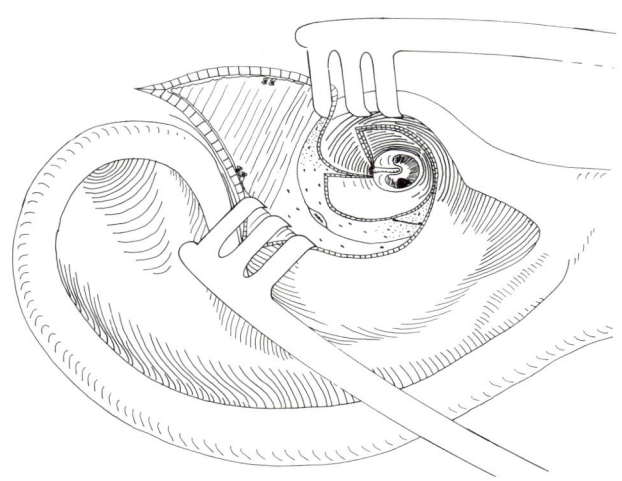

Fig. **328** Harvesting the ear-canal skin for large perforations (Plester), leaving the superior vascular strip intact. The lateral circumferential incision is carried out from the 12-o'clock position right round to the 2-o'clock position, where the radial incision is placed. The skin can be removed together with the drum remnant of the perforation

Myringoplasty with Canal Skin

Plester and his associates have continued to use meatal skin grafts, but in a special way, and with a different philosophy from that of the sandwich grafts. He places small pieces of canal skin as a double graft exactly on the uncovered fascia or perichondrium, which has been placed as an underlay graft. This skin is taken from the anterior canal wall at the end of the operation, and placed exactly at the borders of the epithelium of the drum remnant. The epithelialization of the myringoplasty is faster (Fig. **329**).

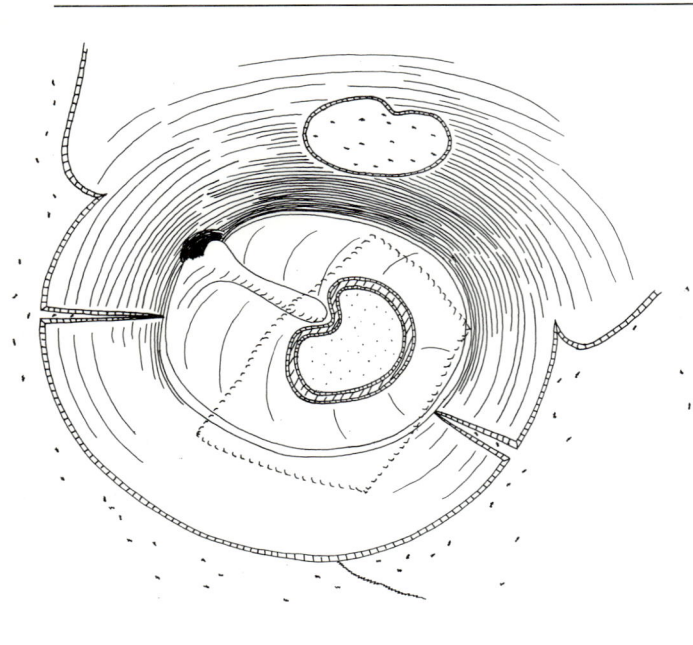

Fig. 329 Closure of the inferior perforation using double grafts with ear-canal skin taken from the anterior wall of the meatus. After elevation of the tympanomeatal flap, excision of the edges of the perforation, scarification of the mucosa under the perforation, placement of the fascia and underlay graft, and replacement of the tympanomeatal flap in its original position, a small piece of meatal skin is excised in the anterior meatal wall and brought to cover the exact size of the perforation

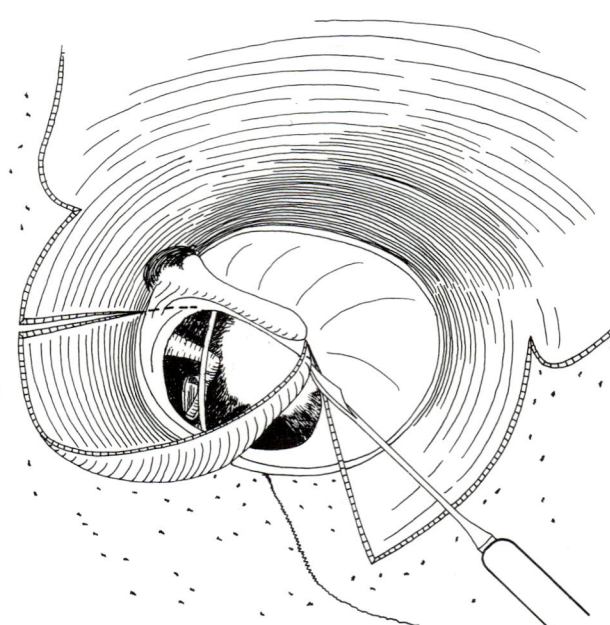

Fig. 330 Use of posterior tympanomeatal flap for closure of a posterior perforation with double grafts. The flap is elevated together with the epithelium of the drum remnant

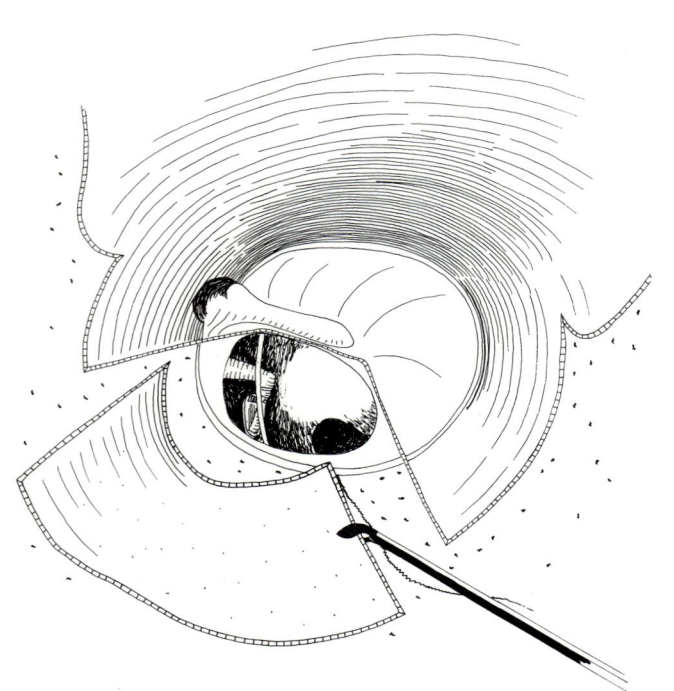

Fig. 331 The entire tympanomeatal flap is removed

Very often, Plester removes the posterior tympanomeatal flap, in order to replace it at the end of the myringoplasty over the fascia. In the endaural approach, either with an ear speculum or with a Heermann or a Lempert incision, the tympanomeatal flap and the skin from the drum remnant are removed (Figs. **330, 331**). Fascia is placed as an underlay graft to cover the perforation (Fig. **332**). The skin from the tympanomeatal flap is placed carefully over the fascia (Fig. **333**).

In very small posterior perforations, meatal skin is the only graft. After a Rosen incision and formation of a small tympanomeatal flap at the level of the perforation, and removal of the epithelium from the drum remnant around the perforation (Fig. **334**), the tympanomeatal skin graft is applied exactly to the deepithelialized edges of the perforation (Fig. **335**).

Ear-Canal Skin   123

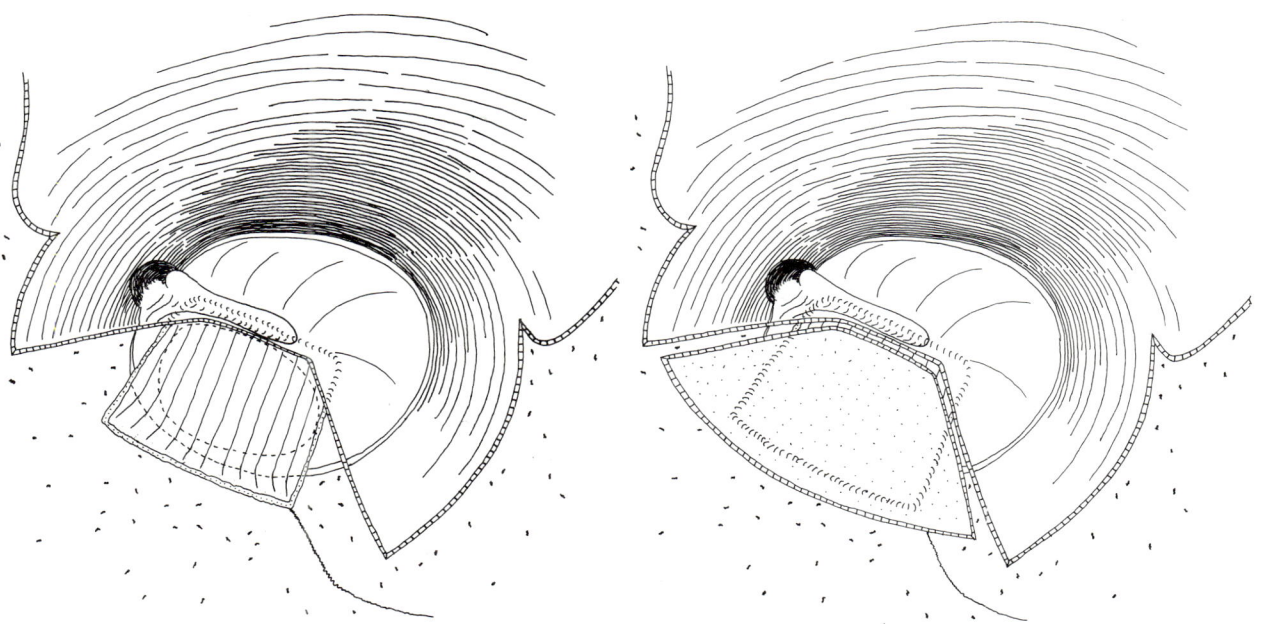

Fig. **332**   The fascia is placed as an underlay graft just under the malleus handle

Fig. **333**   The skin is replaced, covering the entire perforation. It is well adapted to the edges of the skin

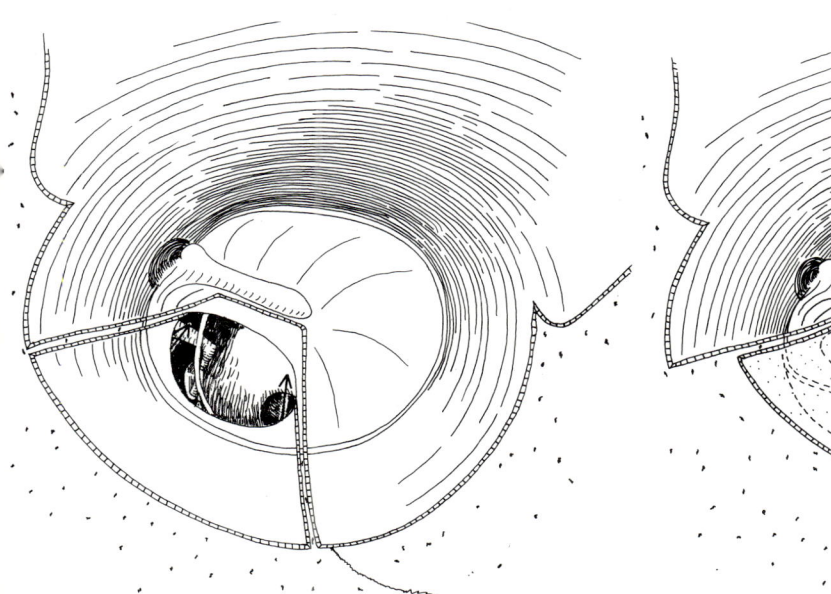

Fig. **334**   Closure of a small posterior perforation with meatal skin (Plester) after deepithelialization of the anterior edges of the perforation. The tympanomeatal skin flap will be moved anteriorly (arrow)

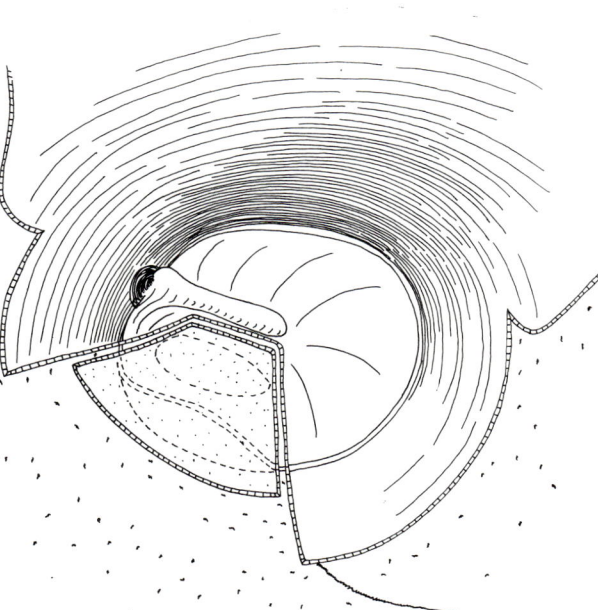

Fig. **335**   The tympanomeatal flap is moved anteriorly, and the canal skin covers the perforation

8 Graft Materials

Heterotopic Skin

Autogenous skin harvested outside the ear canal is termed "heterotopic." Heterotopic skin was introduced into modern myringoplasty by Wullstein and Zöllner at the beginning of the 1950s. It was, advocated by Wullstein for a relatively long period, even in the 1960s, after the fascia and perichondrium grafts had been introduced. Skin is today used for special purposes, and still has its place in middle-ear surgery. It is used in the form of full-thickness grafts and split-thickness grafts.

Full-Thickness Grafts

Full-thickness skin grafts have been widely used by Wullstein and others to cover mastoid cavities, and can still be advocated today in selected cases for that purpose. The skin to be used should not be thick, and should not contain deep hair follicles or sebaceous glands. Retroauricular skin just at the retroauricular fold is most often used as a full-thickness graft.

The first skin incision starts at the superior attachment of the auricle, and runs inferiorly about 7 mm behind the retroauricular fold towards the inferior attachment of the auricle. The second incision runs on the auricle relatively close to the retroauricular fold (Fig. 336). A skin strip 1.5 cm wide can easily be obtained, but larger pieces can also be harvested by placing the incision more posterior to the retroauricular fold. The remaining skin is elastic, and there is no problem with closing the incision.

The same technique is used in retroauricular approaches, or when performing a separate retroauricular incision when using an endaural approach. The skin is elevated by surgical forceps, and the subcutis is carefully resected away with a pair of scissors (Fig. 337). Sometimes, e.g., in reconstruction of congenital atresia and major reconstruction of the entrance of the ear canal, a larger piece or an additional piece of full-thickness skin graft may be used, and in these cases skin from the upper arm (the middle third of it) is used. A long, oval incision through the skin and subcutaneous tissue is necessary to avoid broad ugly scars due to the elasticity of the skin.

Cleaning the full-thickness skin graft can be performed by placing it on a plastic plate, fixing it with a finger, and removing the subcutaneous tissue piece by piece with a pair scissors (Fig. 338). Skin taken from the upper arm is more elastic, and will roll together, creating difficulties in cleaning and, later on in exact positioning of the graft. When the

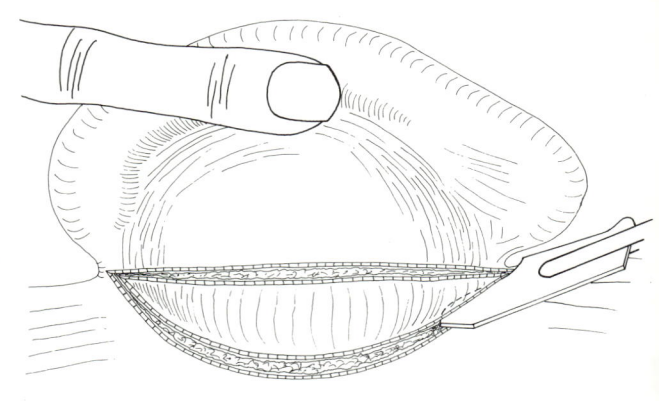

Fig. **336** An oval retroauricular incision for harvesting full-thickness skin graft

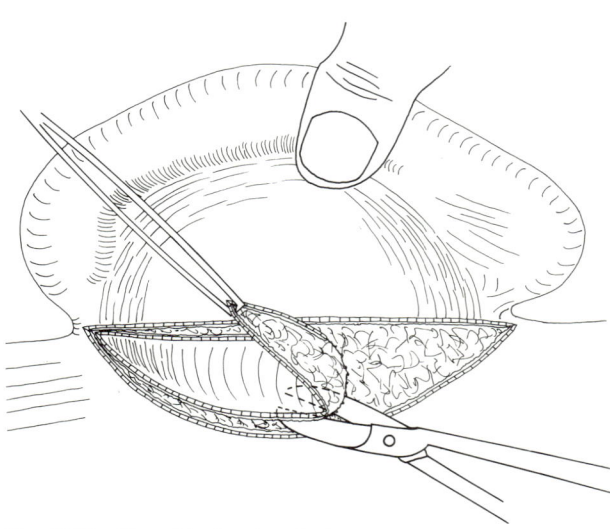

Fig. **337** The skin is elevated

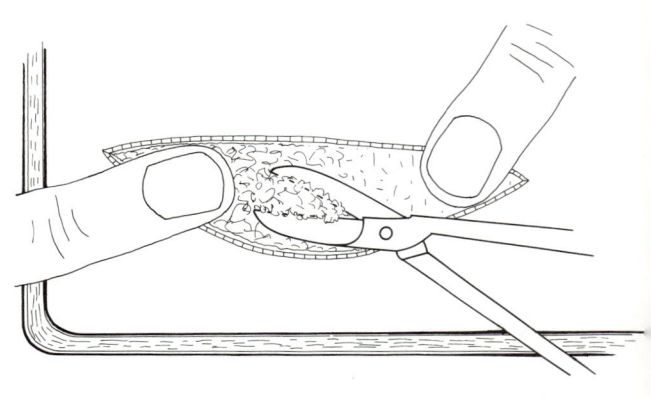

Fig. **338** With the skin flap placed on a plate, the subcutaneous tissue is removed using a pair of scissors

graft is placed on the index finger and hold with a thumb, removal of the subcutis is easier in rolled grafts (Fig. 339).

The author uses a retroauricular full-thickness graft in reconstructing the entrance of the ear canal, in congenital atresia, and in severe acquired stenosis of the ear canal, e.g., postoperative stenosis. The full-thickness skin graft is carefully sutured to the remaining skin.

Split-Skin Grafts

Split-skin grafts do not include the entire thickness of the skin. Only a layer of varying thickness is used. Thick split-skin grafts, including two-thirds or three-quarters of the skin thickness, are seldom used in middle-ear surgery. Usually, thinner grafts, especially the Thiersch graft, are used.

The Thiersch flap is the thinnest split-skin graft. It is cut through the germinative layer of the skin, and has a thickness of 0.1–0.05 mm. The advantages of the Thiersch flap are the following:

1. Larger areas can easily be harvested (i.e., several cm^2).
2. There are no scars on the surface.
3. There are no cutting scars.
4. It is easily adaptable on smooth, solid surfaces.

The Thiersch flap needs a solid surface, such as bone, fascia, or periochondrium. The hair follicles are crosscut in the Thiersch flap, resulting in many microperforations that may entail a risk of the epidermis growing into the tympanic cavity. It should therefore not be used as the only graft covering the holes. Even covering of small air cells in a mastoid cavity using a Thiersch graft may create deep retractions, with poor selfcleaning.

The Thiersch flap is today used at any point where denuded bone needs to be covered:

1. In large mastoid cavities when no mesodermal grafts are available, in order to facilitate faster healing and avoid formation of the granulations arising from the denuded bone.
2. In the ear canal and on the drum with larger epithelial defects, e.g., after surgery for blunting, acquired postinfectious atresia, exostoses, postoperative atresia, and postoperative ear-canal stenosis. In such cases, a recurrent atresia may be prevented when the bone is covered with a Thiersch flap.
3. In congenital atresia, large Thiersch flaps are needed.

Harvesting a Thiersch flap depends on the size needed. If a small piece of skin is needed, the inner surface of the upper arm is a good place. The author prefers the upper leg. The Thiersch flap is harvested using various dermatomes. It is important that the donor site is completely flat, and this is achieved by stretching the skin with two plates, one being pulled by an assistant in the superior direction, and the other being pulled by the surgeon's left hand in the inferior direction. The harvested piece of Thiersch flap is rolled together slightly, and put on a plastic plate covered with a sheet of gauze moistened with hydrocortisone–tetracycline cream. The outer surface of the graft is placed on the gauze, and the graft is rolled out using a Freer's rugine (Fig. 340). The graft will stick to the moistened surface of the gauze, and will remain folded out (Fig. 341). After the graft is folded out, the uneven edges are cut off with a large knife, and pieces of graft and gauze of an appropriate size are cut to be ready for placement on the bone (Fig. 342). To avoid renewed curving during adaptation of the graft, the Thiersch flap is brought to the bone together with gauze, and the gauze is removed just before the final adaptation of the graft to the edges of the skin (Fig. 343). After removal of the gauze, the Thiersch flap is fixed by some Gelfoam balls, and the new graft can be placed on the remaining denuded bone (Fig. 344). If the gauze is not too stiff, it can easily be brought into the ear canal through the ear speculum, as shown in Figure 342 in a case of acquired postinflammatory atresia. Usually, such major surgery on the ear canal will be performed using the retroauricular approach.

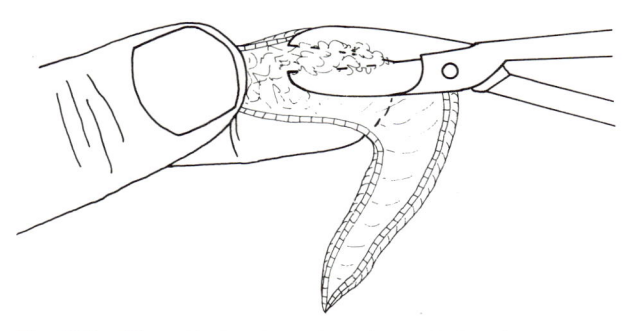

Fig. 339 The skin is placed on the pointing finger, and the subcutis is removed

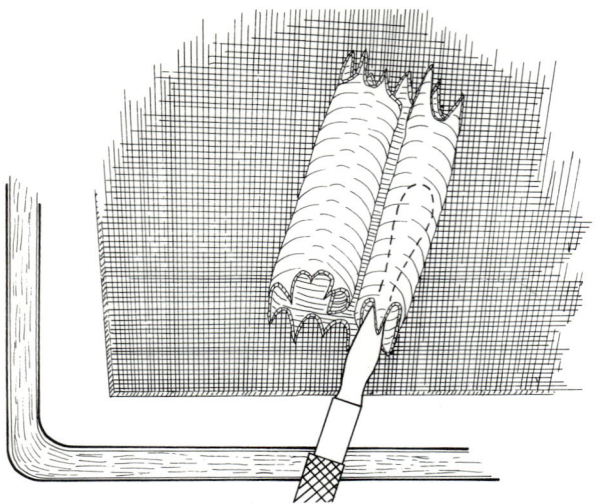

Fig. **340** The Thiersch flap is placed on a piece of gauze

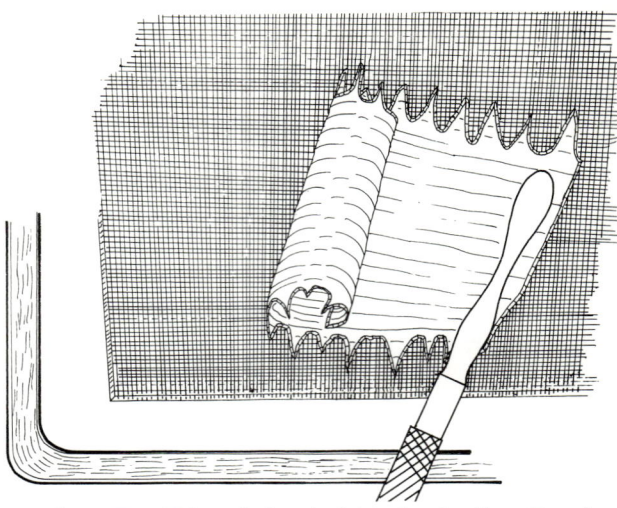

Fig. **341** The Thiersch flap is folded out with a Freer's rugine

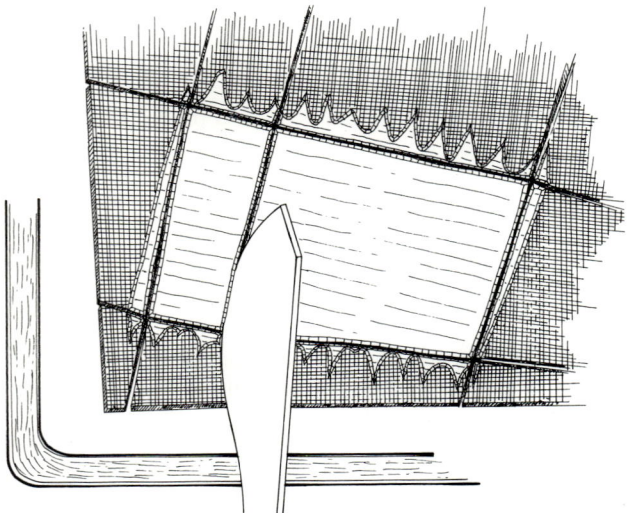

Fig. **342** The Thiersch flap is cut at the edges, and suitable pieces are cut together with the gauze

Allogenous Grafts

Over the last thirty years, several allogenous grafts have been introduced in myringoplasty, but the majority of them have been used only by a few surgeons and for a short period of time. Only the following grafts will be mentioned here: amnion (Wullstein 1952), cornea (Holewinski 1958, Forman 1960), dura (Preobrazhenski 1961), peritoneum (Birch 1961), pericardium (Trombetta 1963), aorta valves (Cornisch 1965), large veins (Nickel 1963), perichondrium (Jansen 1962), cartilage (Jansen 1963, Overbosch 1971), fascia (Hildmann and Steinbach 1970). Apart from allogenous cartilage and fascia, which are still used sporadically today, none of the grafts mentioned is in use today.

The present author has never used allogenous grafts. In myringoplasty it has always been possible to harvest enough autogenous graft material, which is always better than allogenous. Another problem today is AIDS. Regulations do not permit us to use allograft unless it has been sterilized, which is good enough for ossicles, but boiled, soft autografts cannot be used.

Allogenous Ear Drum

Chalat (1964) was the first to transplant fresh allogenous ear drum. Marquet (1966) used otimerate sodium (Cialit) to conserve allogenous ear drum, and popularized this method, which was used during the late 1960s and 1970s in several places and by many surgeons. Betow (1970) used frozen total blocks, consisting of drum and all three

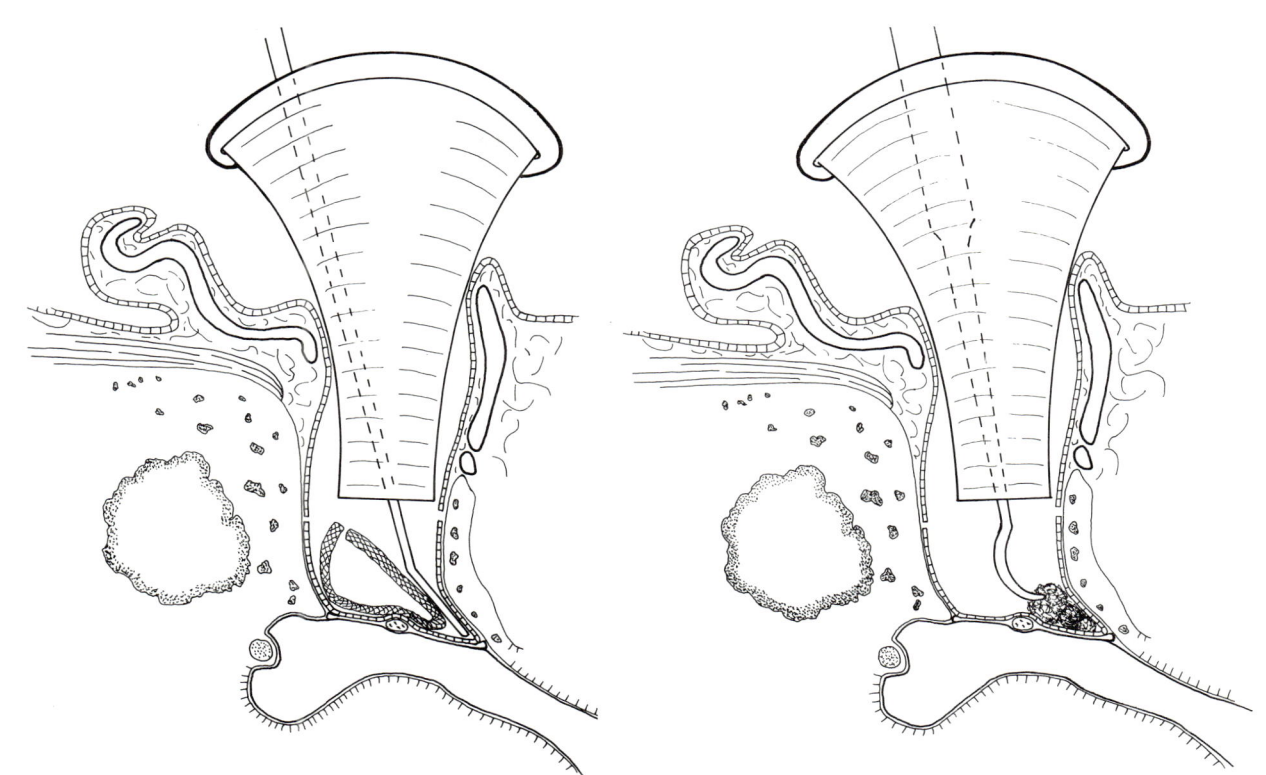

Fig. 343 The Thiersch flap and the gauze are placed in the ear canal and the drum to cover the denuded bone after removal of an acquired atresia. The gauze is elevated from the Thiersch flap

Fig. 344 After removal of the gauze, the first flap is fixed by Gelfoam, and the next flap can be placed on the denuded bone

ossicles. Glasscock and House (1968) used 70% alcohol for preservation of total blocks, and Perkins (1970) used formaldehyde. Today, only few centers are using allogenous ear drum myringoplasty (pupils of Marquet, Lesinski, Wehrs, Magnan, and some others).

Lyophilized Dura

Lyophilized dura is a commercially available allogenous dura which has been subjected to freeze-drying, so that antigenicity has been minimized or lost. In myringoplasty, lyophilized dura was introduced by Kup in 1967. Pfaltz et al. (1975) performed drum reconstructions using lyophilized dura as a sandwich technique. Palva et al. (1978) used lyophilized dura for many years, at first in myringoplasty as an underlay graft. However, the lyophilized dura was stiff and thick, and it was impossible to make in conform with the conical shape of normal drum. Palva later used lyophilized dura as sheeting for the denuded bone instead of Silastic. Lyophilized dura was also used in nonadhesive pieces to prevent adhesions, e.g., on the promontory under the interposed incus, and on the facial nerve at the level of the footplate, to support an incus columella on the footplate. Lyophilized dura has also been used as an additional support for the soft new ear-canal wall placed behind the fascia in reconstruction of the ear canal, especially after previous radical cavity surgery. Although it was used by many surgeons some years ago, lyophilized dura is very little used today because of the risk of Creutzfeldt-Jakob disease, which was reported in one case.

Xenogenous Grafts

There have been some experiments with xenogenous fascia (Hildmann and Steinbach 1970). Jansen (1973) used bovine peritoneum in tympanoplasty, and bovine drum. Zini et al. (1985) constructed an artificial drum out of bovine jugular vein. This Parma-Tymp is commercially available from the Xomed-Zimmer company.

9 Myringoplasty: General Aspects Definitions

Definitions

Myringoplasty is the term for closure of any drum perforation. It can be part of a major reconstruction of the entire middle ear and ear canal, or part of a tympanoplasty with ossicular reconstruction, or only a repair of a perforation, without any work in the tympanic cavity. In the literature, there are many classifications of myringotympanoplasties. Some of these are minor modifications of the original Wullstein classification, while others take the size of the perforation into consideration, using the term "myringoplasty" only for the act of closing small perforations. Others again take the approach to the tympanic cavity into consideration, using the term "myringoplasty" only in cases with an endaural approach. Yet others take the condition of the middle ear mucosa into consideration, defining myringoplasty only as closure of a dry perforation.

"Myringoplasty" is used here to refer to closure of an ear-drum perforation without any other work in the tympanic cavity or mastoid process. This definition is unrelated to the size of the perforation, the approach, the condition of the mucosa, or tubal function.

Classification of Perforations

Anatomically, the pars tensa is divided into four quadrants, the posterosuperior, anterosuperior, posteroinferior, and anteroinferior. Perforations could possibly be classified in relation to the four quadrants, but only small perforations are located exclusively in one of the quadrants. The vast majority of perforations in chronic otitis media, especially medium-sized and large perforations, usually border on, or involve, the neighboring quadrants, making the description of perforations in terms of quadrants complicated.

In the author's epidemiological and pathogenetic research on drum perforations and drum pathology, a simplified classification of perforations, which takes into account both surgical aspects, and research on the functional results of middle-ear surgery, has developed over the years. The perforations are classified (Figs. **345, 346**) into:

Anterior perforation
Inferior perforation
Posterior perforation
Total or subtotal perforation

Anterior perforations can extend inferiorly, as can posterior perforations (Fig. **345**). A large inferior perforation can extend superiorly, involving the posterosuperior and anterosuperior quadrants, and become a subtotal perforation. There is a gradual transition between a subtotal perforation and a total perforation (Fig. **346**), but surgically this is not of great importance. The techniques used to treat subtotal perforations are usually the same as those for total perforations, and many subtotal perforations are, after excision of the edge of the perforation, converted to a total perforation.

Description of the surgical techniques here will distinguish between anterior, inferior, posterior, and total perforation.

Pathogenetic Aspects

Our epidemiological studies of secretory otitis and drum pathology in childhood, conducted by following several cohorts of otherwise healthy children from birth to their teens with repetitive tympanometries and otomicroscopies, as well as long-term studies of clinical material from children treated for recurrent suppurative otitis media and after surgically treated secretory otitis, have led us to the following conclusions (Tos 1990).

1. Atrophies of the pars tensa, either diffuse or localized to some particular parts of the pars tensa, are common sequelae after long-lasting secretory otitis or chronic tubal dysfunction in childhood. Atrophy represents a constant risk for permanent perforation of the drum caused by a trivial acute otitis or trauma later in life. The majority of dry drum perforations are due to the following causes:

A. Secretory otitis and chronic tubal dysfunction during childhood.
B. Atrophy of the drum.
C. A commonplace episode of acute otitis in adulthood, or a slight trauma to the drum, caused for example during swimming, diving, flying, by a blow, while cleaning the ear of cerumen, etc.

Fig. **345** Anterior, posterior, and inferior perforations of the pars tensa, with possible extensions of the perforations (dotted lines)

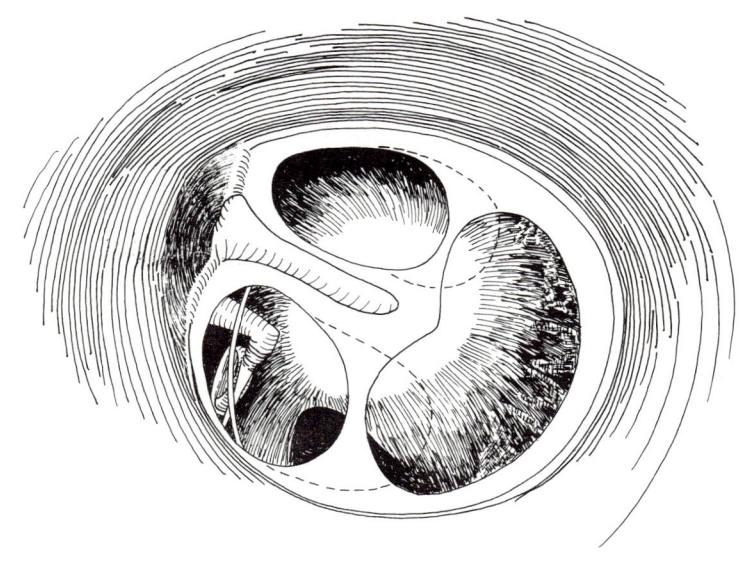

Fig. **346** Subtotal and total (dotted line) perforations

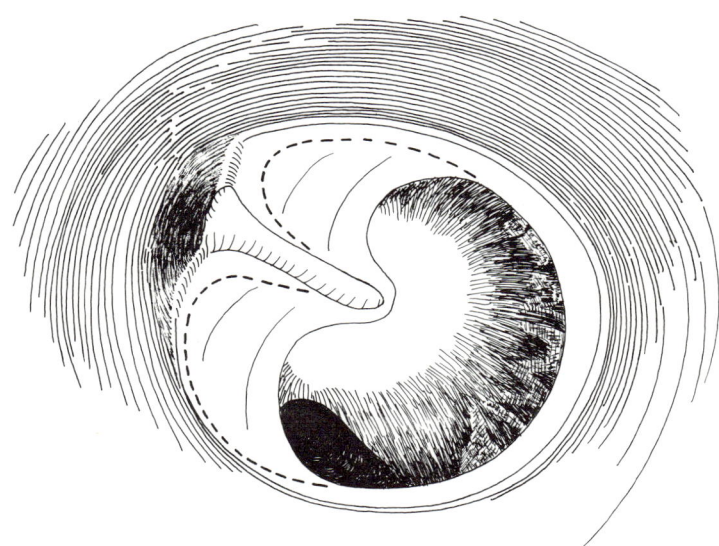

D. Perforation of the atrophic part.
E. Poor healing due to poor vascularization of the atrophic part.
F. Permanent perforation.
G. Secondary infection resulting in active chronic otitis.

2. Atrophy is a consequence of long-lasting retraction of the drum resulting from long-lasting negative middle-ear pressure, with stretching and disappearance of the fibrous and elastic fibers in the lamina propria, which becomes thin and nonelastic, and can disappear totally (Fig. **347**). In such cases, the drum consists only of keratinized squamous epithelium on the ear-canal side, and flat middle-ear mucosa epithelium on the inner side. Dissection of such a thin drum, with removal of keratinized squamous epithelium in an onlay technique, or

ATROPHY

MYRINGOSCLEROSIS

Fig. **347** Atrophy of the pars tensa: normal drum at the right side, with a gradual decrease in the thickness of the lamina propria until it totally disappears at the left. Varying degrees of myringosclerosis of the pars tensa: normal thickness of lamina propria at the right side

removal of mucosal layer in an underlay technique, is technically very difficult, and sometimes impossible.

3. Retraction of an atrophic drum occurs easily with negative middle-ear pressure, and the retracted, atrophic drum can adhere to the long process of the incus—myringoincudopexy (Fig. **348**). The long process of the incus can be resorbed, and the drum will adhere to the head of the stapes—myringostapediopexy (Figs. **349**, **350**). Permanent posterior retraction of the atrophic drum onto the incudostapedial joint was found in 10% of ears after actively treated secretory otitis (Tos 1990). In addition, posterior atrophy with retraction and adhesion to the medial walls of the posterior tympanum—adhesive otitis—was found in an additional 4% of ears after secretory otitis. Retraction of a diffuse atrophic drum to the promontory results in atelectasis. Posterosuperior retraction can extend to the sinus tympani, cause resorption in the stapes, and progress to sinus cholesteatoma. Diffuse atro-

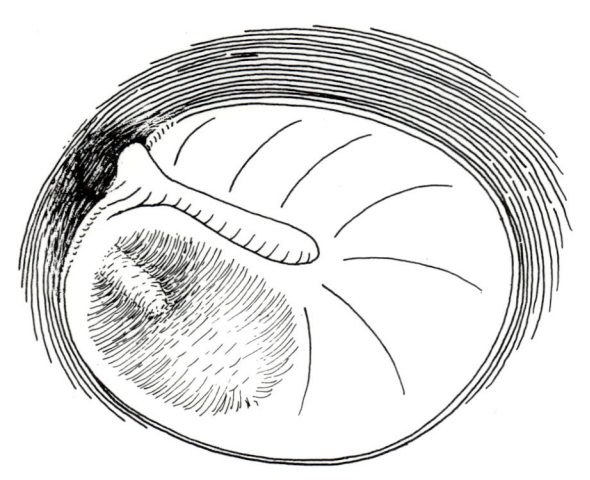

Fig. **348** Posterior atrophy of the pars tensa, with retraction onto the long process of the incus: myringoincudopexy

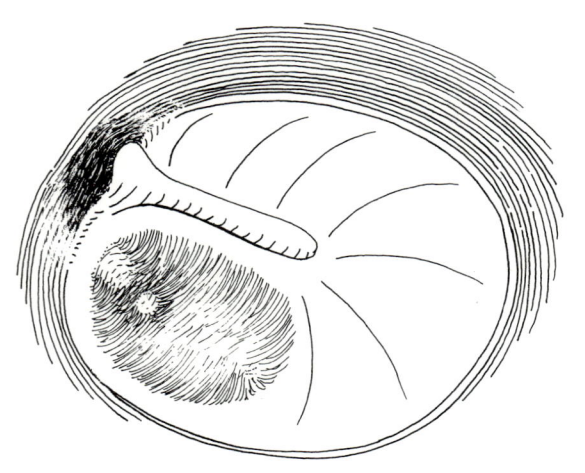

Fig. **349** Posterior atrophy, with retraction and resorption of the long process of the incus, and adhesion to the head of the stapes: myringostapediopexy

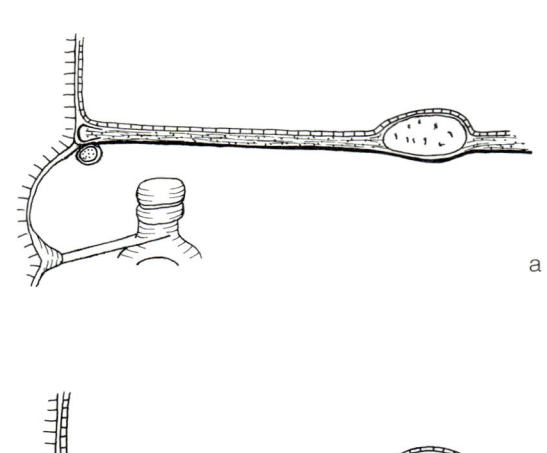

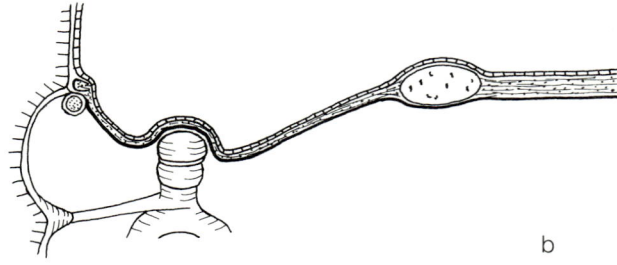

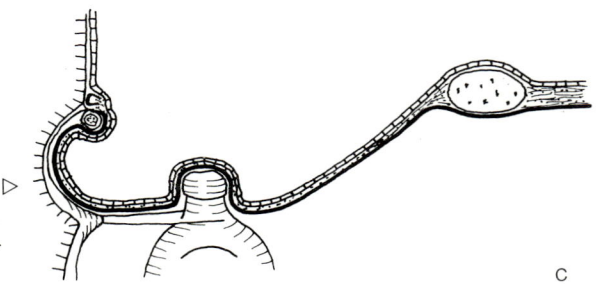

Fig. **350 a** Normal position of pars tensa.
b Posterior atrophy, retraction and myringoincudopexy.
c Posterior atrophy and retraction in myringostapediopexy

phy with retraction and atelectasis can progress to tensa-retraction cholesteatoma. A common pathological situation is posterior retraction with a permanent perforation of the atrophic membrane (Figs. 351, 352). Such ears may have excellent hearing because of establishment of a myringoincudopexy or myringostapediopexy, and good ventilation of the middle ear through the perforation.

The logical explanation for membranes of keratinized squamous epithelium "growing" down onto the ossicles, is the initial posterior atrophy of the drum with retraction, myringoincudopexy, or myringostapediopexy, and subsequent perforation and disappearance of the major part of the atrophic membrane, except in some places around the ossicles, resulting in remnants of keratinized squamous epithelium and illuminating adhesions covered with keratinized squamous epithelium (Fig. 353).

4. Atrophy often appears together with myringosclerosis—another common sequela after secretory otitis. Myringosclerotic plaques are often located in one or two quadrants, and atrophy in another (Figs. 354, 355). Based on our epidemiological research on secretory otitis, our general conclusion is that secretory otitis and chronic tubal dysfunction in childhood are the primary causes of all chronic middle-ear diseases in adults. Secretory otitis results in sequelae in the drum, especially atrophy and retraction that can later progress to cholesteatoma or perforation, causing noncholesteatomatous chronic otitis (Table 1). Secretory otitis appears at least once in 90% of children of preschool age. Even if it resolves spontaneously in the majority of children without any major sequelae, 10% of children still suffer some

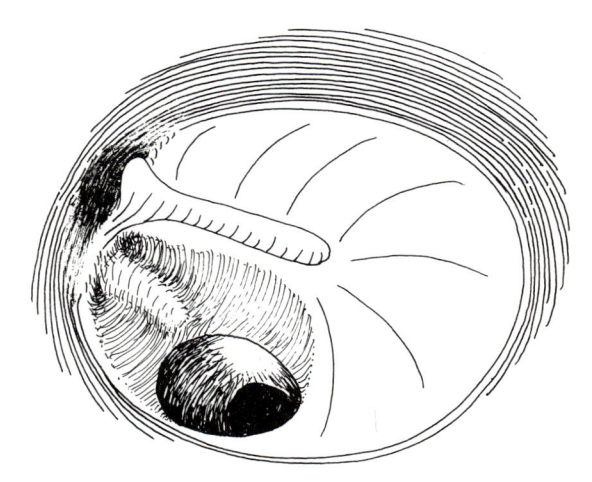

Fig. 351 Posterior atrophy with retraction, and myringoincudopexy with "peripheral" posterior perforation of the atrophic membrane

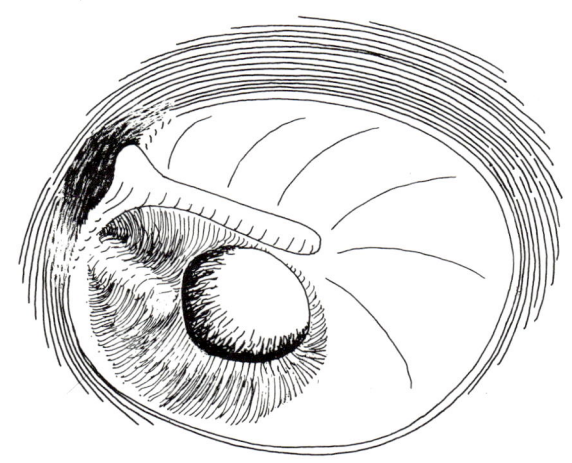

Fig. 352 Posterior atrophy and retraction of the pars tensa, with myringoincudopexy and perforation of the atrophic membrane

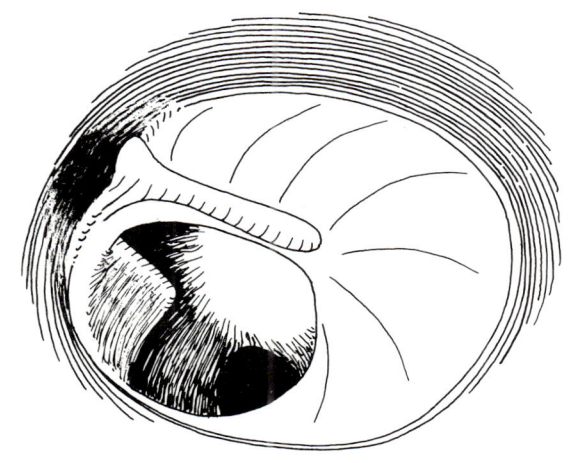

Fig. 353 Posterior perforation of an atrophic membrane with myringoincudopexy, imitating adhesions to the incus

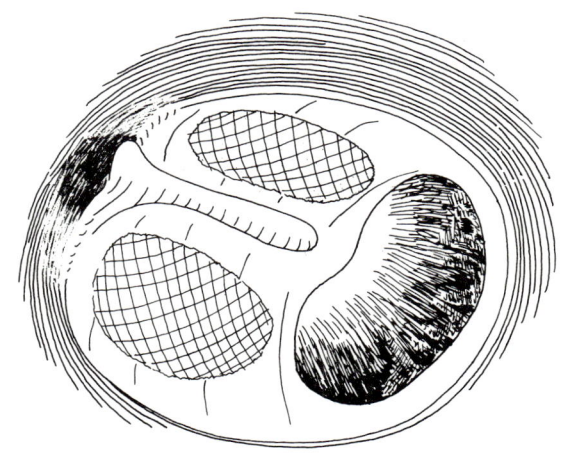

Fig. 354 Inferior perforation, with anterior and posterior tympanosclerotic plaques

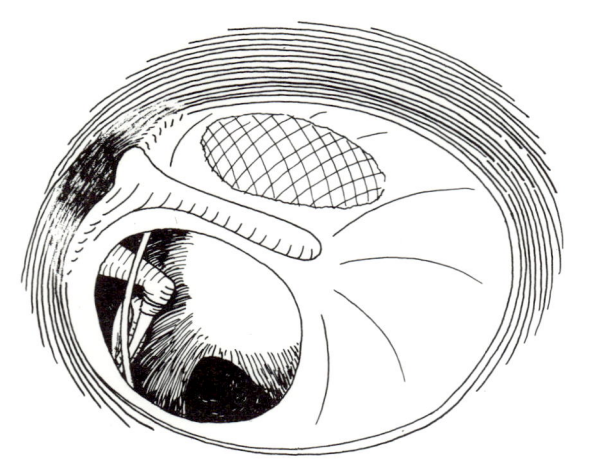

Fig. 355 Posterior perforation, with tympanosclerotic plaque anteriorly

sequelae in the drum. In long-lasting and severe cases, 55% will have sequelae in the drum despite active surgical treatment (Table **1**).

The pathogenetic aspects of chronic middle-ear diseases are significant when considering the indications for surgery and the choice of the surgical method to be used in each particular pathological condition.

Classification of Myringoplasty Techniques

Over the years, many techniques have been published in the literature, and all of these are still in use, either routinely or sporadically. Some are used by certain surgeons in any pathology, while others are used in special pathological conditions. Here, a classification is attempted in relation to:

The placement of the graft
The epithelial covering of the graft
The approach to the undersurface of the drum
The suspension of the graft

In relation to the *placement* of the mesodermal graft over or under the lamina propria of the drum remnant and of the fibrous annulus, myringoplasty is mostly divided into a) onlay or overlay techniques, and b) underlay techniques.

In relation to the management of the epithelium of the drum remnant and annulus skin, the *onlay techniques* are subdivided into techniques involving:
A. Removal of the drum-remnant epithelium without covering the graft.
B. Elevation and outward dissection of the drum-remnant epithelium and ear-canal skin, creating various skin flaps and covering the graft edges with these elevated skin flaps. The mesodermal

Table **1** The prevalence of abnormalities of the pars tensa at various ages in a cohort of healthy children and in two clinical groups of secretory otitis cases treated by adenoidectomy and grommet insertion (groups I and II)

Type of pathology	Randomized cohort age (years)		Treated secretory otitis (years postoperatively)			
			I			II
	7 n = 444 (%)	10 n = 470 (%)	3–8 n = 527 (%)	10–16 n = 362 (%)	½–7 n = 178 (%)	11–18 n = 178 (%)
Atrophy	6.3	8.1	21.3	11.4	30.3	14.6
Atrophy + pexis	2.0	2.3	3.2	4.7	2.8	10.1
Adhesive otitis	–	–	2.5	2.2	2.8	3.9
Sinus cholesteatoma	–	–	–	0.3	–	–
Atrophy + perforation	0.2	0.2	–	–	1.7*	1.7
Atrophy + tympano-sclerosis	1.4	2.3	9.1	10.8	2.2	9.6
Tympanosclerosis alone	7.2	5.1	18.8	25.7	7.3	18.5
Abnormal pars tensa	17.1	18.0	54.8	58.1	47.2	58.4
χ^2 test, $p < 0.001$			n.s.		$p < 0.05$	

* Closed by tympanoplasty.   n.s. = not significant.

graft is thus partly placed under the skin flaps in this technique, which is also described as the intermediate technique, or inlay technique.
C. Sandwich techniques, with complete removal of drum-remnant epithelium and ear-canal skin, placement of the fascia on the annulus, and covering of the fascia with ear canal skin.

Underlay techniques are further subdivided into:
A. Techniques without tympanomeatal flaps. The graft is placed under the drum through the perforation, without tympanotomy.
B. Techniques with tympanomeatal flaps, and tympanotomy—either posterior tympanotomy, inferior tympanotomy, anterior tympanotomy, or total elevation of the fibrous annulus.
C. Sandwich techniques, with the graft placed under the fibrous annulus and the drum remnant, and the perforation covered with ear-canal skin in a manner similar to the onlay sandwich technique.

General Principles of Myringoplasty Techniques

Whether an onlay or an underlay technique is used, some general principles have to be used to avoid failures:

1. Keratinized squamous epithelium should be removed from the edges of the perforation. This can be achieved either by a) excision of the perforation edge, b) excision of a major part of the drum remnant, or c) dissection of the squamous keratinized epithelium from the edges.
2. No remnants of keratinized epithelium should be left between the graft and the outer surface of the drum remnant in onlay techniques, and between the graft and the undersurface of the drum remnant in underlay techniques.
3. The size of the graft should be carefully fitted to the deepithelialized area of the drum, and should not overlap the keratinized epithelium. This problem is seen only in onlay techniques.
4. The graft should have firm contact with the undersurface of the drum, either by suspension to the drum remnant using special measures, or by pressing it up under the drum remnant with solid Gelfoam packing of the tympanic cavity.

Excision of the Edges of the Perforation

This procedure always precedes the underlay techniques, but it is not always necessary in onlay techniques. Excision can be performed by a sickle knife (Figs. **356, 357**), cutting through all three layers of the drum, starting on one side of the perforation, and continuing to the other side (Fig. **358**) until the edge of the entire circumference of the perforation is excised. Cutting the drum edge with a sickle knife can be technically difficult, especially in a tympanosclerotic and fibrotic drum. After the knife has been introduced through all three layers, it should be moved from that point forward and backward, with care being taken not to remove too much of the lamina propria. By introducing the sickle knife obliquely through the drum, a large piece of the keratinized epithelium can be removed, and the lamina propria preserved.

Removal of squamos epithelium from the edges of the perforation can be performed with curved double-cup forceps all the way around the perforation (Fig. **359**). By careful pulling of the edge, the border between the keratinized epithelium and the mucosa can be observed. The author prefers to remove the perforation edge with a curved double-cup forceps, as it allows one to remove the keratinized epithelium and the epithelial junction without removing the lamina propria or enlarging the perforation.

A third method of removing the perforation edges is by making small holes with a curved needle all around the edge of the perforation (Fig. **360**). With double-cup forceps, the edge is gradually removed (Fig. **361**). The needle can also act as a knife luxating the edge between to two holes, away from the drum remnant (Fig. **362**).

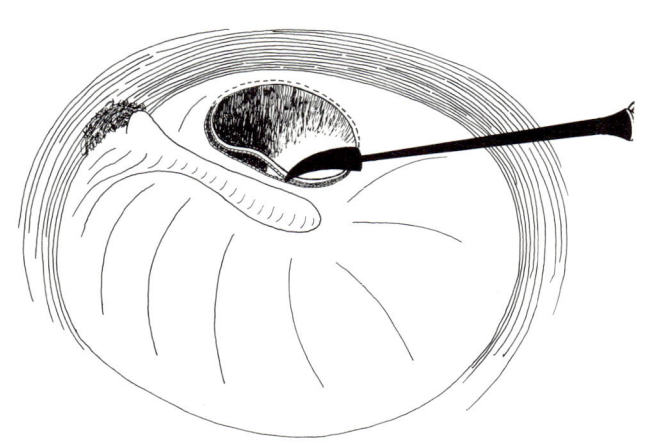

Fig. **356** Excision of the edge of an anterior perforation

9 Myringoplasty: General Aspects Definitions

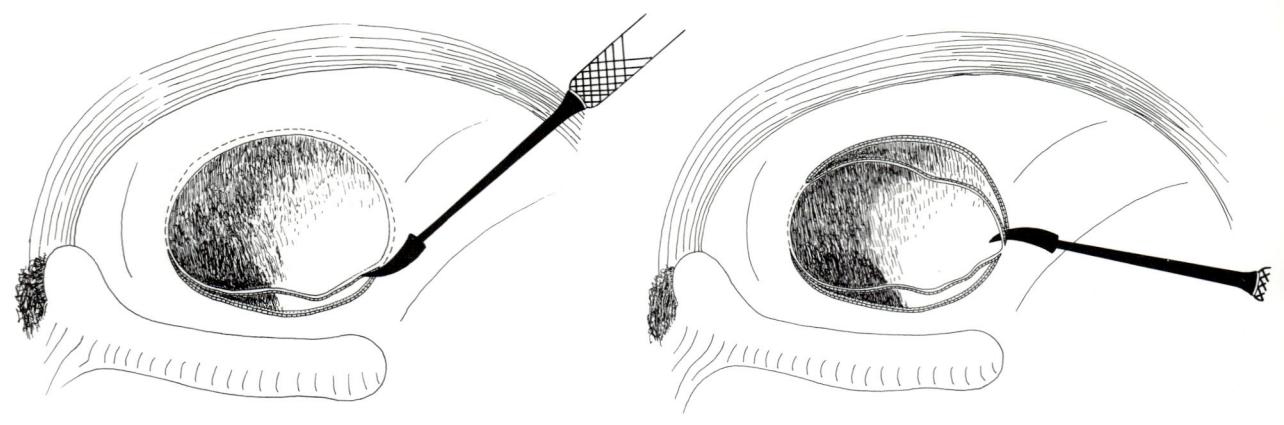

Fig. 357 Part of the edge is excised with a sickle knife

Fig. 358 Continuous excision around the entire edge

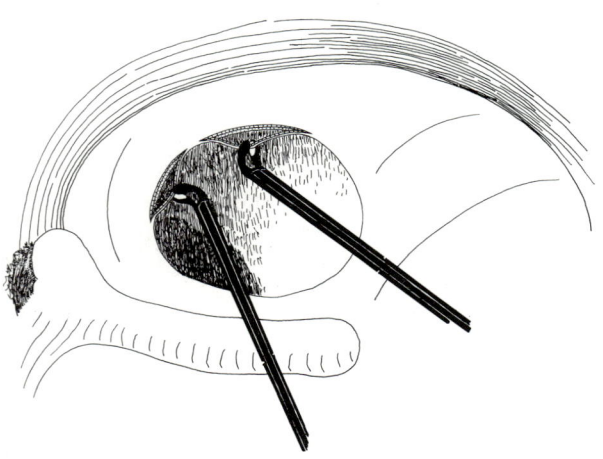

Fig. 359 Excision of the edge of the anterior perforation using a double-cup forceps

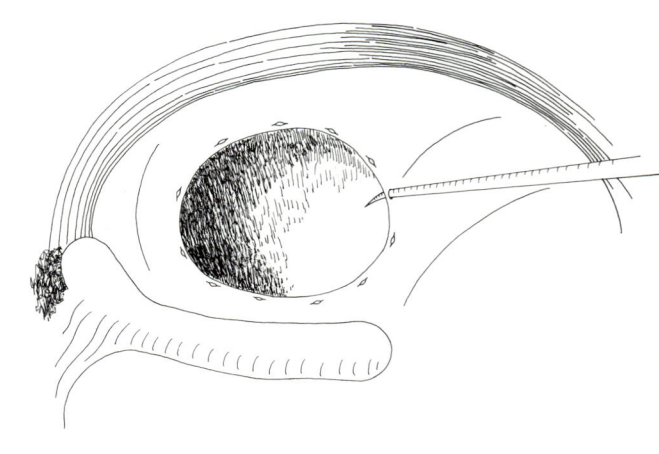

Fig. 360 Several holes are made with a curved needle around an anterior perforation

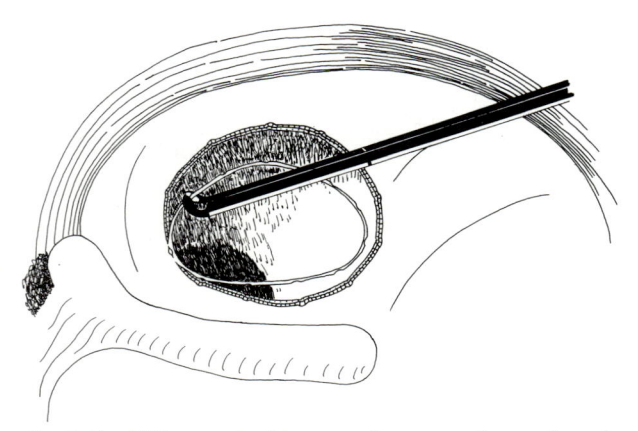

Fig. 361 With a double-cup forceps, the edge is pulled out in toto

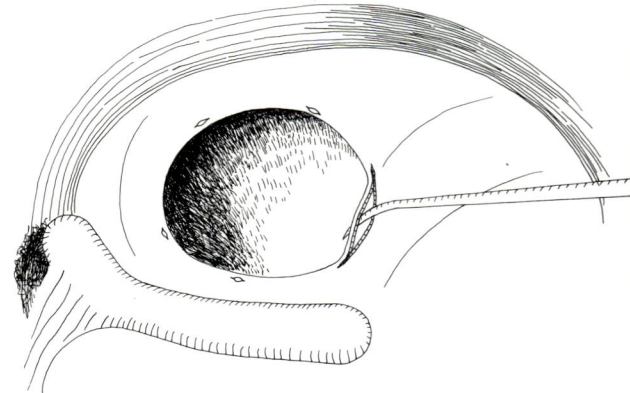

Fig. 362 The edge of the perforation is luxated from the drum remnant between the two holes

The problem with excising the edge is that the thickness of the drum remnant is seldom normal. Usually, part of the edge consists of tympanosclerosis and an atrophy remnant without lamina propria. It is difficult to cut tympanosclerotic plaque, and an atrophic drum can tear in places other than those desired, considerably enlarging the perforation. In addition cutting the drum is not possible on the retracted part.

Dissection on the Perforation Edge

In onlay techniques, it is always preferable to elevate the keratinized epithelium from the edge of the perforation, leaving the lamina propria intact. The epithelium is incised 0.5–3 mm peripheral to the edge of the perforation, and elevated towards the perforation edge (Fig. 363). This can be performed by a rugine, a round knife, the back of a sickle knife, or a curved double-cup forceps. The epithelium is elevated all around the edge, providing good visibility of the epithelial junction between the keratinized epithelium and the mucosa. With a thin suction tip, the mucosa is perforated (Fig. 364) and torn, and the keratinized epithelium is removed together with the epithelial junction. The mucosa can also be cut by the sickle knife or a needle, or the keratinized epithelium can simply be suctioned out by controlling the epithelial junction (Fig. 365). The epithelial junction is usually clearly visible as a transition from white membrane to a bluish membrane. Preferably, the epithelium can be removed with a curved double-cup forceps, still controlling the epithelial junction (Fig. 366).

Elevation of the keratinized epithelium can be performed very easily from the tympanosclerotic plaques, and in atrophic parts of the drum, elevation can also be carried out without tearing the drum remnant.

In many perforations, the keratinized epithelium not only covers the edge, but also extends beneath the drum. This is often the case in tympanosclerotic drums (Fig. 367). By carefully elevating the keratinized epithelium all around the edge, and elevating the epithelium under the edge (Fig. 368), the junction between the keratinized and the mucosal epithelium can be located, and the mucosa can then be further elevated from the undersurface of the drum (Fig. 369) and the keratinized epithelium safely removed all the way around the perforation (Fig. 370) without cutting the lamina propria or enlarging the perforation.

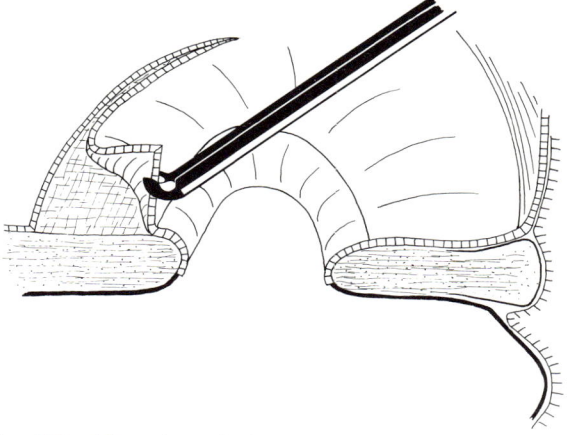

Fig. 363 Elevation of the squamous epithelium from the thick tympanosclerotic drum remnant

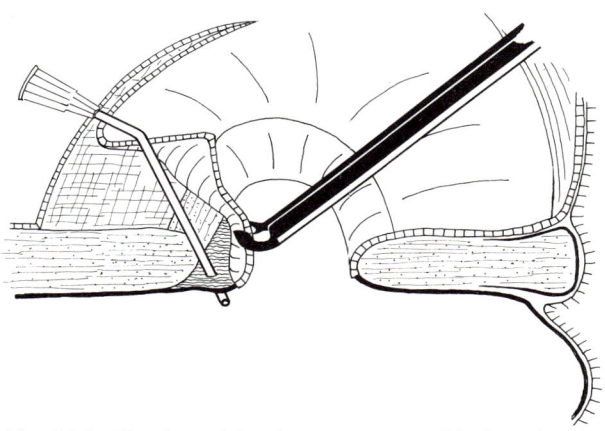

Fig. 364 The keratinized squamous epithelium is elevated, and the junction with the mucosal epithelium is visualized. The mucosa is perforated with a sucker, and torn

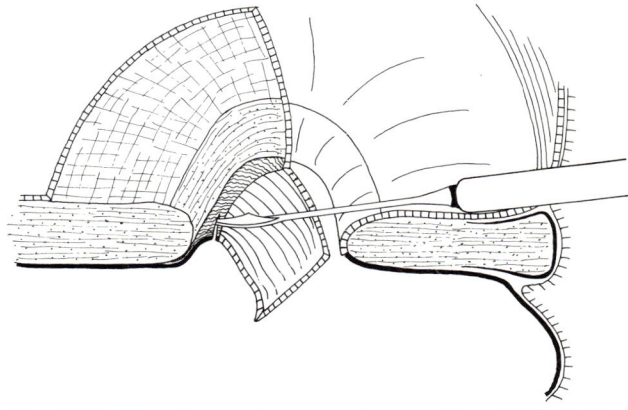

Fig. 365 The elevated mucosa is cut with a sickle knife

9 Myringoplasty: General Aspects Definitions

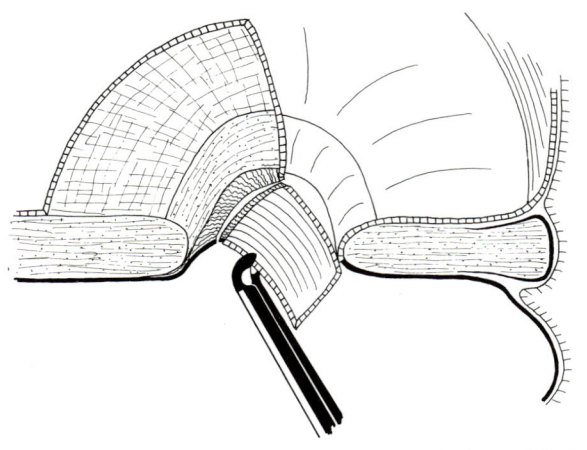

Fig. 366 The keratinized epithelium and the epithelial junction are removed

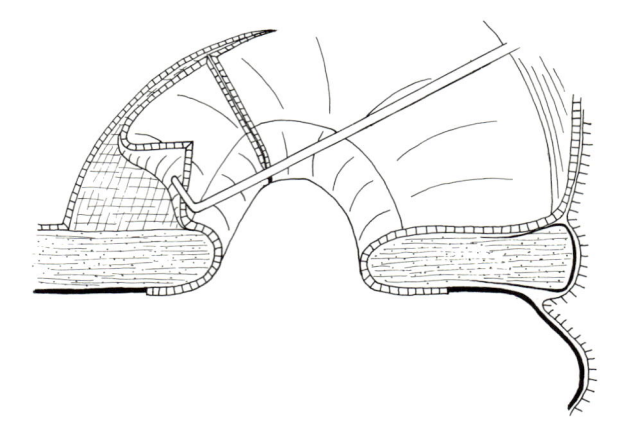

Fig. 367 The keratinized epithelium extends far under the edge of the perforation

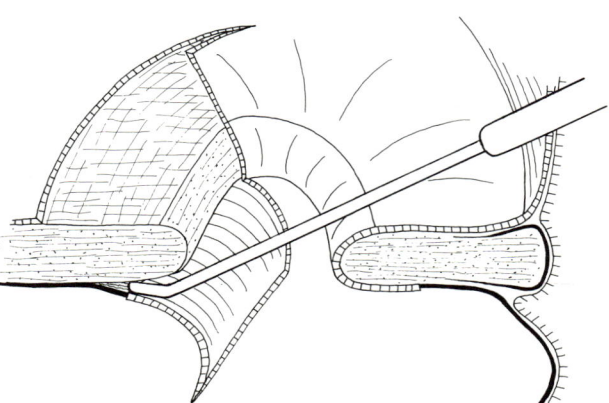

Fig. 368 The keratinized epithelium is elevated from the lamina propria around the edge of the perforation

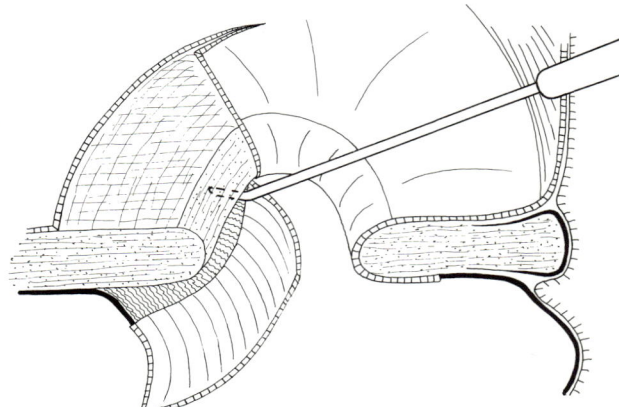

Fig. 369 The mucosa is elevated

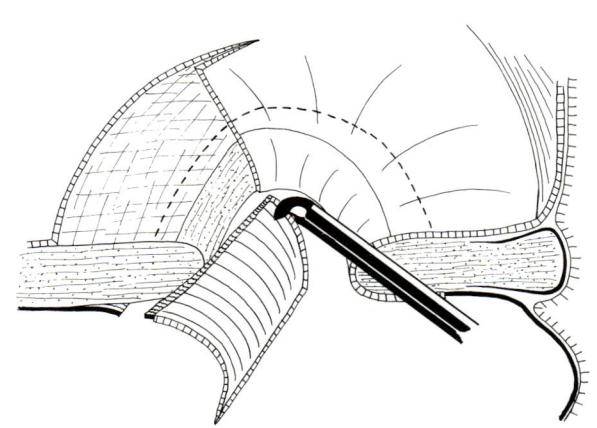

Fig. 370 The keratinizing squamous epithelium is removed

Dissection of the Perforation Edge

The elevation technique can also be used in underlay methods, requiring removal of the mucosa under the perforation edges. The incision of the squamous epithelium is performed close to the edge of the perforation (Fig. 371). The keratinized epithelium is elevated around the edge, together with the mucosa epithelium far under the drum remnant (Fig. 372). The elevated mucosa, together with the keratinized epithelium, can easily be removed by a curved double-cup forceps (Fig. 373), and the perforation is ready for underlay grafting without being enlarged.

In cases with pronounced extension of keratinized epithelium under the drum (often associated with myringosclerosis), and in cases where the epithelial junction cannot be located, an excision of the drum remnant is necessary (Fig. 374) all around the perforation, which is thereby enlarged (Fig. 375). Further dissection after excision of the drum depends on whether an underlay or onlay graft technique is preferred.

The presence of the keratinized squamous epithelium under the drum remnant is usually caused by retraction (Fig. 376) or the remnants of a retraction. In intact retractions, it is important to place the instrument behind the retraction and dissect the membrane away from the medial wall of the tympanic cavity (Fig. 377), and from the undersurface of the drum (Fig. 378). The entire membrane can be gradually elevated from the edge of the perforation and removed with double-cup forceps (Fig. 379).

Where there are remnants of keratinized epithelium under the drum remnant, it can sometimes be elevated by drawing a curved rugine (Fig. 380) towards the edge of the perforation, and then removed (Fig. 381). The risk of leaving keratinized epithelium behind the drum is considerable, and excision of drum remnant is often necessary.

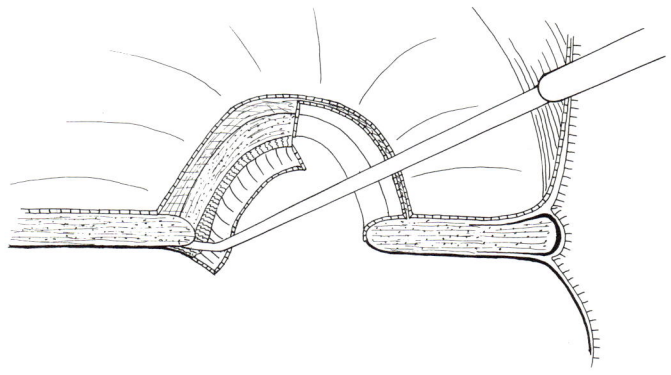

Fig. 371 Elevation of the epithelium together with the mucosa, in underlay graft methods. Squamous epithelium is incised close to the edge of the perforation and elevated as far as the mucosal junction

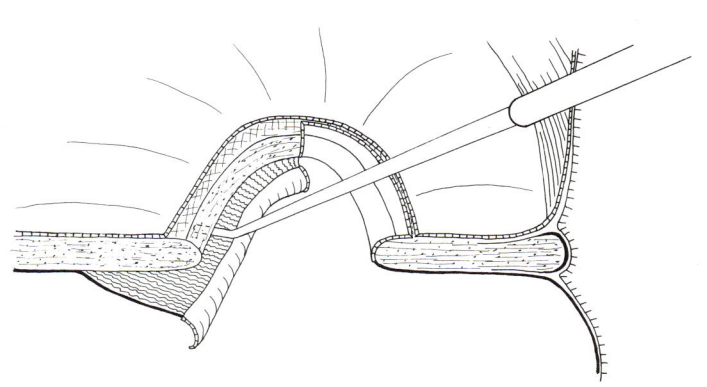

Fig. 372 Further elevation of the mucosa from the lamina propria

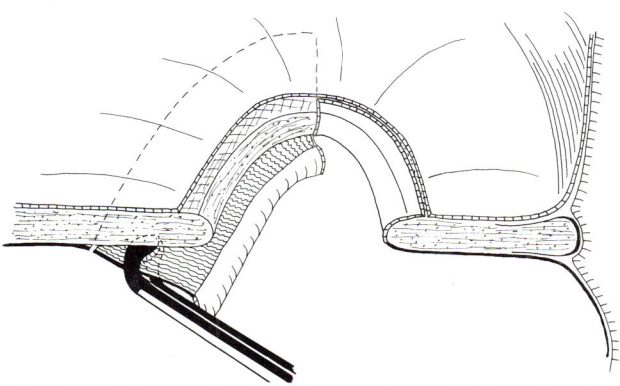

Fig. 373 Removal of a large piece of the elevated mucosa, together with the keratinized epithelium, from the edge of the perforation

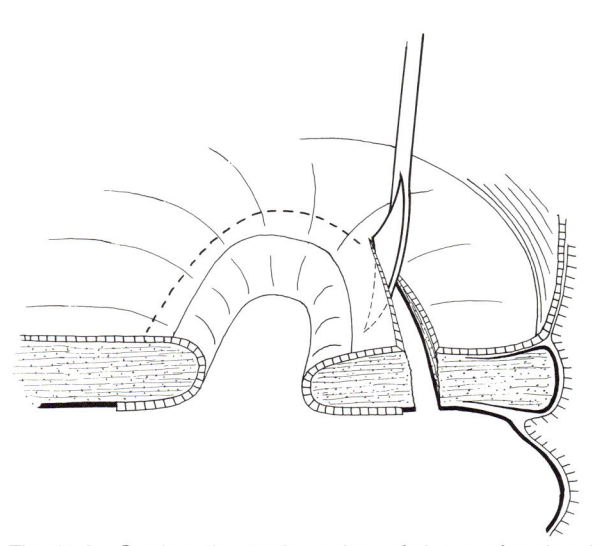

Fig. 374 Cutting the entire edge of the perforation in cases with tympanosclerosis and keratinized epithelium under the drum remnant

9 Myringoplasty: General Aspects Definitions

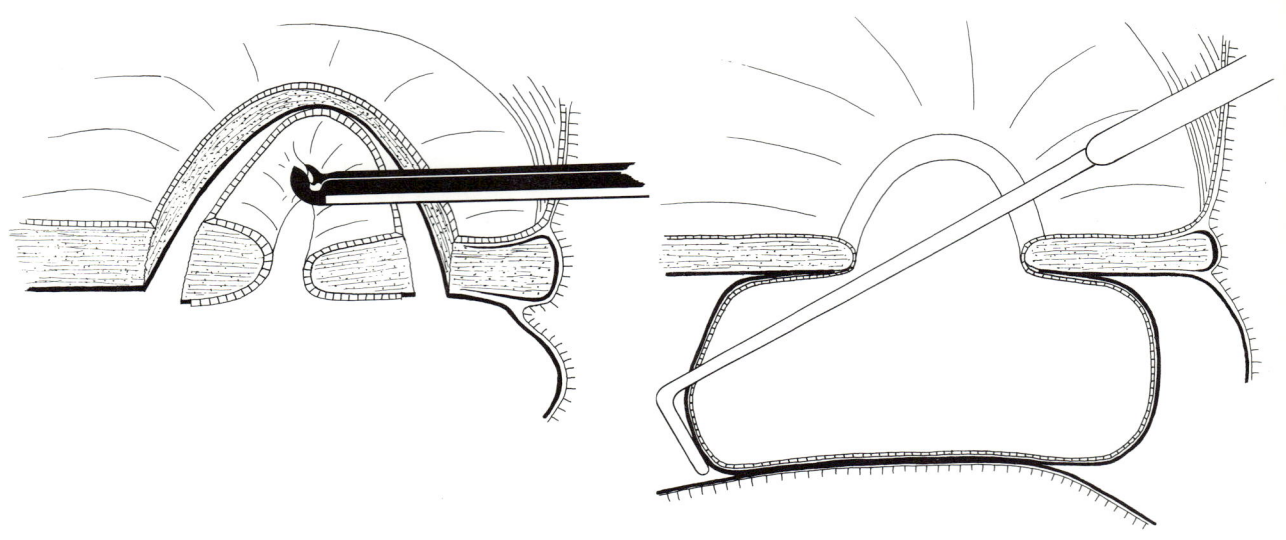

Fig. 375 The edge is removed, and the perforation is considerably enlarged

Fig. 376 Keratinized epithelium under the drum remnant, caused by retraction

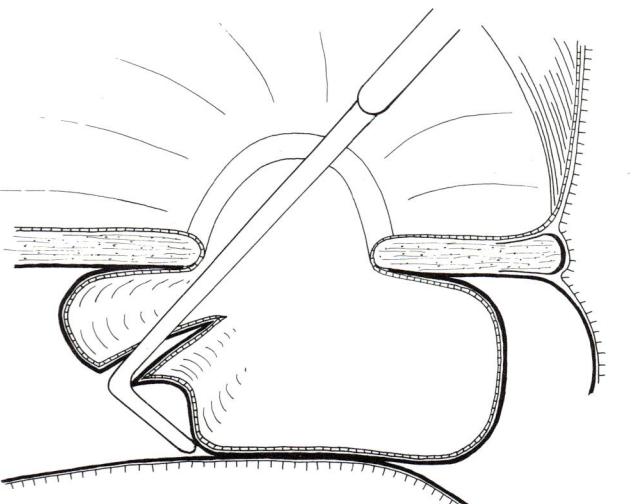

Fig. 377 The retraction is elevated from behind, and the membrane is loosened from the promontory

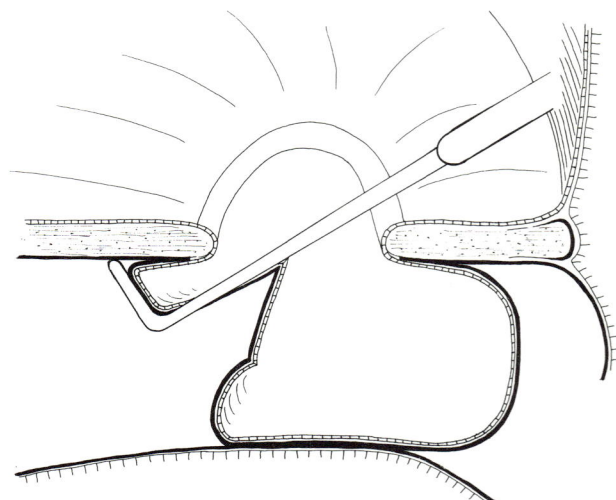

Fig. 378 The retracted membrane, attached to the undersurface of the drum, is elevated

Removal of the Drum Epithelium

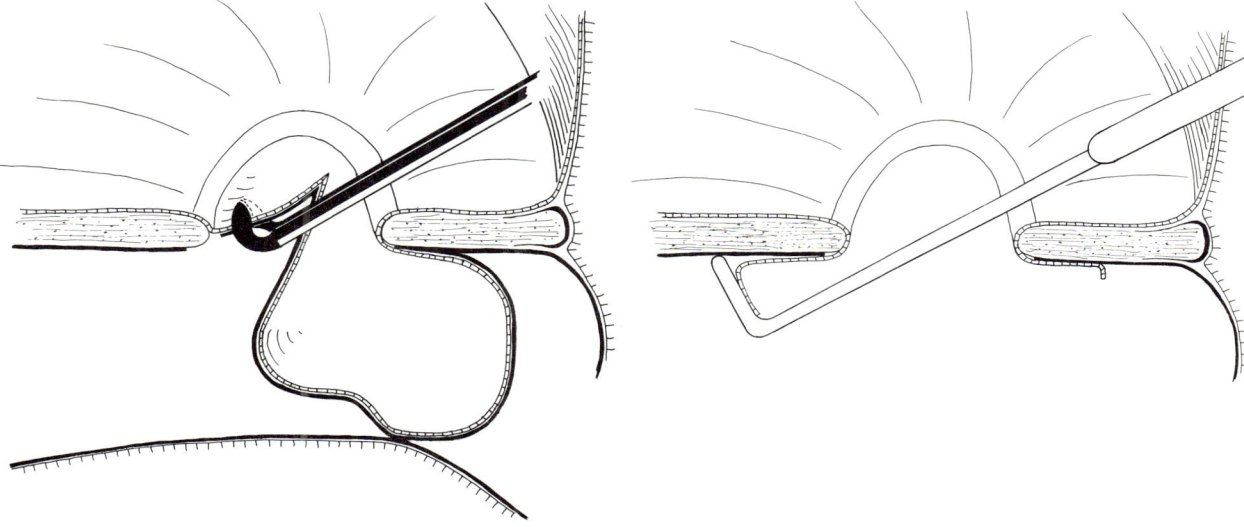

Fig. 379 The posterior half of the retracted membrane is totally elevated, and can be removed with forceps

Fig. 380 Elevation of a remnant of the retracted membrane under the edge of the perforation

Management of Drum-Remnant Epithelium

The fastest and safest epithelialization of the graft in onlay techniques will be achieved if:

1. The denuded area of the drum an ear canal is as small as possible.
2. There is enough denuded drum remnant left to receive the graft.
3. The graft is of the exact size, not too small to be displaced into the tympanic cavity, and too large to overlap the keratinized epithelium.
4. No keratinized epithelium is left under the graft.
5. The small epithelial flaps are placed exactly over the graft.

In onlay myringoplasty, the surgeon usually has to compromise between these demands.

Removal of the Drum Epithelium

After resecting the edge of the perforation (Fig. 356) or preferably after elevating the keratinized epithelium from the edge of the perforation (Fig. 365), the epithelium is removed from the drum remnant. The epithelium is incised with a sickle knife, elevated from all sides, and removed with a double-cup forceps (Fig. 382).

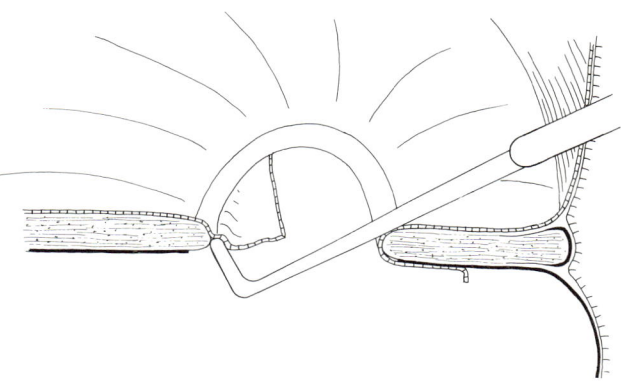

Fig. 381 The keratinized epithelium is elevated, and can be removed

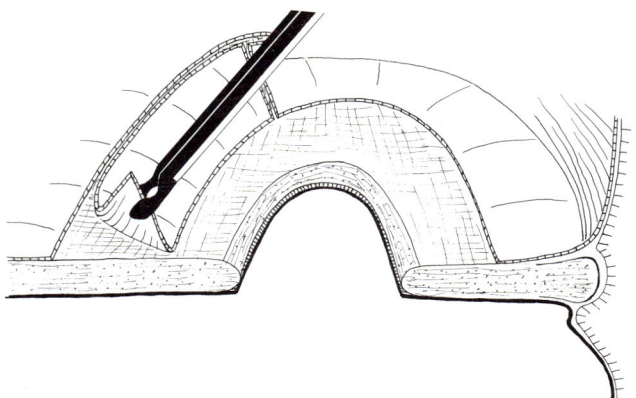

Fig. 382 Onlay myringoplasty on a normal lamina propria. The epithelium of the edge of the perforation has been dissected away, as shown previously, without enlarging the perforation. The epithelium is incised and elevated

9 Myringoplasty: General Aspects Definitions

Further removal of the epithelium can be performed by a new incision 1 mm lateral to the annulus (Fig. **383**). The drum epithelium and ear-canal skin are elevated from all sides and removed (Fig. **384**). The drum remnant is now carefully cleared of all epithelial remnants, and is ready to be covered with a wet or a dry fascia graft (Fig. **385**). The exact size of the graft needed to cover the denuded drum remnant can be measured by a perpendicularly curved instrument (Fig. **386**). The fascia is adapted to cover the drum remnant only (Fig. **387**), and fixed by semiwet Gelfoam balls (Fig. **388**). By pressing the balls into the tympanomeatal angle one by one, firm adherence of the graft can be obtained, especially if the drum remnant is large and thick enough. Even if the fascia only covers the annulus and not the denuded bone, the fixation can be effective, and the new epithelium will soon cover the bone and the graft.

In cases with total perforation, the fascia can be placed on the denuded bone, close to the ear-canal skin (Fig. **389**). The first Gelfoam balls will be orientated towards the annulus, with solid fixation of the graft (Fig. **390**). Epithelialization of the graft from the ear canal will occur without any blunting.

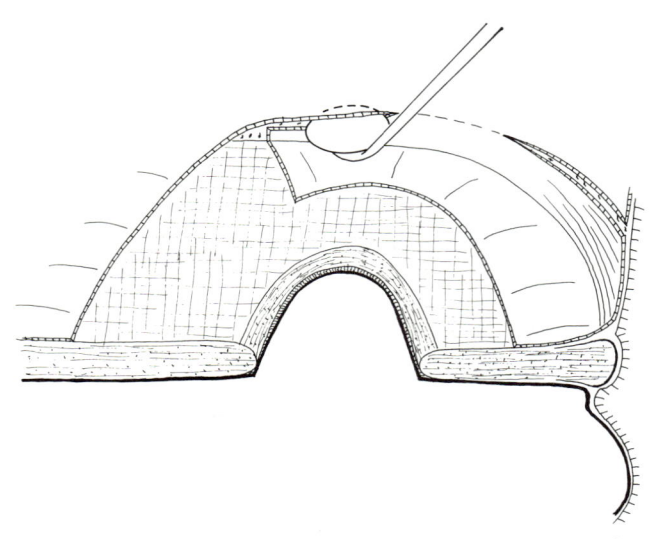

Fig. **383** The epithelium is removed, and an incision is made in the ear-canal skin no more than 1 mm lateral to the annulus

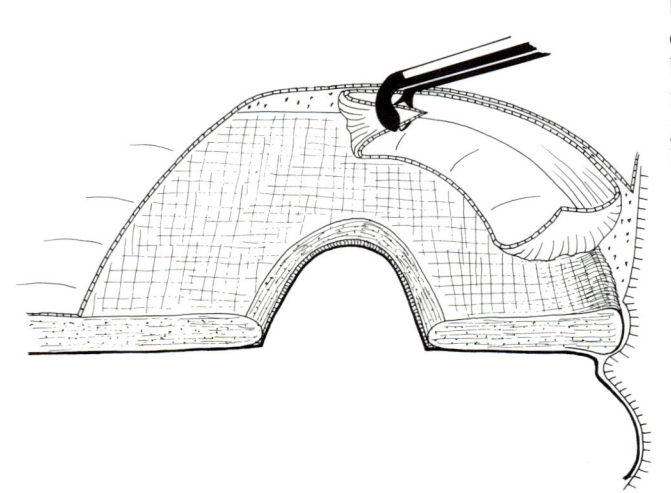

Fig. **384** The epithelium elevated from all sides

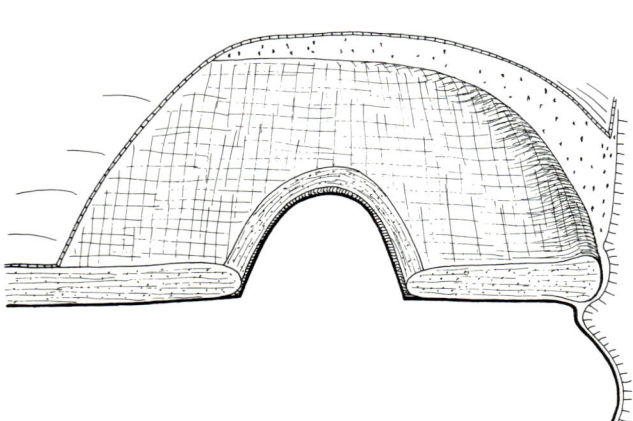

Fig. **385** The drum remnant is carefully cleared of all remaining epithelium

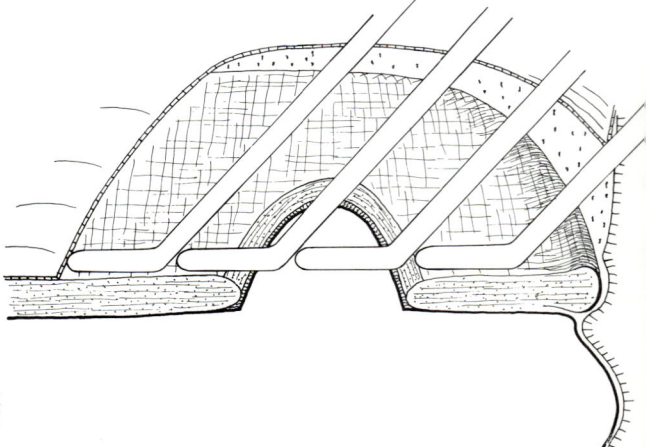

Fig. **386** The size of the area of the denuded epithelium is measured with a curved instrument

Epithelial Flaps

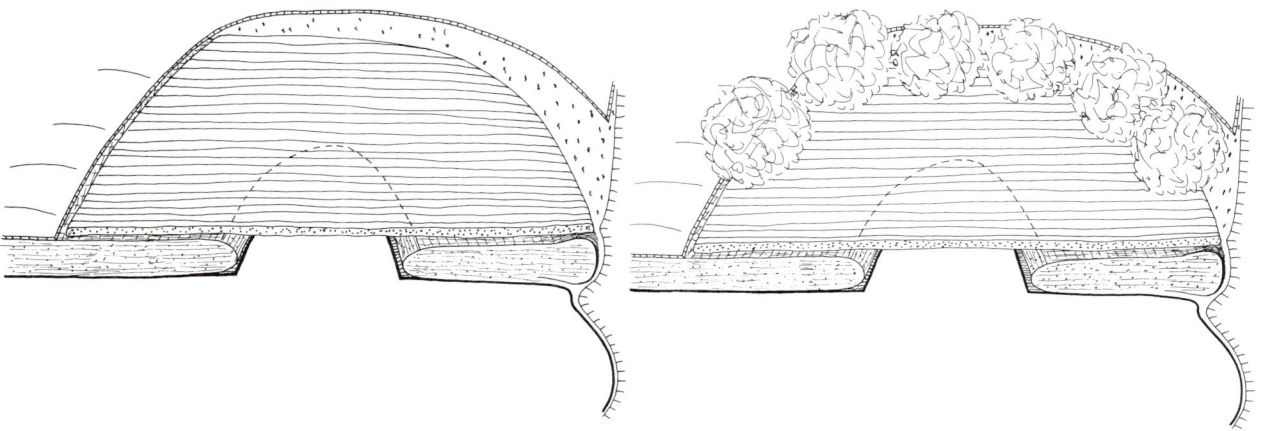

Fig. 387 The wet fascia is approximated to the denuded area of the drum

Fig. 388 The fascia is fixed with semiwet Gelfoam balls, firstly in the anterior tympanomeatal angle

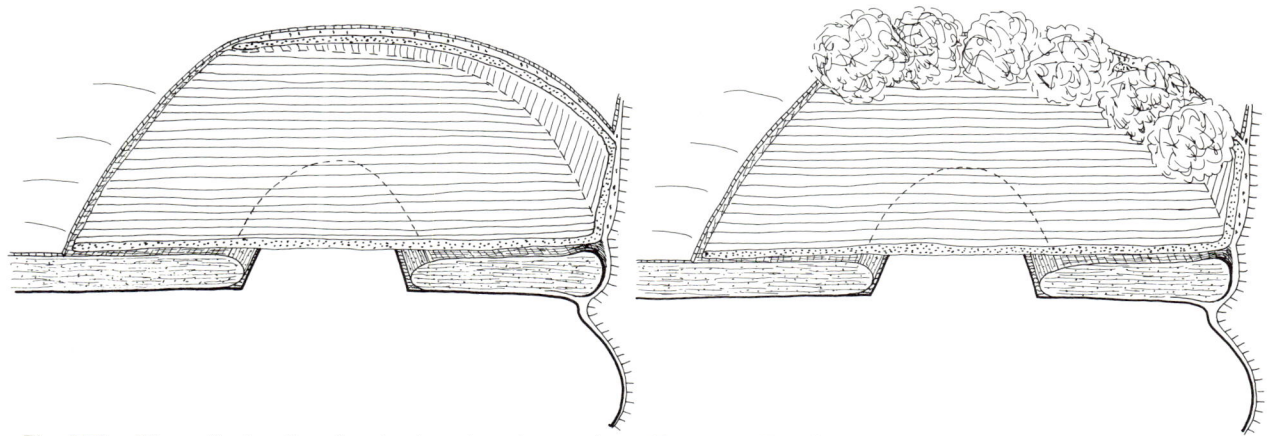

Fig. 389 Alternatively, the fascia is placed on the denuded ear-canal bone and the drum remnant

Fig. 390 The fascia is fixed by pressing the Gelfoam balls toward the bone and the annulus

Epithelial Flaps

Instead of removing the keratinized epithelium of the drum remnant, flaps can be made by elevating the epithelium from the lamina propria (Fig. 391). This is often tempting, and is very easy to perform, especially in ears with a tympanosclerotic or fibrous drum remnant. The flaps cover the fascia, and are fixed by Gelfoam (Fig. 392). The great advantage of the epithelial flaps is the security provided, in that the fascia does not overlap the keratinized epithelium. Sometimes the surgeon will regret all the epithelial flaps which were made during the de-epithelialization of the drum, however, for the following reasons:

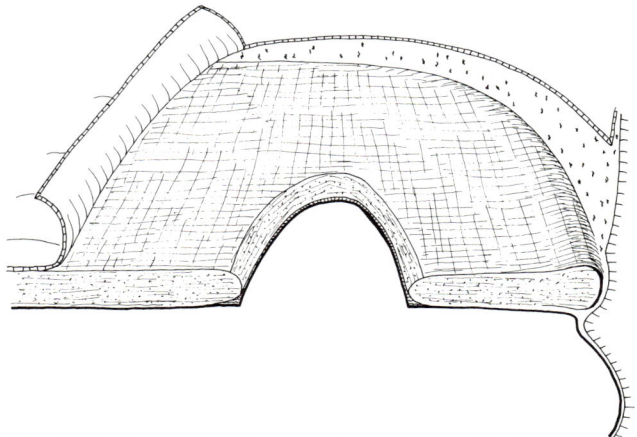

Fig. 391 Instead of removing the epithelium, an epithelial flap is created by elevating it

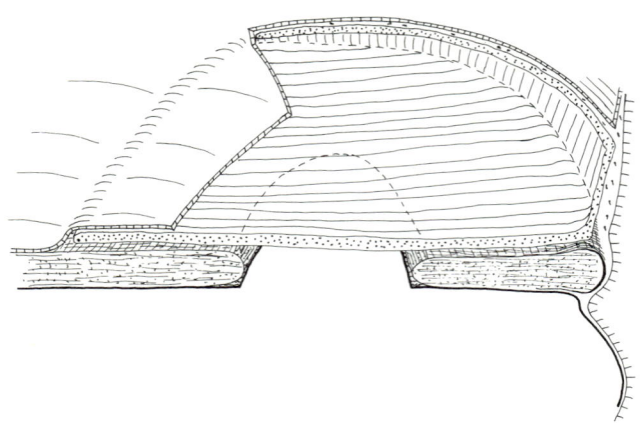

9 Myringoplasty: General Aspects Definitions

Fig. 392 After positioning, the fascia is covered by the epithelial flap

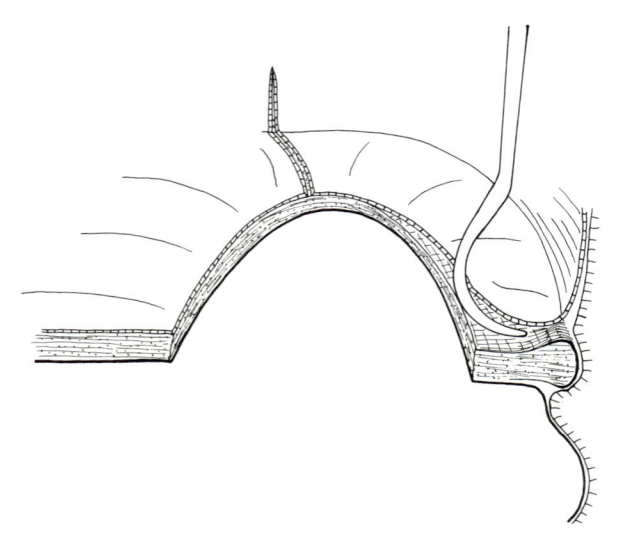

Fig. 393 An epithelial flap in the anterior tympanomeatal angle. After excision of the edge of the perforation and a radial incision of the epithelium, the epithelium of the annulus and the ear-canal skin are elevated

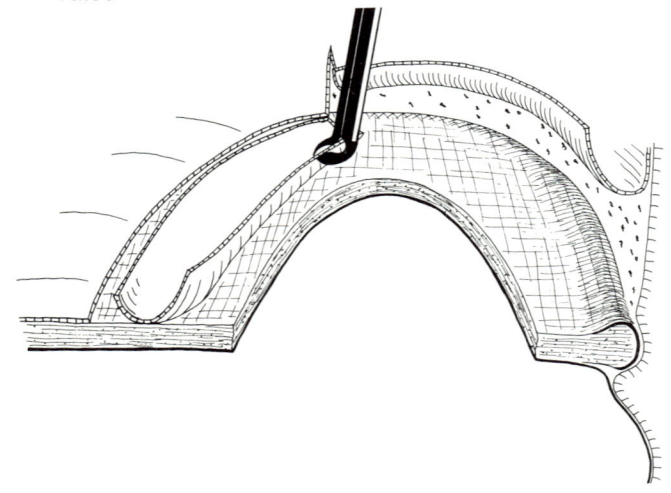

Fig. 394 The small skin flap is elevated, and the remaining epithelium is removed

1. The flaps can dry an shrink. Before replacement, they ought to be moistened with wet Gelfoam balls.
2. It is very difficult to place the fascia under a small, dry flap. Sometimes it is better to remove a dry flap.
3. The fascia should be of a proper size to fit exactly under the flap; folding of the edges of the fascia will make it too thick, and the flap will not be able to cover it.

Nevertheless, the flaps can be very useful to cover the graft at the annulus, and we use flaps very often in onlay techniques.

After the epithelial flap is elevated at the annulus (Fig. 393), the elevation is extended towards the ear canal (Fig. 394), and a small canal-skin flap is established. After removing epithelium from the surface of the drum (Fig. 395) the fascia is placed on the annulus (Fig. 396) and the flap is returned (Fig. 397). The flap is fixed using Gelfoam.

The fascia can cover the denuded bone in the tympanomeatal angle (Fig. 398), and it will be safely covered by the epithelial flap (Fig. 399). The flap is fixed by solid pressure of small Gelfoam balls on the annulus (Fig. 400). There are no problems with blunting of the tympano-meatal angle. The epithelialization of the flap will be fast, and the drum will not be thickened. The tympanomeatal angle will not be changed by this technique. In atrophic drum remnants with a very thin, or completely absent, lamina propria, the removal of the epithelium and onlay technique can be difficult, and perforation of the mucosa can occur (Fig. 401). Small perforations can be ignored and covered by fascia. If a small perforation occurs peripherally in the deepithelialized area, the edge of the fascia can be pressed into the perforation (Fig. 402). In such situations, it is good to have some epithelial flaps covering the weak points (Fig. 403).

Epithelial Flaps 143

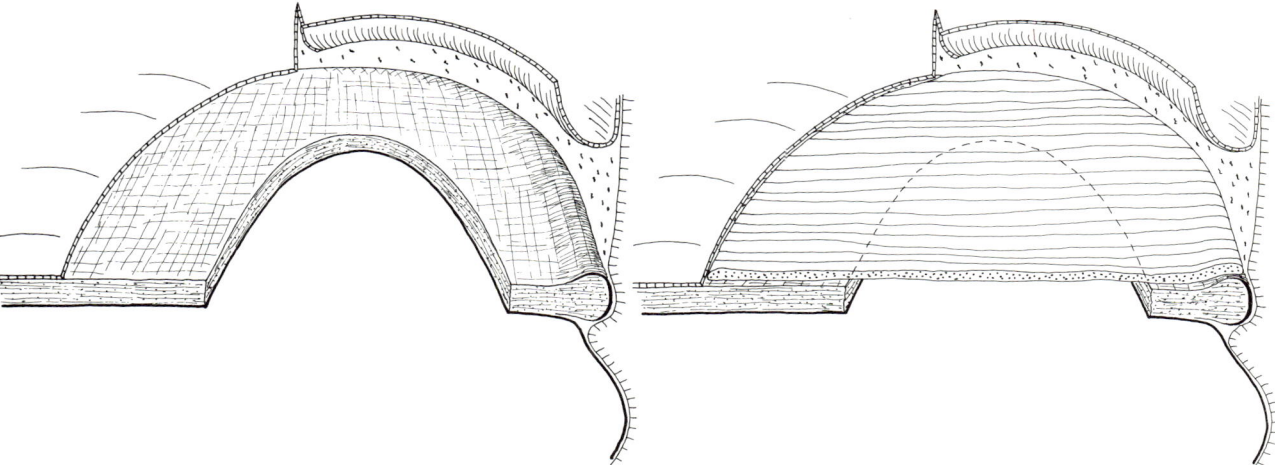

Fig. 395 The drum remnant is cleaned, and is now ready for the onlay graft

Fig. 396 The fascia is positioned, but does not cover the bone

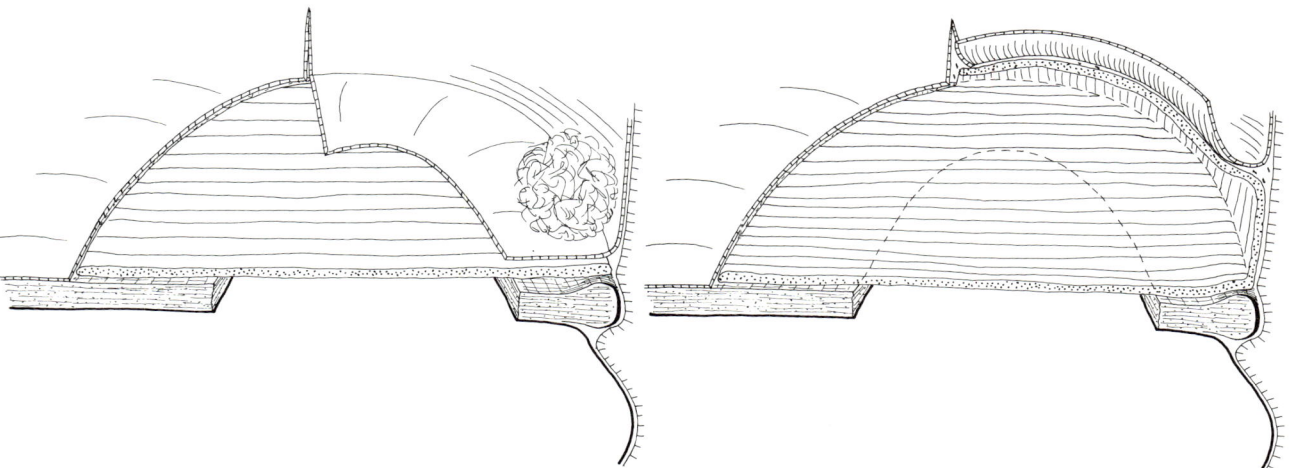

Fig. 397 The epithelial flap is returned and fixed with Gelfoam balls, providing firm closure

Fig. 398 Alternatively, the fascia can also cover the denuded bone

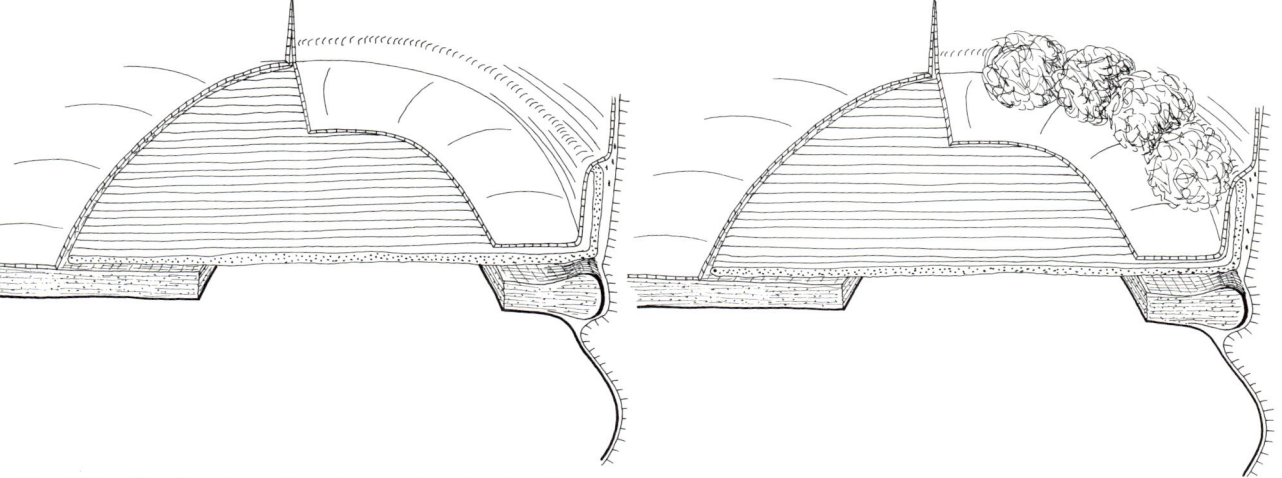

Fig. 399 The flap is replaced, covering the fascia

Fig. 400 The flap is carefully fixed with Gelfoam balls pressed onto the annulus

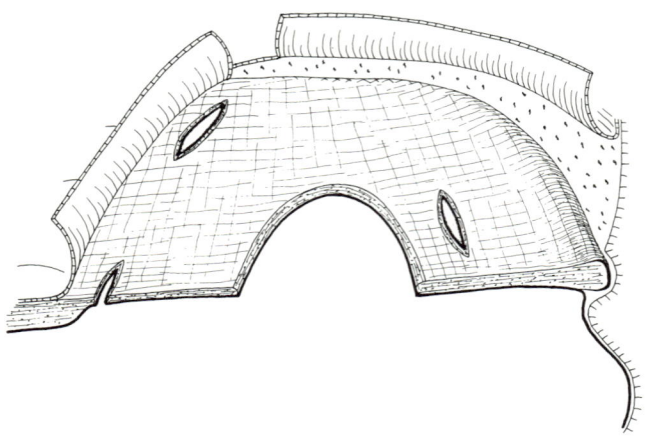

Fig. 401　During elevation of the keratinized epithelium from the thin atrophic drum, some perforations of the lamina propria and the mucosa can occur

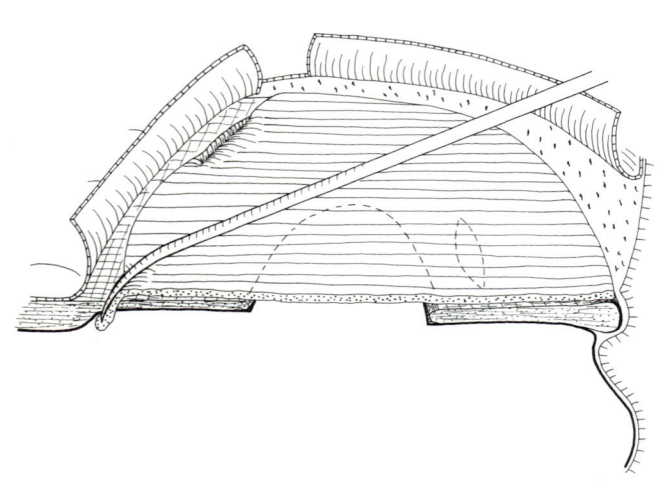

Fig. 402　An edge of the fascia is placed in the perforation

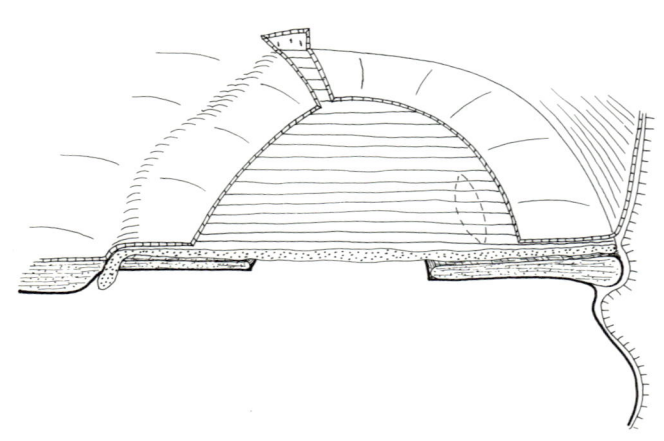

Fig. 403　The epithelial flaps are returned

Fixation of the Underlay Graft under the Drum Remnant

The mucosa of the undersurface of the drum remnant around the perforation should either be elevated from the lamina propria or removed.

Elevation of the mucosa can be performed together with elevation of the keratinized epithelium covering the edge of the perforation, as shown in Figures **365** and **366**. The mucosal edges can be further elevated (Fig. **369**), and removed together with the keratinized epithelium using curved double-cup forceps (Fig. **370**).

Elevation of the mucosa is important under the antrior and inferior edges of the perforation, especially under the fibrous annulus. With a curved elevator, the mucosa can be detached from the undersurface of the annulus (Fig. **404**). The elevation is continued around the annulus, making a plane of cleavage (Fig. **405**) for placement of the fascia as an underlay graft between the mucosa and the annulus (Fig. **406**). This method can be used if a posterior tympanotomy is performed. The fascia is brought through the tympano and pushed forward towards the anterior and inferior parts of the annulus. This will be the case in total or subtotal perforations. After placement of the fascia, the mucosal flap is supported by firm packing with Gelfoam balls.

Some surgeons recommend extended elevation of the mucosa under the annulus and from the hypotympanic bone, using a large, curved elevator. The bone anteriorly and inferiorly under the annulus is denuded (Fig. **407**), and fascia is placed on the denuded bone in the hypotympanum. The mucosa is replaced, and held in place by Gelfoam balls (Fig. **408**). This method is especially recommended at the tympanic orifice of the Eustachian tube. By elevating the mucosa from the lateral wall of the Eustachian tube far towards the isthmus (Fig. **409**), the bone is denuded, and the fascia is placed on the denuded bone (Fig.**410**). Fascia is supported by firm packing of Gelfoam balls in the orifice of the Eustachian tube (Garcia-Ibanez et al. 1986).

Elevation of a mucosal flap under the annulus and removal of the flap (Fig. **411**) is an easier method. Using curved double-cup forceps, the mucosa can be pulled off in small pieces until the denuded bone under the annulus is palpated (Fig. **412**). The fascia is placed under the annulus and pushed towards the denuded bone (Fig. **413**). The fascia should be supported by Gelfoam balls.

Fixation of the Underlay Graft under the Drum Remnant   145

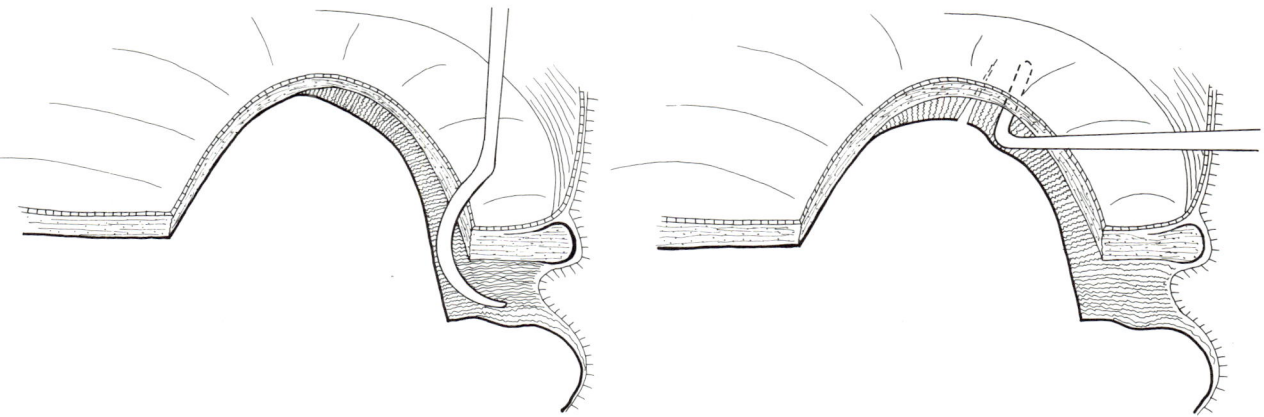

Fig. 404 Fixation of the underlay graft. The perforation edges are excised, and the mucosa is elevated from the annulus

Fig. 405 The mucosa under the drum remnant and annulus is elevated anterior to the bone

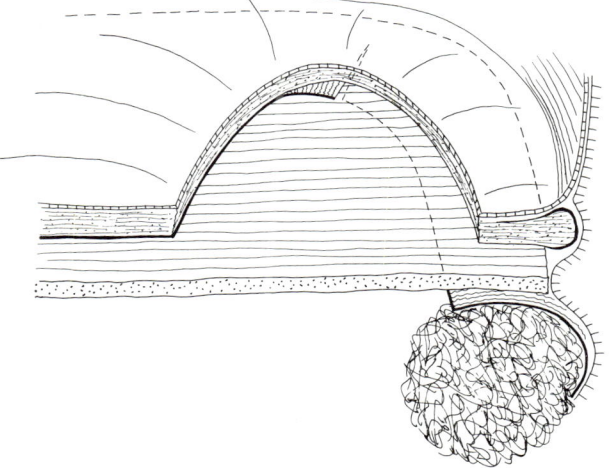

Fig. 406 The fascia is placed under the annulus and on the mucosal flap, which is pressed up to the annulus and held in place by Gelfoam

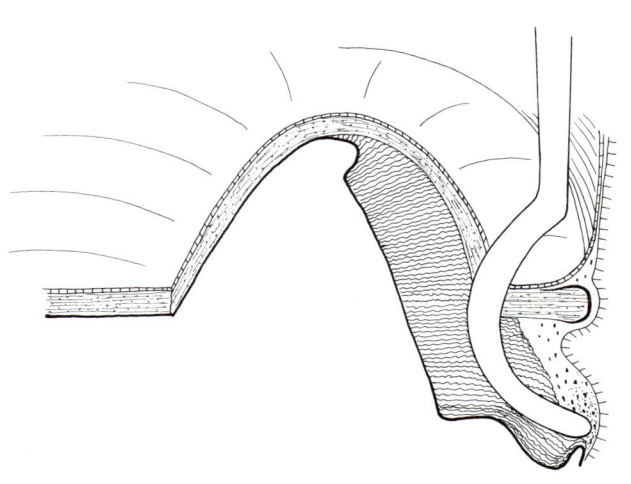

Fig. 407 Extensive elevation of the mucosa under the annulus and from the hypotympanic bone. With a large curved elevator, the mucosa is elevated from the annulus and the bone

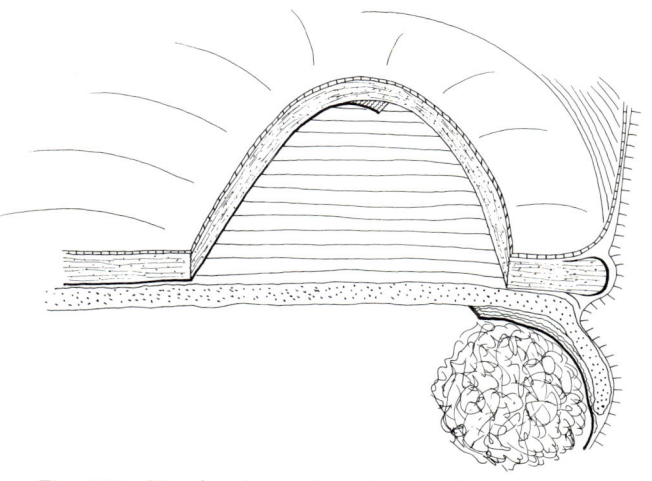

Fig. 408 The fascia is placed under the annulus and on the denuded bone. The mucosal flap is returned onto the fascia and held in place by Gelfoam

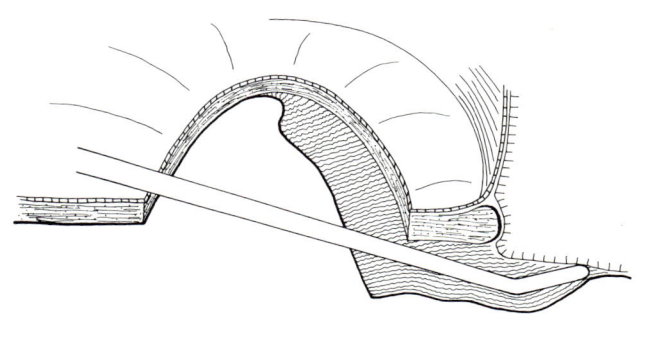

Fig. 409 Extended dissection of the mucosa under the annulus and from the lateral bony wall of the Eustachian tube in the region of the tympanic orifice of the tube. The mucosa is elevated with a curved elevator

9 Myringoplasty: General Aspects Definitions

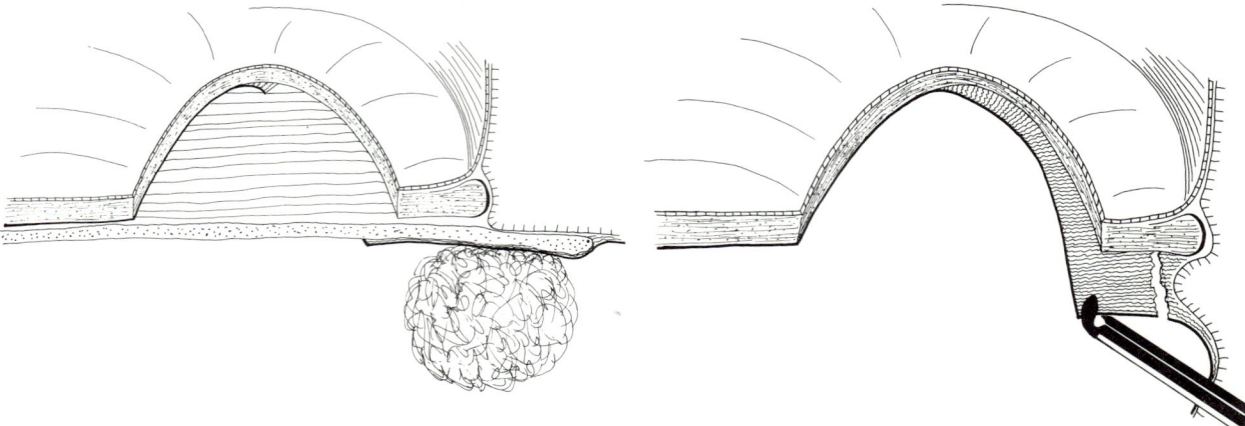

Fig. **410** The fascia is placed on the bone of the lateral wall of the Eustachian tube, and supported by the returned mucosal flap and Gelfoam

Fig. **411** Excision of the elevated mucosa from the anterior remnant of the drum. The edge of the perforation is excised, and the mucosa is elevated and removed using a forceps

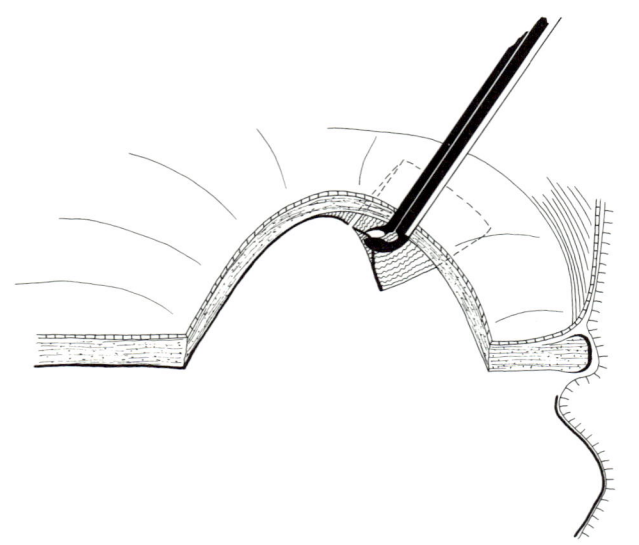

Fig. **412** Further removal of the elevated mucosa under the annulus

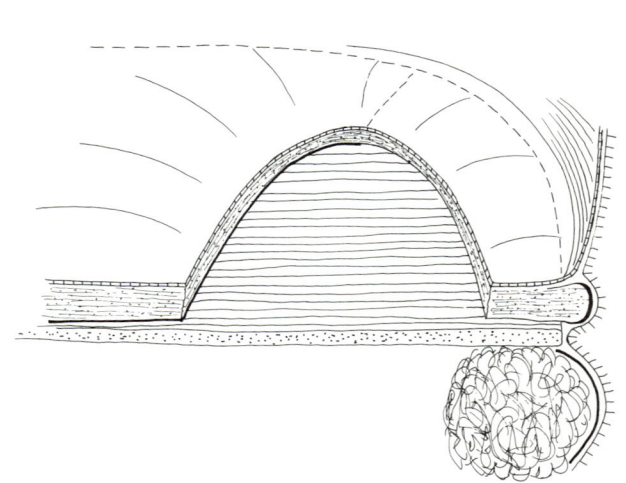

Fig. **413** The fascia is placed under the drum, in contact with the denuded bone. The fascia is supported by Gelfoam balls

A sophisticated, and technically difficult, method of fixating the graft is to pull the fascia edges into the ear canal through a hole made between a subluxated fibrous annulus and the bony annulus. After excision of the edges of the perforation, a small incision of the ear-canal skin just lateral to the annulus is performed. A sharp instrument is pushed through the skin incision along the bone, and into the tympanic cavity, subluxating the fibrous annulus (Fig. **414**). After elevation of the mucosa with a curved elevator, the fibrous annulus is further subluxated from inside, an attempt being made to push the elevator through the same hole (Fig. **415**). With a tip of the suction or another instrument, the opening between the bone and the annulus is enlarged, allowing the edge of the fascia to be pushed or pulled through the hole into the tympanomeatal angle of the ear canal (Fig. **416**). If necessary, a similar hole is made at another point on the annulus (Fig. **417**). The fascia is brought through the posterior tympanotomy from behind under the annulus. With a courved rugine, it is pushed into the ear canal through the hole (Fig. **418**), and further pulled by forceps into the ear

Fixation of the Underlay Graft under the Drum Remnant

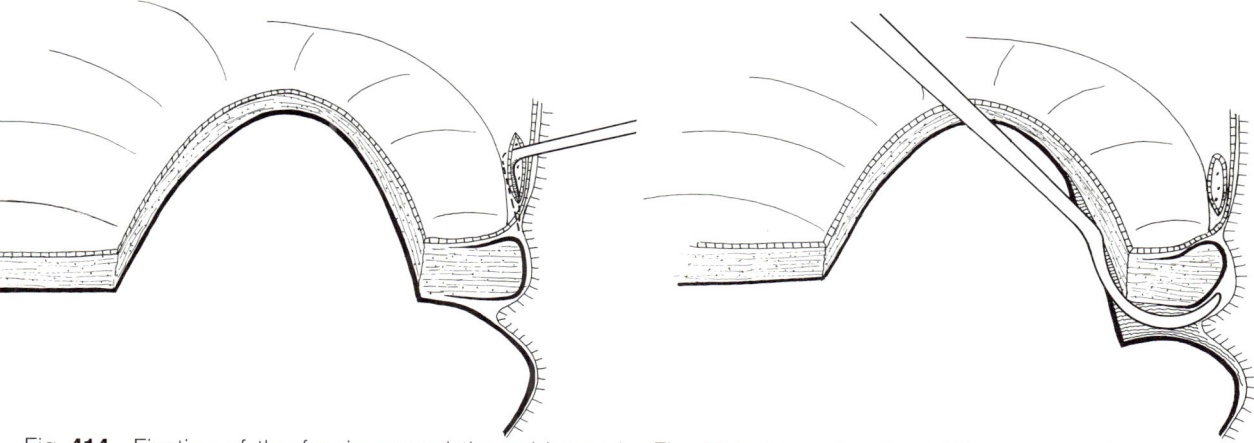

Fig. 414 Fixation of the fascia around the subluxated annulus. After excision of the perforation edges, a hole is made with a hook between the bony annulus and the fibrous annulus

Fig. 415 After elevation of the mucosa, the annulus is further subluxated with a curved elevator, which is pushed toward the previous hole

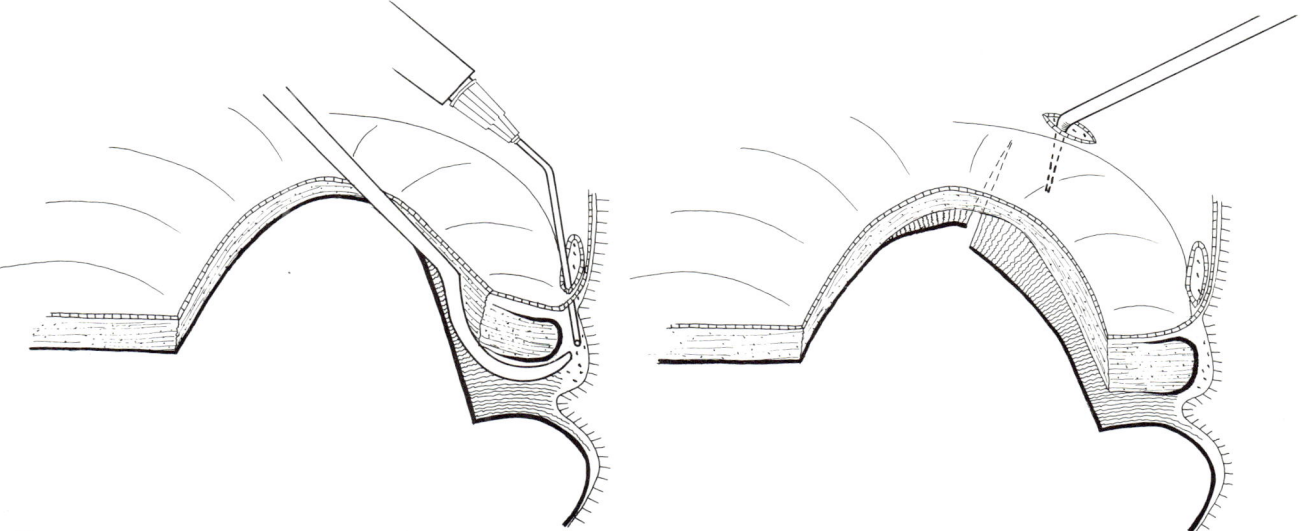

Fig. 416 With suction, the two instruments connect through the performed opening

Fig. 417 A new perforation is made with a hook

canal (Fig. 419). If two or three holes are used (Fig. 420), further support of the fascia by Gelfoam is not necessary.

The original idea of pushing the fascia through holes created in the drum remnant was described by Gerlach (1975). The method is suitable for inferior perforations with a relatively thin drum remnant. After excision of the edge of the perforation and removal of the mucosa under the drum remnant, holes are made 1.0–1.5 mm peripheral to the edge of the remnant using the sickle knife or a needle (Fig. 421). The fascia is placed under the drum remnant, and the edges of the fascia are pulled through the holes, either by a small hook, or a double-cup forceps. When the forceps are passed through the hole, it is widened (Fig. 422), and a small edge of the fascia can be grasped and pulled through the perforation, thus fixing the fascia under the drum (Fig. 423). This method is suitable in inferior perforations (Fig. 424), but the Gerlach principles can be used in many situations in which fixation of the fascia is desired, but filling of the tympanic cavity with Gelfoam needs to be avoided.

9 Myringoplasty: General Aspects Definitions

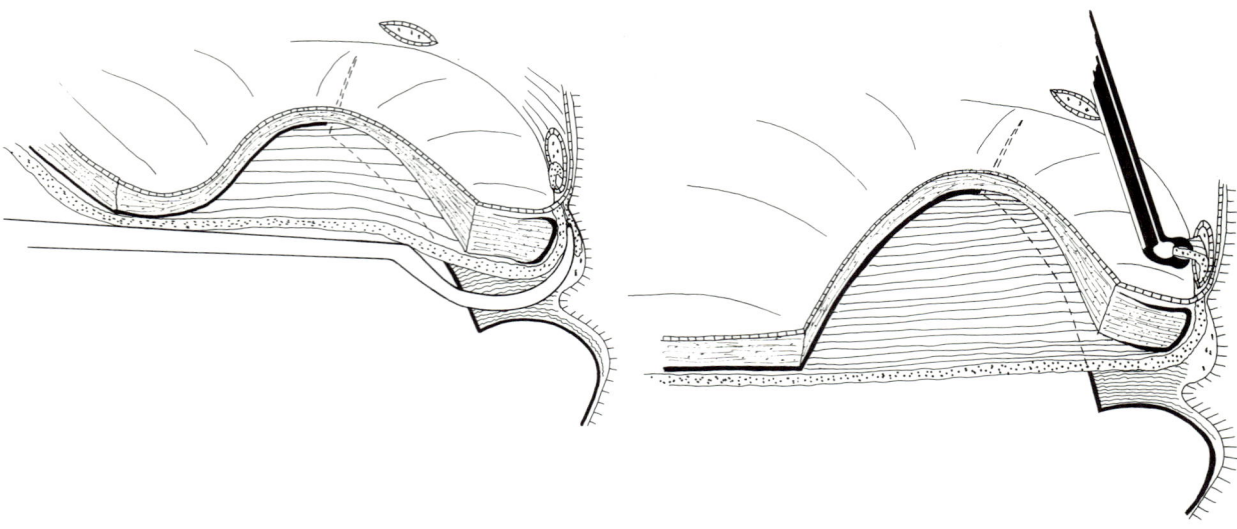

Fig. 418 The fascia is placed under the drum from behind, and pushed through the hole, using a curved elevator

Fig. 419 With a double-cup forceps, the edge of the fascia is pulled out of the hole

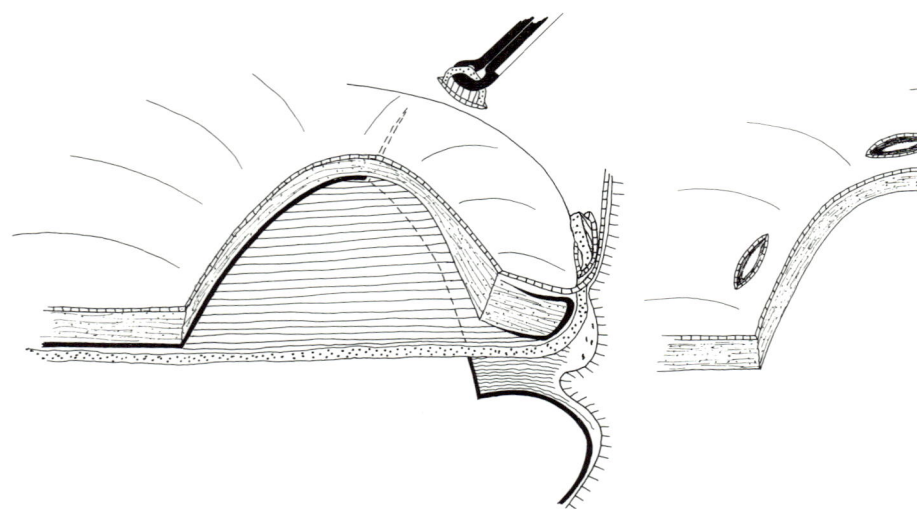

Fig. 420 The fascia is firmly fixed under the drum with two holes in the ear-canal skin

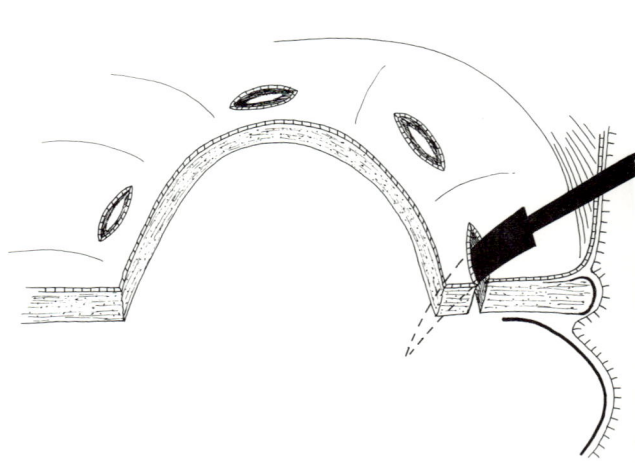

Fig. 421 Gerlach suspension of the underlay graft from the drum, using holes made through the drum remnant. After excising the perforation edge and removing of the mucosa from the undersurface of the drum, several holes are made through the drum remnant using a sickle knife

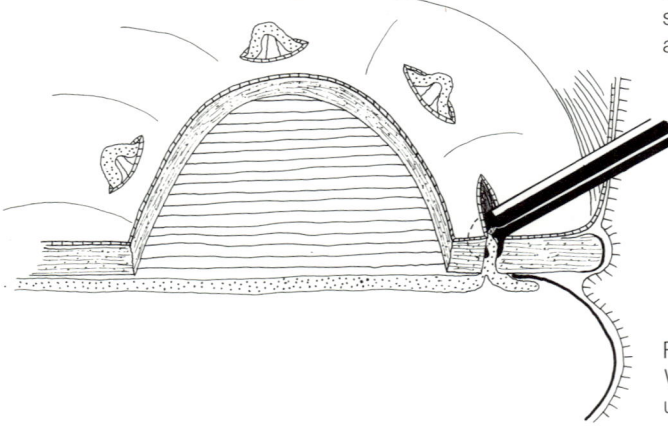

Fig. 422 The fascia is placed under the drum remnant. With curved forceps, an edge of the fascia is caught under the drum

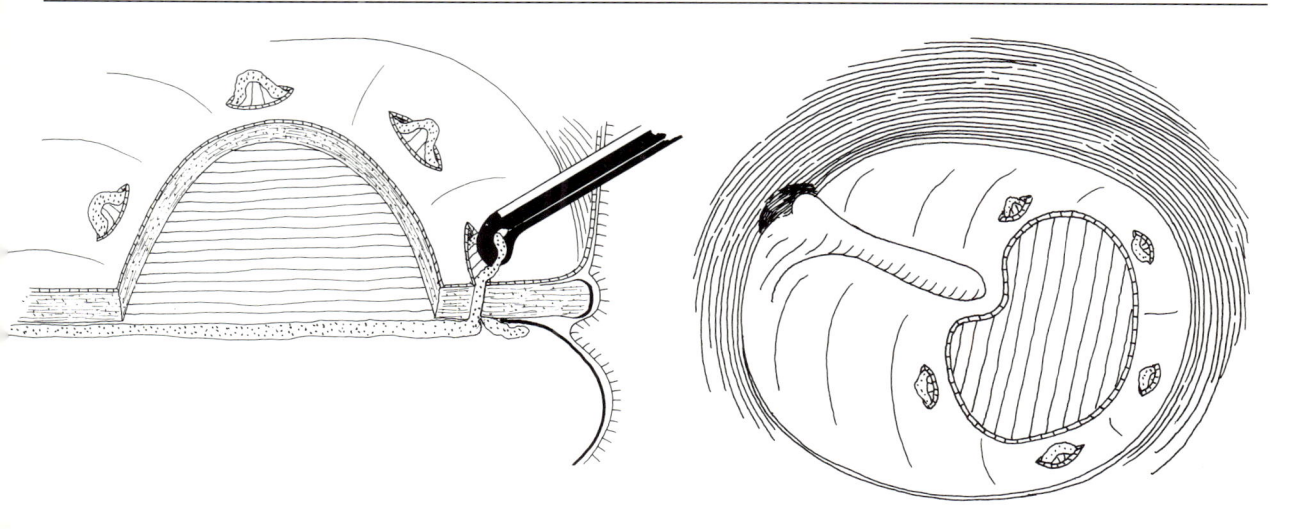

Fig. 423 The edge of the fascia is pulled through the hole, thus fixing the drum

Fig. 424 A typical situation in an inferior perforation, with an underlay graft suspended from the drum with the Gerlach technique

Fibrin Glue in Tympanoplasty

Two types of surgical adhesives have been used in tympanoplasty: Hystoacryl and fibrin glue. The synthetic cyanoacrylate adhesive Hystoacryl was used for a short period during the 1970s, but was soon abandoned because of tissue damage, including bone destruction. The present author used it only in two cases, in both of which treatment failed.

Fibrin glue can be either autogenous or allogenous. Autogenous fibrin glue is produced from the patient's own blood. There are several techniques for isolating fibrinogen from human plasma, but all of them are time-consuming and complex. The principle is to produce a clot from the patient's own plasma so that the fibrin of the coagulum will keep the graft in place.

Autogenous Fibrin Glue

Everberg was the first to use fibrin glue in otology and myringoplasty. He claimed high take rates in myringoplasties performed in 1975 and 1976 using autogenous fibrin glue. During 1977, Everberg and the author performed a controlled randomized prospective study on autogenous fibrin glue, comparing his method of fibrin-glue graft fixation with the author's method of Gelfoam fixation. Each of us performed 15 myringoplasties with autogenous fibrin glue and 15 with Gelfoam in a total of 60 patients. Three months after the operation, there was no significant difference in the take rates between the two methods, which were fairly high with both (Everberg et al. 1977).

The following method is used (Tos et al. 1987). Three 4.5-mL portions of venous blood are withdrawn, and 0.5-mL 3.1% sodium citrate is added to each. The blood is centrifuged for three minutes at room temperature to yield a thrombocyte-rich citrated plasma. Sixty units of thrombin are dissolved in 0.6-mL sterile water. To this is added 1.8-mL sterile calcium levulinate (0.1 gram per mL). In a sterile syringe, 0.5-mL of thrombocyte-rich plasma is taken up. Immediately after this 0,05-mL of the thrombin–calcium mixture is taken up in the syringe. This is mixed quickly and efficiently, and can now be applied to the fascia graft which has just been placed in position (Fig. **425**). After 15-10 seconds, the mixture of plasma and thrombin–calcium begins to coagulate. The coagulum covers the whole tympanic membrane and the inner third of the ear canal (Fig. **426**). Apart from hydrophobic cotton, no further packing is needed. The coagulum is removed after three weeks. In order to prevent fibrinolysis, an antifibrinolyticum is applied immediately before surgery; a slow intravenous injection of 2 g tranexamic acid (Cyclokapron) is given. Postoperatively, 1 g Cyclokapron is given in tablets three times daily for four weeks.

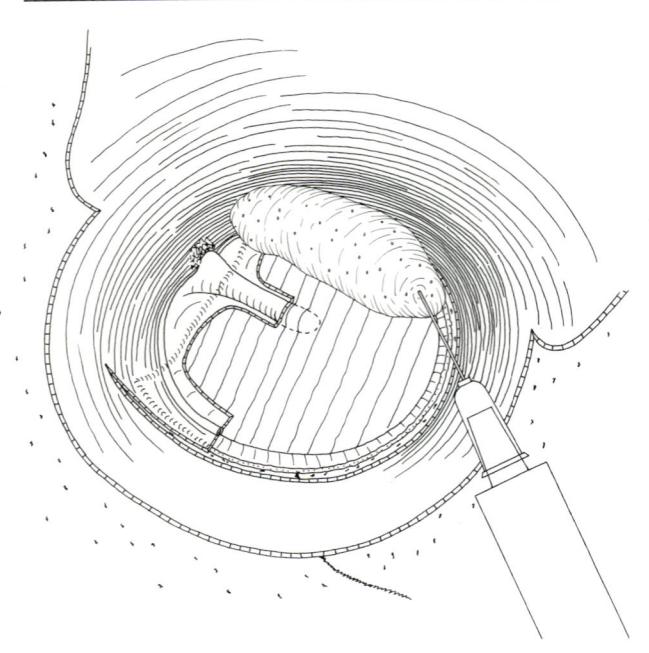

Fig. 425 Autogenous fibrin glue fixation onlay fascia graft in a total perforation

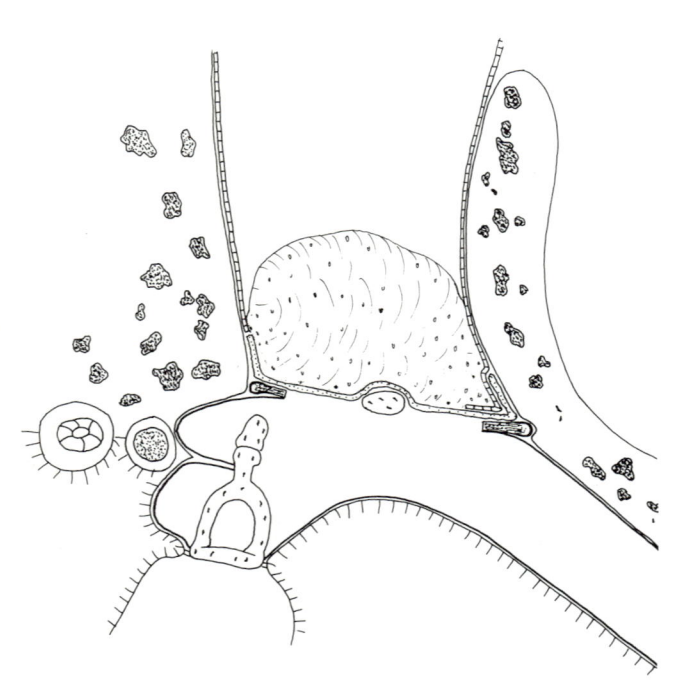

Fig. 426 A side view illustrates the autogenous fibrin glue clot covering the medial third of the ear canal

Allogenous Fibrin Glue

Commercially available allogenous fibrin glue (Tisseel or Tissucol, Immuno Company, Vienna) was later introduced into tympanoplasty (Panis et al. 1978, Panis and Rettinger 1979) with favorable results for graft take rates (Strauss 1979). The two components of the commercially available fibrin sealant are mixed before use, and can be applied separately using two separate syringes, one containing a Tisseel–aprotinin solution, and the other a thrombin–calcium chloride solution. The advantage of this method is that the graft is not glued before the second mixture is applied. Another possibility is using a specially-constructed double-syringe system (Duploject) (Fig. 427). The two components come together in a common application needle, and the fibrin glue attaches the fascia to the edge of the perforation immediately after application.

Fibrin glue is especially popular in underlay techniques for fixation of the anterior part of the graft to the anterior edge of the perforation, or to the anterior annulus (Fig. 428). In fixation of the underlay fascia using fibrin glue placed in the ear canal, placement of Gelfoam in the tympanic cavity can be totally avoided, which is an advantage.

The use of fibrin glue has been reported in every aspect of tympanoplasty: for fixation of the drum and ossicles or grafts, for fixation of the flaps in reconstruction of the ear canal, in cavity obliteration, and in mixtures with bone pate, bone chips, or hydroxyapatite granules. Some of these applications are mentioned in the second volume of this book.

Yuasa et al. (1922) use subcutaneous tissue and fibrin glue to close small drum perforations as a simple ambulatory myringoplasty method. Connective tissue obtained from the retroauricular region is placed inside the perforation, and pulled out in order to ensure complete coverage of the perforation. The graft is fixed with fibrin glue (Figs. 429, 430). Since no packing is necessary either in the middle ear cleft or in the external ear canal, the air–bone gap decreases immediately after the operation. The overall take rate for these small perforations was 79%.

Since it was already shown in 1977 that results with fibrin glue are no better than with Gelfoam graft fixation, the present author has not used fibrin glue in tympanoplasty. We use it routinely for closure of the dura in acoustic neuroma surgery, but here, too, we have found no statistically significant reduction in postoperative CSF leakage using fibrin glue in comparison with other methods (Tos and Thomsen 1985).

Fibrin Glue in Tympanoplasty

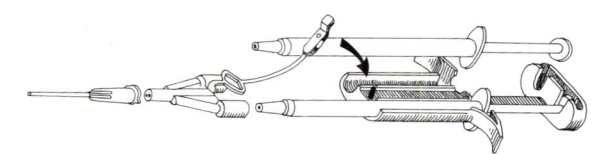

Fig. 427 The Duploject system, with two syringes and one application needle

Allogenous fibrin glue is biologically compatible, and has adequate tensile strength. It is isolated from pooled plasma, so that the risk of viral hepatitis and acquired immune deficiency syndrome (AIDS) cannot be entirely excluded. For this reason, the use of Tissucol has not been approved in the United States. Some American otologists therefore use autogenous fibrin glue, and the previously used method of preparing autogenous fibrin glue has once again become current.

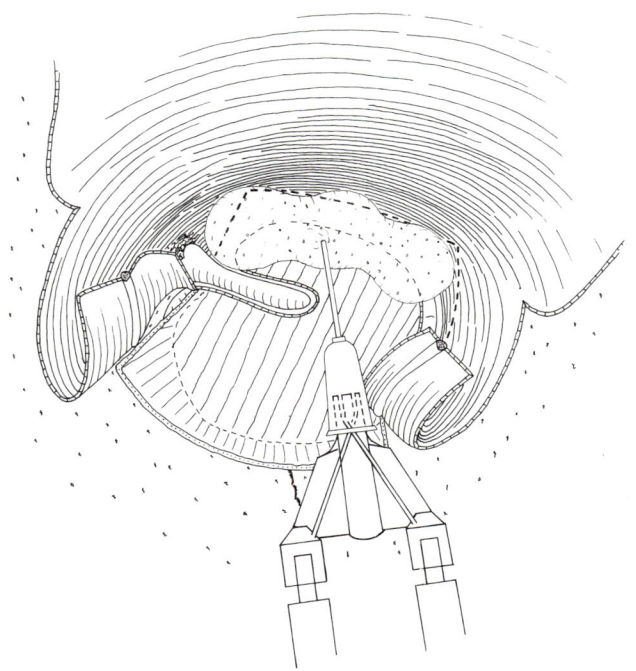

Fig. 428 Fixation of an underlay-placed fascia to the edges of the perforation in the anterior tympanomeatal angle, using allogenous Tisseel

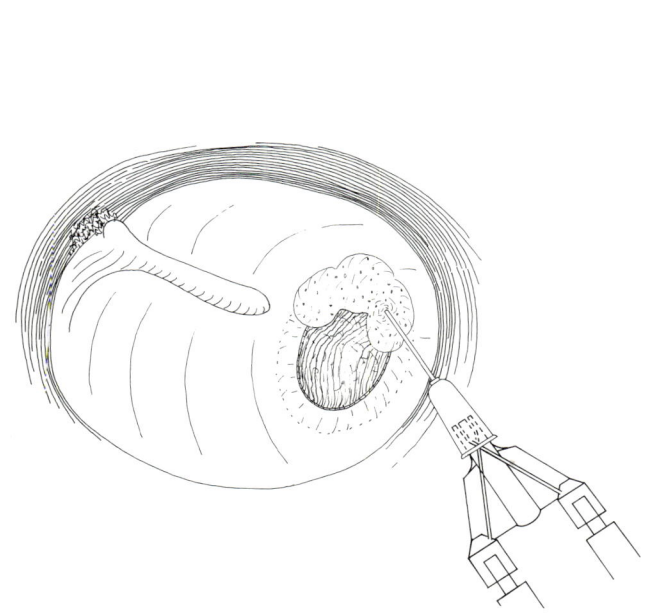

Fig. 429 **The Yuasa method** of underlay grafting for small perforations, with subcutaneous tissue pulled out of the perforation and fixed using allogenous fibrin glue

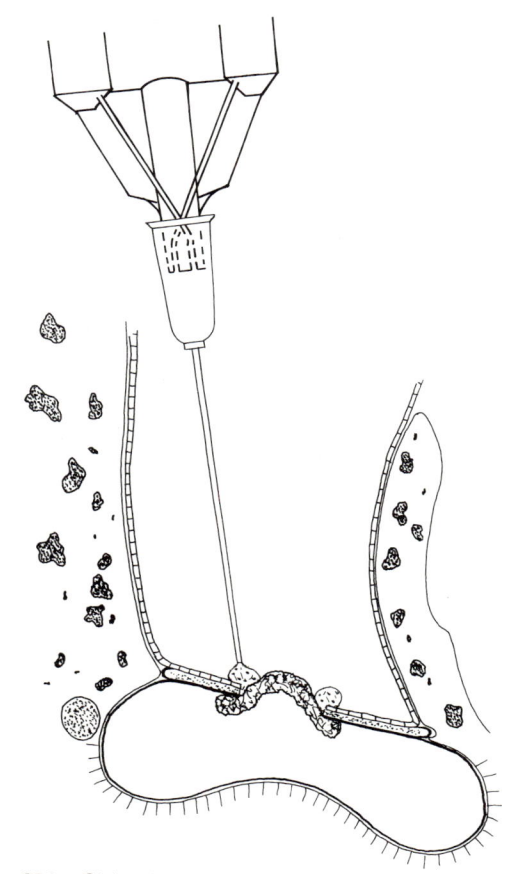

Fig. 430 Side view, illustrating the position of the graft

10 Onlay Techniques

As mentioned above, onlay techniques can be divided into:

1. Techniques with removal of the epithelium without covering of the graft.
2. Techniques with skin flaps covering the grafts.
3. Sandwich techniques.

Techniques with Removal of the Epithelium

In the early period of myringoplasty, using split-skin grafts and ear-canal skin grafts, only onlay techniques were employed, and these involved total removal of the drum epithelium. With increasing use of mesodermal grafts, a combination of removal of the keratinized epithelium and epithelial flaps has increasingly been used, but the principles of total removal of the epithelium are still used in some types of perforation.

Anterior Perforation

All the epithelium around the perforation, along with a small strip of ear-canal skin just lateral to the annulus, is removed, starting with elevation of the epithelium just behind the malleus handle (Fig. 431). The malleus handle is cleaned, and the epithelium is elevated toward the edge of the perforation (Fig. 432). The epithelium is dissected from the edge of the perforation without excising the edge, and without enlarging the perforation (Fig. 433). In the anterior ear-canal wall 1 mm lateral to the annulus, an incision is performed in the canal skin, and the flap is elevated down to the annulus. With double-cup forceps, the remnant of the epithelium and the elevated skin flap are removed completely (Fig. 434). The perforation is covered with semiwet or dry fascia, exactly fitted to the denuded area of the drum and the ear canal. The fascia is fixed using small Gelfoam balls (Fig. 435). There is no need for gelfoam in the tympanic cavity.

This technique can be used in the endaural approach with an ear speculum if the anterior ear canal is not prominent, and the anterior edge of the perforation is visible. If this is not the case, Heer-

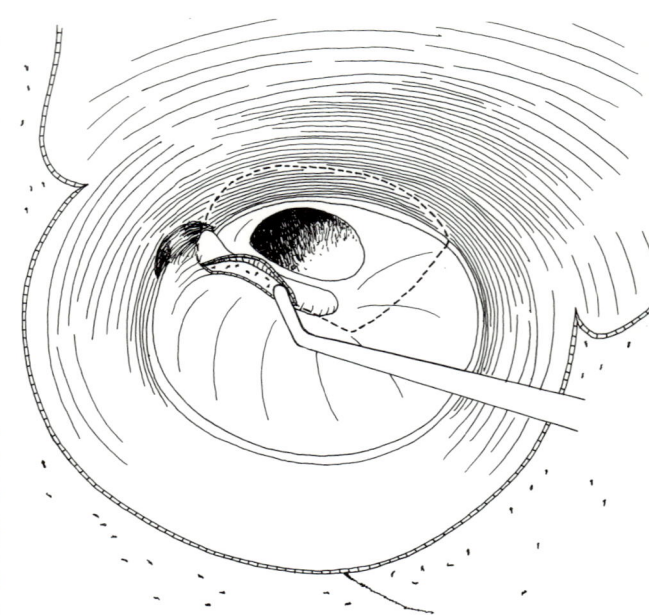

Fig. **431 Onlay technique with removal of the epithelium in an anterior perforation.** The drum epithelium is elevated from the malleus handle. The incision line is indicated by a dotted line

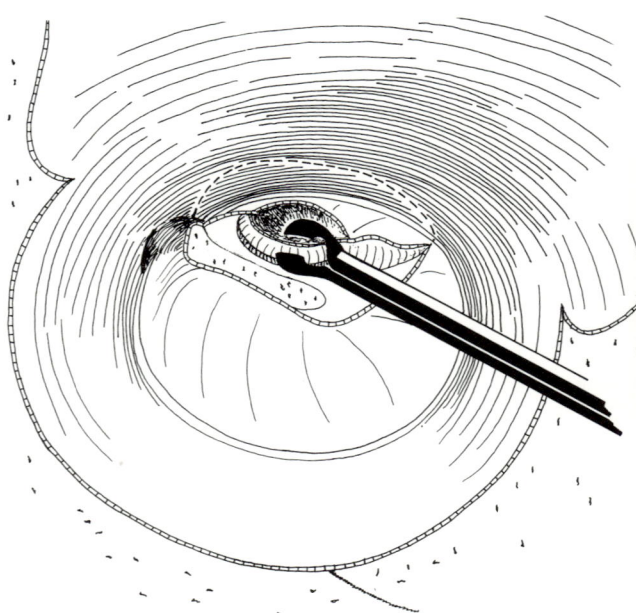

Fig. **432** The epithelium is elevated towards the posterior edge of the perforation, and the epithelial junction is visualized

Techniques with Removal of the Epithelium

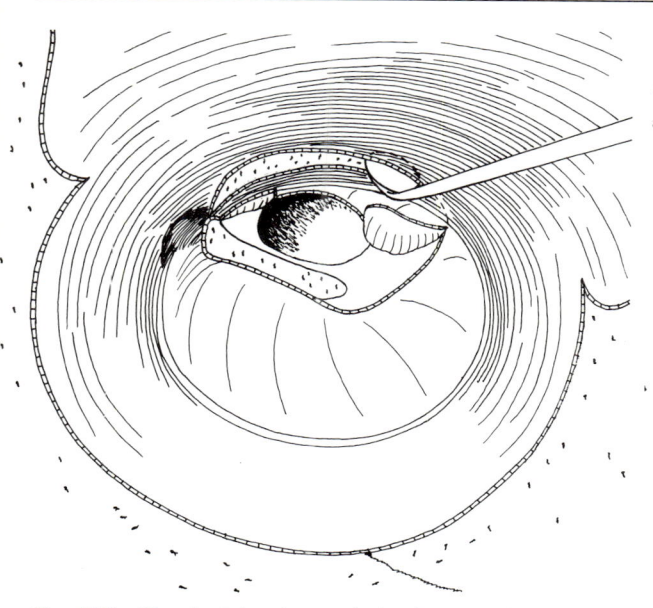

Fig. 433 The incision is made in the canal skin 1 mm lateral to the annulus, and the epithelium is elevated further

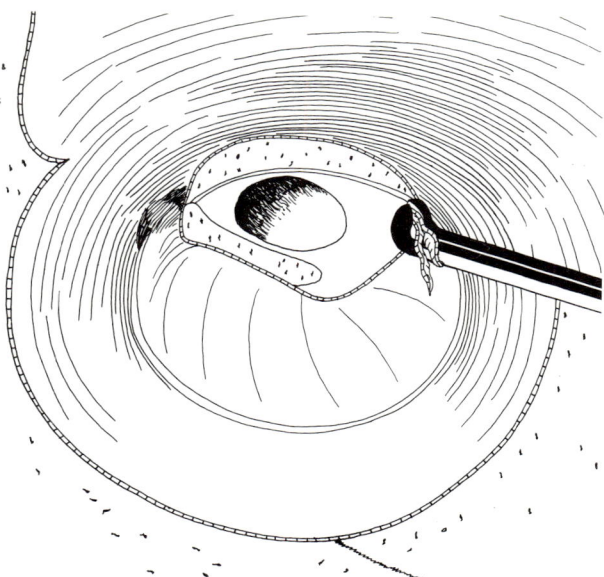

Fig. 434 All of the drum epithelium is removed

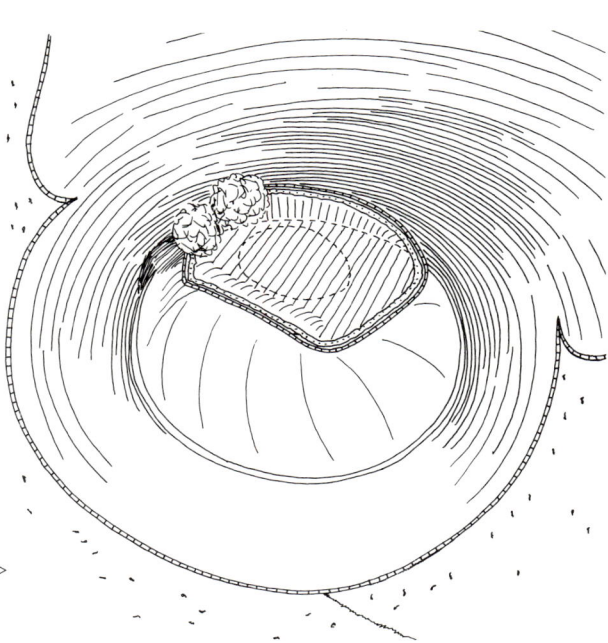

Fig. 435 The perforation and the denuded area around it are covered by fascia, carefully adapted to the epithelial edges

mann or other endaural incisions or, of course, the retroauricular approach can be carried out.

Inferior Perforation

The onlay technique with removal of the epithelium is an easy and safe technique in cases with inferior perforation and no need for inspection of the ossicular chain.

After an incision in the ear-canal skin 1 mm lateral to the annulus, the skin flap, together with the keratinized epithelium from the inferior drum remnant, is elevated. The epithelium is dissected from the edge of the perforation without resection of the lamina propria or enlargement of the perforation (Fig. 436). The epithelium is then elevated from the superior drum remnant (Fig. 437), as well as from the malleus handle. Finally, the epithelium

154   10   Onlay Techniques

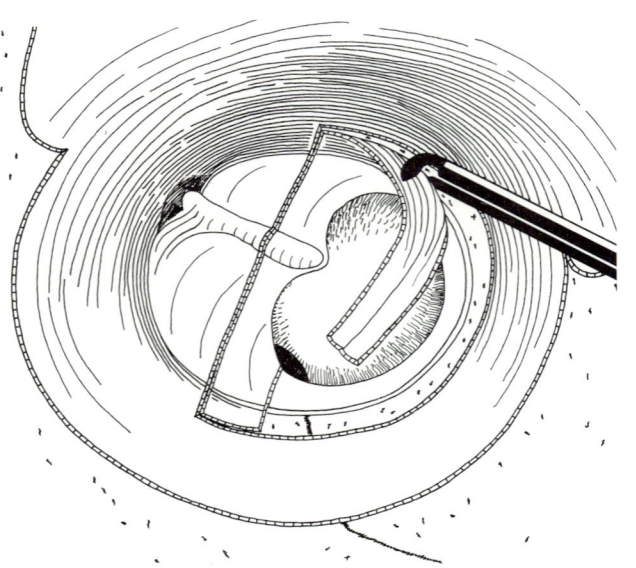

Fig. 436 **Onlay technique with removal of the drum epithelium in a large inferior perforation.** The skin is incised 1 mm lateral to the annulus. The skin flap and the epithelium from the drum remnant are removed

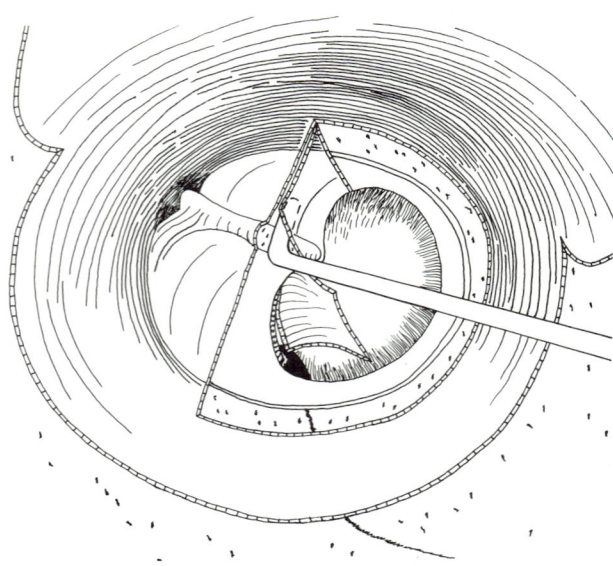

Fig. 437 The drum epithelium is removed from the posterosuperior area of the drum, and the epithelium is elevated from the malleus handle and umbo

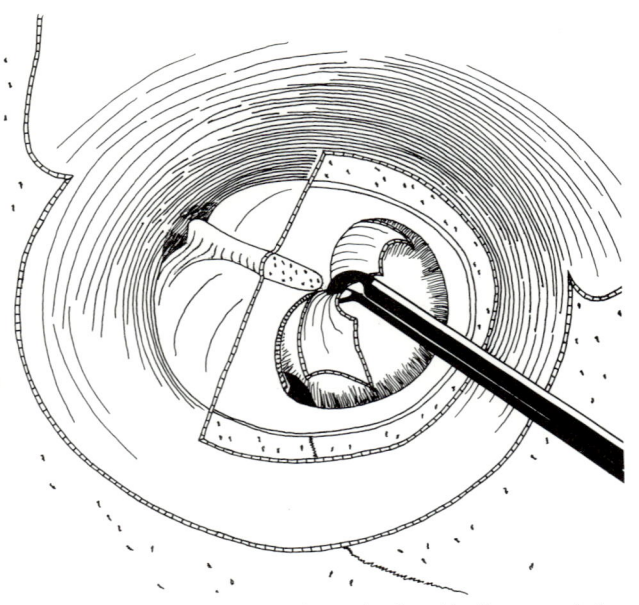

Fig. 438 The umbo is cleared of epithelium, and the epithelium is removed from the anterosuperior edge of the perforation with forceps

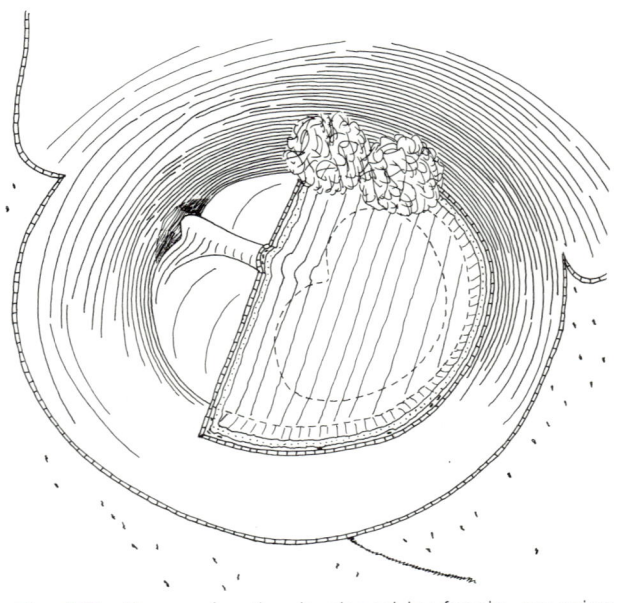

Fig. 439 The perforation is closed by fascia, covering the annulus and the denuded bone and carefully adapted to the epithelial edges. The fascia is covered with Gelfoam balls

is carefully cleaned and removed from the umbo (Fig. **438**), and the undersurface of the umbo is inspected for possible remnants of keratinized epithelium. The perforation is covered by an onlay fascia graft (Fig. **439**), and fitted to the annulus and to the skin incision around the annulus. The fascia is fixed with Gelfoam balls, starting anterosuperiorly in the tympanomeatal angle. There is no need for Gelfoam packing of the tympanic cavity if the perforation is not too large.

These techniques can be performed with any approach, but the simplest approach is an endaural one with an ear speculum. Larger inferior perforations or subtotal perforations can be managed in the same way. In cases with smaller inferior perforations, there is no need to perform an incision in the ear-canal skin. It is enough to elevate and remove the epithelium around the perforation as far as the fibrous annulus, but an incision in the epithelium just at the annulus will be very helpful to get into the proper cleavage plane between the lamina propria and the epithelium.

Total Perforation

Techniques with total removal of the skin in total perforations are nowadays seldom used. Incisions are made in the ear-canal skin all the way around the drum, about 1 mm lateral to the annulus (Fig. 440). The ear-canal skin flap and the epithelium from the drum remnant are elevated and removed, as is Shrapnell's membrane (Fig. 441). The malleus handle is carefully cleared of keratinized epithelium on both sides, and the incudostapedial joint is inspected. After the tympanic cavity has been filled with Gelfoam balls, the wet fascia is placed on the malleus handle and on the denuded bone (Fig. 442). Care should be taken to cover the Shrapnell's membrane area with the fascia. The fascia is fixed with small, solid Gelfoam balls placed on the border between the skin and the fascia, starting anterosuperiorly in the tympanomeatal

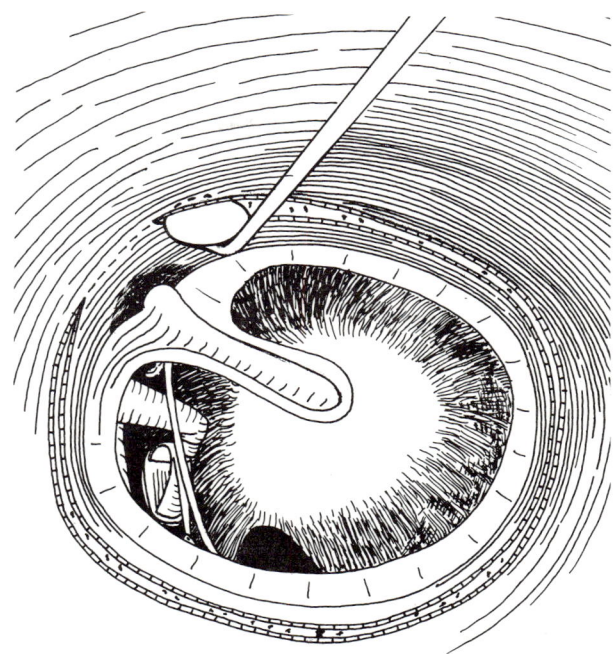

Fig. 440 **Onlay technique with removal of the drum epithelium in a total perforation.** The incision is made all the way round about 1 mm lateral to the annulus. The incision is continued to the attic region, about 1 mm lateral to Shrapnell's membrane

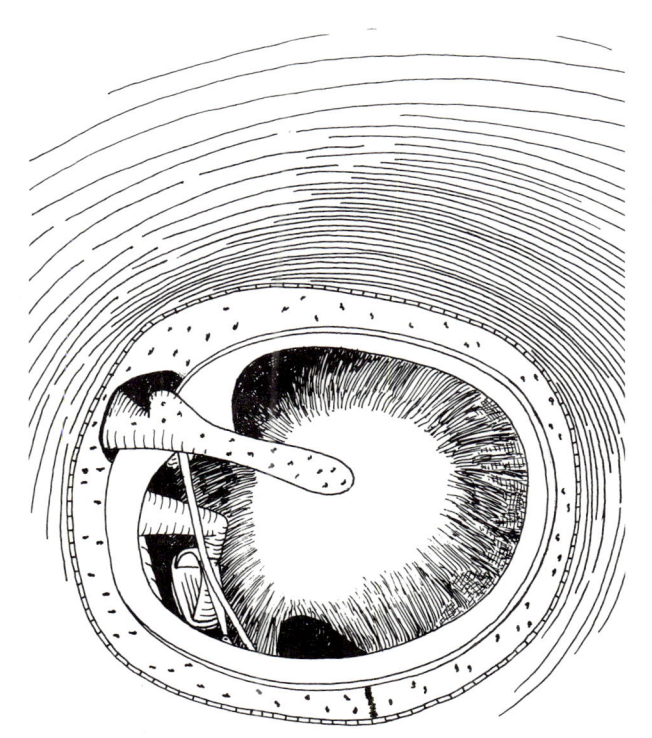

Fig. 441 The annulus, drum remnant, and malleus are cleared of keratinized epithelium, as well as the Shrapnell's membrane region

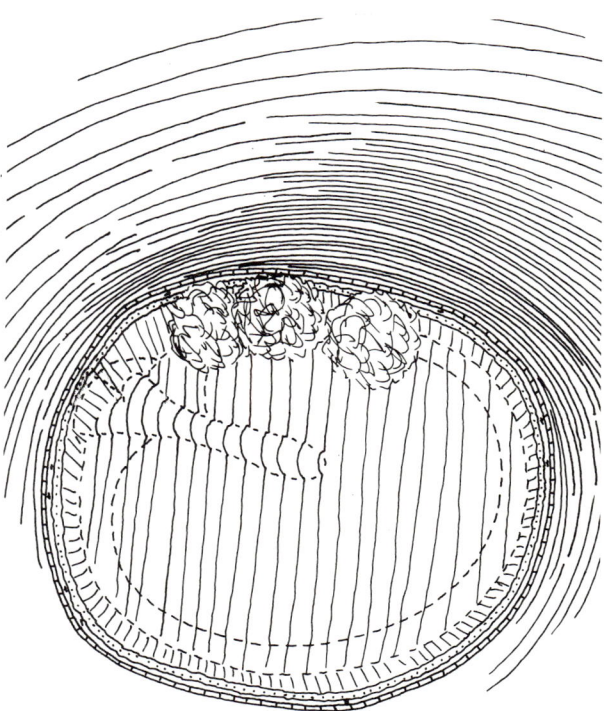

Fig. 442 All the drum region, including the annulus and the bone, are covered by fascia, approximated to the epithelial edges. Fascia is placed on the malleus, carefully fixed with Gelfoam balls

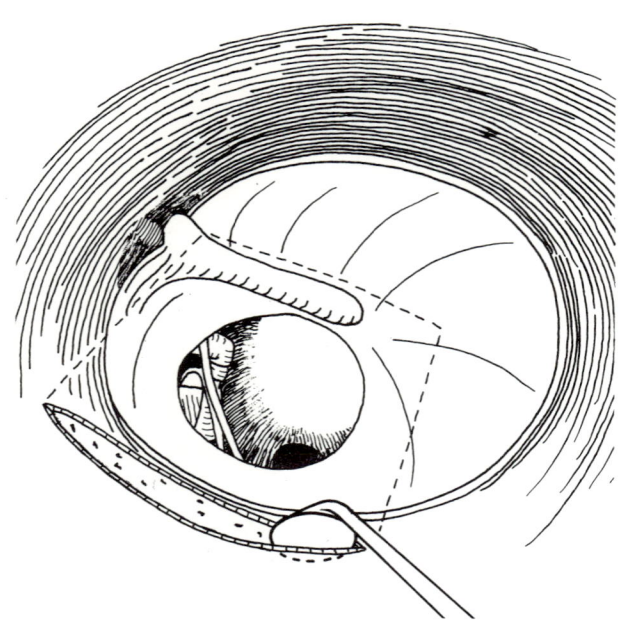

Fig. 443 **Onlay technique with removal of drum epithelium in a posterior perforation.** The incision is 2 mm lateral to the annulus. The course of the epithelial incision on the drum is indicated by a dotted line

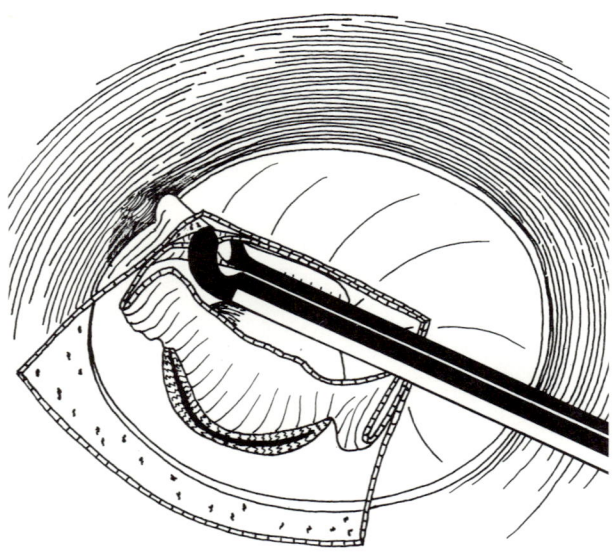

Fig. 444 The skin from the posterior bony annulus is elevated as far as the posterior edge of the perforation, and the epithelial junction is visible

angle, and continuing all around the ear canal. Firm pressure on the umbo with a Gelfoam ball should prevent lateralization of the graft.

This method is a relic of myringoplasty with split-thickness skin grafts, which was the first myringoplasty operation performed. Today, the author would definitely use small skin flaps superiorly (the method described below, pp. 170–173) instead of removal of the epithelium around the anterior and posterior malleolar folds and Shrapnell's membrane.

Posterior Perforation

The onlay technique is relatively seldom used in posterior perforations, mainly because of the risk of leaving keratinized epithelium behind the graft. Since the posterior perforation most often occurs in atrophic retracted drums, remnants of the retracted membrane will still adhere to the incudostapedial joint, or there may be pexis to the stapes. In addition, a retraction may extend around the chorda tympani and along the posterior wall of the tympanic cavity. The remnants of previous retractions will still be present, and may not be discovered using an onlay technique.

Under special conditions, e. g., in a small recurrent posterior perforation, using the onlay technique with removal of the epithelium may be reasonable. Incision of the canal skin is performed 1 mm lateral to the annulus (Fig. 443). The ear-canal skin is elevated as far as the annulus, and elevation is continued towards the drum remnant and towards the posterior edge of the perforation (Fig. 444). It is important to inspect the junction between the keratinized epithelium and the mucosal epithelium to see whether there is a retraction or not. Often, the posterior edge of the perforation has to be excised in order to be certain of removing all the keratinized epithelium. Removal of the epithelium is continued from the malleus handle, elevating the epithelium with a small elevator or a double-cup forceps. Finally, the epithelium all around the perforation is removed (Fig. 445), and the perforation can be closed using dry or wet fascia placed on the malleus handle, denuded drum remnant, and denuded posterior bony annulus (Fig. 446). The fascia is fixed by Gelfoam balls, and reepithelialization is fast, provided no squamous epithelium has been left behind.

Closure of the posterior perforation is very much a procedure for the endaural approach with an ear speculum.

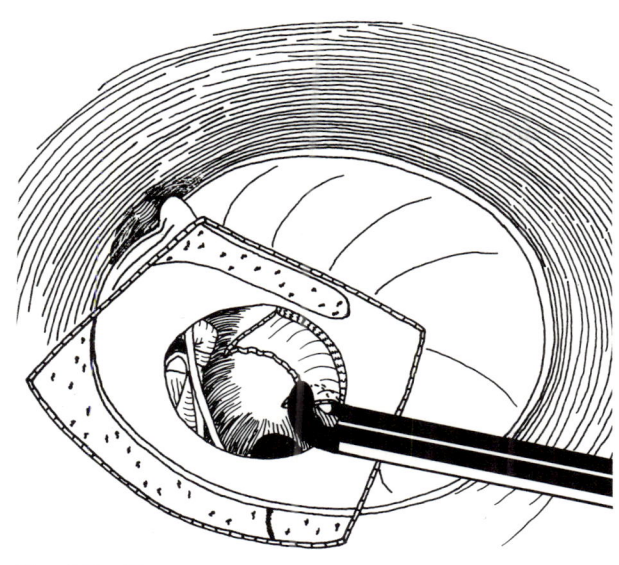

Fig. 445 The epithelium from the malleus handle is removed. The superior edge of the perforation is cleaned, and the epithelium at the inferior edge of the perforation is elevated

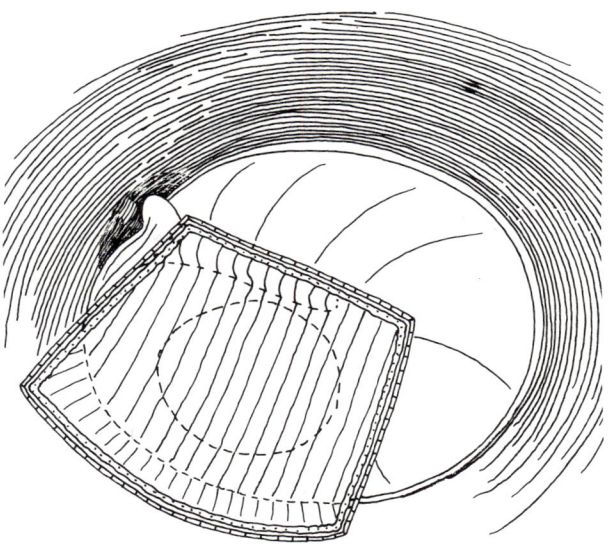

Fig. 446 The fascia covers the denuded area of the drum, including the bone

Onlay Techniques with Epithelial Flaps

In some techniques, the majority of the keratinized squamous epithelium is removed, and only a small epithelial flap is used. In other techniques, several epithelial flaps are made, and only a small part of the epithelium from the drum remnant is removed. The onlay technique with flaps always requires some improvisation in the procedure, but the intention of reducing the area to be epithelialized and securing proper epithelialization of the flap is clear. The author has always used, and will continue to use, the epithelial flap methods in all onlay techniques.

Anterior Perforation

The method used in anterior perforations is based on an *anterosuperior epithelial flap and a malleus flap*. The incision starts 1 mm lateral to the annulus (Fig. 447). Superiorly, the anterosuperior flap and the malleus flap are created. Inferiorly, the epithelium is elevated and removed. The elevation of the epithelium is directed towards the edges of the perforation (Fig. 448). With double-cup forceps, the epithelium is gradually removed from the edge of the perforation, with constant control of the epithelial junction. After cleaning of the inferior half of the perforation, the epithelium is elevated

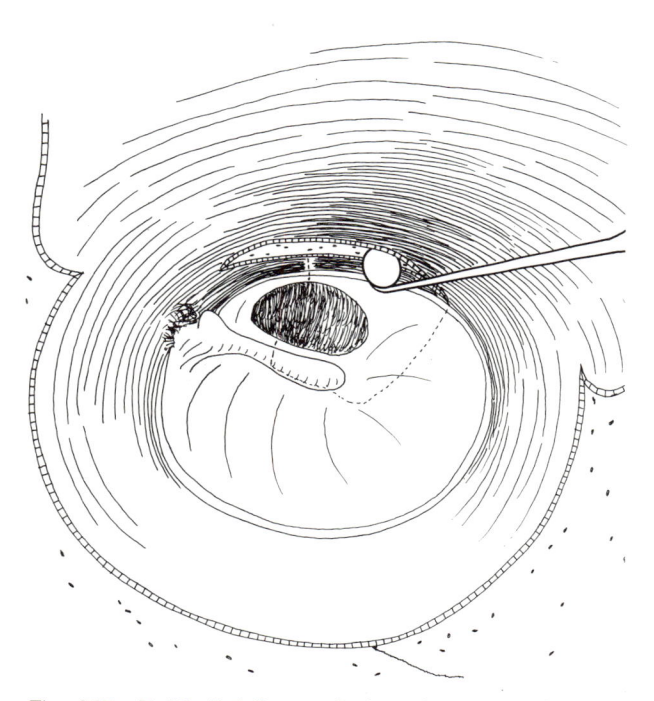

Fig. 447 **Epithelial flap technique in an anterior perforation.** An incision is made 1 mm lateral to the annulus

10 Onlay Techniques

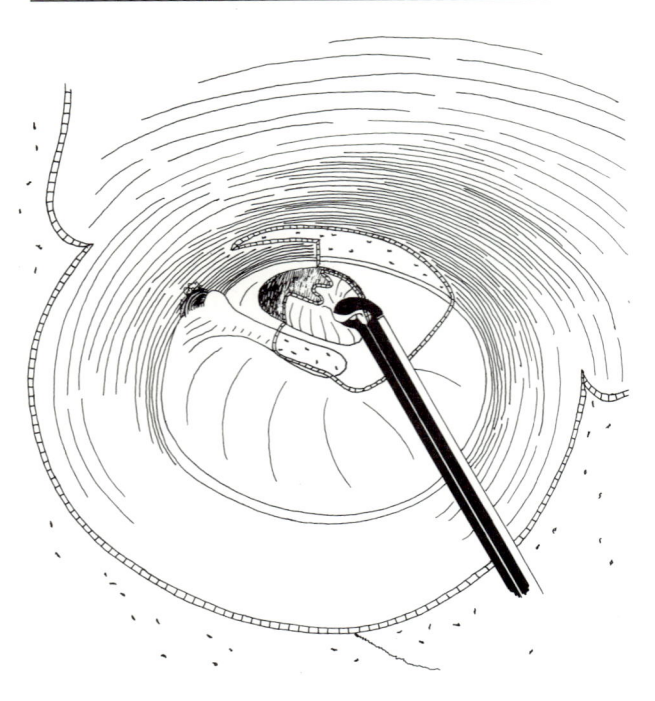

Fig. 448 The epithelium is elevated from the inferior part of the drum and the malleus handle, as well as from the inferior edge of the perforation

superiorly (Fig. 449), creating the malleus flap. The ideal situation is that both flaps, the anterosuperior skin flap and the malleus flap, are intact and large, and that the area of the denuded drum around the perforation, including the malleus handle, is large enough to support the graft (Fig. 450). The perforation is covered by a semiwet or dry fascia, fitted to the edges of the epithelium (Fig. 451). With a double-cup forceps, the superior flap and malleus flap are pulled over the fascia. Fixation of the flap is started superiorly with a Gelfoam ball, gently pressed in the inferior direction, providing further attachment of the fascia to the annulus (Fig. 452). The next Gelfoam ball is placed in the same way, gradually filling all the tympanomeatal angle and fixing the entire flap. The fixation of the malleus flap is performed by pushing Gelfoam balls from the short process of the malleus in an inferior direction, along the flap and malleus handle (Fig. 453).

Another onlay flap method is based on a large anterior meatal skin flap and *elevation of the flap together with the epithelium* from the drum remnant, creating a large epithelial flap. The skin incision is performed 4–6 mm lateral to the annulus (Fig. 454), depending on the approach to the ear

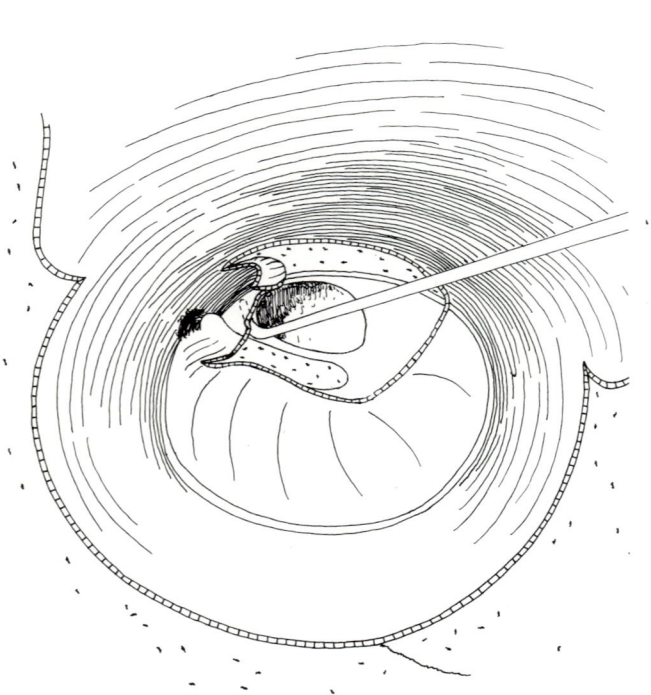

Fig. 449 The anterosuperior skin flap is elevated, and the epithelium from the anterior malleus fold is elevated

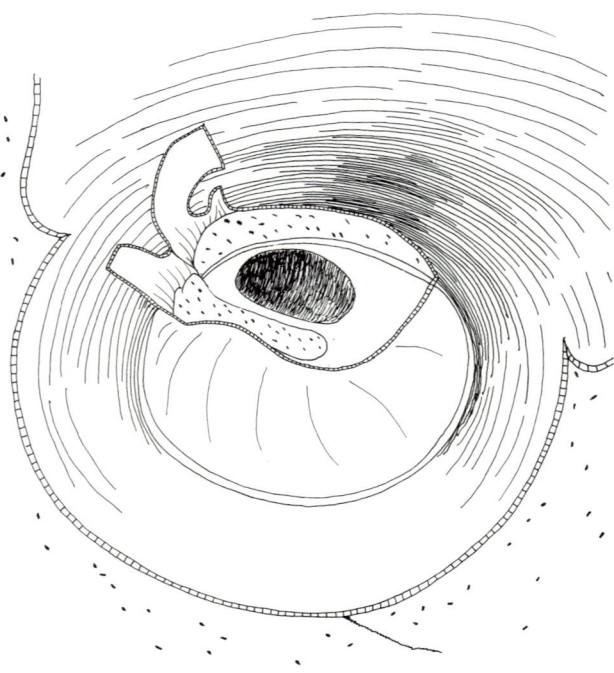

Fig. 450 The malleus flap and the anterosuperior skin flap are elevated, and the perforation is ready to be covered

Onlay Techniques with Epithelial Flaps 159

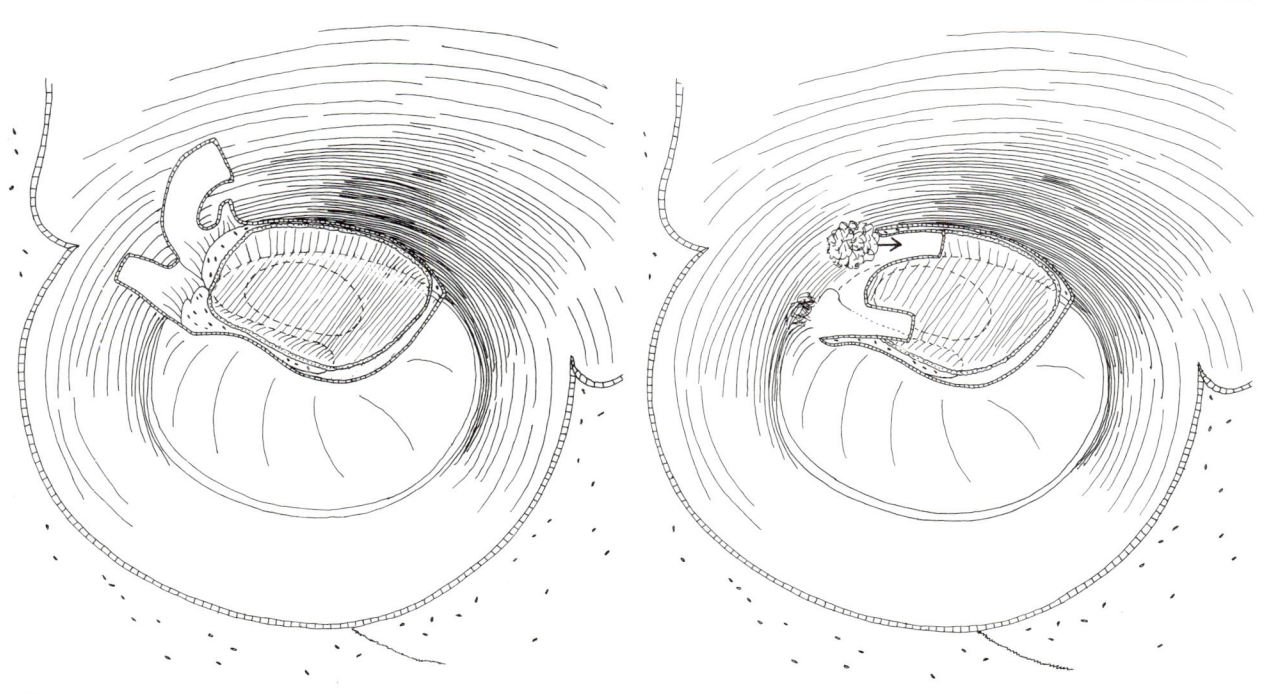

Fig. **451** Fascia is placed on the denuded area of the drum and bone

Fig. **452** The flaps are returned, and the anterosuperior flap is fixed with a Gelfoam ball, pressed in the inferior direction

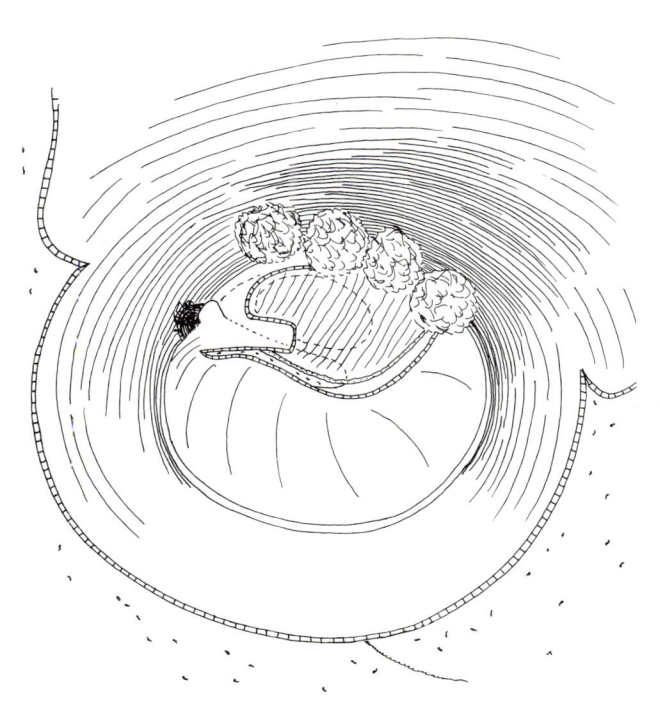

Fig. **453** Several Gelfoam balls fixing the fascia in the anterior tympanomeatal angle

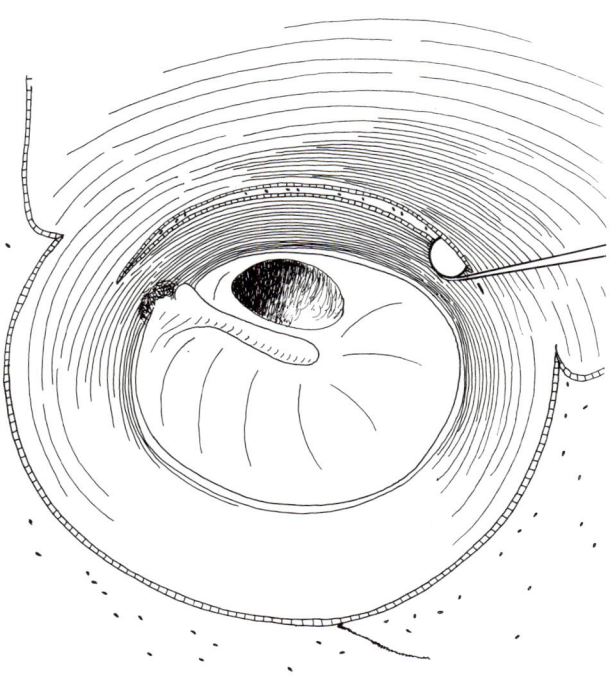

Fig. **454 Onlay technique with elevation of all epithelium in an anterior perforation.** A circumferential incision is made several millimeters lateral to the annulus

10 Onlay Techniques

canal used. The anterior tympanomeatal flap is elevated together with the epithelium of the drum (Fig. 455). Care is taken when dissecting the epithelium around the perforated edges, by visualizing the epithelial junction. With further elevation of the epithelium from the posterior edge of the perforation and the malleus handle, a sufficient area of the drum remnant is denuded (Fig. 456). The perforation and the denuded area are covered by the fascia. If the epithelial flaps are intact and large enough, the fascia does not need to be large (Fig. 457). The flaps are replaced (Fig. 458), and the fascia is covered and fixed by Gelfoam balls in the same way as described above (Fig. 453). The fixation along the anterior annulus should be firm, preventing any bluting.

The third technique is based on *cutting the anterior meatal skin flap,* a kind of anterior swing-door technique. After incision in the anterior wall 4-6 mm lateral to the annulus, the meatal skin flap is elevated to the anterior annulus (Fig. 459), and cut, leaving the drum epithelium remnant in place. The skin flap is then divided into an inferior and a superior flap (Fig. 460). This swing-door maneuver facilitates proper elevation and removal of the epithelium around the perforation, and further elevation of the epithelial flap from the malleus handle.

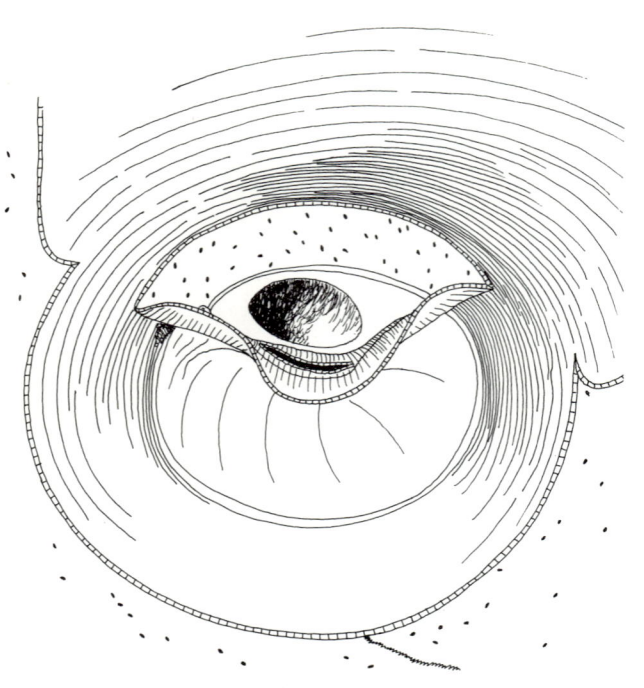

Fig. 455 The meatal flap is elevated together with the epithelium from the anterior half of the drum

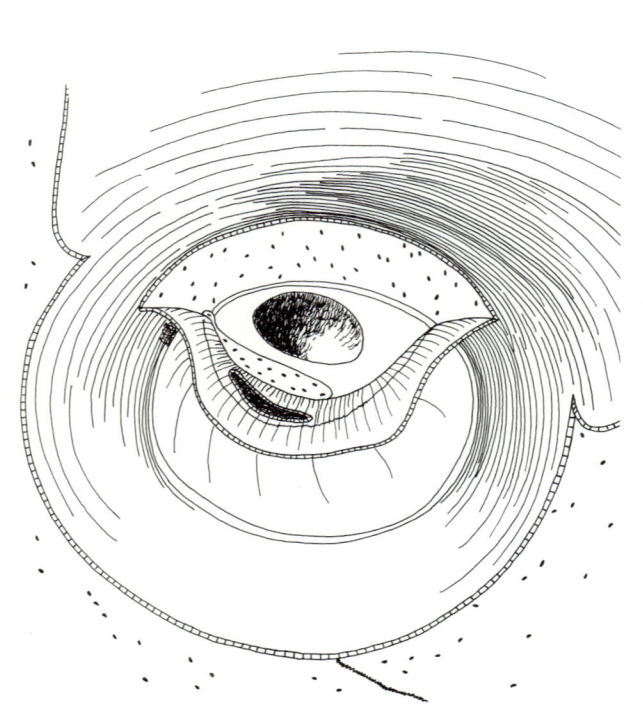

Fig. 456 The epithelium from the malleus handle is elevated, and the perforation is ready to be covered by fascia

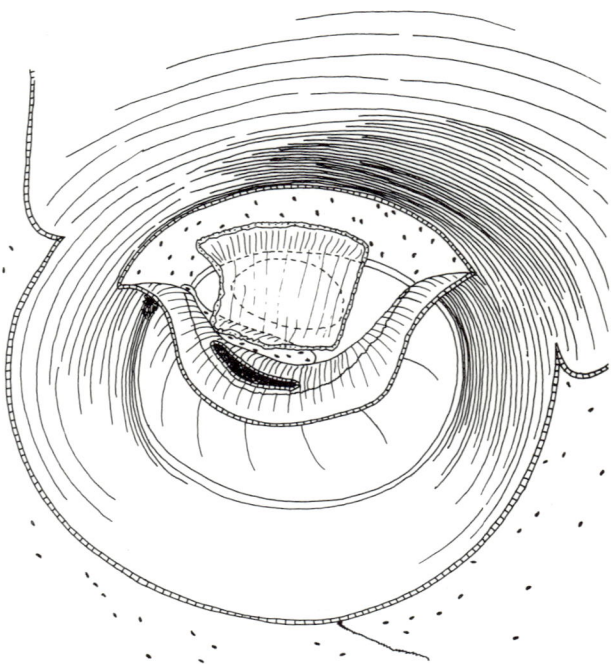

Fig. 457 The fascia covers the perforation

Onlay Techniques with Epithelial Flaps

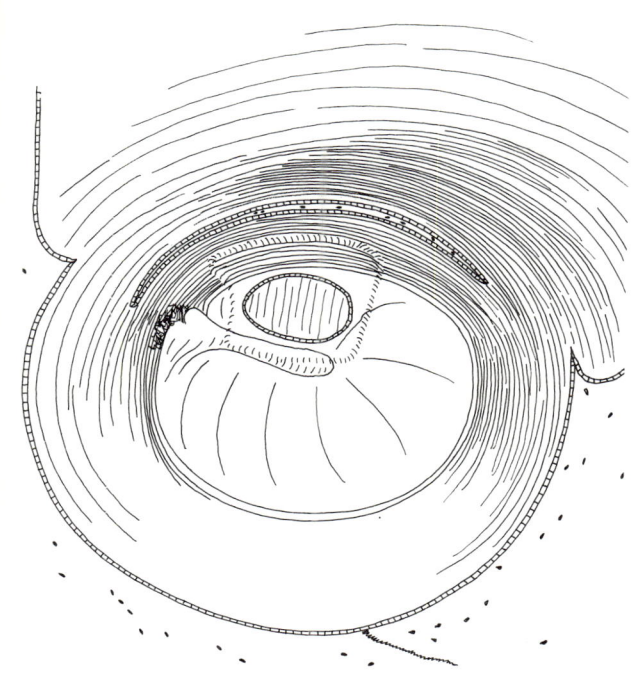

Fig. **458** The flaps are returned

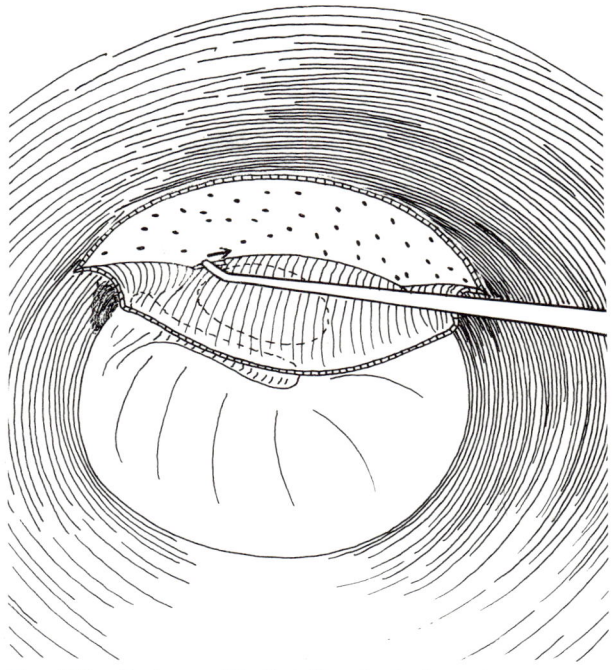

Fig. **459 Onlay epithelial flap technique in an anterior perforation.** A lateral incision of the canal skin is performed, and the meatal skin flap is elevated down to the annulus

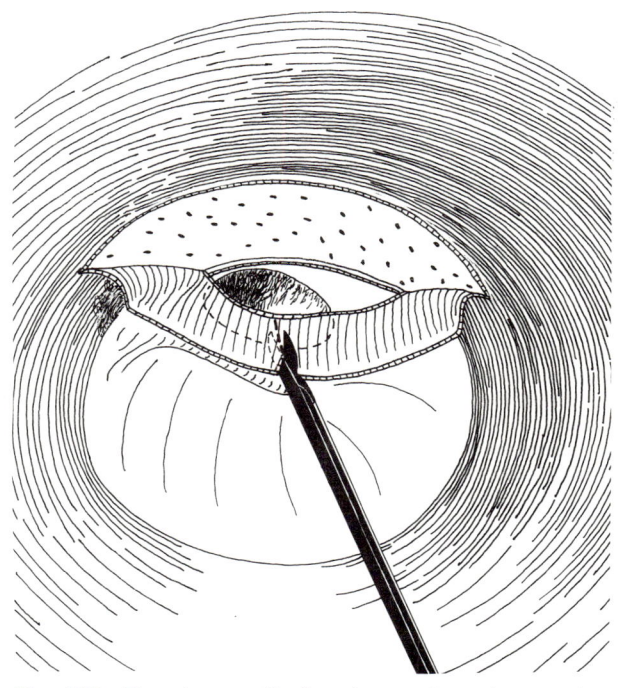

Fig. **460** The drum epithelium is cut along the annulus, and the skin flap is divided into a superior and an inferior flap

The perforation is covered by a small semiwet piece of fascia (Fig. **461**), and the flaps are turned back (Fig. **462**) and fixed by Gelfoam balls in a way similar to that described above.

In another modification, *the meatal skin flap is elevated* (Fig. **463**), *divided into a superior and an inferior part,* and all the epithelium from the drum and around the perforation is elevated and preserved as flaps (Fig. **464**). After the fascia has been placed, the flaps are returned (Fig. **465**) and fixed by Gelfoam balls. The difference between this method and the others is the extent of the removal of the epithelium around the perforation.

This method, with a large meatal flap, can be used in cases with a prominent anterior ear-canal wall with poor visualization of the anterior edge of the perforation. After removal of the prominent bone with a diamond burr, visualization can be improved. In cases with a prominent ear-canal wall, another method is described (Fig. **466**) with *outward elevation of the meatal skin flap* together with the drum-remnant epithelium, starting with a radial incision at the 11-o'clock and 4-o'clock positions, elevating the epithelium from the inferior part of the drum, continuing with elevation of the drum all around the perforation, and elevating the epithelium from the malleus handle (Fig. **467**), creating a poste-

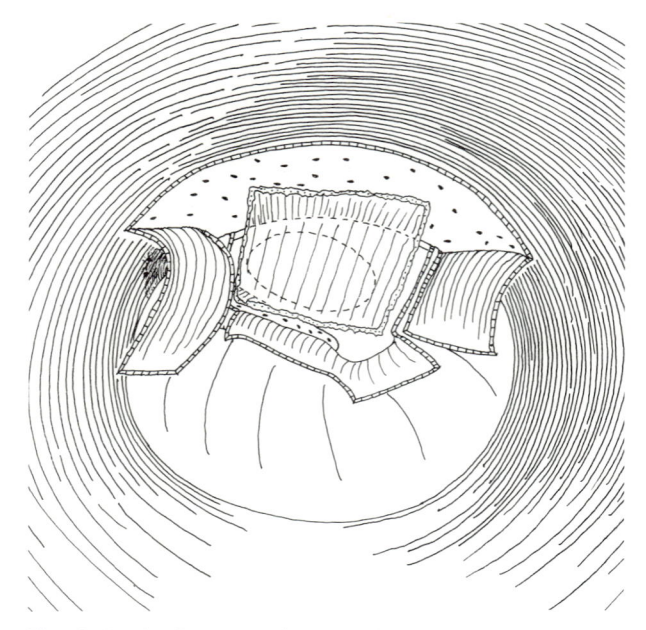

Fig. **461** A flap anterior to the malleus handle is created, and the epithelium is removed around the perforation, which is covered by a fascia graft

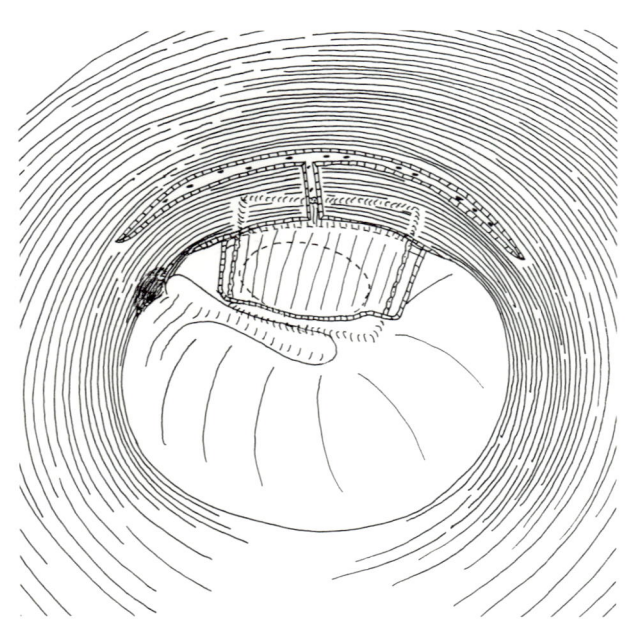

Fig. **462** The flaps are returned, covering the fascia

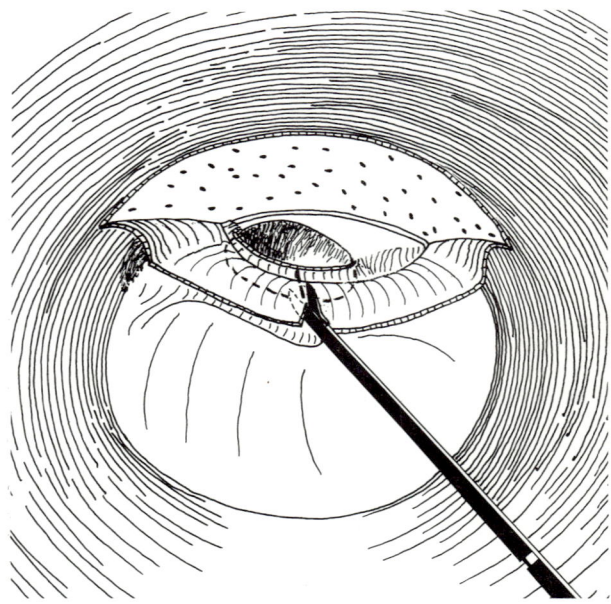

Fig. **463 Another modification of the onlay epithelium flap technique in an anterior perforation.** After elevating the meatal skin flap together with the epithelium from the drum remnant, the flap is divided into a superior and an inferior flap

Onlay Techniques with Epithelial Flaps

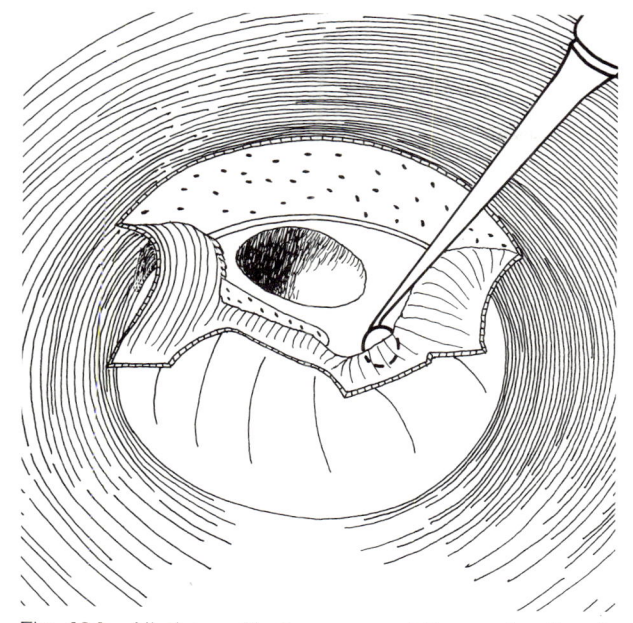

Fig. **464** All the epithelium around the perforation is elevated, and the edges of the perforations is cleaned

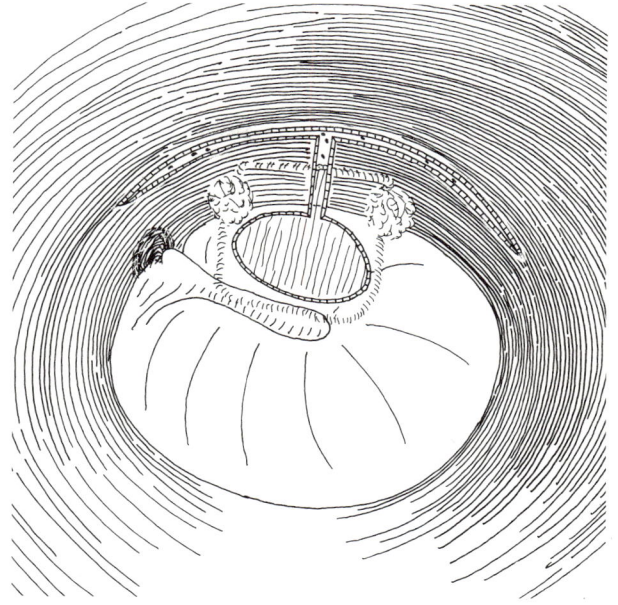

Fig. **465** The fascia covers the perforation, and the flaps are returned

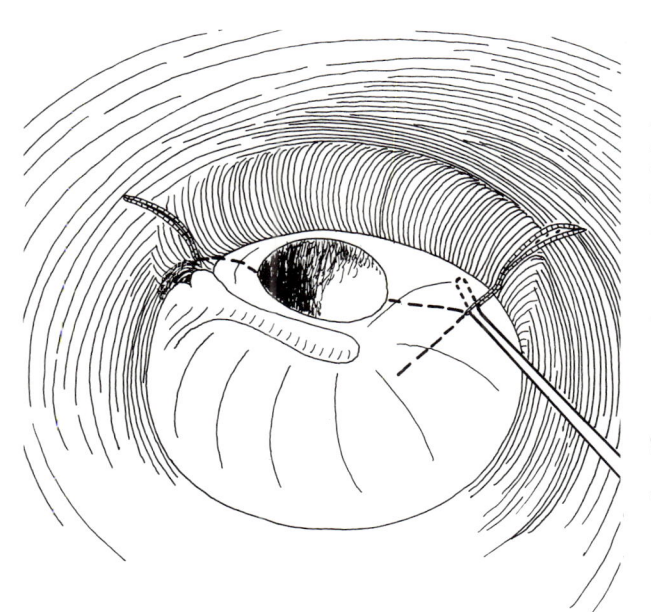

Fig. **466 Outward elevation of the skin flap in an anterior perforation.** Two radial incisions are performed, one at the 1-o'clock position, and the other at the 5-o'clock position. Epithelial incisions on the drum are indicated by dotted lines

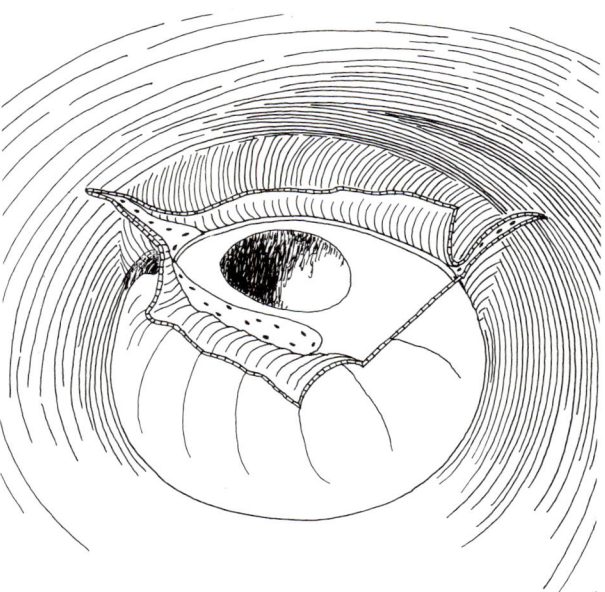

Fig. **467** The epithelium around the perforation is elevated, and the malleus handle is exposed

rior flap. The meatal skin flap is now further elevated outward, exposing the prominent ear-canal wall, which can be drilled with a diamond burr (Fig. **468**). After cleaning all the epithelium around the perforation, the semiwet or dry fascia is placed on the drum remnant, and partly on the denuded bone close to the annulus, and the flaps are turned back (Fig. **469**). They are fixed with Gelfoam balls (Fig. **470**). This method requires good visibility of the anterior edge of the perforation, and the outward elevation of the skin can only be performed with the retroauricular approach. The problems of a prominent ear canal in the endaural approach are illustrated below, and special methods for solving these problems are described.

Inferior Perforation

In inferior perforations, there are in principle two basic methods. One involves *partial removal of the epithelium,* making only posterosuperior and anterosuperior flaps, and the other involves elevating all the epithelium.

In the first method, the incision goes from the 9-o'clock to the 3-o'clock position 1 mm lateral to the annulus (Fig. **471**). The skin from the annulus and the posteroinferior drum remnant are carefully elevated and removed (Fig. **472**). Care is taken to visualize the epithelial junction, and the keratinized

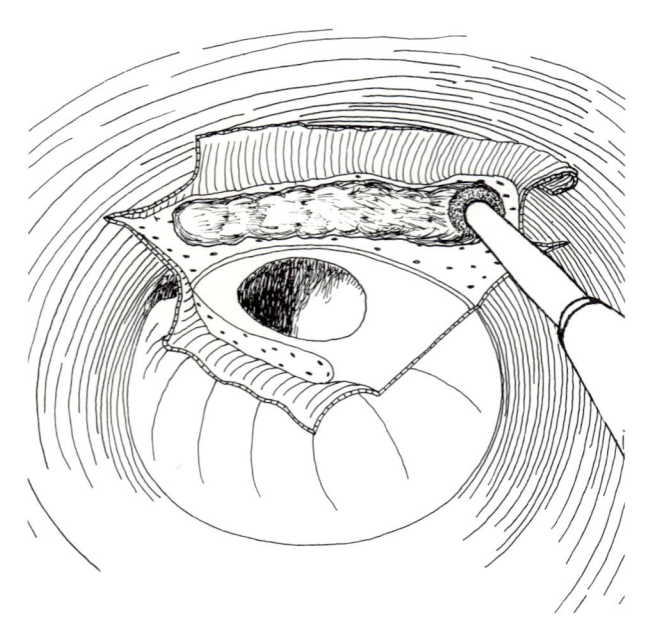

Fig. **468** The anterior canal skin is elevated, and the bulging bone is drilled away using a diamond drill

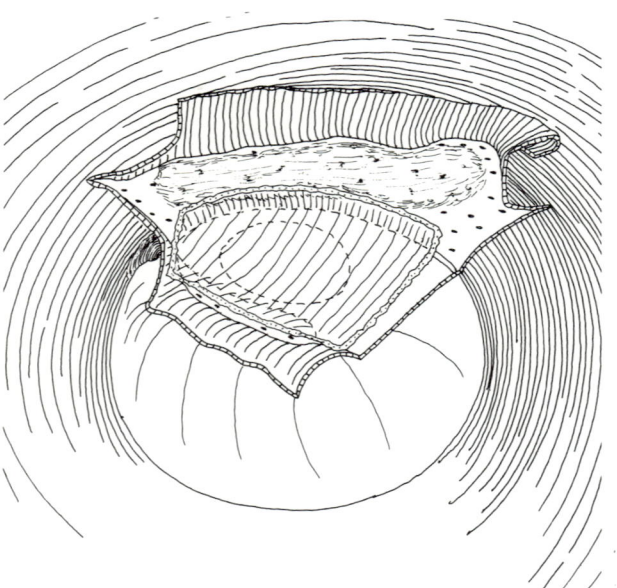

Fig. **469** The onlay graft covers the perforation

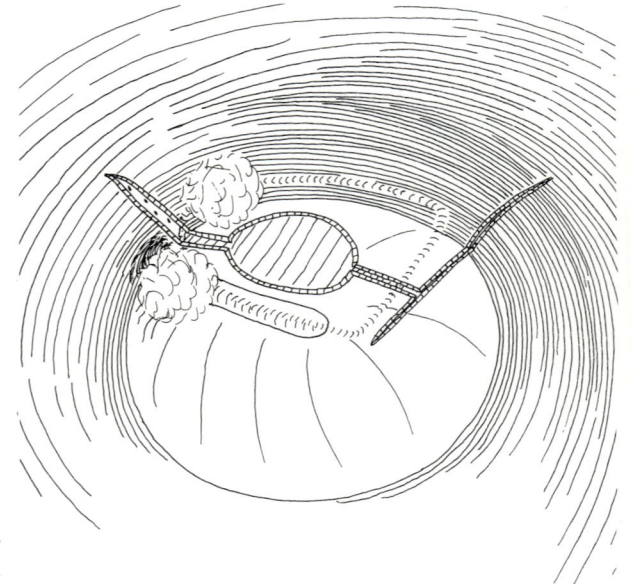

Fig. **470** The flaps are returned to the original position, and are fixed with Gelfoam balls

Onlay Techniques with Epithelial Flaps

epithelium is removed with a pair of curved double-cup forceps. All the annulus and the inferior drum remnant is cleared of keratinized epithelium. Superiroly, the epithelial flaps are created, as is a malleus flap (Fig. **473**). The size of the flaps varies, depending on the quality of the epithelium to be elevated and the thickness of the lamina propria. In large inferior perforations, some Gelfoam balls can be placed in the tympanic cavity. In smaller perforations, Gelfoam is not necessary. The perforation and denuded area of the drum is covered by fascia (Fig. **474**). The fascia is first fixed inferiorly by Gel-

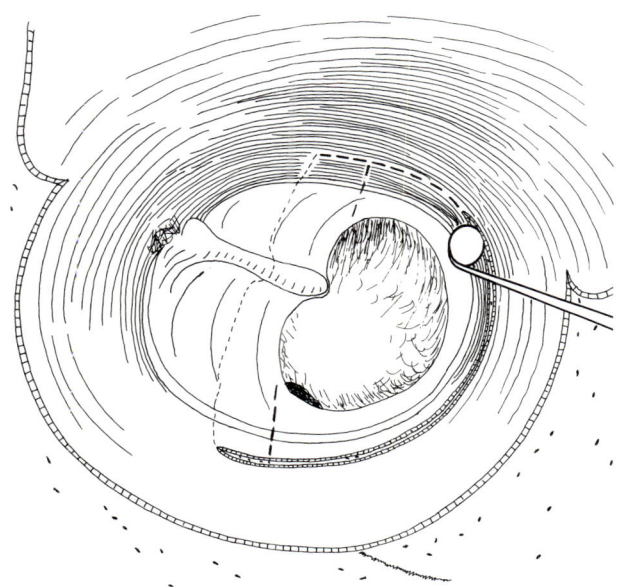

Fig. **471 Onlay epithelium flap technique in a large inferior perforation.** The skin is incised 1 mm lateral to the annulus from the 9-o'clock to the 3-o'clock position. The thin dotted line indicates the superior level of epithelial elevation, the thick dotted lines show the incisions of the drum epithelium

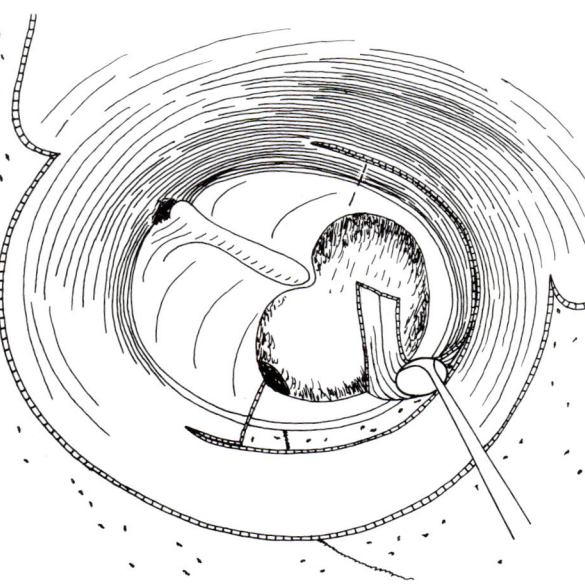

Fig. **472** The skin from the annulus and the bone, as well as the inferior drum remnant, is removed. The edge of the perforation is cleaned

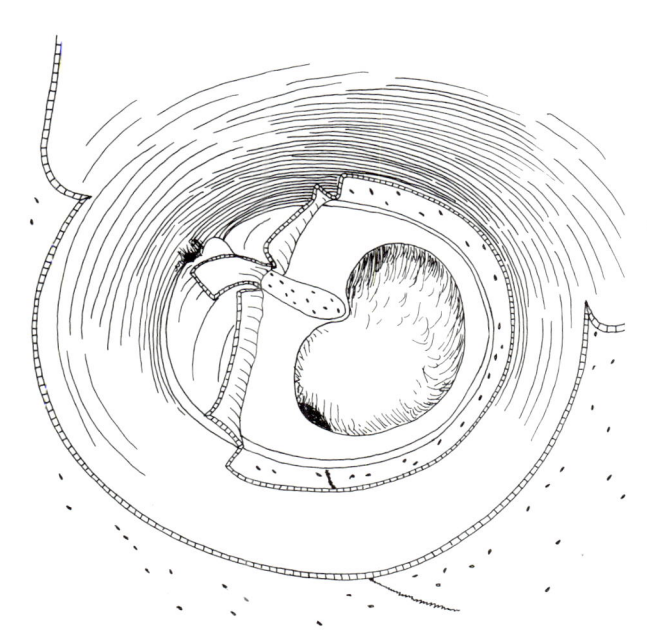

Fig. **473** Superiorly, the epithelium is elevated by creating two epithelial flaps

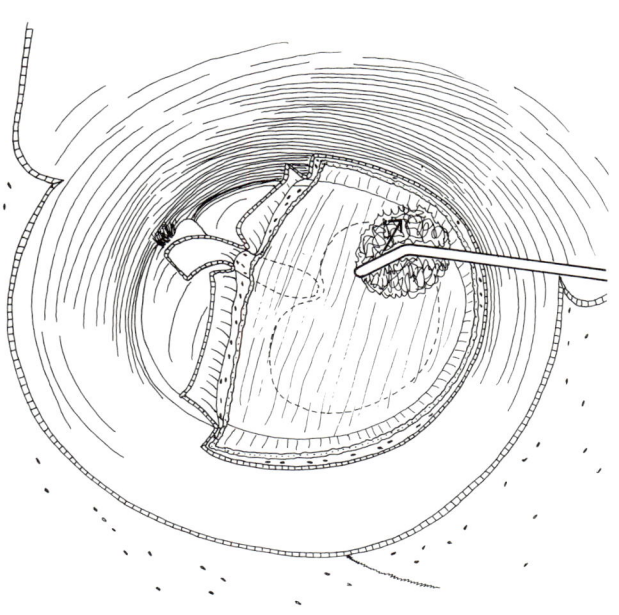

Fig. **474** The perforation is covered with a fascia graft

foam balls pressed onto the annulus and denuded bone. The flaps are then returned and fixed with further Gelfoam balls (Fig. **475**). After fixation of the anterior part of the fascia, a larger, firm Gelfoam ball is pressed onto the region of the umbo (Fig. **476**). Finally, the posterior half of the fascia is fixed.

This method is preferably performed with the endaural approach through the ear-canal speculum, but it can also be performed through other endaural approaches, or retroauricular approaches.

Another method is *elevation of a large meatal skin flap*, together with elevation of all the drum-remnant epithelium. An incision is made from the 9-o'clock to the 3-o'clock position at least 5 mm lateral to the annulus (Fig. **477**). A large meatal skin flap is elevated, and the bone is exposed. The epithelium from the drum remnant is elevated, with careful dissection of the epithelium around the perforation. Usually, there is no need for excision of the perforation edge. The epithelium around the perforation can easily be dissected away and an epithelial junction observed. The epithelium is further elevated superiorly from the malleus handle and the umbo (Fig. **478**). The fascia is placed on the annulus and drum remnant (Fig. **479**), and the epithelial flap, together with the meatal flap, is returned (Fig. **480**). The flaps are fixed by pressing Gelfoam balls along the annulus and along the edge of the perforation. In addition, a firm Gelfoam ball is pressed onto the umbo, providing good contact between the fascia and the umbo (Fig. **481**).

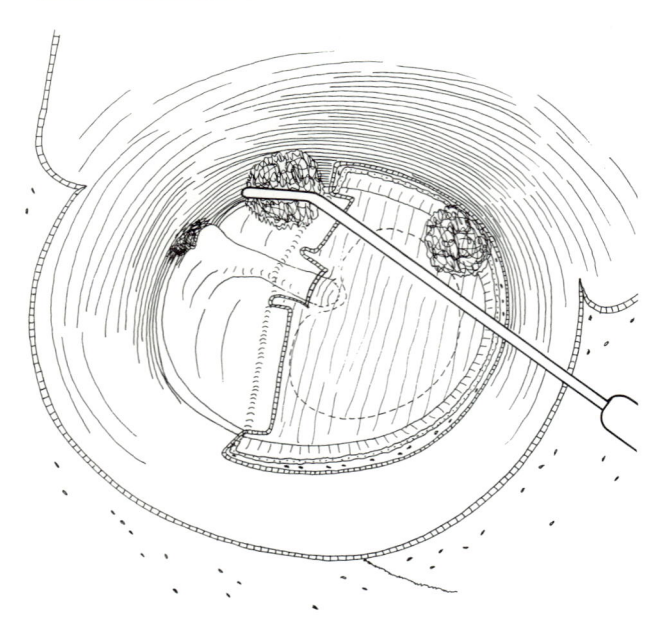

Fig. **475** The flaps are returned and fixed by Gel-foam balls

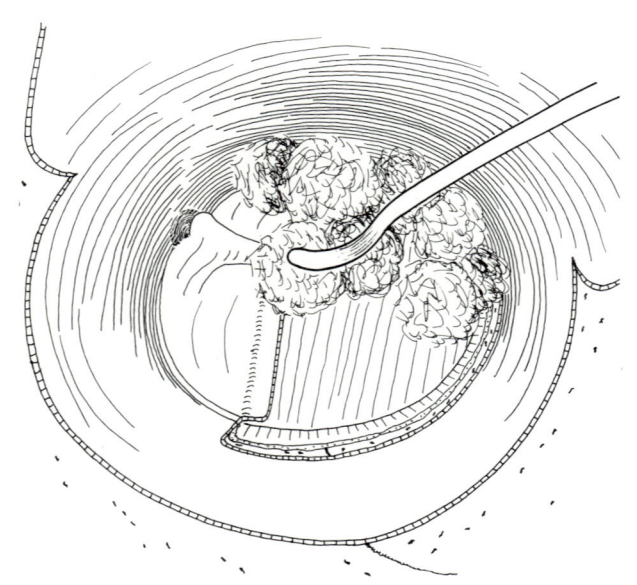

Fig. **476** Several Gelfoam balls are fixing the fascia in the tympanomeatal angle, and a large Gelfoam ball is pressing on the umbo

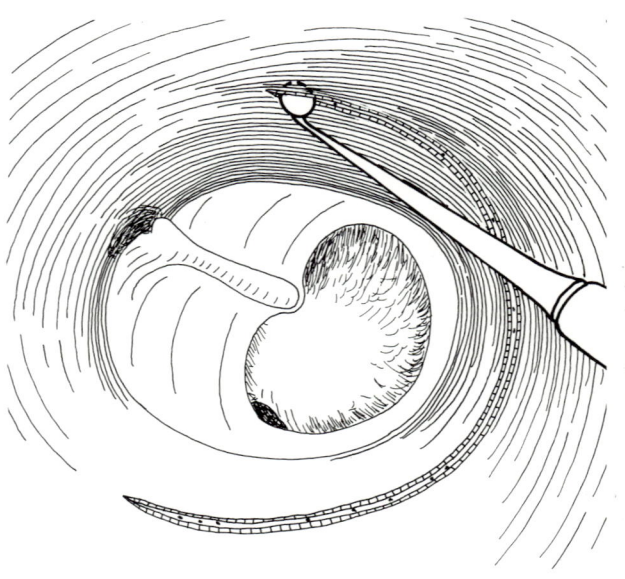

Fig. **477 Onlay epithelial flap technique with a large tympanomeatal flap.** An incision is made from the 9-o'clock to the 3-o'clock position several millimeters lateral to the annulus

Onlay Techniques with Epithelial Flaps

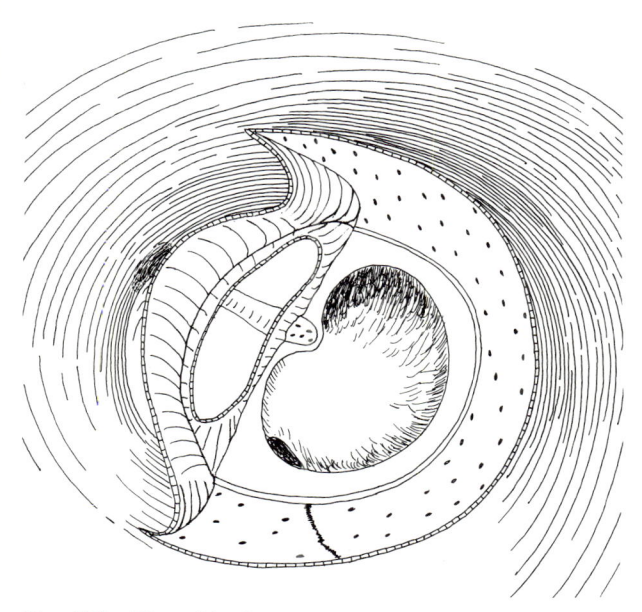

Fig. **478** The skin flap is elevated together with the epithelium from the inferior half of the drum. The umbo and the edge of the perforation are cleared of keratinized epithelium

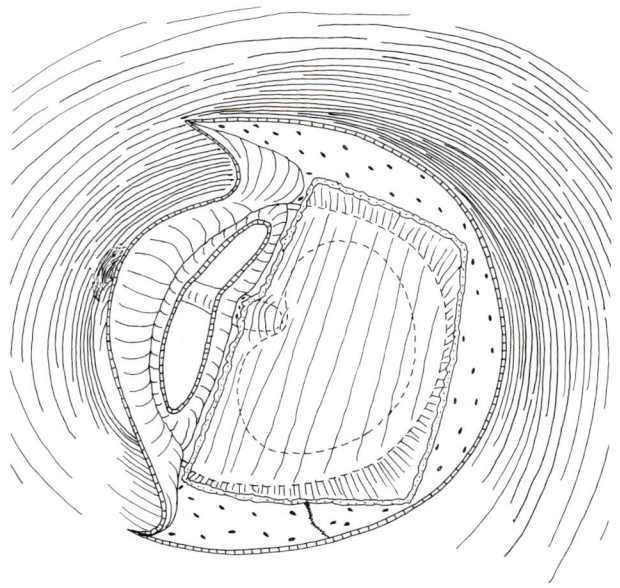

Fig. **479** Fascia covers the perforation and the denuded drum remnant

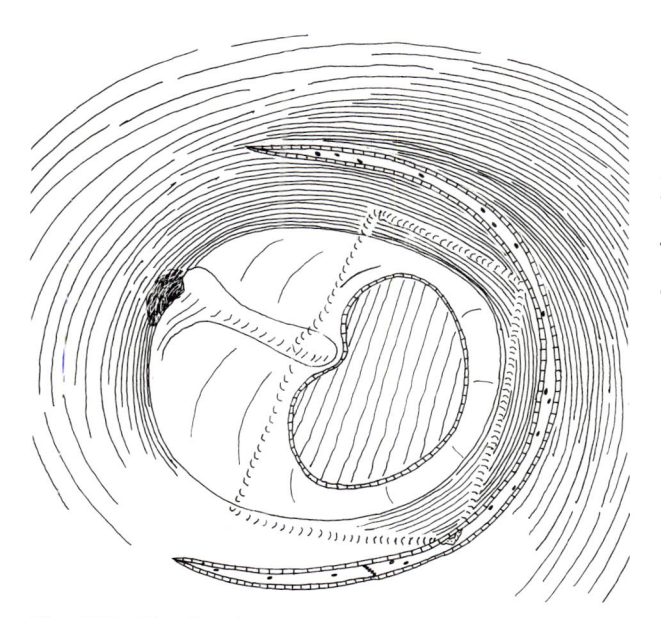

Fig. **480** The flap is returned

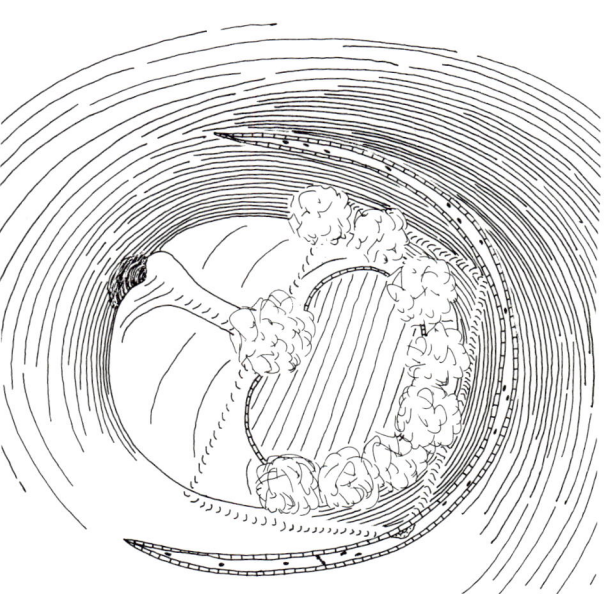

Fig. **481** The flap is fixed around the annulus with Gelfoam balls

10 Onlay Techniques

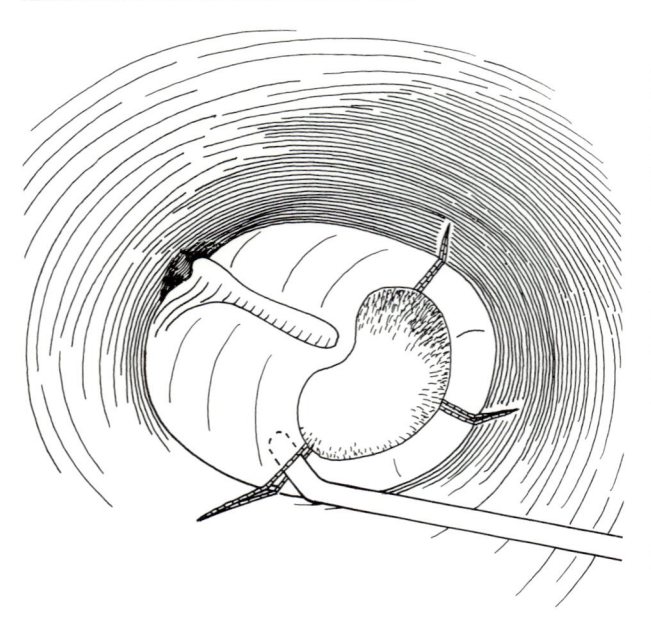

Fig. **482** **A technique with outward elevation of the epithelium in an inferior perforation.** Three radial incisions are performed, and the epithelium is elevated superiorly

A third method is *outward elevation* of the drum epithelium and the canal skin. With a sickle knife, radial incisions are made at the 9-o'clock, 6-o'clock, and 3-o'clock positions. The incisions run from the edge of the perforation to about 2 mm lateral to the annulus. With a small elevator, elevation of the skin flap superiorly is started (Fig. **482**), with care being taken when dissecting the epithelium from the edge of the perforation, especially at the umbo. After a large superior flap has been created (Fig. **483**), the outward elevation of the posteroinferior epithelial flap is started by a round knife. Finally, the anteroinferior skin flap is elevated outward by placing a curved rugine under the epithelium, and taking care over the edge of the perforation. The epithelium from the edge of the perforation should be elevated with the epithelial junction being controlled. The junction is first torn, and the epithelial flap is then elevated towards the annulus and further outward from the annulus (Fig. **484**). After outward elevation of all the flaps, the perforation edge is cleaned (Fig. **485**), and the perforation is covered by fascia and placed on the drum remnant and partly on the denuded bone (Fig. **486**). The flaps are returned to their original position, and can be fixed with several Gelfoam balls pressed onto the annulus all the way round the circumference of the drum (Fig. **487**). With this method, the usual elevation of the epithelium from the annulus toward the edge of the perforation is not possible. An excision of the perforation edge as a first step is therefore recommended.

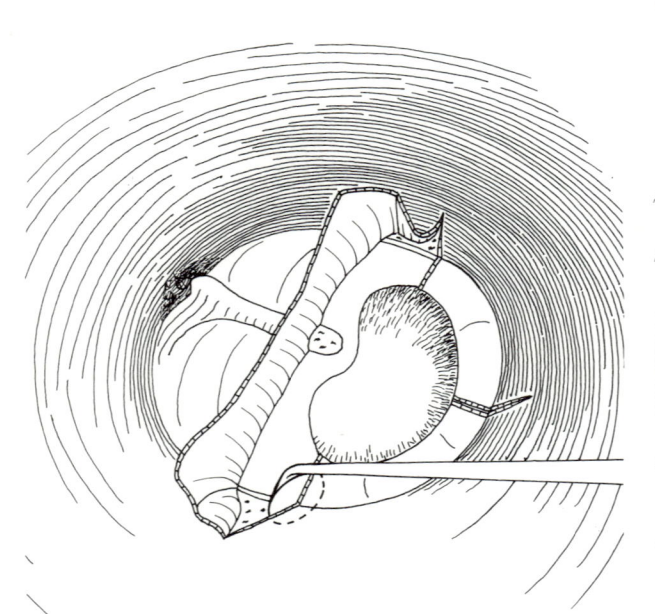

Fig. **483** Superiorly, the epithelium, with the skin, is elevated. Outward elevation of the inferior meatal skin is initiated with the round knife

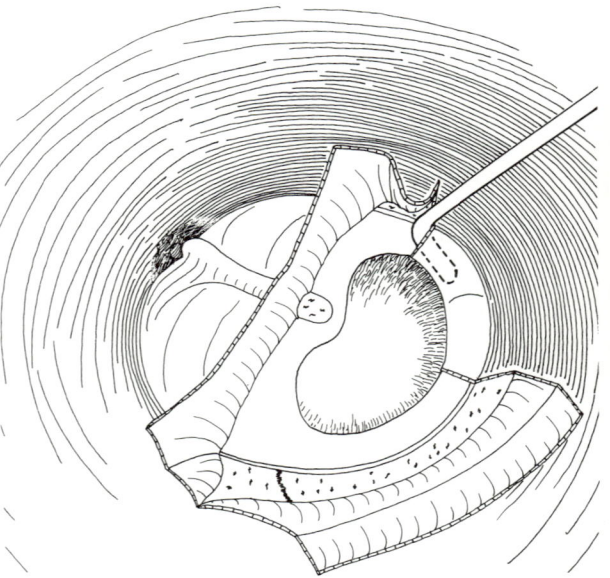

Fig. **484** Elevation of the posteroinferior canal skin is completed. The inferior anterior skin is elevated with a curved elevator

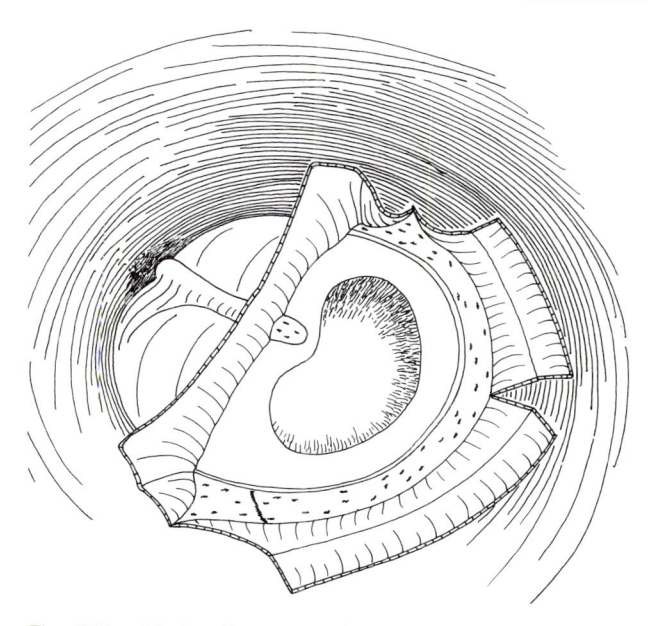

Fig. 485 All the flaps are elevated outward, and the edges of the perforation are cleaned

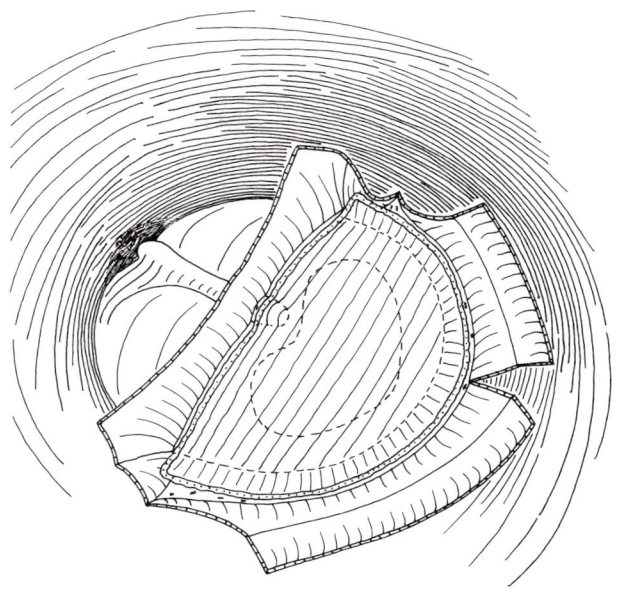

Fig. 486 The perforation is covered with fascia placed on the annulus

Total Perforation

In total perforations, a transition from the onlay flap technique to the underlay technique is seen. When the posterosuperior epithelial flap is being created, the thickness of these flaps and the original pathology will decide whether the annulus is to be cut at the 9-o'clock position, and the flap is also to include the annulus, or whether the flaps will only include the epithelium. In the inferior part of the perforation, the epithelium is removed all round the annulus. The onlay flap technique is the author's technique of choice in total perforations, and these operations are preferably through an ear-canal speculum. However, this technique can also be performed with any other endaural or retroauricular approach.

The incision starts at the 11-o'clock position about 2 mm lateral to the annulus, and continues towards the annulus. It is about 1 mm lateral to the annulus at the 9-o'clock position. The incision then continues at this level all round the annulus to the 10-o'clock position, where it turns more laterally into the ear canal (Fig. 488). The purpose of this incision is to create the superior epithelial flaps. At the 10-o'clock position, the epithelium is cut, preserving the annulus intact, and the posterosuperior skin flap is elevated (Fig. 489). The malleus handle is cleared of epithelium. The keratinized epithelium

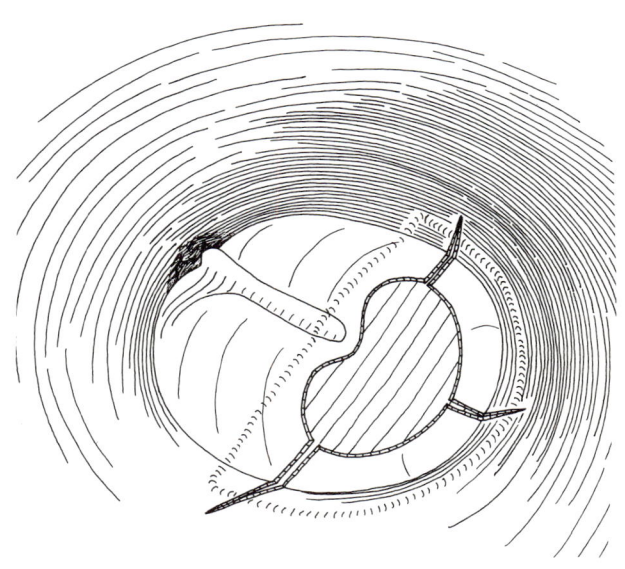

Fig. 487 The skin flaps are returned to their original positions, and will be fixed by Gelfoam balls

10 Onlay Techniques

is removed from the inferior part of the malleus handle and the undersurface of the umbo with forceps. After further elevation of the skin posterosuperiorly, the malleus flap is created by elevating the epithelium from the malleus, pushing it upwards towards the short process (Fig. **490**). After elaborating the superoposterior flap and the malleus flap, the anterosuperior epithelial flap is created by elevating the epithelium from the anterior malleus fold (Fig. **491**). Cleaning of the annulus now starts by elevating the skin and the epithelium all round the annulus (Fig. **492**). Finally, all the epithelium from the annulus and drum remnant is removed, and the perforation is ready te be closed by fascia (Fig. **493**).

Another commonly employed version of this technique is that the annulus is cut at the 9-o'clock position and elevated, and the thin annulus is included in the posterosuperior flap. This means that this technique, by definition a posterosuperior one, is an underlay technique (Fig. **494**).

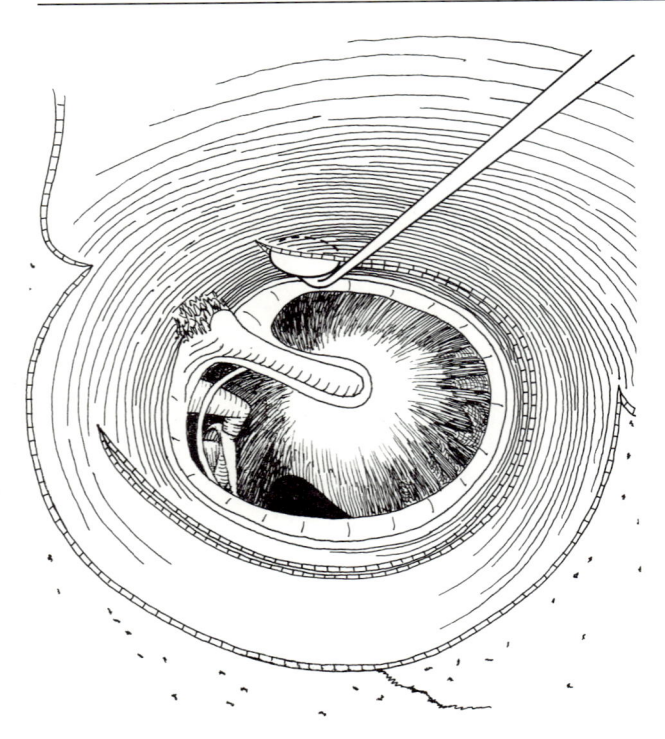

Fig. **488** **Onlay technique with epithelial flaps in a total perforation.** A skin incision is made from the 11-o'clock to the 1-o'clock position, about 1 mm lateral to the annulus

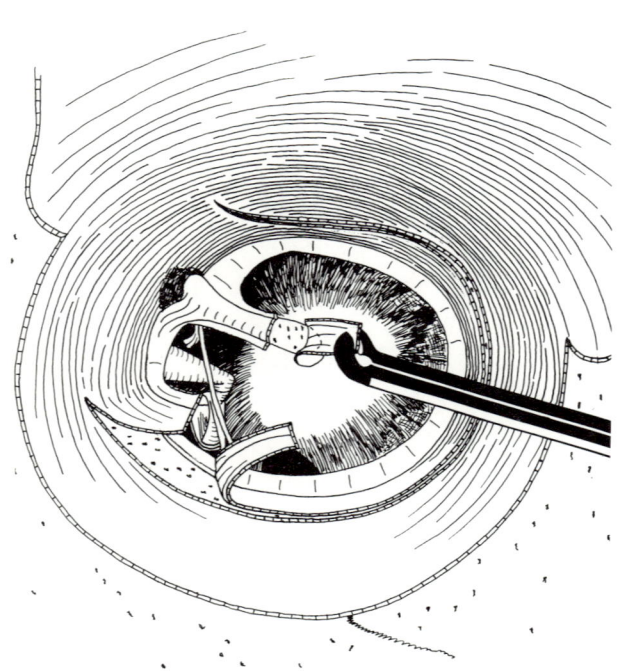

Fig. **489** The inferior parts of the malleus and umbo are cleared of keratinized epithelium. A superior skin flap is elevated

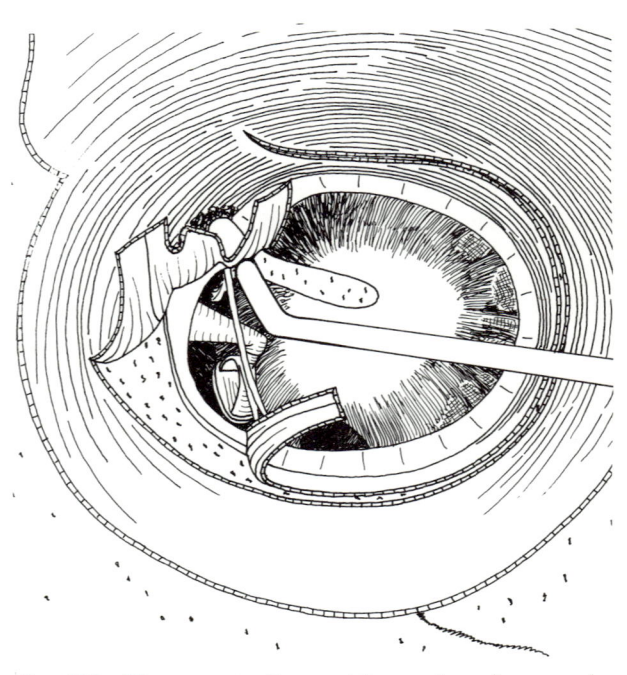

Fig. **490** The superior flap and the malleus flap are elevated

Onlay Techniques with Epithelial Flaps 171

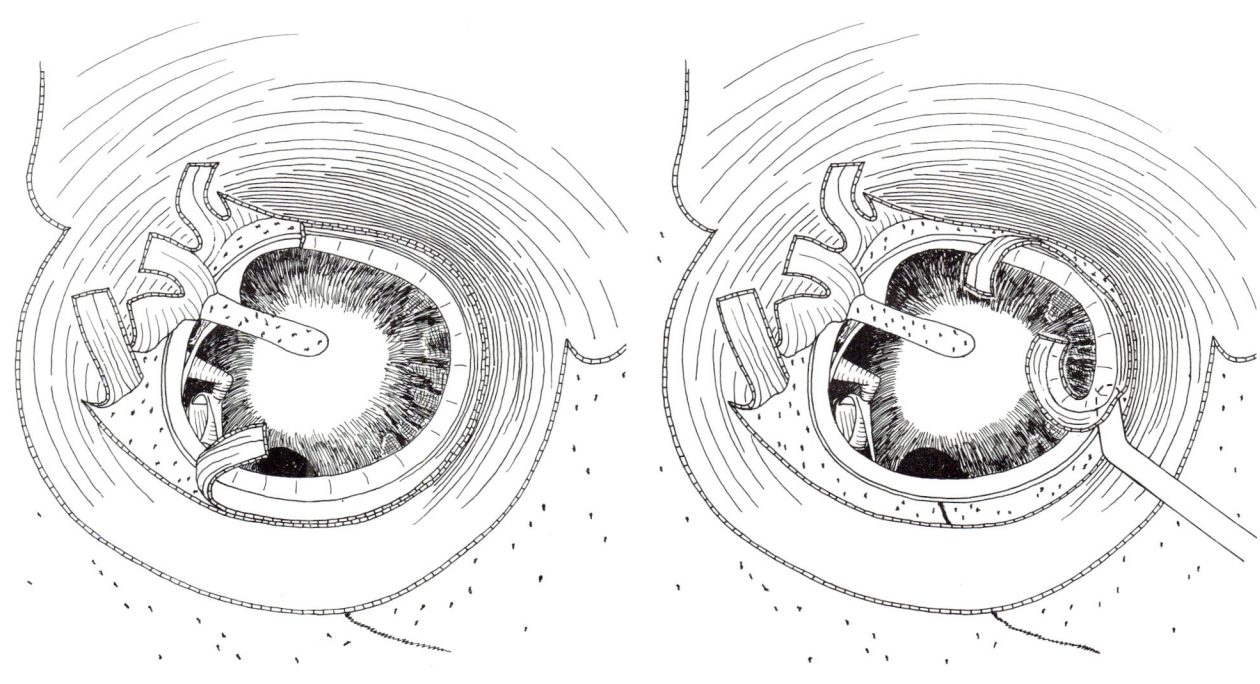

Fig. **491** All three superior flaps are elevated. The annulus is intact all the way round

Fig. **492** The skin and epithelium from the drum remnant are elevated and removed

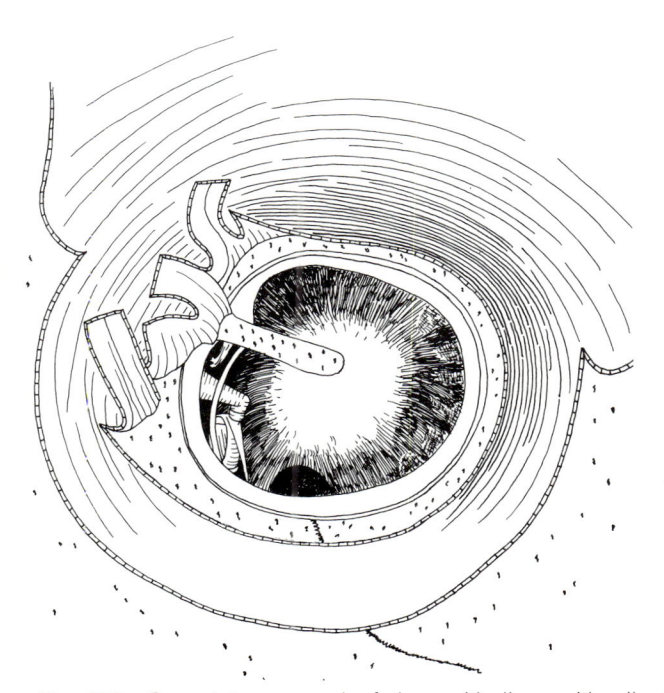

Fig. **493** Complete removal of the epithelium with all three epithelial flaps. The annulus is not resected

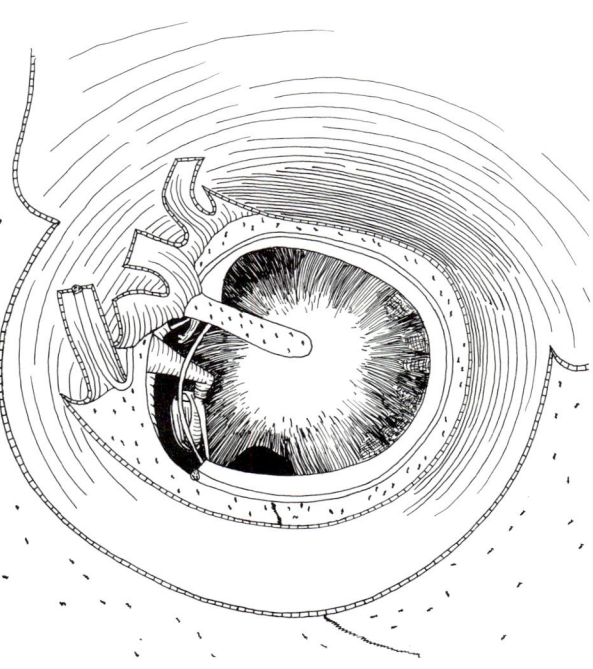

Fig. **494** The same situation as in Figure **493**, except that the annulus has been resected at the 9-o'clock position and elevated as in the underlay technique

10 Onlay Techniques

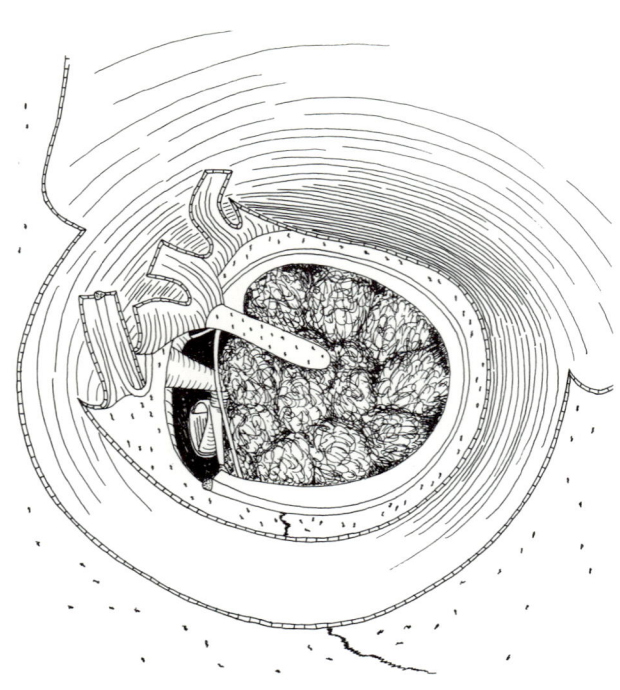

Fig. 495 The tympanic cavity is filled with moistened Gelfoam balls

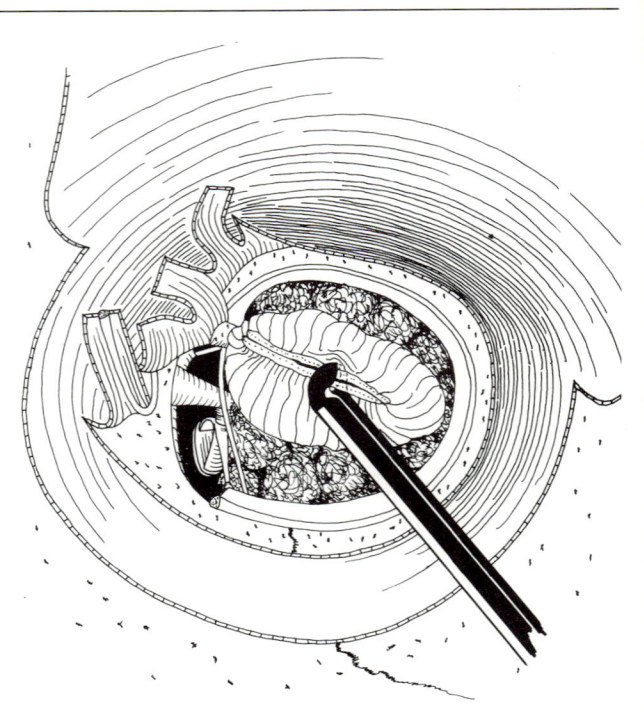

Fig. 496 The fascia bag, containing one or two Gelfoam balls, is placed on the malleus handle

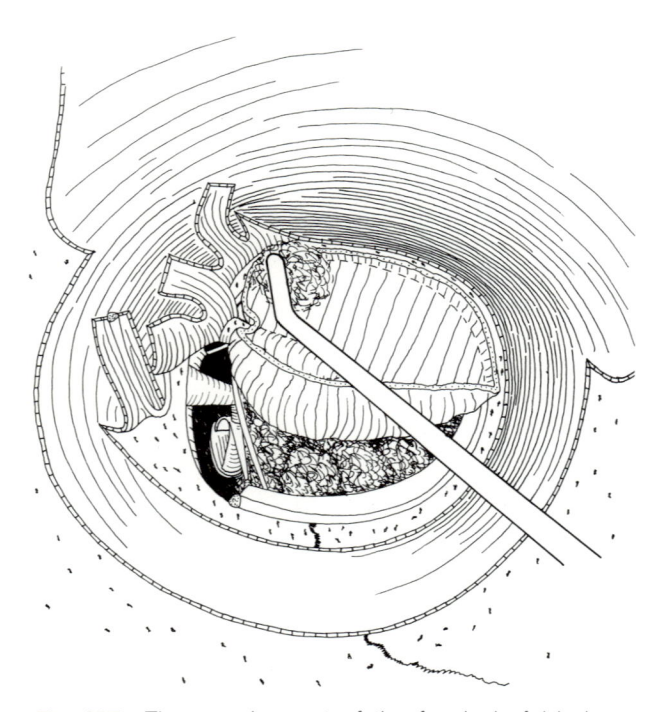

Fig. 497 The anterior part of the fascia is folded out and adapted to the annulus with a Gelfoam ball

The tympanic cavity is filled with some pieces of Gelfoam, moistened in ampicillin (Fig. 495). As little Gelfoam as possible should be placed in the middle ear, but in total perforation, Gefloam is necessary to support the fascia during placement. The cleaned fascia is cut to the appropriate size (Figs. 236, 237), and a bag is prepared to bring the fascia into the ear canal (Fig. 239). The fasciabag, containing one or two Gelfoam balls, is placed on the malleus handle (Fig. 496). With a curved double-cup forceps, the anterior part of the fascia is folded out and placed on the fibrous annulus. With a curved rugine, the Gelfoam ball is rolled towards the anterosuperior part of the fascia (Fig. 497), and adapted carefully to the annulus all the way round (Fig. 498). Finally, the posterior half of the fascia is placed on the annulus, leaving a niche open posterosuperiorly to allow gases to escape (Fig. 499).

Finally, the fascia is carefully adapted under the skin flaps (Fig. 500), and the flaps are turned back: first, the anterosuperior flap, and then the malleus flap. The anterosuperior flap is fixed with a Gelfoam ball, which is pressed in the inferior direction (Fig. 501), as are the subsequent balls, fixing the fascia all round the anterior and inferior annulus

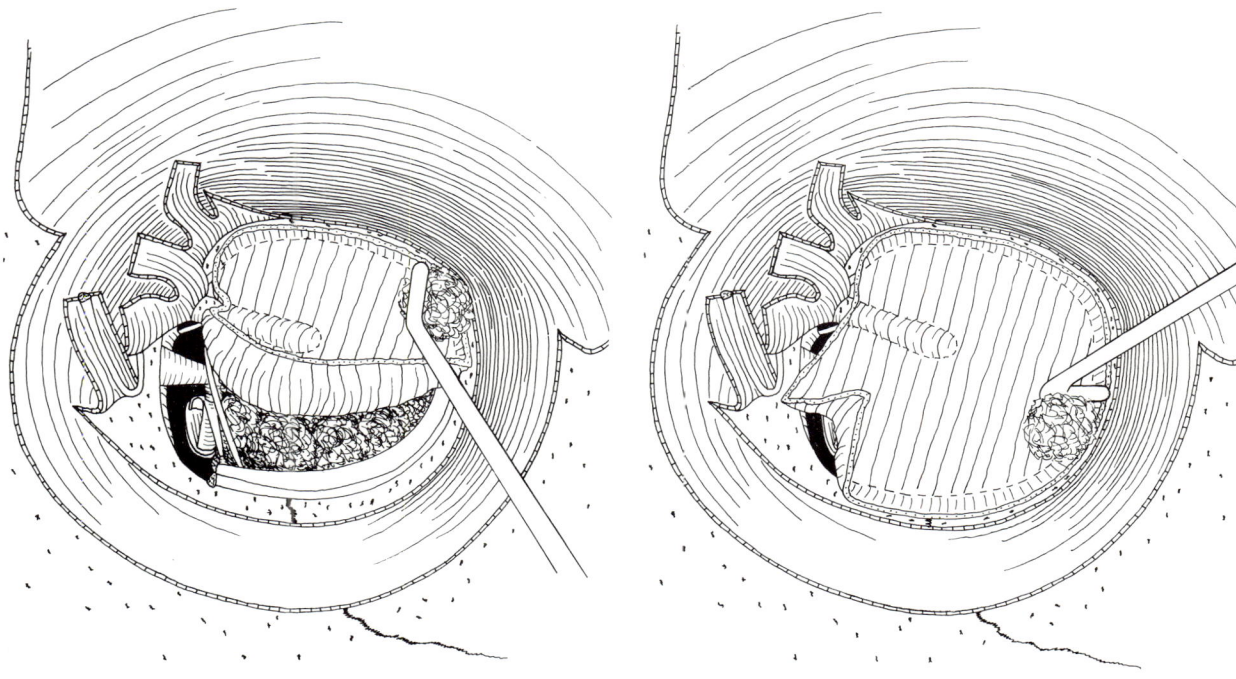

Onlay Techniques with Epithelial Flaps 173

Fig. **498** With the same Gelfoam ball, the fascia is adapted to the skin all the way round

Fig. **499** The posterior half of the fascia is folded out on the annulus and adapted

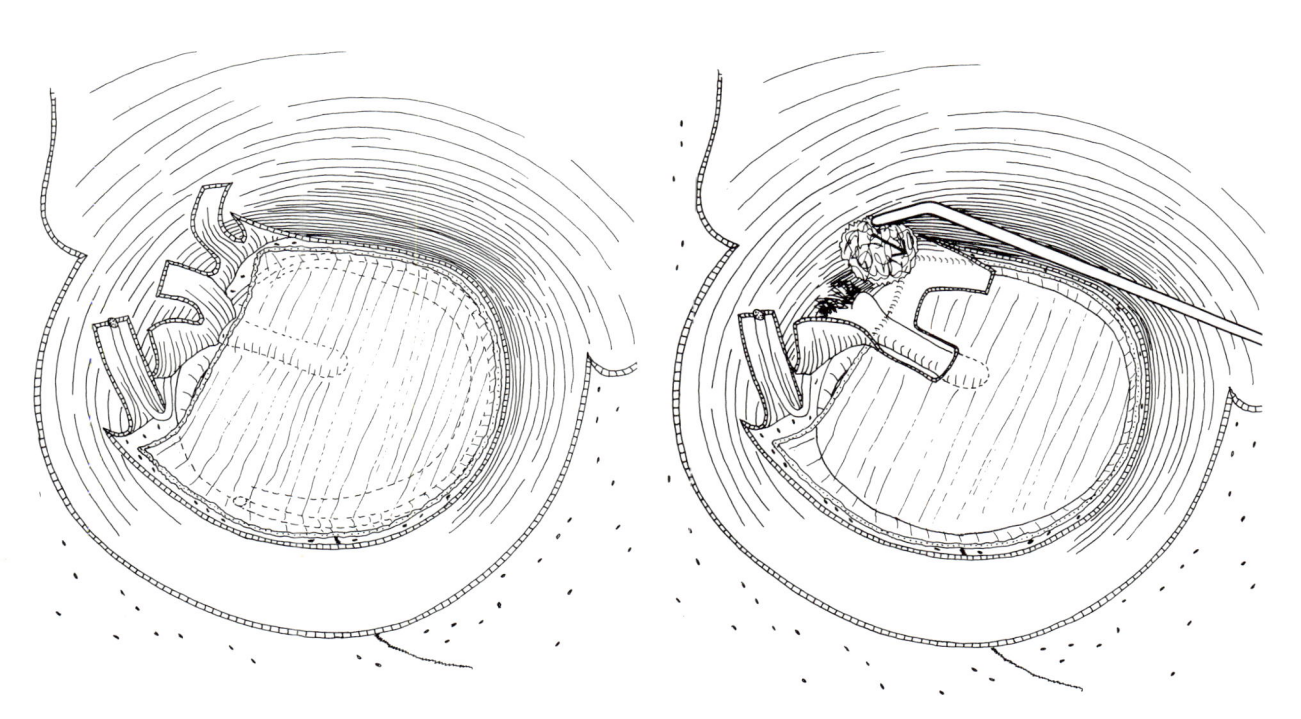

Fig. **500** The fascia is placed on the annulus all the way round, except from the 9-o'clock to the 11-o'clock positions

Fig. **501** The flaps are returned, beginning with the anterosuperior and malleus flaps. The flap is fixed with Gelfoam balls pushed in the inferior direction

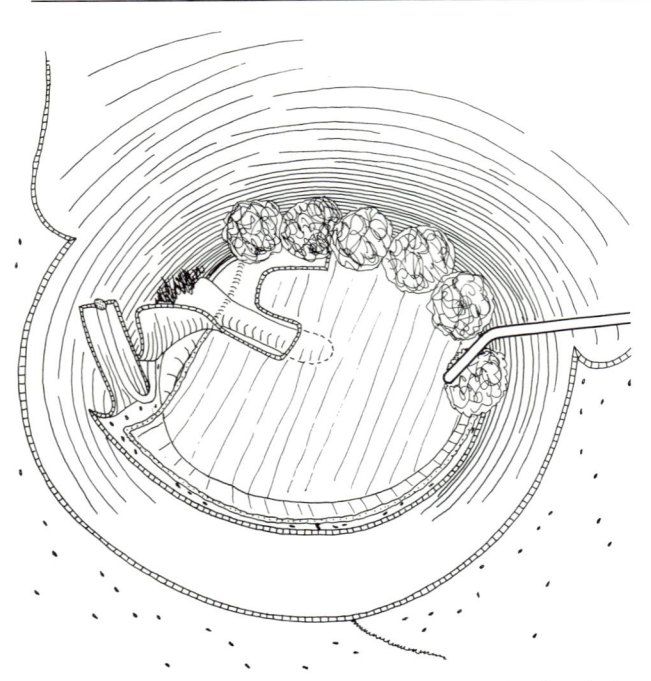

Fig. 502 Several Gelfoam balls are fixing the fascia in the tympanomeatal angle all the way round

(Fig. 502). After the fascia has been fixed to the annulus all the way round, the posterosuperior flap is turned back and fixed with Gelfoam balls (Fig. 503). Finally, some firm balls are placed on the malleus handle, and especially on the umbo, holding the fascia in a concave position. This part of the packing is very important, and prevents lateralization of the ear drum (Fig. 504). Using this technique for all total perforations, the author has not seen any problems of blunting. Problems of lateralization at the umbo do exist, but with careful packing and careful placement of the fascia on the umbo, lateralization can be avoided.

Another technique in total perforation starts with a *lateral circumferential incision* more than 5 mm lateral to the annulus at the 11-o'clock position, and continues all the way round to the 1-o'clock position (Fig. 505). A large meatal skin flap is elevated down to the annulus, and then all the epithelium from the drum remnant, as well as from the malleus handle, is elevated. The short process of the malleus is totally denuded, and Shrapnell's membrane is also elevated (Fig. 506). The fascia is placed on the annulus, on the malleus handle and its short process, on Shrapnell's membrane region, and on the ear-canal bone (Fig. 507). The flap is returned to the original position, and fixed with Gelfoam balls or other packing, initially at the anterior tympanomeatal angle (Fig. 508). In this

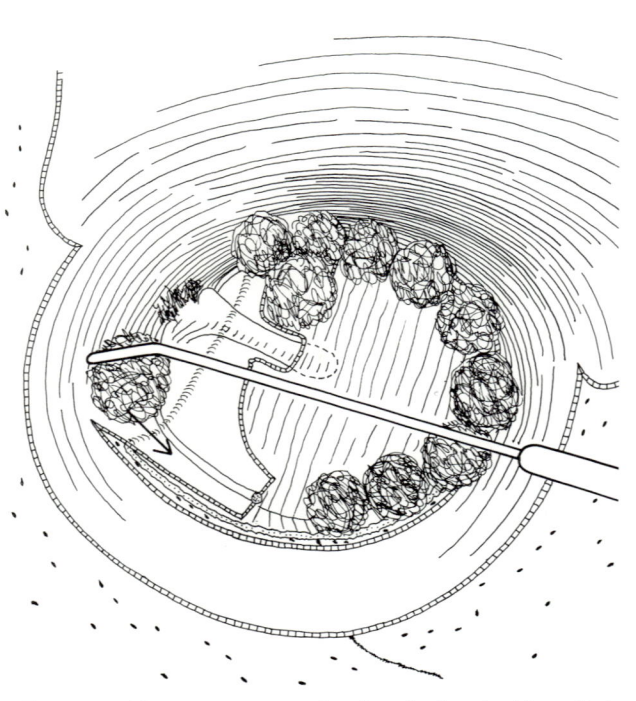

Fig. 503 The posterosuperior flap is fixed with a Gelfoam ball, pushed in the inferior direction

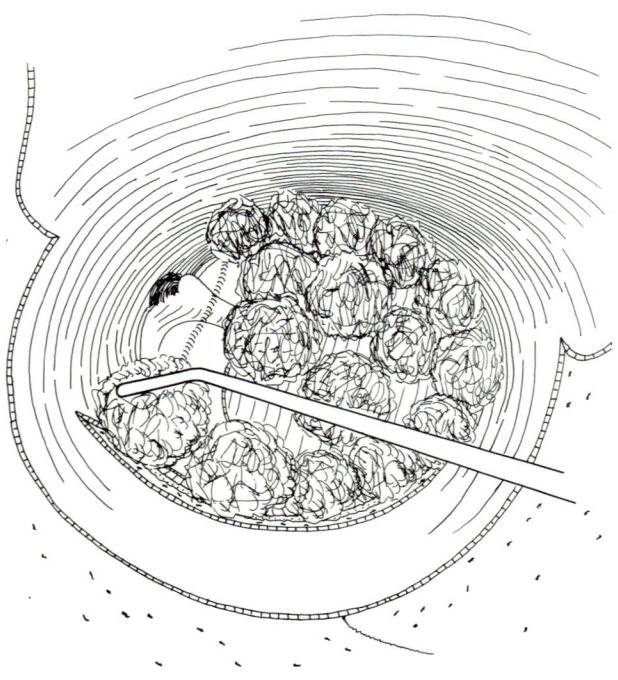

Fig. 504 Finally, a large Gelfoam ball is placed on the umbo, preventing lateralization of the drum

Onlay Techniques with Epithelial Flaps 175

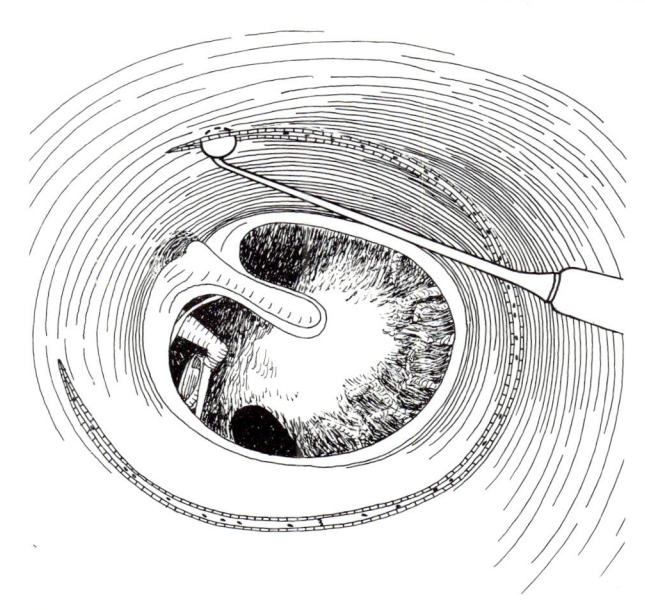

Fig. **505 Onlay technique with a large epithelial flap in a total perforation.** An incision is made several millimeters lateral to the annulus from the 11-o'clock to the 1-o'clock positions

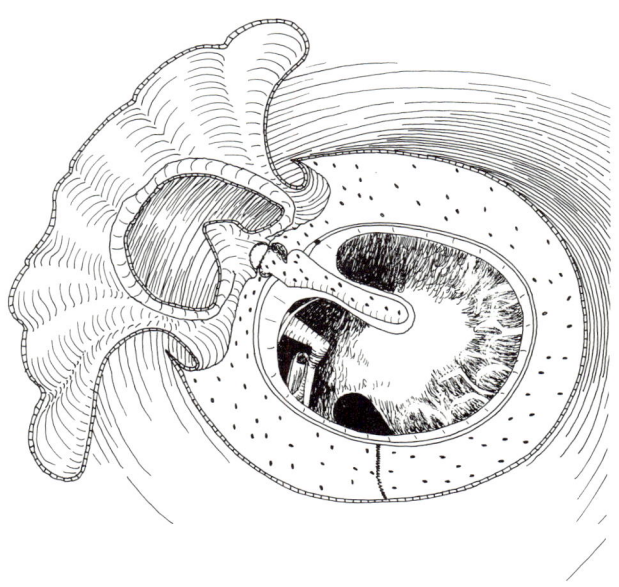

Fig. **506** The entire meatal skin flap, together with the epithelium from the drum remnant, is elevated, as well as the epithelium from the malleus handle

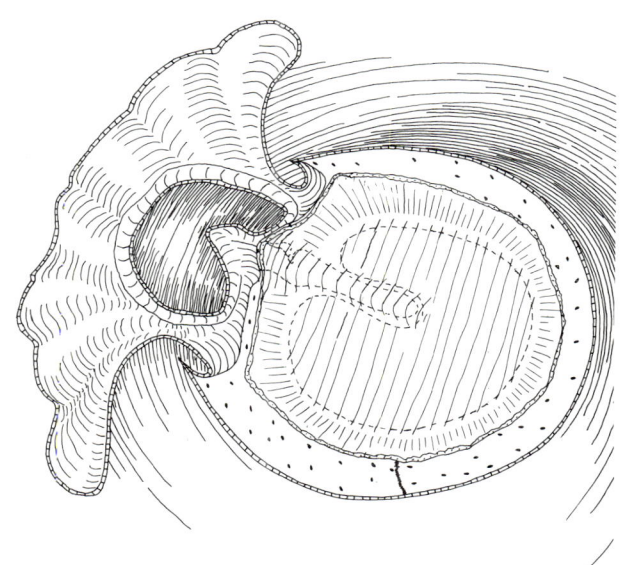

Fig. **507** The fascia is placed on the annulus, the denuded bone, and on the malleus handle

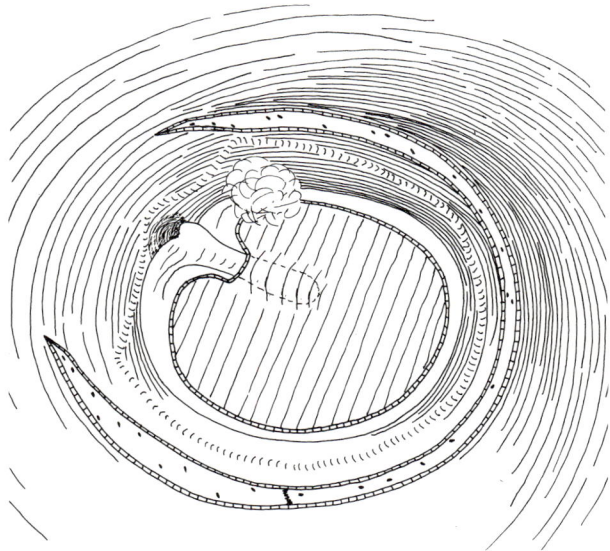

Fig. **508** The flap is returned, and will be fixed with Gelfoam balls

176   10 Onlay Techniques

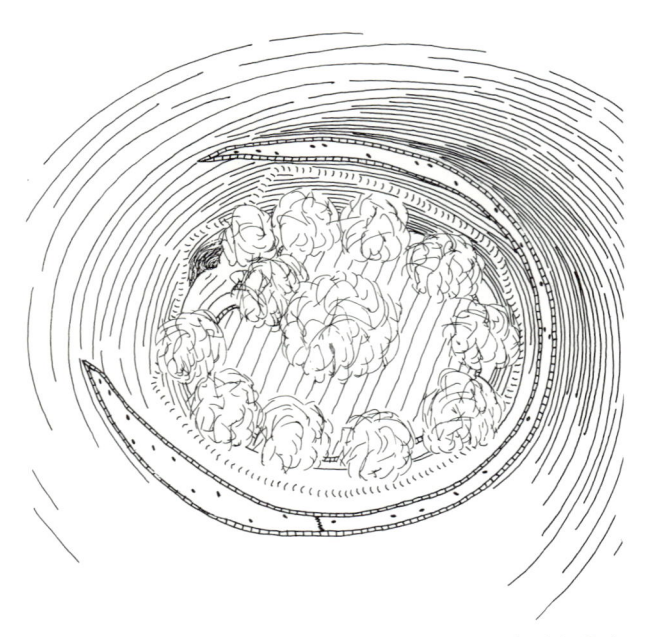

Fig. 509 The tympanometal angle is packed with Gelfoam balls. A large ball is placed on the umbo

technique, firm packing of the tympanomeatal angle and around the annulus is very important in order to maintain the tympanomeatal angle and prevent fibrosis and thickening of the drum at this point. Firm pressure on the umbo is also necessary to prevent lateralization of the new drum away from the umbo. Also, the conical shape has to be maintained (Fig. 509).

A third method was published by Calcaterra in 1972, based on *outward elevation of the pedicled ear-canal skin flaps*, conserving as much of the canal-skin epithelium as possible, and promoting rapid epithelialization of the tympanic membrane graft. The operation starts with an excision of the perforation edge, and careful elevation of the squamous epithelium around the edge. This can be done using a sickle knife or small elevator, or by double-cup forceps, and should be performed all the way around (Fig. 510). The malleus handle is then cleaned by removing the epithelium from the inferior half of the malleus handle and the umbo. The canal skin is incised at the 10-o'clock, 5-o'clock, and 1-o'clock positions several millimeters laterally (Fig. 511). The superior flap is now carefully elevated from the posterior region, from the malleus and Shrapnell's membrane regions, and from the anterior malleus fold. Elevation of this flap is the most delicate and difficult; elevation of the other two flaps is easier, and takes place together

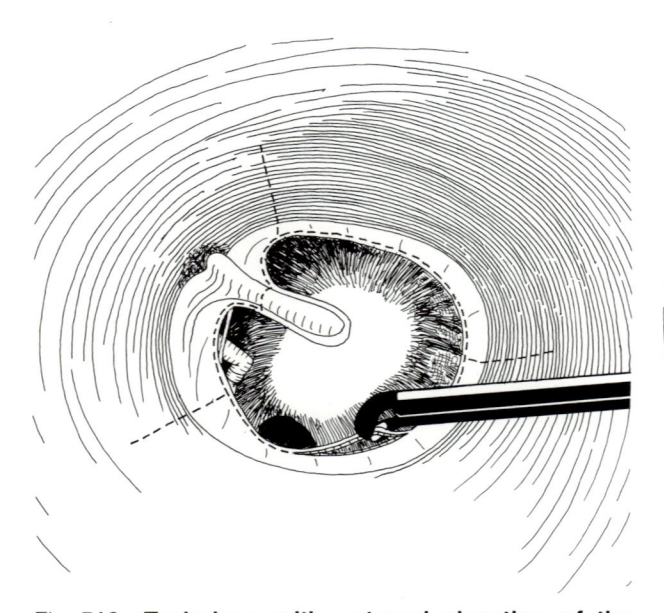

Fig. 510 **Technique with outward elevation of the drum epithelium and ear-canal skin in a total perforation.** Excision of the epithelium from the edge of the perforation is started with a cup forceps. The radial incisions are indicated by dotted lines

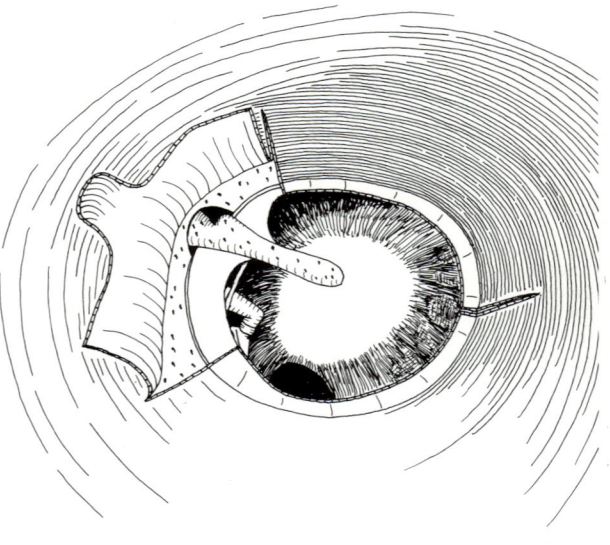

Fig. 511 The superior flap is elevated, as is Shrapnell's membrane

Onlay Techniques with Epithelial Flaps

with the elevation of the epithelium (Fig. 512). The final situation is a clearly visible annulus, some denuded bone around the annulus and the drum remnant, with the malleus totally cleared of keratinized epithelium. After the middle-ear cavity has been filled with some Gelfoam, the fascia covers the Shrapnell's membrane, the malleus handle, and the annulus. The fascia is carefully positioned on the annulus into the tympanomeatal angle (Fig. 513). The skin flaps are rolled back and fixed to the annulus all the way round (Fig. 514). The problems with this method are possible blunting and lateralization, but with careful packing this can be avoided. This technique can be performed through an endaural approach, but is usually with the retroauricular approach.

The fourth flap method is *outward elevation of the pedicled ear-canal skin* of the *anterior* tympanomeatal angle. This method was already recommended by Wullstein in the retroauricular approach. Through the retroauricular approach, the canal skin from the posterior half of the ear canal is elevated. Elevation includes the drum-remnant epithelium and the malleus-handle epithelium, as well as Shrapnell's membrane. Radial incisions with a scalpel are performed at the 1-o'clock and 5-o'clock positions (Figs. 515, 516). The elevated skin is held away by a long selfretaining retractor (Fig. 110), or sutured outward (Fig. 111), allowing

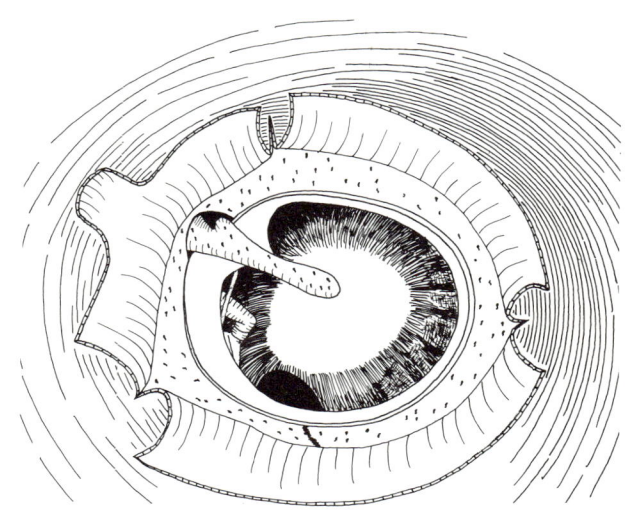

Fig. 512 Both inferior flaps are elevated outward, and the perforation is ready for fascia covering

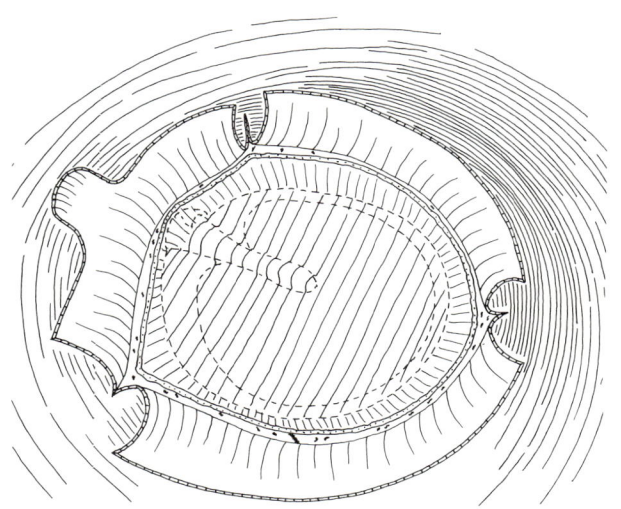

Fig. 513 Fascia is placed on the annulus and on the malleus handle

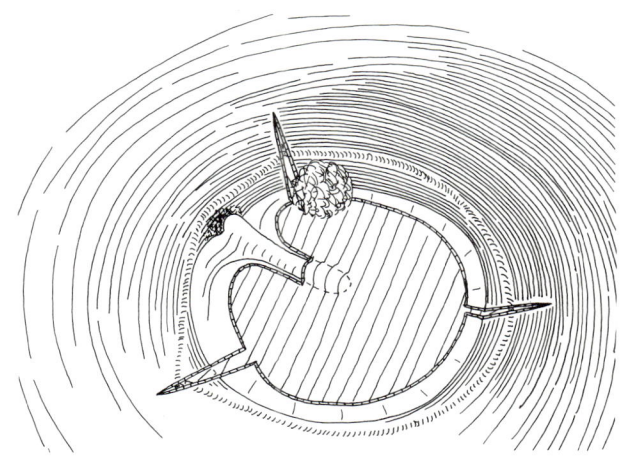

Fig. 514 The flaps are returned, and will be fixed along the tympanomeatal angle and on the malleus with Gelfoam balls

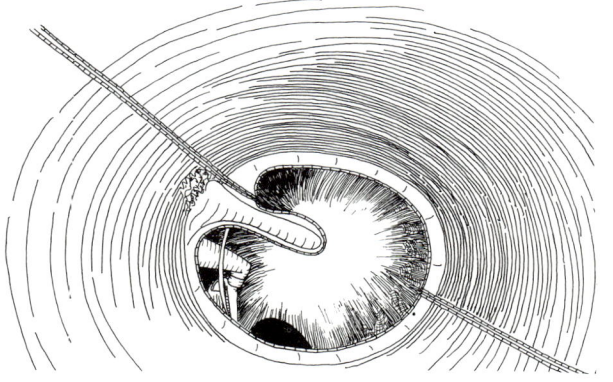

Fig. 515 **The onlay epithelium flap method, with outward elevation of the pedicle ear-canal skin of the anterior tympanomeatal angle.** In a retroauricular approach, the two radial incisions at the 11-o'clock and 5-o'clock positions are indicated

10 Onlay Techniques

a good view of the anterior tympanomeatal angle. The epithelium from the drum remnant is elevated outward, together with the canal skin. This elevation is started at the 5-o'clock and 1-o'clock positions. (Fig. **517**), and continued in an anterior direction, gradually elevating the skin from the entire anterior tympanomeatal angle (Fig. **518**). After careful cleaning of the annulus, the drum remnant, and the malleus handle for keratinized squamous epithelium possibly left behind during the elevation, an onlay fascia graft is placed either under or on the malleus handle. In placing the fascia under the malleus handle, lateralization of the graft should be avoided (Fig. **519**). A slit is cut into the upper part of the fascia, to facilitate its placement under the malleus handle. The upper anterior edge of the fascia is pulled posteriorly, covering the Shrapnell's membrane region (Fig. **520**). The anterior canal skin and the drum-remnant epithelium is replaced and fixed by Gelfoam balls. Finally, the upper posterior edge of the fascia is pulled anteriorly for further covering of the Shrapnell's membrane region. The posterior canal-skin flap, with the drum epithelium, is replaced after removal of the selfretaining retractor (Fig. **521**). The ear canal is packed with Gelfoam and gauze.

This method is very popular in the retroauricular approach, and can be adapted to several variations of it which are described in Chapter 4. The principle of outward elevation of the ear-canal skin of the anterior tympanomeatal angle can also be adapted to the endaural approach.

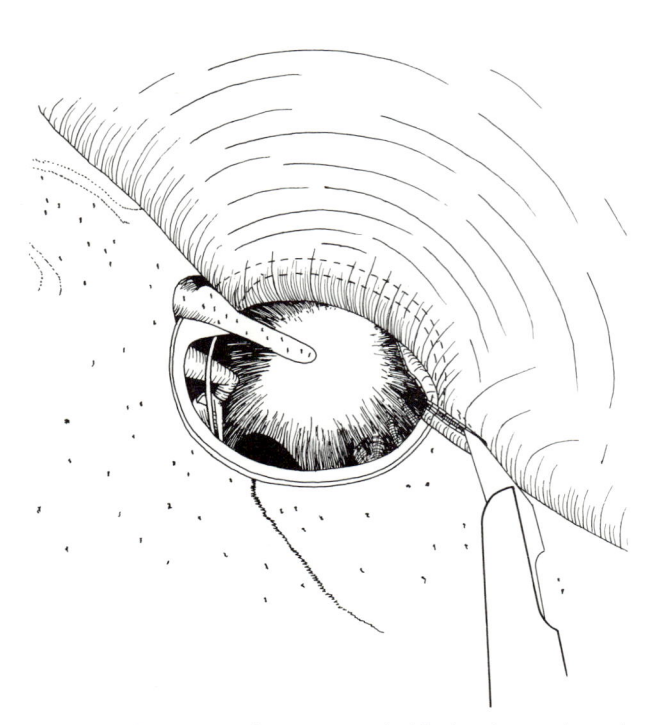

Fig. **516** The posterior ear-canal skin is elevated, and the inferior radial incision is made with a scalpel at the 5-o'clock position

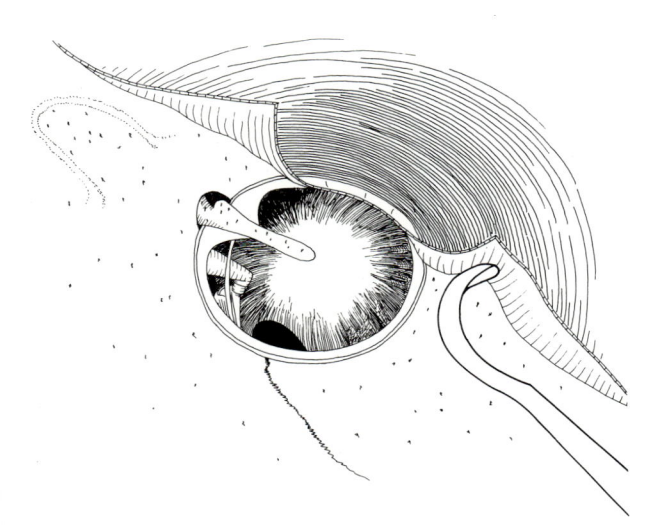

Fig. **517** The drum epithelium and the epithelium from the annulus are elevated outward starting at the 11-o'clock and 5-o'clock position

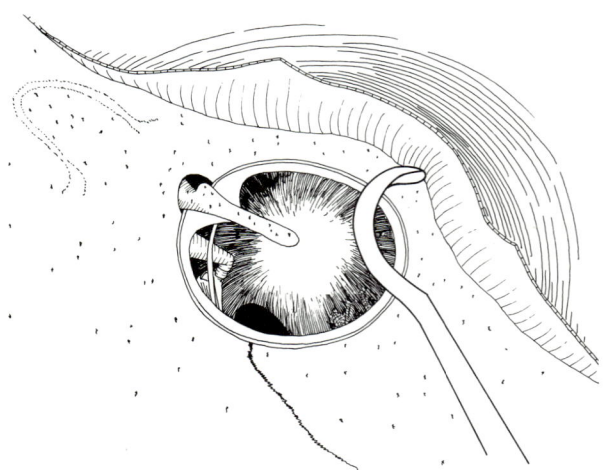

Fig. **518** The keratinized epithelium from the anterior half of the drum remnant and the anterior annulus, and the skin from the tympanomeatal angle, are elevated outwards

Onlay Techniques with Epithelial Flaps   179

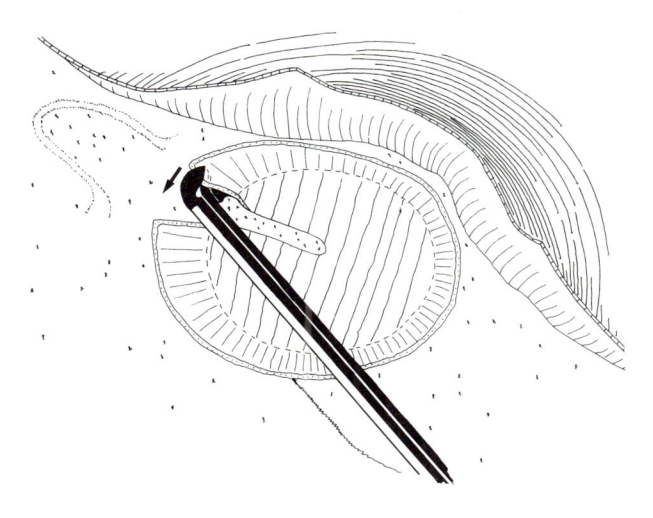

Fig. 519 Fascia is placed on top of the annulus and bone but below the malleus handle. A slit is made superiorly in the fascia. The anterosuperior edge of the fascia is pulled posteriorly (arrow)

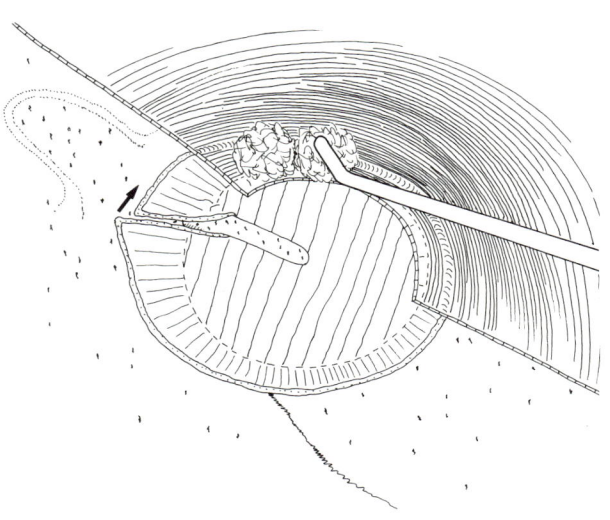

Fig. 520 The Shrapnell's membrane region is covered with the fascia, pulled in anterior direction (arrows). The epithelium from the anterior tympanomeatal angle is replaced and fixed with Gelfoam balls

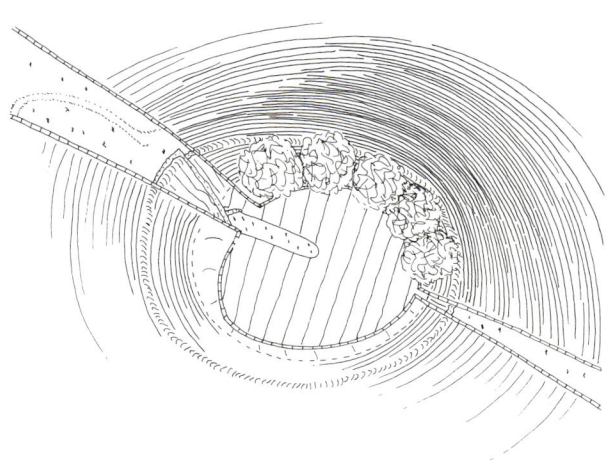

Fig. 521 The posterior edge of the fascia covers the Shrapnell's region, and the skin from the posterior half of the ear canal is replaced

Posterior Perforation

In posterior perforations, the incision is performed about 2 mm lateral to the annulus (Fig. 522). The superior flap, including elevation of the keratinized epithelium from the border of the perforation, is elevated. The epithelium from the malleus handle and the umbo is elevated (Fig. 522). The inferior skin flap is created, and the epithelium from the inferior area around the perforation is removed by cup forceps (Fig. 523). The perforation is now ready to be covered by fascia onlay. The fascia is placed on the lamina propria (Fig. 524), and the epithelial flaps are returned. They are fixed with Gelfoam balls. This operation can easily be performed through the speculum (Fig. 525).

10 Onlay Techniques

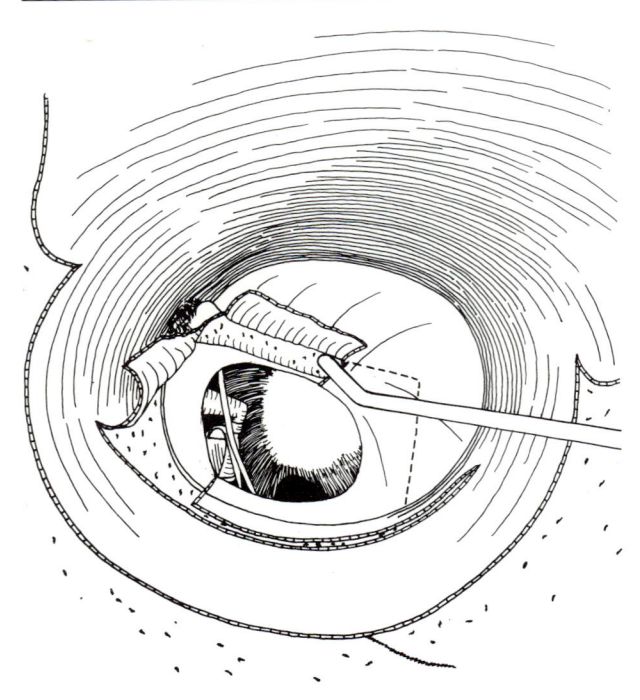

Fig. 522 **Onlay flap technique in a posterior perforation.** An incision is made 2 mm lateral to the annulus. The skin flap and the epithelium from the superior drum remnant are elevated. The epithelium from the malleus handle is also elevated

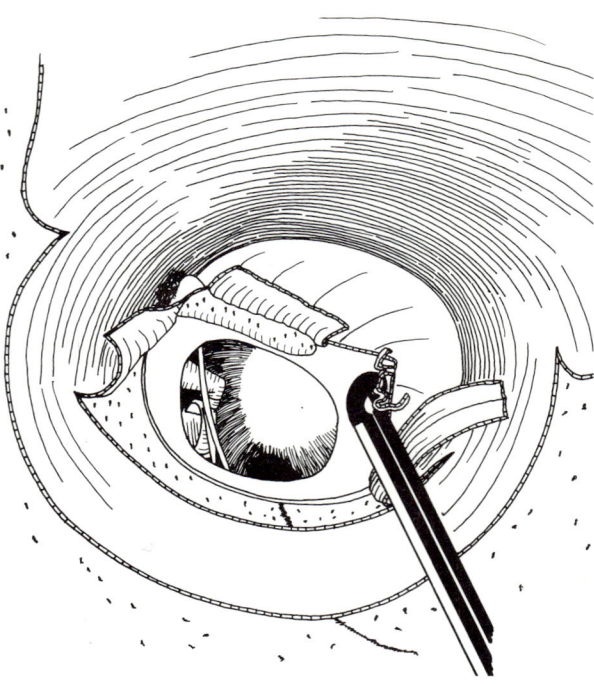

Fig. 523 The inferior skin flap is elevated, and the drum epithelium from the inferior edge of the perforation and the inferior area of the drum is removed

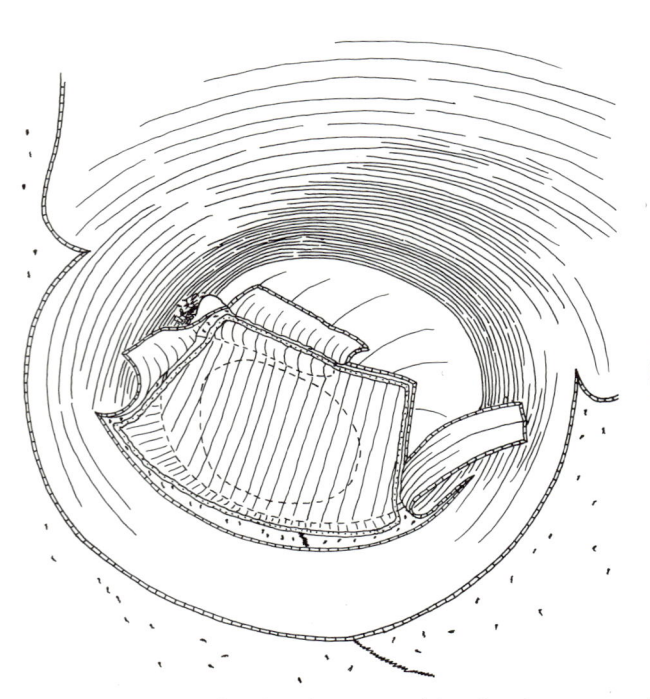

Fig. 524 The perforation is covered by fascia as an onlay graft

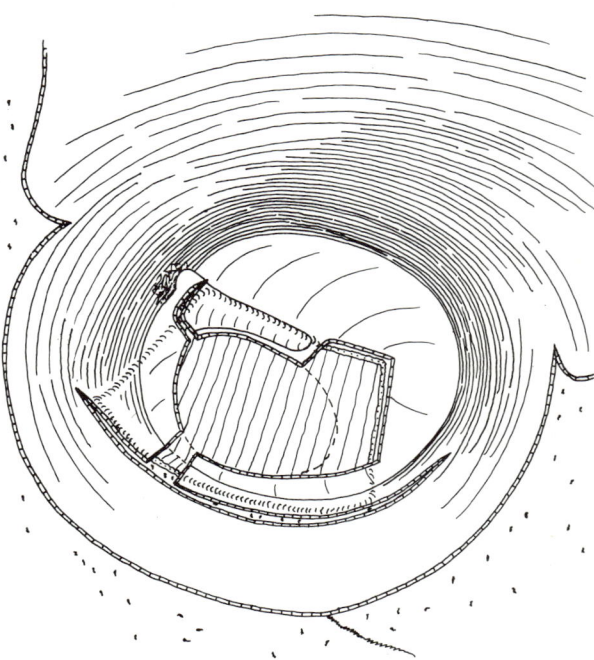

Fig. 525 The skin flaps are returned, and will be fixed with Gelfoam

The Onlay Sandwich Technique

This technique is advocated and practised by Sheehy and the House group. The principle is to remove a large part of the ear-canal skin by a circumferential incision in the outer third of the ear canal, together with the drum-remnant epithelium. A relatively large fascia graft is placed on the de-epithelialized annulus and drum remnant, as well as on part of the denuded ear canal bone. The fascia is then partly covered by the ear-canal skin. Sheehy uses the same technique in all kinds of perforations, including small inferior and small posterior perforations, as well as total perforations. Different sizes of fascia are used to cover the perforation. The smallest size is 0.75–1.50 cm, the largest 2.25–3.75 cm.

The Sheehy retroauricular approach to canal wall–up mastoidectomy is described above (Figs. **148–157**). Here, only the method for myringoplasty will be described. A radial incision with a sickle knife is performed at the 12-o'clock position, starting close to the annulus and running laterally. A small circumferential incision running 1 mm lateral to the annulus is performed between the 12-o'clock and 9-o'clock positions. A radial incision is then made starting at the 9-o'clock position and continuing laterally along the tympanomastoid suture to the outer third of the ear canal. Finally, with a beaver knife or a large round knife, a lateral circumferential incision is made between the 9-o'clock and 12-o'clock positions. Elevation of the skin starts posteriorly, and continues all the way round the ear canal. The epithelium from the drum remnant posterosuperiorly is elevated and cut from the remaining skin, and the malleus handle is cleared of epithelium (Fig. **526**). After removal of all skin from the ear canal, and all epithelium from the drum remnant, as well as from the Shrapnell's membrane region, the final cleaning and removal of the epithelium from the malleus handle is performed (Fig. **527**). A large piece of dry fascia, like dry parchment, is trimmed to the correct size, depending on the perforation involved. The fascia is cut with a pair of scissors. A radial incision is performed as far as the center. The fascia is rehydrated, and placed on the annulus in such a way that the malleus handle is outside the fascia. The radial incision facilitates pulling of the fascia under the malleus handle, toward the attachment of the medial ligament (Fig. **528**). Afterwards, the fascia is carefully approximated to the annulus and the bone. The posterosuperior edge of the fascia is pulled anteriorly so as to cover the Shrapnell's membrane region and the anterior malleolar fold (Fig. **529**). The anterosuperior edge of the fascia is then turned posteroinferiorly to cover the entire malleus handle, with the short process and the umbo (Fig. **530**). Before replacing the ear-canal skin, further adjustment of the fascia to tie onto the annulus is performed. Finally, the meatal skin is replaced in such a way that the anterior and inferior meatal angle are covered by skin. Laterally, there will be a defect in

Fig. **526** **The onlay sandwich technique.** The anterior and inferior ear-canal skin is incised from the 12-o'clock to the 9-o'clock positions using a circumferential incision placed in the lateral third of the canal. A small medial circumferential incision placed posterosuperiorly 1 mm lateral to the annulus connects the former incision between the 12-o'clock and 9-o'clock positions. The ear-canal skin and epithelium are elevated from the drum remnant posteriorly, and the elevation of the large skin area is indicated laterally

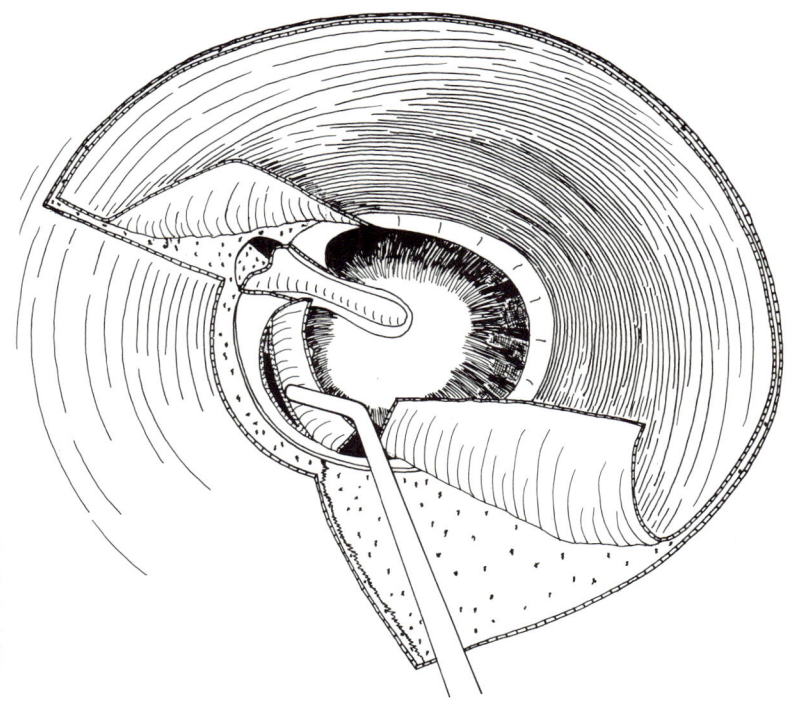

10 Onlay Techniques

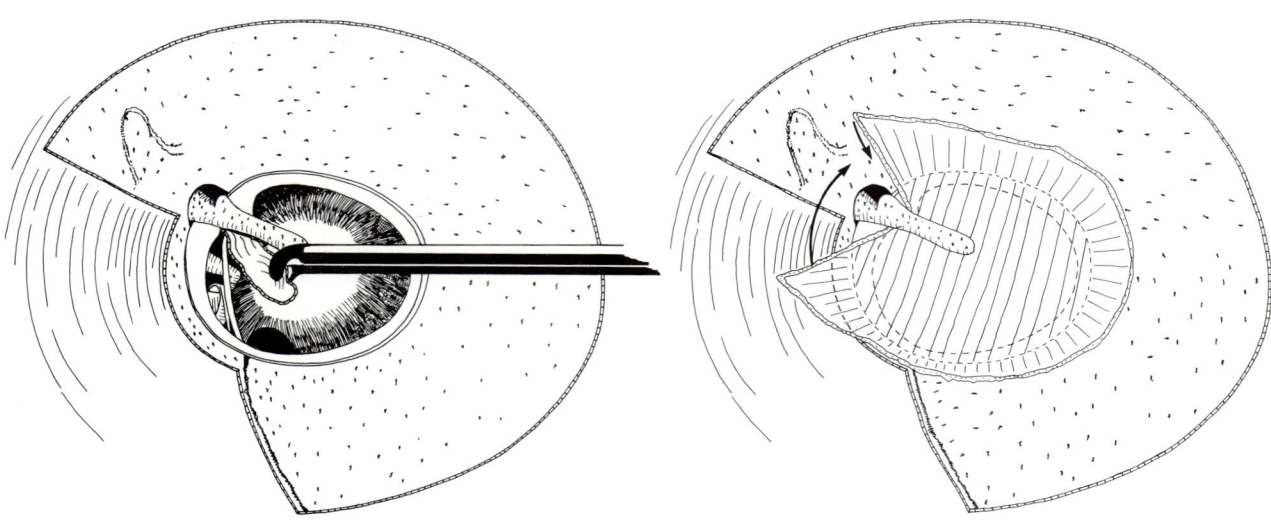

Fig. **527** All the ear-canal skin is elevated together with the drum remnant except from the malleus handle, which is now cleaned, and the last part of the epithelium is removed using a double-cup forceps

Fig. **528** A 4 mm long slit is cut superiorly on a large, dry fascia graft. The fascia is placed on top of the annulus and the denuded bone, but under neath the malleus handle. The fascia is pulled far superiorly under the handle. The end of the slit is located at the tendon of the tensor tympani muscle

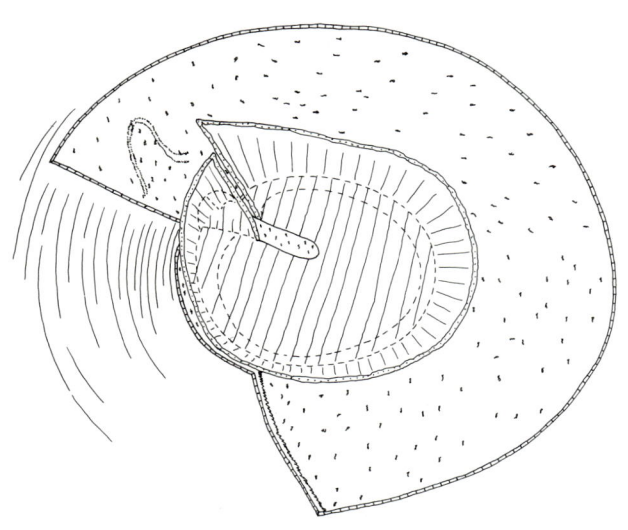

Fig. **529** The posterior edge of the fascia is pulled in an anterior direction, to cover the Shrapnell's membrane region and the short process of the malleus

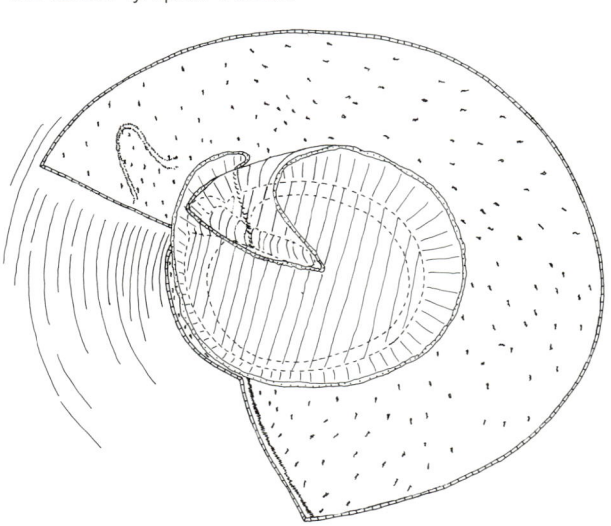

Fig. **530** The anterior edge is pulled posteroinferiorly, to cover the malleus handle and the umbo

the covering of the bone, which will later epithelialize spontaneously (Fig. **531**). A firm pack of Gelfoam balls and gauze is provided, so as to prevent lateralization of the graft and blunting (Fig. **532**). The epithelium can be turned during the removal, and small epithelial pearls can be formed after replacing of the epithelium.

The onlay sandwich technique is used by several surgeons, and nearly all of them remove the ear-canal skin (Farrior 1968, Wolfermann 1971). The present author's view is that, in the majority of cases, removal of the ear-canal skin is unnecessary. After total removal of the skin, such replacement can never be precise, and the method is unphysiological. Reepithelialization will be delayed, and proper migration may later be disturbed. Other problems in this method are blunting due to excessive thickness of the graft in the anterior tympanomeatal angle, lateral traction of the malleus handle, lateralization of the drum, and epithelial crusts resulting from the inability of the epithelium to remove keratin.

The Onlay Sandwich Technique 183

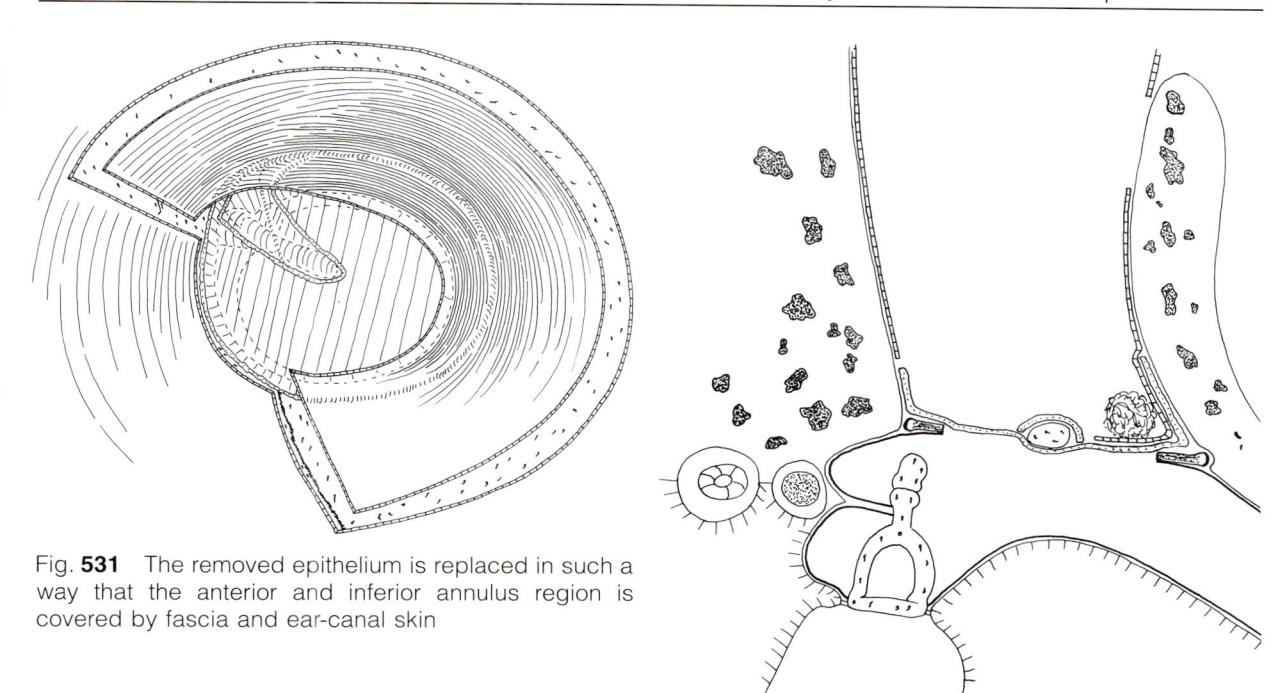

Fig. 531 The removed epithelium is replaced in such a way that the anterior and inferior annulus region is covered by fascia and ear-canal skin

Fig. 532 Side view of the placement of the fascia on both sides of the malleus handle and replacement of the canal-wall skin in the onlay sandwich technique

11 Underlay Techniques

The underlay technique is defined as placement of the graft under the drum, or under the fibrous annulus. Underlay techniques are very popular, and are used in nearly all retroauricular approaches. Three types of underlay techniques are described here: techniques without tympanomeatal flaps; techniques with tympanomeatal flaps; and sandwich techniques.

Techniques Without Tympanomeatal Flaps

The graft in this type of myringoplasty is placed through the perforation under the drum remnant, without tympanotomy, usually without inspection of the tympanic cavity or ossicular chain. This technique is usually used in anterior perforations and minor inferior perforations.

Anterior Perforation

The edge of the perforation is removed all the way round (Fig. 533) with a curved rugine or a pair of double-cup forceps. The mucosa from the undersurface of the drum is removed a couple of millimeters peripheral to the edge. Removal of the mucosa from the undersurface of the drum is especially important anteriorly under the annulus. A curved double-cup forceps can be introduced towards the annulus and the mucosa removed piecemeal (Fig. 534). Under the posterior edge of the perforation, scarification of the mucosa along the malleus handle can be performed with a right-angled curved elevator (Fig. 535). The tympanic cavity is firmly filled with Gelfoam, and the fascia is first placed under the anterior edge as far towards the annulus as possible (Fig. 536). The fascia is held under the drum by the Gelfoam, and then the fascia is pushed under the posterior edge of the perforation and spread under the malleus handle (Fig. 537). Finally, adjustment of the fascia placement is made all round the perforation. The precise placement of Gelfoam balls is important in the underlay technique, because pressure on the fascia should be avoided. The first balls should be placed exactly on the edge of the perforation. These press the edge towards the fascia. The

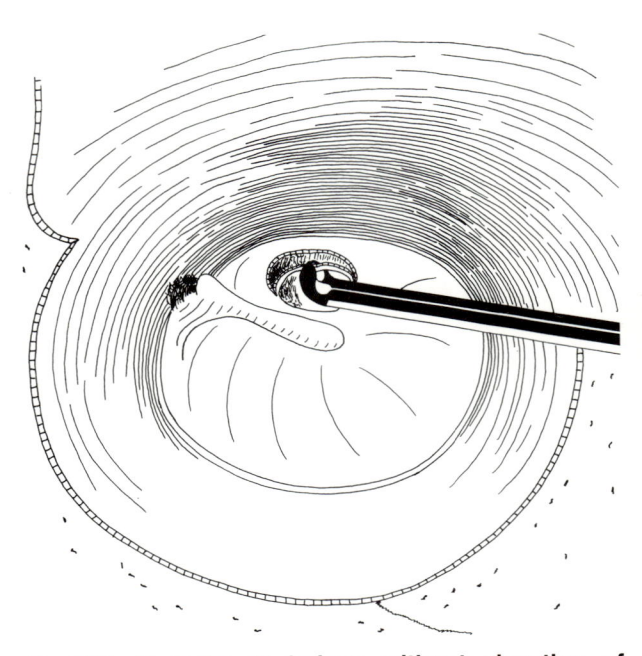

Fig. **533** **Underlay technique without elevation of the tympanomeatal flap in an anterior perforation.** The edge of the perforation is excised

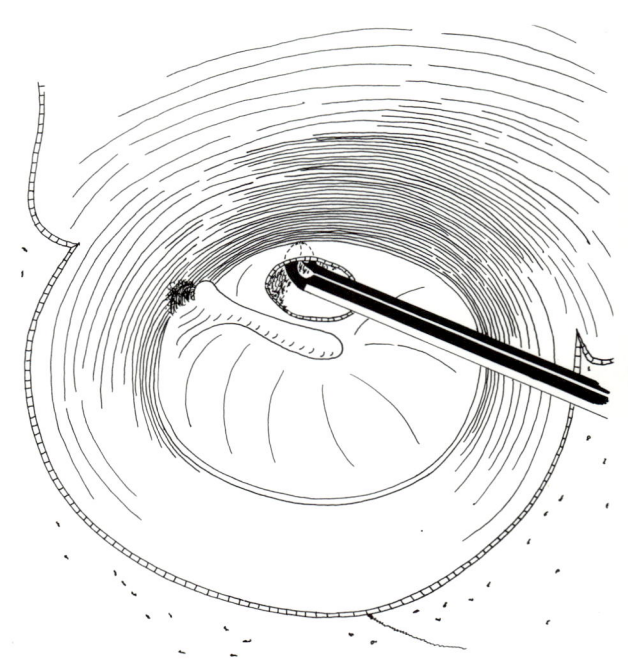

Fig. **534** The mucosa from the undersurface of the anterior annulus is removed

Techniques Without Tympanomeatal Flaps

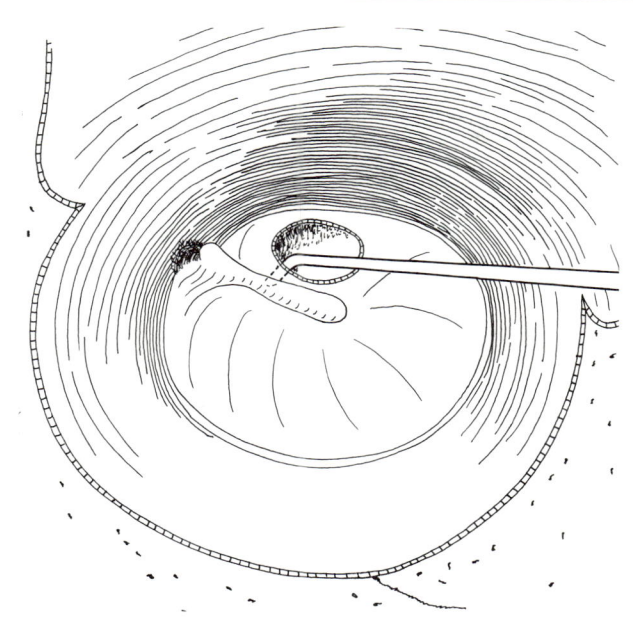

Fig. 535 The mucosa from the undersurface of the malleus handle is removed

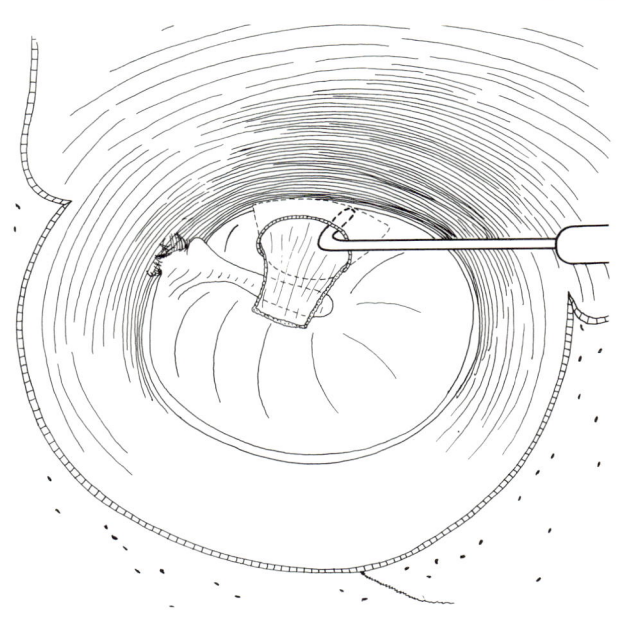

Fig. 536 The fascia is brought through the perforation and positioned anteriorly

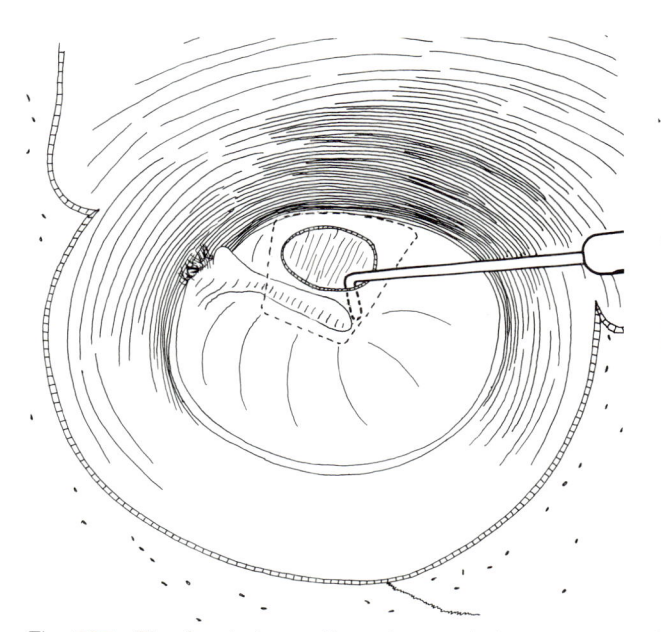

Fig. 537 The fascia is positioned posteriorly

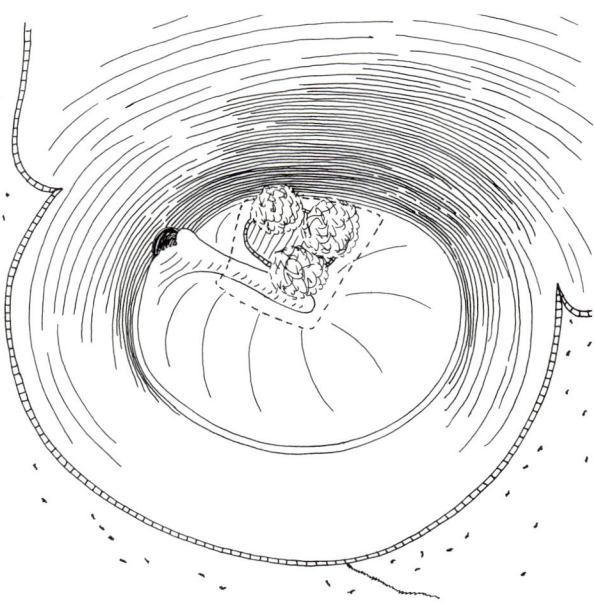

Fig. 538 The fascia is fixed with Gelfoam balls placed at the edge of the perforation. Gelfoam of semi-wet consistence will adhere to the fascia and the epithelium at the edge of the perforation

Gelfoam balls also adhere to the fascia and hold it in place. Placement of the balls is performed all the way round the perforation (Fig. 538). In the majority of cases, this will be enough. Alternatively, fixation of the fascia can be achieved using the Gerlach technique, or by fixation around the annulus as described above (pp. 148–149).

This procedure can be performed through an endaural approach with an ear speculum, with any other endaural incision, or with any retroauricular approach.

11 Underlay Techniques

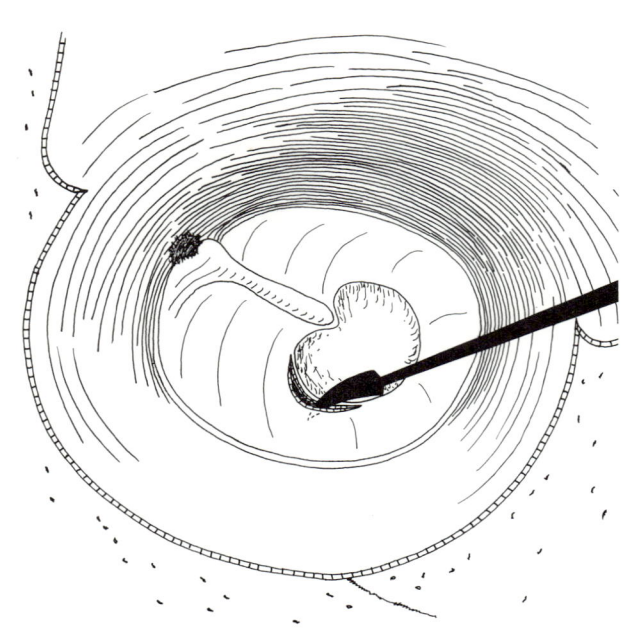

Fig. 539 **Underlay technique without tympanotomy in an inferior perforation.** The edge of the perforation is excised

Inferior Perforation

As with anterior perforation, the perforation edge is excised (Fig. **539**), or keratinized epithelium from the edge is elevated without excision of the lamina propria. At the umbo, special care should be taken, and the keratinized epithelium should be elevated here both on the outer and the inner surfaces (Fig. **540**). Removal of the mucosa under the drum remnant can be performed using a curved instrument (Fig. **541**), or it can be pulled out by curved cup forceps (Fig. **542**). After firm filling of the tympanic cavity with Gelfoam (Fig. **543**), the fascia is placed on the perforation, and pushed under the drum remnant using a long curved rugine, first anteriorly (Fig. **544**), then superiorly, inferiorly, and posteriorly. Fixation of the graft can be performed by Gelfoam balls placed at the edge of the perforation all the way round, pushing only on the drum remnant, not on the fascia (Figs. **545, 546**). With firm filling of Gelfoam in the tympanic cavity, the graft should not fall into the tympanic cavity. The graft can also be fixed using the Gerlach technique, or with fibrin glue.

Larger inferior perforation, subtotal perforation, total perforation, and posterior perforation are usually not managed by techniques without tympanotomies.

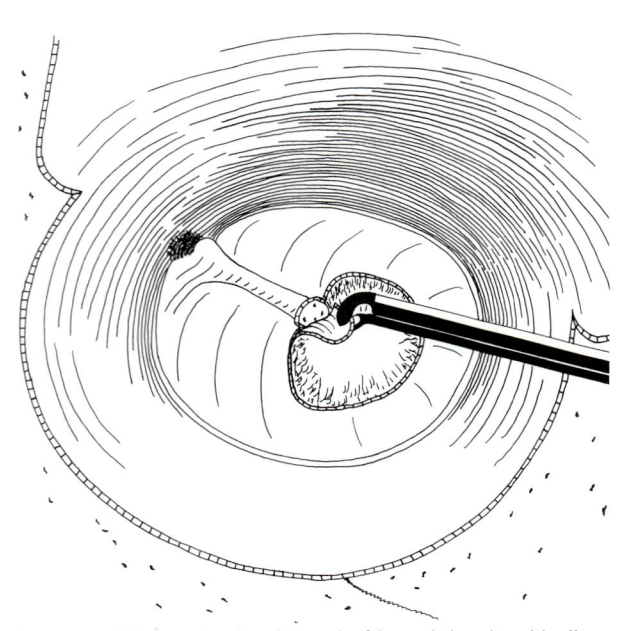

Fig. **540** The umbo is cleared of keratinized epithelium

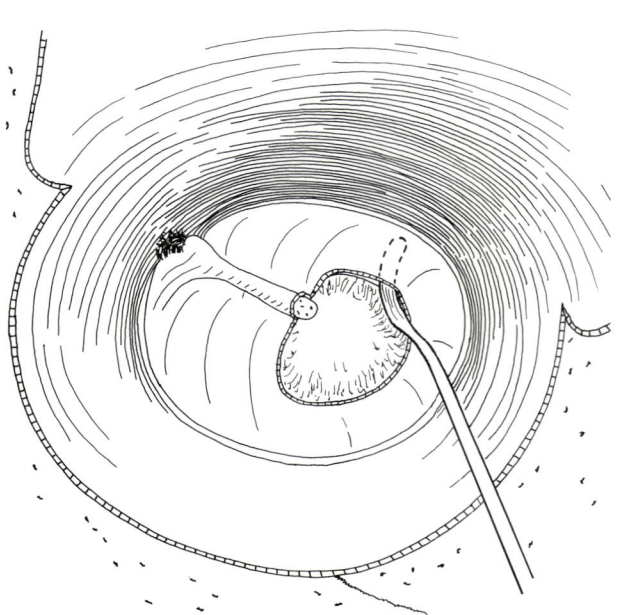

Fig. **541** The mucosa from the undersurface of the drum remnant is elevated

Techniques Without Tympanomeatal Flaps 187

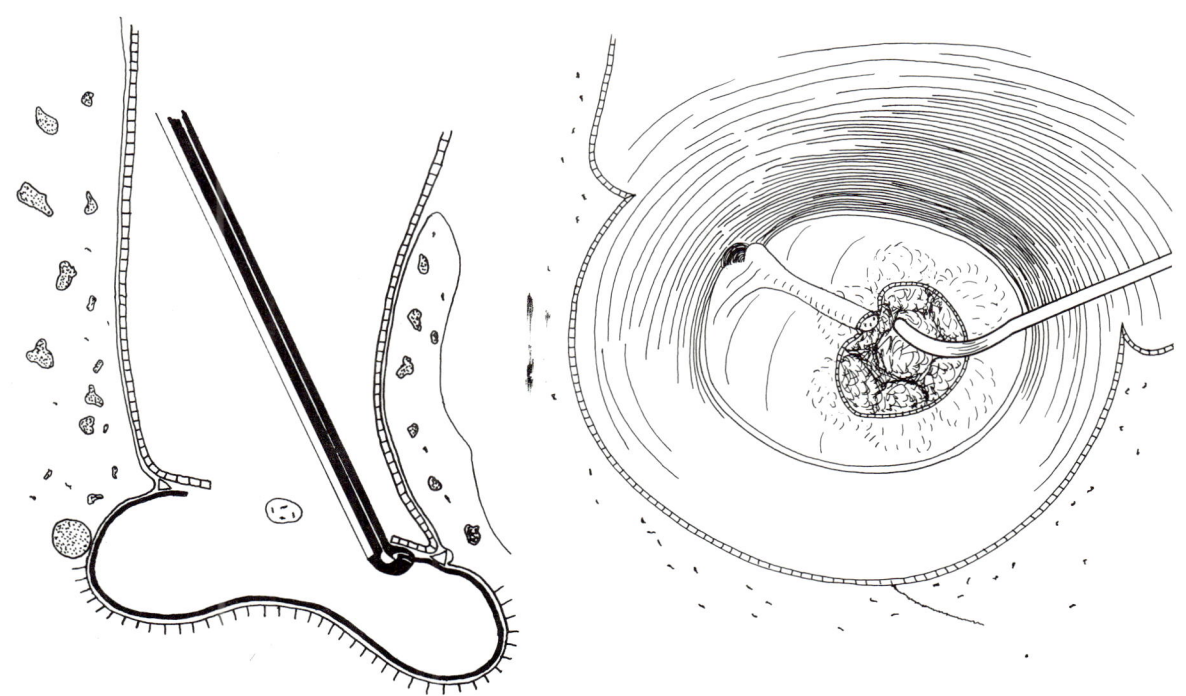

Fig. 542 The mucosa is removed using curved forceps, seen here in a side view

Fig. 543 The tympanic cavity is filled with Gelfoam balls

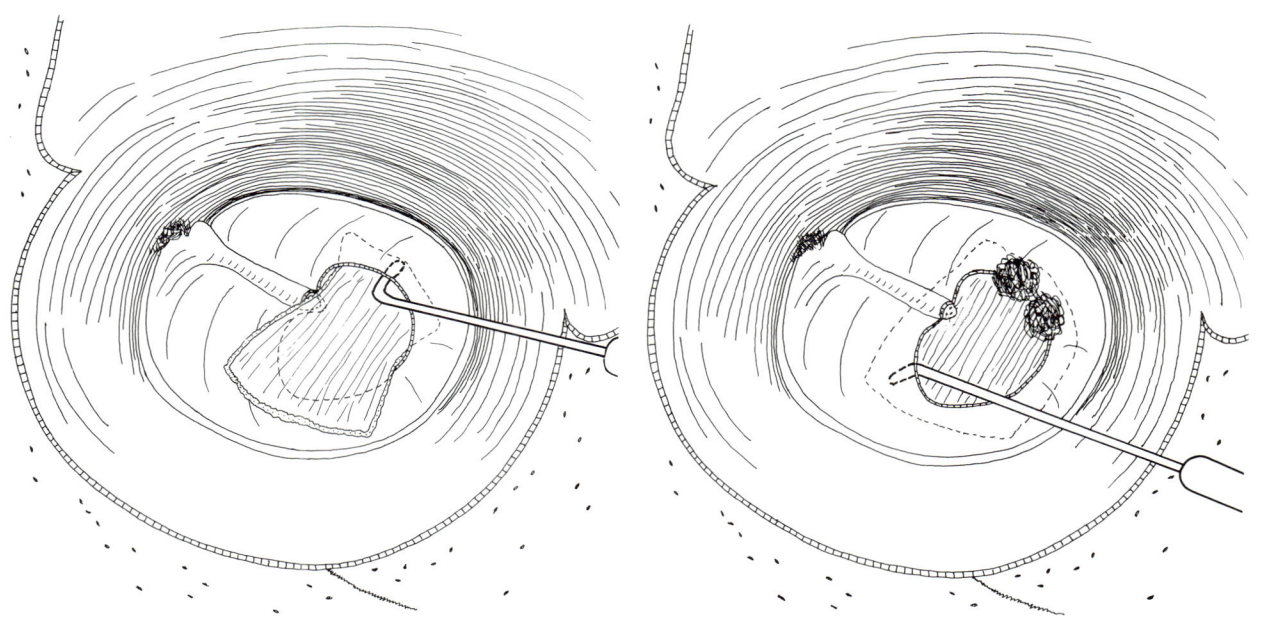

Fig. 544 The fascia is brought under the anterior drum remnant

Fig. 545 The fascia is positioned around the edge of the perforation and fixed with Gelfoam balls

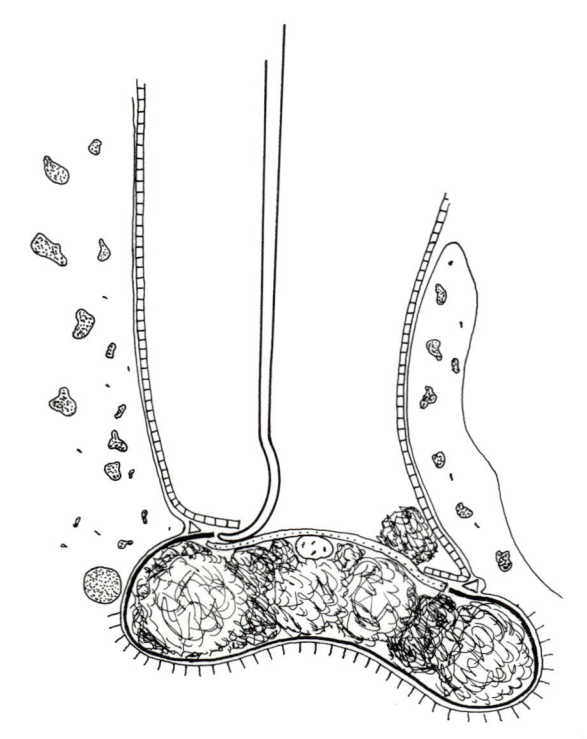

Fig. 546 The side view, illustrating the placement of the fascia

Techniques with Tympanomeatal Flaps

Techniques involving elevation of the tympanomeatal flap and the annulus are in fact tympanotomy techniques. Tympanotomy techniques can be performed using any approach, and can be applied in any perforation. Their greatest advantage is that the tympanic cavity can be inspected. The size of the tympanomeatal flap can vary from 2 mm to 15 mm, depending on the location of the circumferential incision and the approach used. In an endaural approach with a speculum, the tympanomeatal flap will be small, and the circumferential incision is placed in the medial half of the bony ear canal. In some retroauricular approaches, the circumferential incision is placed at the level of the suprameatal spine, and the tympanomeatal flaps are very large. The tympanomeatal flap (usually a posterior one) can be cut at the 9-o'clock position, resulting in swing-door techniques, or remain intact as a large flap.

Swing-Door Technique

Palva (1963) introduced the swing-door technique in the early 1960s. By cutting a small or large posterior flap at the 9-o'clock position and elevating and pushing the superior and inferior flaps aside, a good view of the tympanic cavity is achieved, both of the sinus tympani, with a posterior perforation, and of the hypotympanum, with an inferior perforation. In total perforation, the swing-door technique allows an excellent view of the tympanic orifice of the Eustachian tube and the anterior tympanum.

Techniques involving posterior tympanotomy with the swing-door technique are commonly used techniques, since nearly all myringoplasties and tympanoplasties can be performed by elevating the posterior tympanomeatal flap.

Posterior Perforation

For treatment of posterior perforation, the author always uses an underlay technique with posterior tympanotomy and the swing-door technique. An incision is performed about 3 or 4 mm lateral to the annulus, resulting in a small flap (Fig. **547**). The tympanomeatal flap is elevated together with the annulus, and a radial incision is made at the 9-o'clock position. The ear-canal skin and the drum remnant are elevated superiorly together with the annulus, forming a superior flap. Any retraction or keratinized epithelium under the drum is controlled, and the edges of the perforation are excised, following the course of the chorda. The elevation is continued towards the neck of the malleus, and the drum remnant attached to the malleus handle is elevated. The mucosa on the posterior side of the malleus handle is scarified. Finally, the inferior tympanomeatal flap with the annulus is elevated (Fig. **548**). The inferior edge of the perforation is excised, still ensuring that no keratinized epithelium is under the drum remnant. The swing-door technique provides an excellent view of the tympanic sinus. It facilitates any drilling of the bony annulus, or ossiculoplasty, that may be necessary. Gelfoam balls are placed in the tympanic cavity, especially in the inferior part. Dry or semiwet fascia is placed in continuity with the malleus handle, and on a possibly interposed ossicle. Inferiorly, the fascia is placed under the drum. It can be pushed between the drum and the umbo to fix it (Fig. **549**). The flaps are returned, and are fixed with Gelfoam balls (Fig. **550**). Especially firm fixation should be provided at the inferior edge of the

Swing-Door Technique

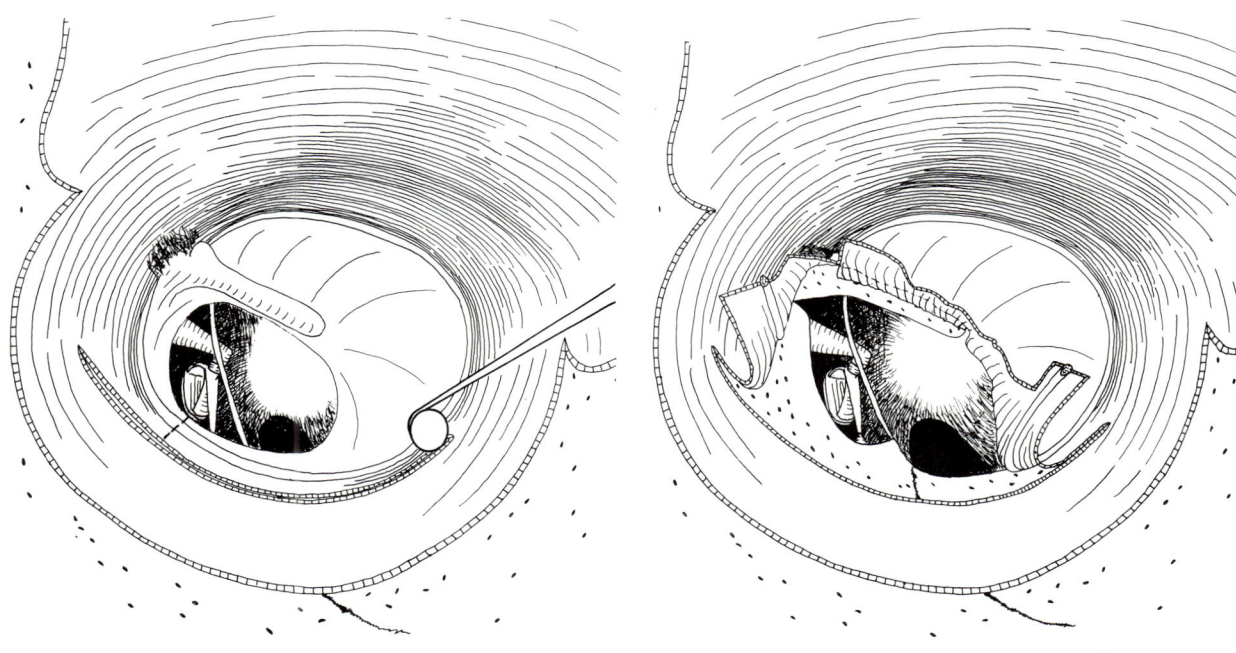

Fig. 547 **Swing-door technique in a posterior perforation.** An incision is made 3 mm lateral to the annulus

Fig. 548 The superior and inferior skin flaps are elevated, together with the drum remnant and the annulus

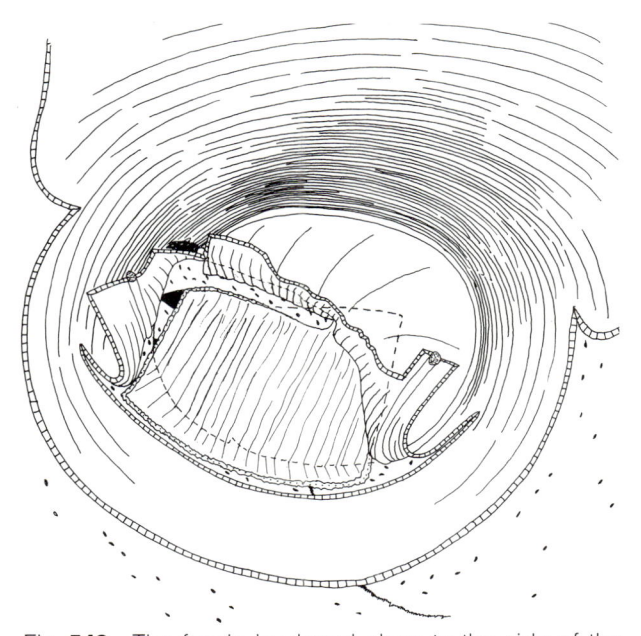

Fig. 549 The fascia is placed close to the side of the malleus handle and under the drum remnant

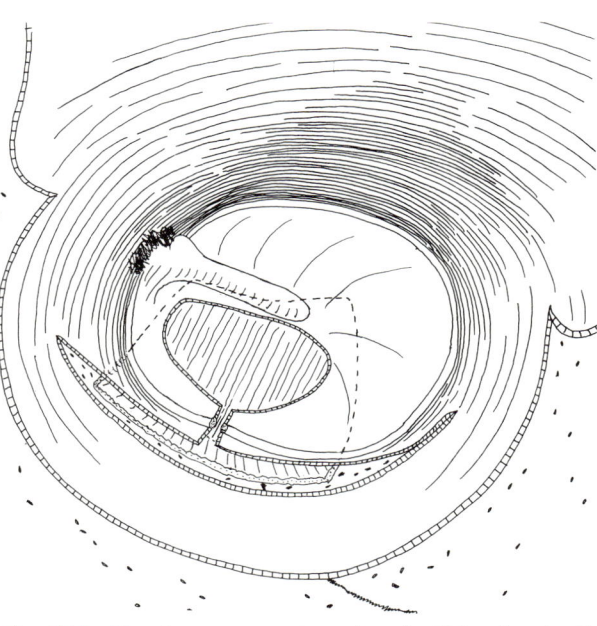

Fig. 550 The flaps are replaced and will be fixed with Gelfoam balls

perforation. The anteroinferior edge of the fascia can be fixed by the Gerlach (1975) technique (Fig. 551).

Fascia can be placed under the malleus handle (Fig. 552) after scarification of the mucosa from its undersurface and placement of Gelfoam.

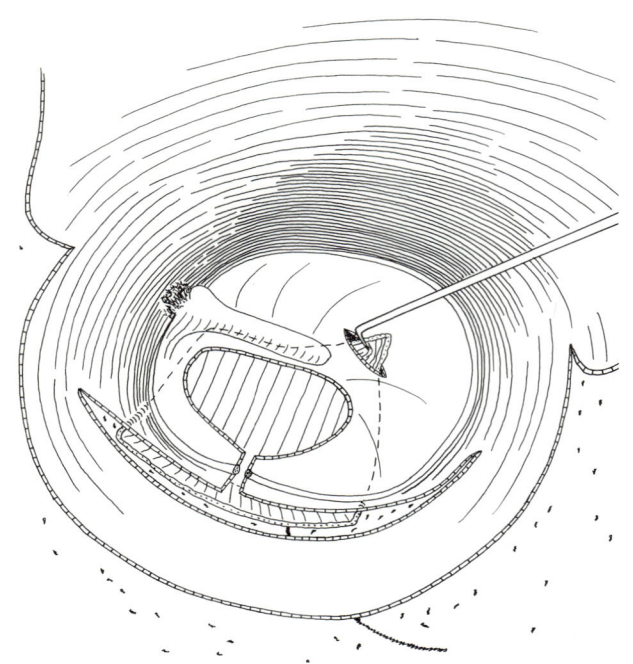

Fig. **551 The Gerlach technique:** through a small hole, the fascia is pulled onto the drum surface using a small hook

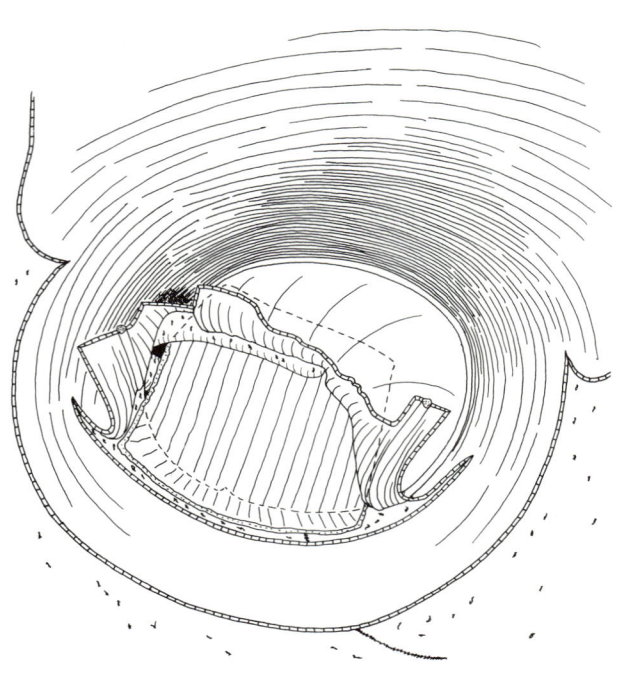

Fig. **552** The fascia is placed under the malleus handle

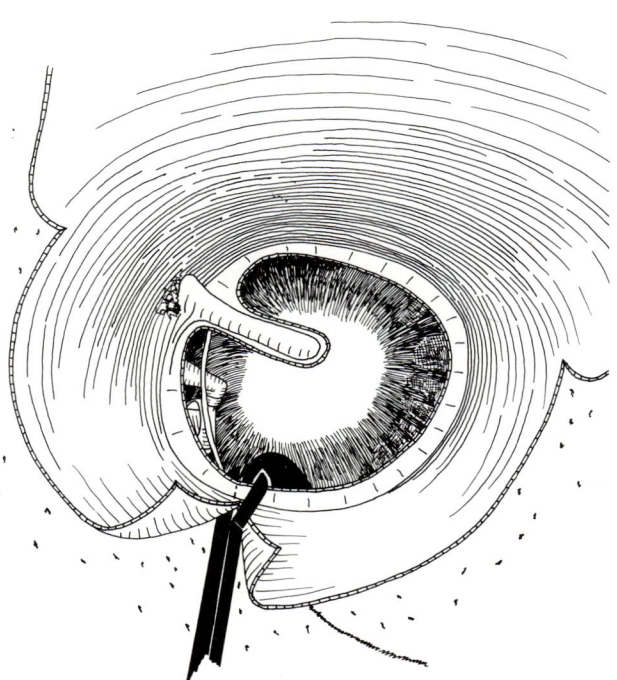

Fig. **553 Swing-door technique in a total perforation.** Epithelium from the edge of the perforation is removed. A large tympanotomy incision is made, and the tympanomeatal flap is elevated and cut at the 9-o'clock position

Total Perforation

After a circumferential incision between the 11-o'clock and 6-o'clock positions at any level 3–15 mm lateral to the annulus (Fig. **553**), and a radial incision at the 9-o'clock position, the edges of the perforations, including the epithelium of the malleus handle, are excised. The tympanomeatal flaps are elevated superiorly and inferiorly (Fig. **554**), separately. The mucosa from the undersurface of the malleus is scarified. The most important part of the operation is to elevate the mucosa under the anterior edge of the perforation and around the annulus. The mucosa should be elevated as indicated before, or removed by a double-cup forceps or around knife all the way round (Fig. **554**). The tympanic cavity is filled with Gelfoam balls, and a large piece of fascia is brought under the malleus handle, and under the fibrous annulus and approximated to the denuded bone all the way round in the anterior tympanum and hypotympanum (Fig. **555**). The flaps are returned (Fig. **556**), and the fascia graft is fixed with Gelfoam balls placed at the edge of the perforation (Fig. **557**). Other methods of fixing the fascia can also be used, e.g., fibrin glue.

Swing-Door Technique

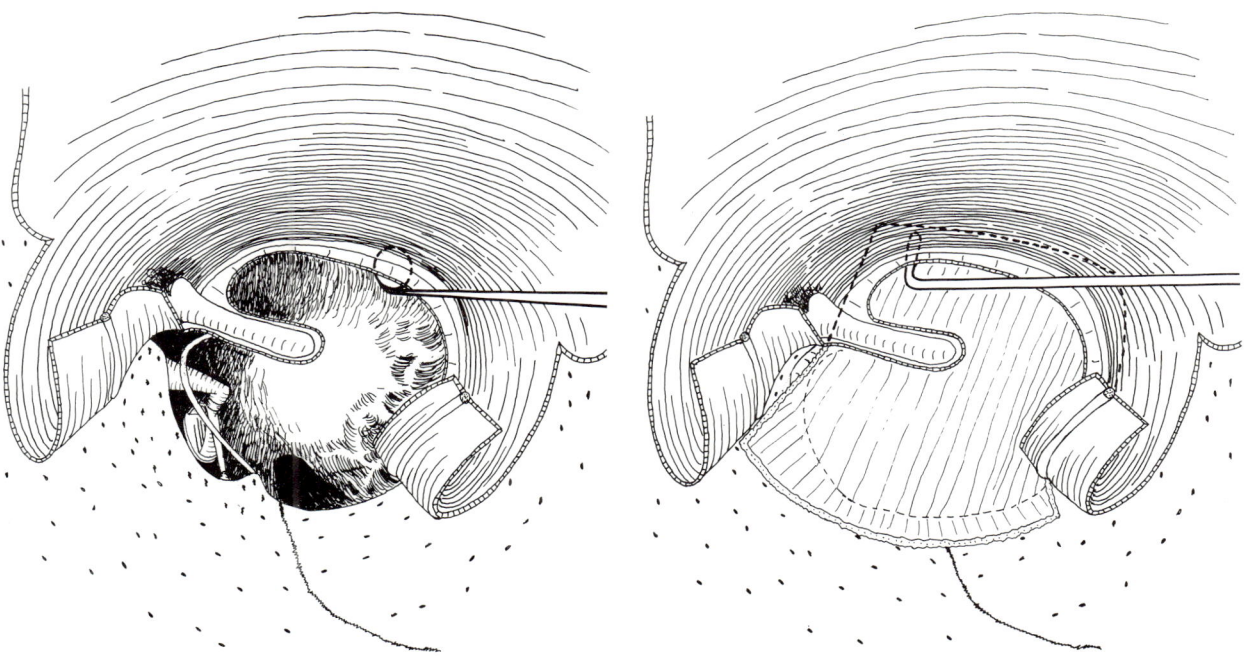

Fig. 554 The superior and inferior tympanomeatal flaps are elevated. The mucosa is elevated from the surface of the annulus anterioroly

Fig. 555 The fascia is placed under the annulus anteriorly and inferiorly, and under the malleus handle

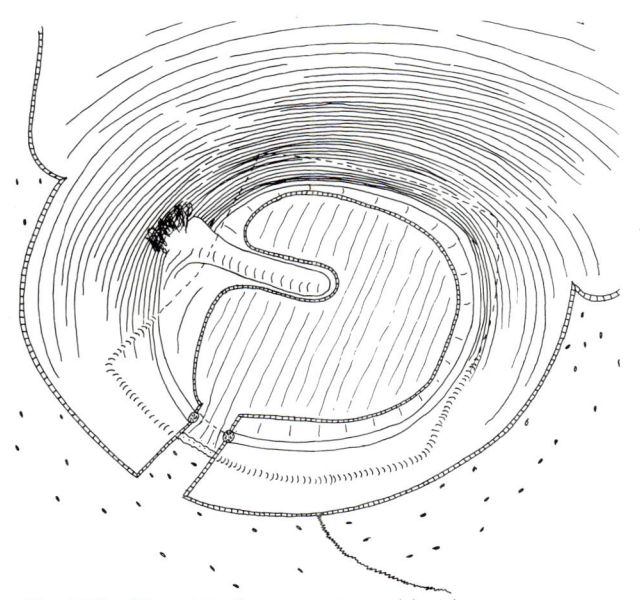

Fig. 556 The skin flaps are turned back

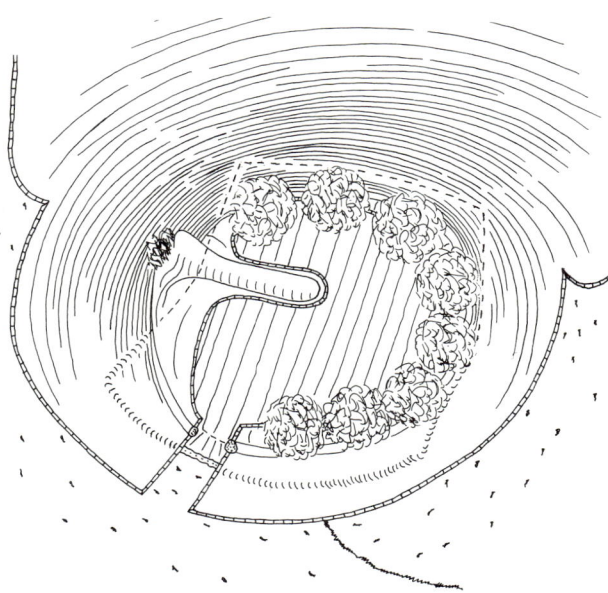

Fig. 557 The skin flaps are fixed with Gelfoam balls

Instead of placing the fascia under the malleus, it can in many cases be an advantage to place it on the malleus, e.g., in cases with a retracted malleus and denuded mucosa at the promontory. The malleus handle is carefully cleared of keratinized epithelium, and the epithelium is removed from the umbo (Fig. 558). Superiorly, at the neck of the malleus, an epithelial flap is created. After the tympanic cavity has been filled with Gelfoam balls, the fascia is placed over the malleus, and the malleus flap is returned (Fig. 559).

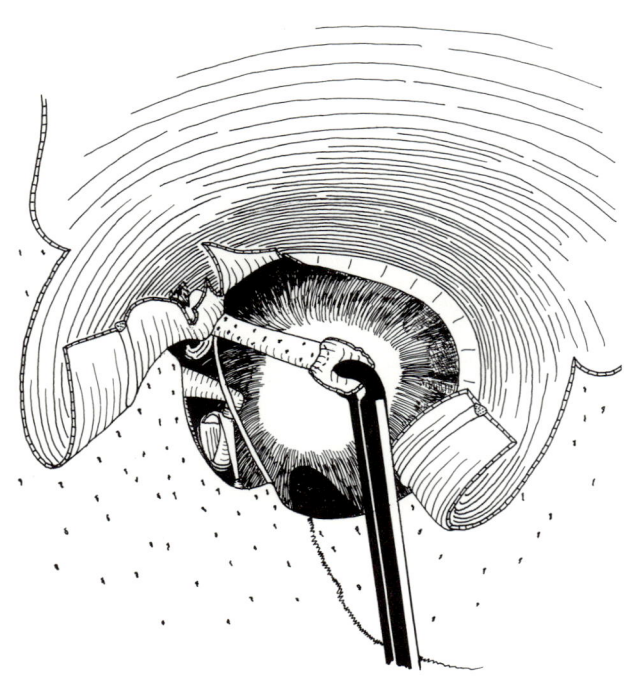

Fig. 558 Placement of the fascia on the malleus handle after cleaning the malleus of keratinized epithelium and creating a small malleus flap

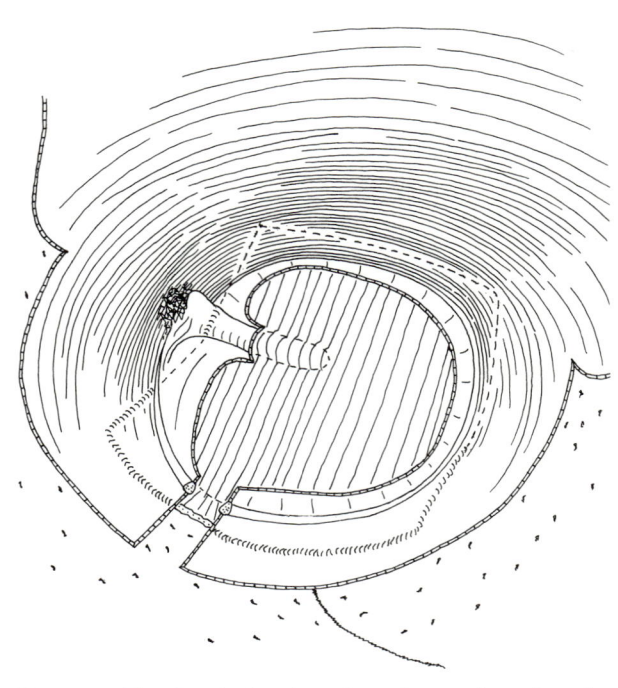

Fig. 559 The fascia is placed on the malleus handle, and the skin flap and the malleus flap are returned

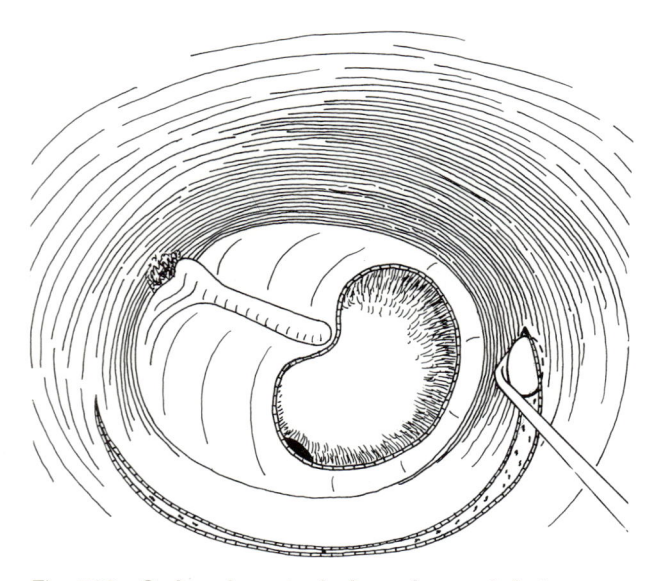

Fig. 560 **Swing-door technique in an inferior perforation.** A tympanotomy incision is performed

Inferior Perforation

A posterior tympanotomy incision with the swing-door technique is an excellent method for underlay closure of an inferior perforation and inspection of the ossicular chain. The incision is performed about 3–4 mm lateral to the annulus, starting at the 10-o'clock position, and continuing down to the 5-o'clock position (Fig. 560). The flap and the annulus are elevated, and the flap is cut at the 8-o'clock position using a pair of scissors. The annulus and the drum remnant are also incised. A superior flap is elevated, exposing the incudostapedial joint, and a large inferior flap is then elevated far anteriorly (Fig. 561). At the beginning of the operation, the epithelial edge of the perforation has been excised, and the mucosa from the undersurface of the drum remnant has been removed. After the flaps have been elevated, an excellent view is provided, facilitating further elevation and excision of the mucosa, and further inspection of the epithelial junction between the keratinized squamous and mucosal epithelium. Under the anterior annulus, mucosa can be excised using a curved double-cup forceps far under the annulus, and the bone can be denuded in this area (Fig. 561). Also, the region under the malleus and the umbo can be cleared of mucosa. After the tympanic cavity has

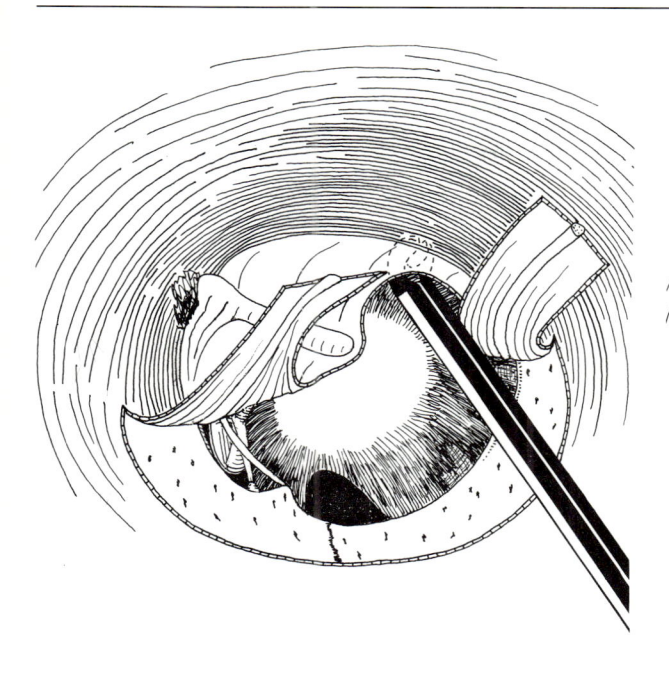

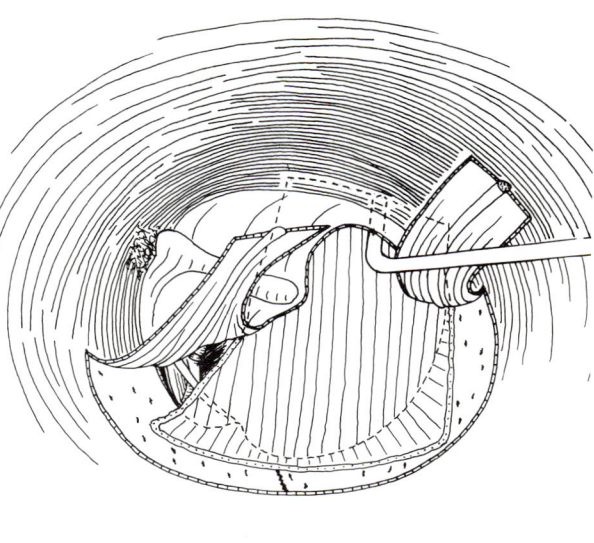

Fig. 561 The tympanomeatal flap is cut at the 8-o'clock positoin. The superior and inferior flaps are elevated. The mucosa from the drum remnant and anterior annulus is removed

Fig. 562 The fascia is placed under the annulus

been packed with Gelfoam, especially anteriorly and inferiorly, an underlay fascia graft is placed (Fig. 562). Care is taken to push the fascia with a curved elevator far anteriorly under the annulus, and superiorly under the malleus. Inferiorly, the edge of the fascia is placed on the bony annulus. The tympanomeatal flaps are returned (Fig. 563), and the fascia is fixed with Gelfoam balls, first placed around the annulus, and then around the border of the perforation.

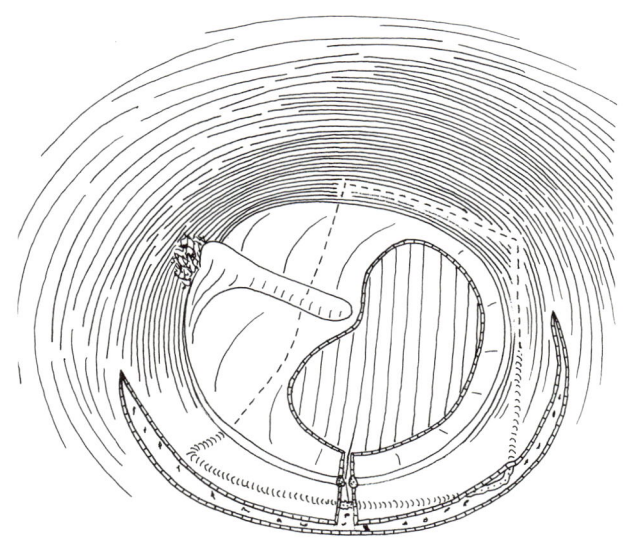

Fig. 563 The tympanomeatal flaps are returned

The Large Tympanomeatal Flap Techniques

The tympanomeatal flap remains in continuity, and is usually large. These technique are popular, especially in the retroauricular approach, which can be combined with a lateral circumferential incision or a medial circumferential incision at any site along the ear canal. A large tympanomeatal flap is elevated together with the annulus, and the fascia is placed under the annulus.

Anterior Perforation

Firstly, the edges of the perforation are excised, and mucosa from the undersurface of the drum remnant, especially the anterior annulus, is removed. A large anterior tympanotomy is performed (Fig. **564**) between the 12-o'clock and 6-o'clock positions, and the tympanomeatal flap is elevated (Fig. **565**). The annulus is luxated out of its bony sulcus. The mucosa is incised, and the anterior tympanum is exposed. It is now possible to remove the mucosa under the edge of the perforation (Fig. **566**). For

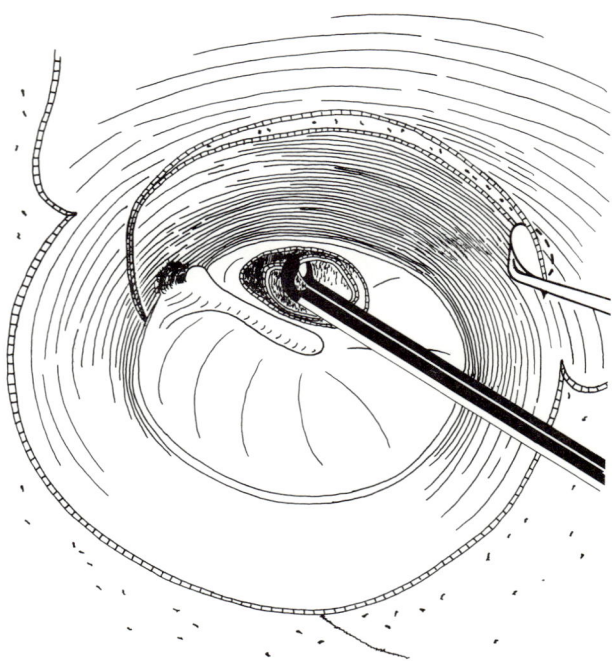

Fig. **564 Anterior tympanotomy in an anterior perforation.** The epithelium from the perforation edge is excised

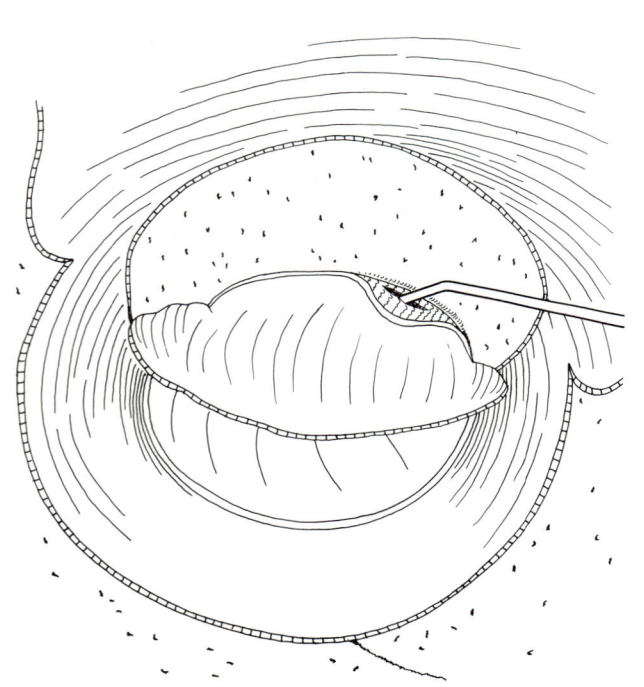

Fig. **565** The large tympanomeatal flap is elevated anteriorly. The annulus is elevated, and the mucosa is perforated

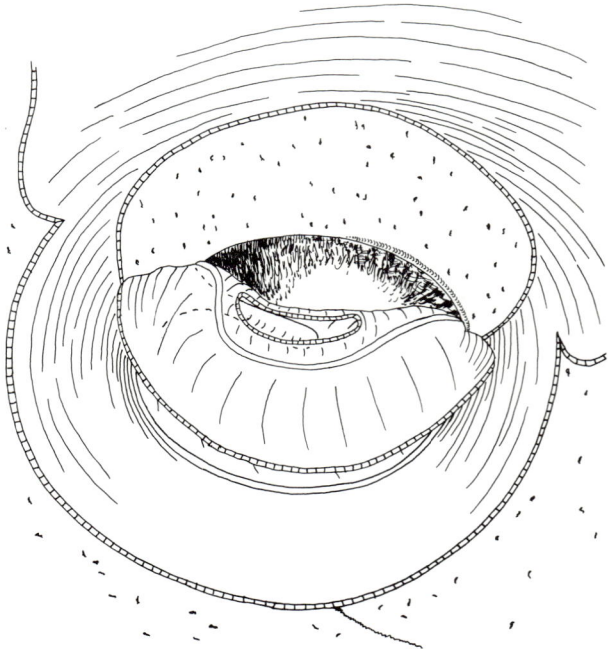

Fig. **566** The anterior annulus, with the drum remnant, is elevated as far as the malleus handle

firm fixation of the fascia posteriorly, the epithelium from the malleus handle is elevated with a small rugine (Fig. 567). The malleus handle is exposed (Fig. 568), and the fascia is placed on the malleus handle and on the denuded bone anteriorly (Fig. 569). The tympanomeatal flap is returned and fixed with Gelfoam balls. Special care is taken to fix the anterior annulus, to prevent blunting or lateralization (Figs. 570 and 571).

Another variation on this method involves placing the fascia under the malleus handle (Fig. 572), and in this case, the fascia should be supported by Gelfoam balls placed in the tympanic cavity.

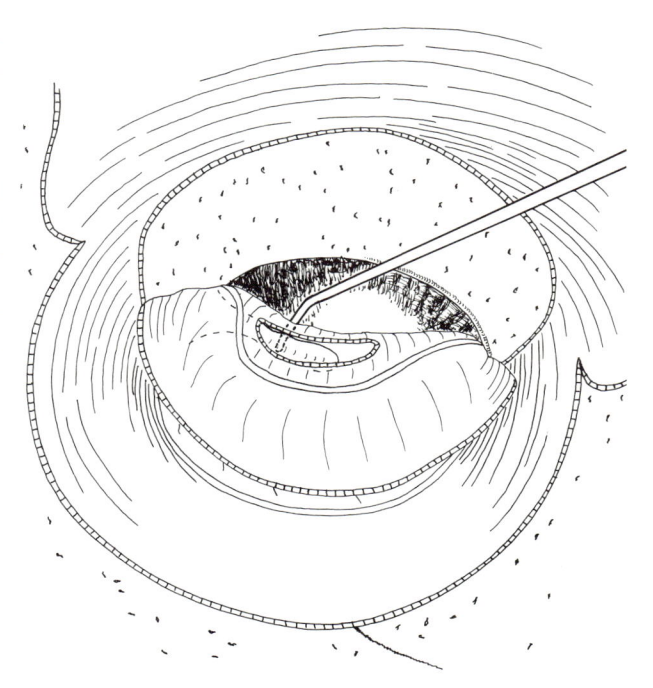

Fig. 567 The epithelium is elevated from the malleus handle

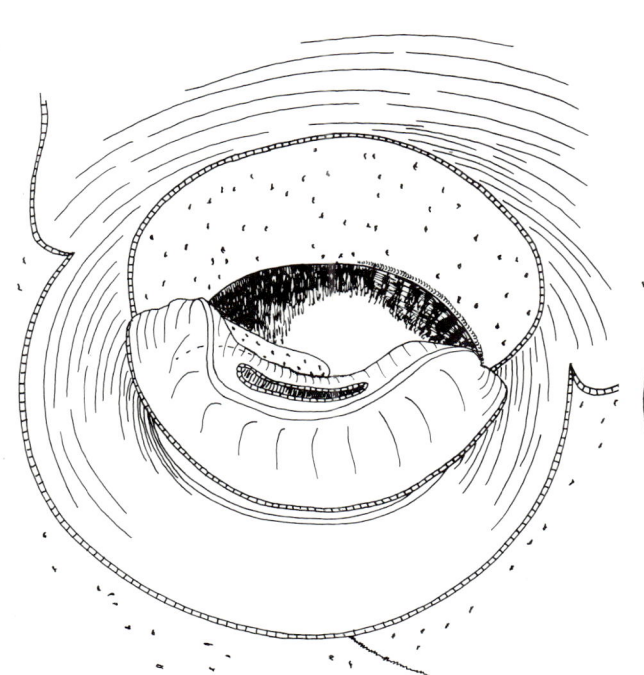

Fig. 568 The malleus handle is exposed

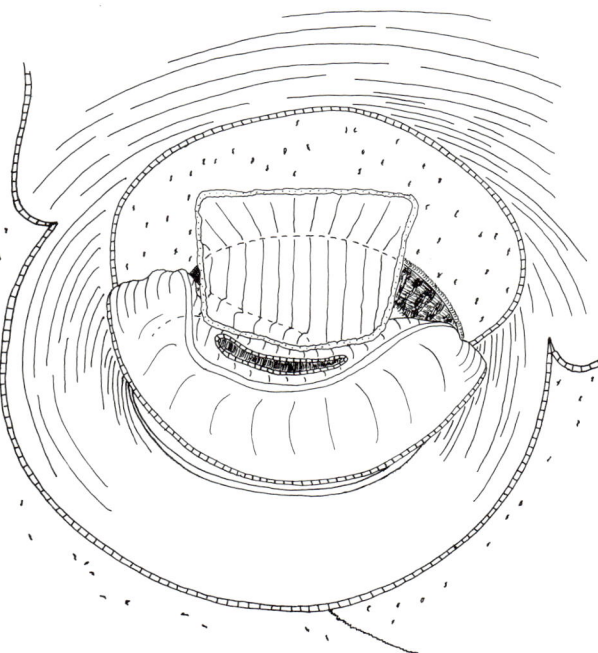

Fig. 569 The fascia is placed on the malleus handle and on the anterior bony annulus

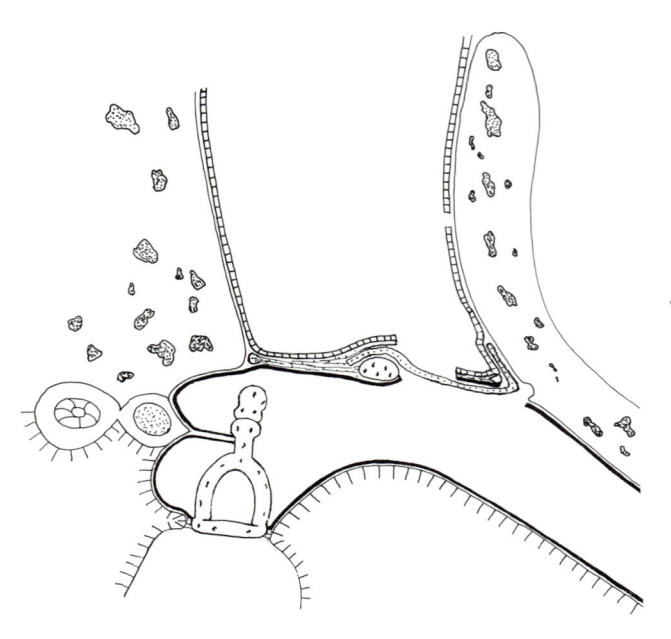

Fig. 570 Side view of the placement of the fascia on the malleus handle. The tympanomeatal flap is returned

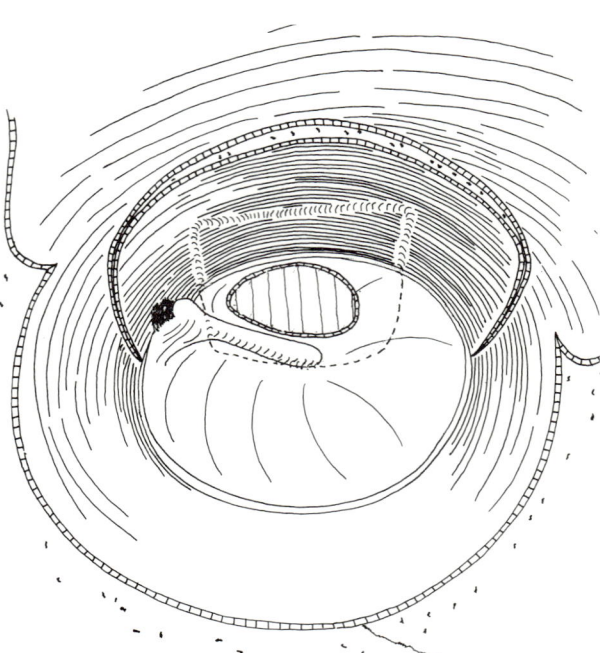

Fig. 571 The fascia is placed under the malleus handle

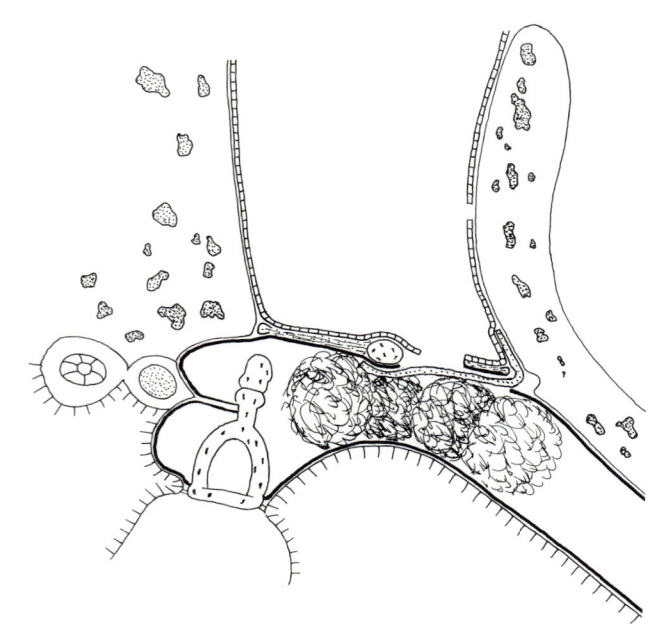

Fig. 572 Side view of the placement of the fascia under the malleus handle. The fascia is supported by Gelfoam balls

Inferior Perforation

After excision of the epithelial edge of the perforation, an extensive skin incision is made between the 10-o'clock and 2-o'clock positions several millimeters lateral to the annulus (Fig. 573). A large inferior tympanomeatal flap is elevated. The annulus is luxated at the 9-o'clock position, perforating the mucosa (Fig. 574). The fibrous annulus is luxated out of its bony sulcus all the way round from the 9-o'clock to the 3-o'clock positions (Fig. 575). The drum remnant is elevated. The mucosa is carefully removed from the undersurface of the drum remnant, and the malleus handle is cleaned. A good view of the inferior half of the tympanic cavity is achieved (Fig. 576). The fascia is placed on the malleus handle and on the bone all round the inferior part of the bony annulus (Figs. 577 and 578). The tympanomeatal flap is replaced (Fig. 579), and is fixed by Gelfoam balls, especially around the annulus.

The fascia can be placed under the malleus handle in order to maintain the conical shape of the drum (Fig. 580).

The Large Tympanomeatal Flap Techniques 197

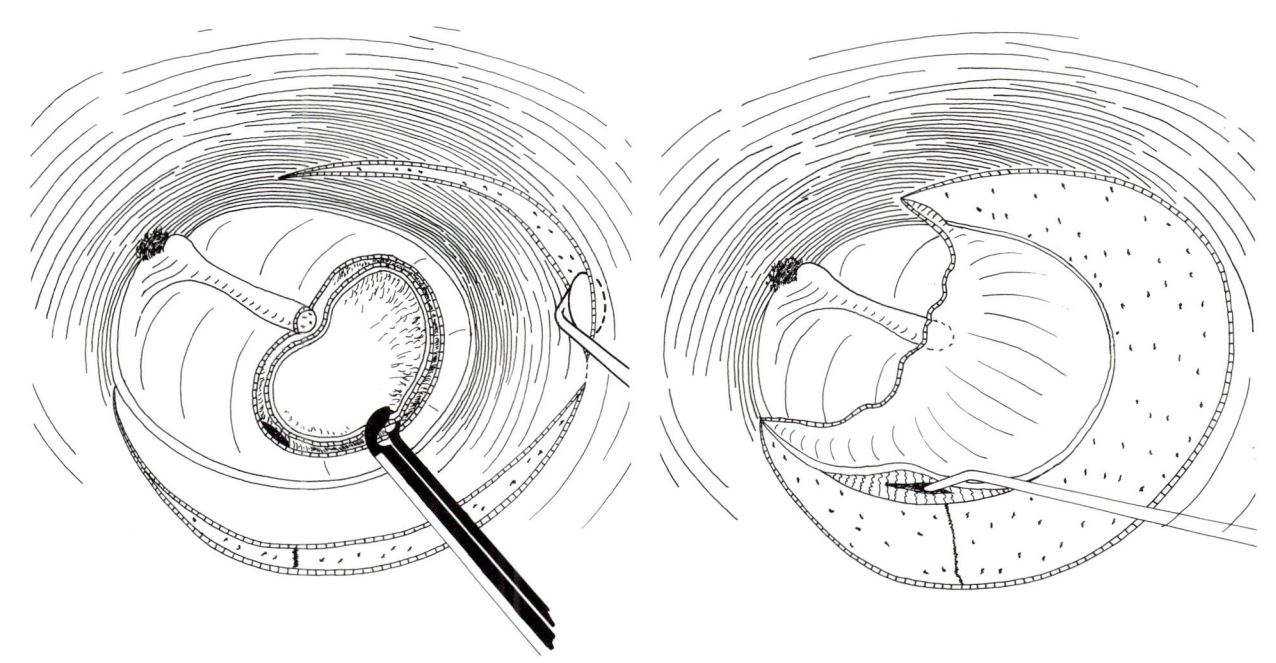

Fig. 573 **Inferior tympanotomy in an inferior perforation.** The edge of the perforation is excised

Fig. 574 A large tympanomeatal flap is elevated, and the mucosa is incised at the 9-o'clock position

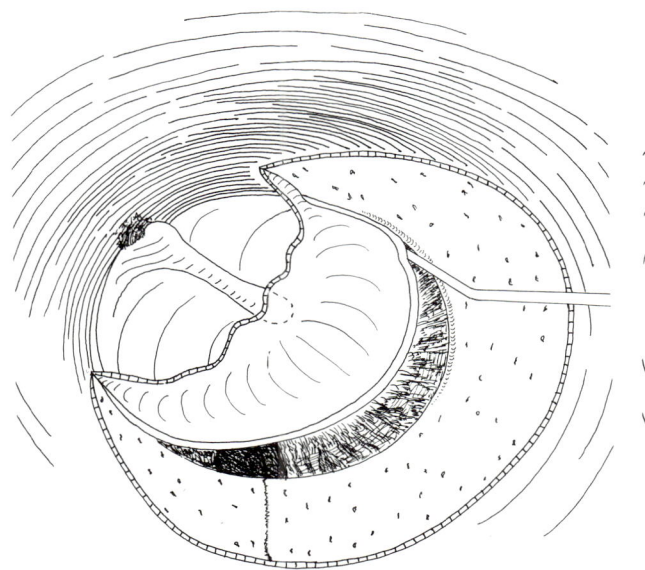

Fig. 575 The annulus is dislocated all the way around

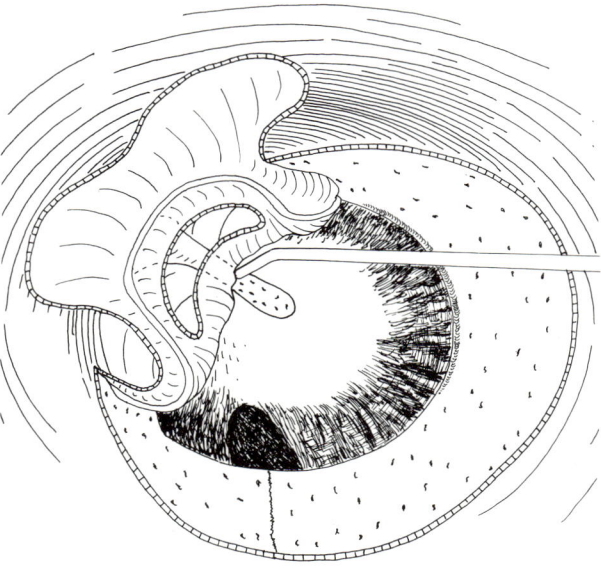

Fig. 576 The large tympanomeatal flap, with the epithelium from the malleus handle, is elevated

198　11　Underlay Techniques

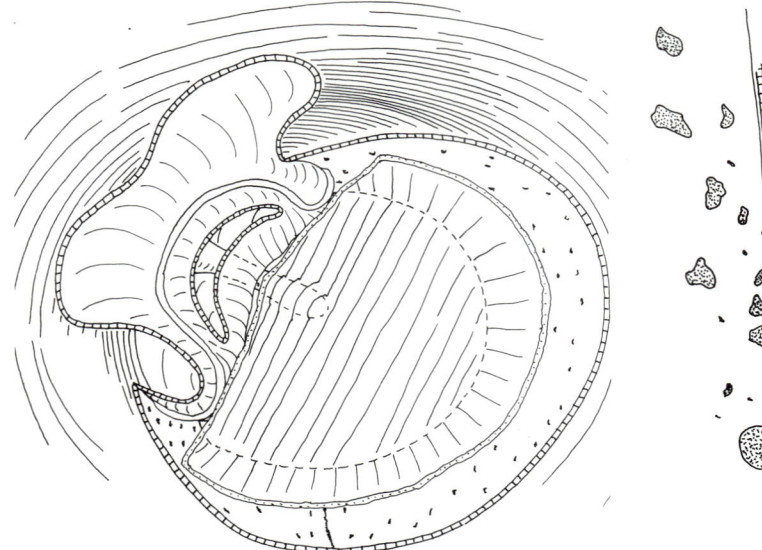

Fig. **577**　The fascia is placed on the malleus handle and denuded bone

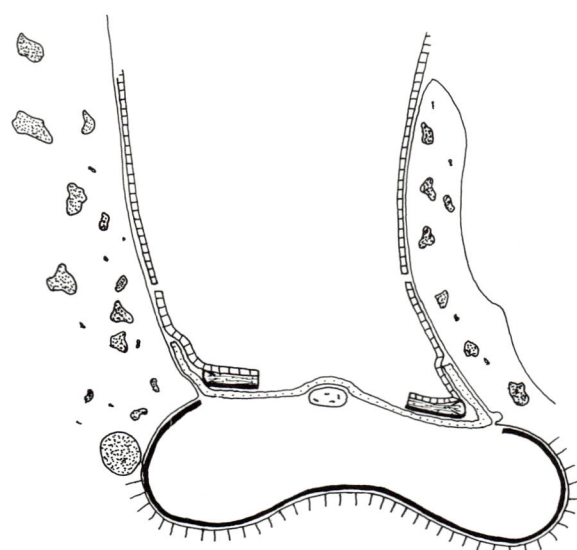

Fig. **578**　Side view of the placement of the fascia on the malleus handle

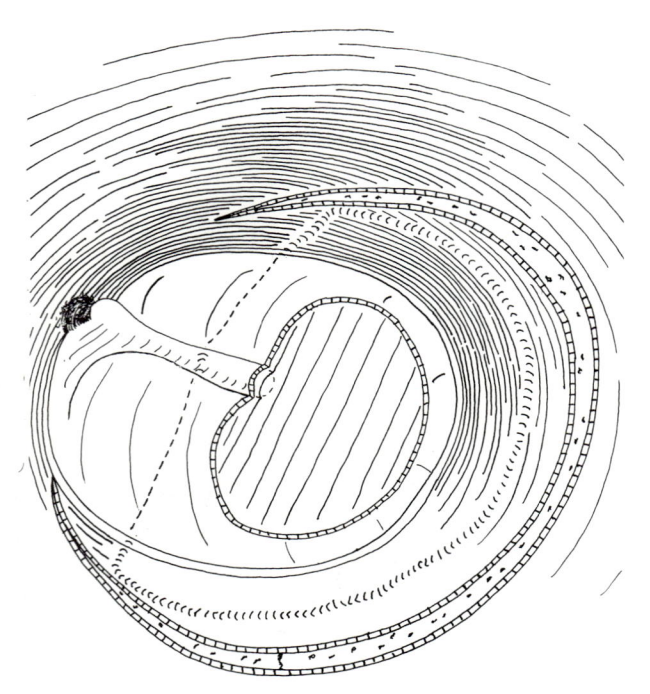

Fig. **579**　The tympanomeatal flaps are returned

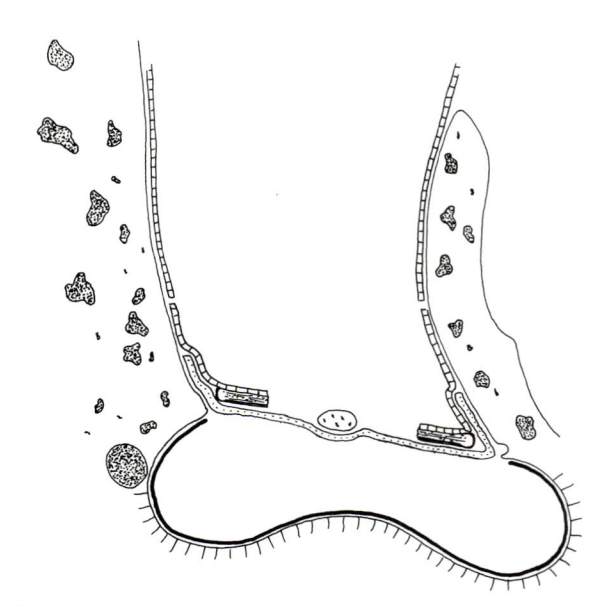

Fig. **580**　Side view of the placement of the fascia under the malleus handle

Posterior Perforation

A posterior tympanotomy incision is performed quite lateral to the annulus. It can be done either through an endaural approach with the ear speculum, or with incisions, or—most often—using a retroauricular approach. The edge of the perforation has been excised (Fig. 581). The tympanomeatal flap, together with the annulus, is elevated far anteriorly, the undersurface of the malleus handle is cleared of mucosa, and the posterior tympanum is exposed (Fig. 582). The tympanic cavity is filled with Gelfoam. A fascia graft is placed under the malleus handle and under the drum remnant, but on top of the bony annulus, and the tympanomeatal flap is replaced (Fig. 583).

Sometimes it is easier and better to place the fascia partly on top of the malleus handle. After elevation of the epithelium from the malleus handle (Fig. 584), the fascia is placed on the posterior side and partly on the lateral side of the malleus (Fig. 585). The flaps are returned (Fig. 586) and fixed with Gelfoam balls.

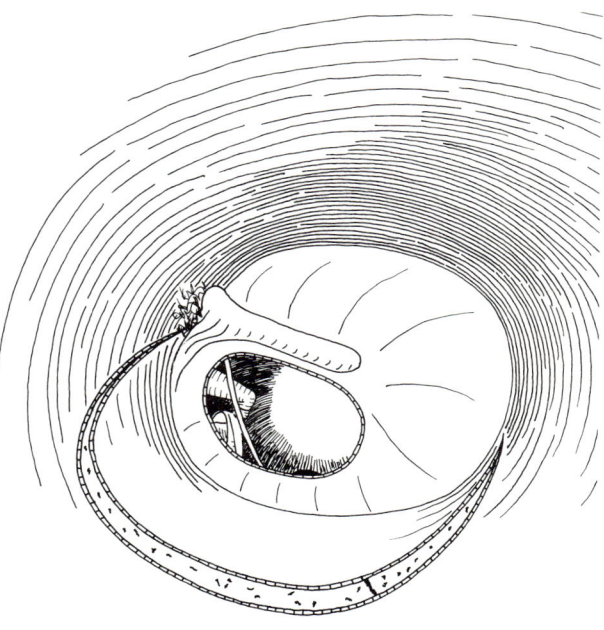

Fig. 581 **Posterior tympanotomy in a posterior perforation.** The edge of the perforation is excised

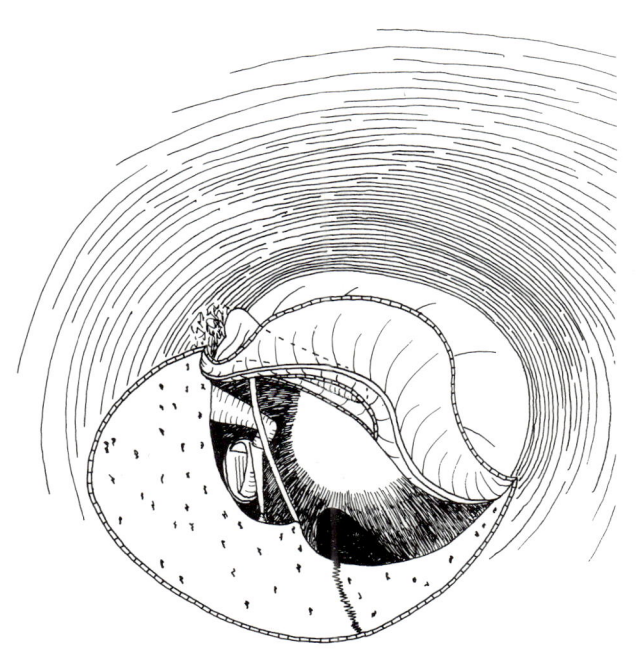

Fig. 582 The large tympanomeatal flap is elevated. The drum remnant is elevated towards the malleus handle

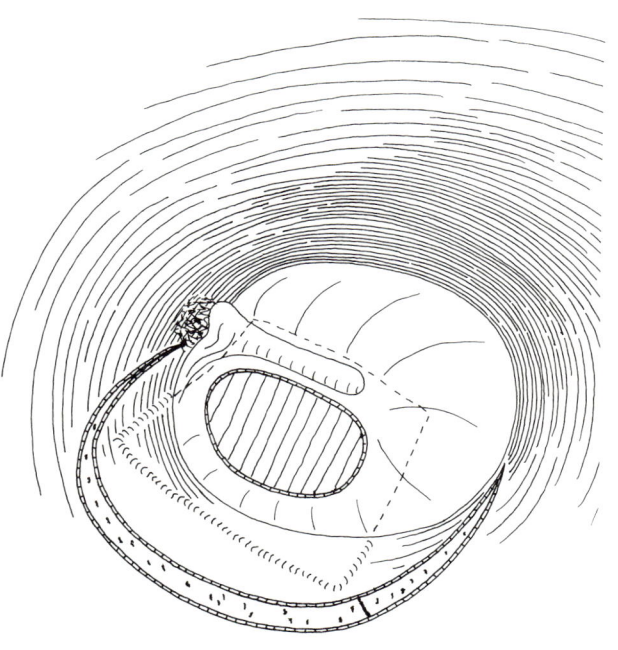

Fig. 583 The fascia is placed under the malleus handle, and the tympanomeatal flap is returned

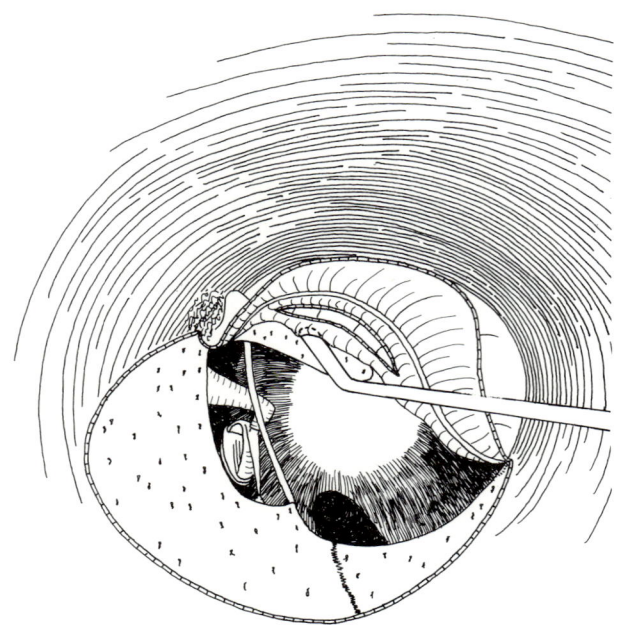

Fig. 584 Placement of the fascia on the malleus handle. The epithelium is elevated from the malleus handle

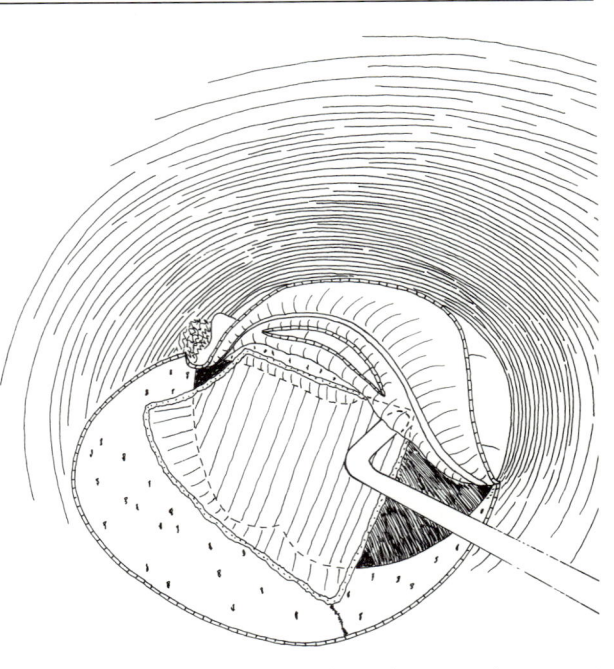

Fig. 585 The fascia is placed on the posterior aspect of the emalleus handle

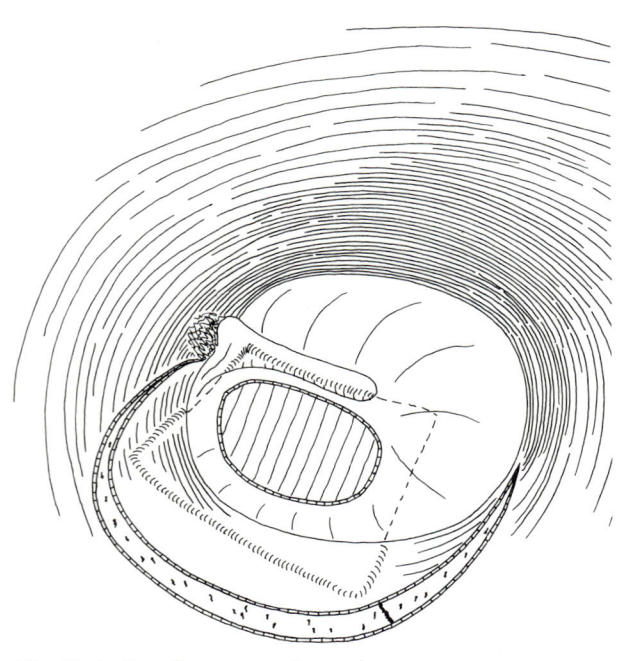

Fig. 586 The flaps are returned

Posterior Tympanotomy in Anterior Perforation

Sometimes it is appropriate to close the anterior perforation through a posterior tympanotomy. This will be necessary when inspection of the incudostapedial joint is required, e.g., in cases with more severe hearing loss than that expected in a simple anterior perforation. It is also appropriate in a defect of the incudostapedial joint, or in myringoincudopexy or myringostapediopexy associated with an atrophic or retracted posterior part of the drum. After excision of the edges of the anterior perforation and removal of the mucosa under the drum remnant around the perforation (Fig. 587), a posterior tympanotomy is performed, and the tympanomeatal flap is elevated together with the atrophic retracted drum. After inspection of the ossicles, a fascia graft is placed under the malleus, pushed through the anterior perforation, and pulled further anteriorly using a forceps (Fig. 588). After the fascia has been positioned, the tympanomeatal flap is returned, and the fascia is pushed under the drum remnant and far anteriorly under the anterior annulus (Fig. 589).

The Large Tympanomeatal Flap Techniques

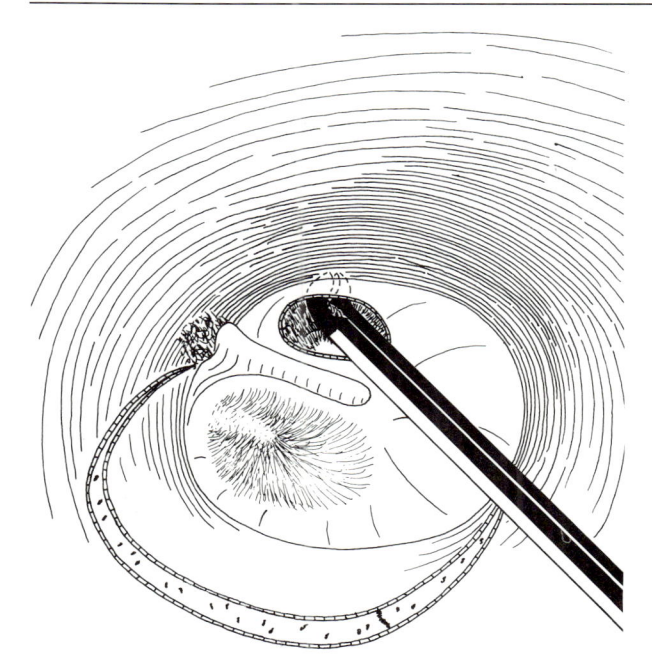

Fig. 587 **Posterior tympanotomy in an anterior perforation and posterior retraction.** The edges of the perforation are excised, and the mucosa is removed from the undersurface of the drum remnant. The large posterior tympanomeatal flap is elevated

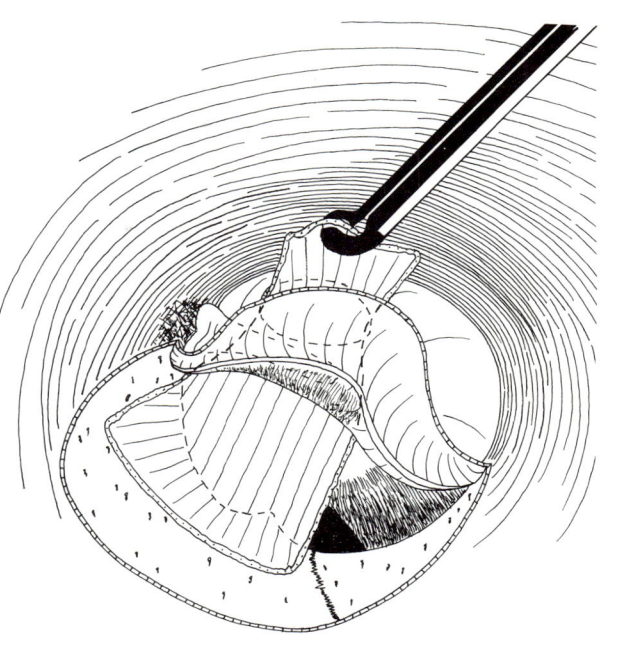

Fig. 588 The fascia is brought under the malleus and pulled into the ear canal through the anterior perforation

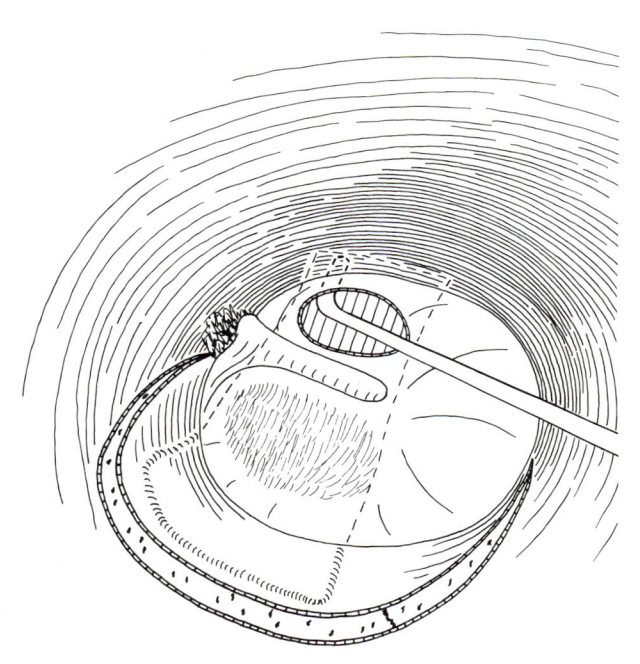

Fig. 589 The tympanomeatal flap is returned, and the fascia is positioned anteriorly

Total Elevation of the Fibrous Annulus

This method is used in total perforation with epithelium under the annulus, and is a popular method in cases using the retroauricular approach. A circumferential incision is performed all round the ear canal from the 2-o'clock to the 4-o'clock positions. The level of the incision can be lateral or medial, depending on the approach. In the retroauricular approach, the circumferential incision is usually placed laterally. The edges of the perforation have to be excised, and the keratinized squamous epithelium is removed all round (Fig. 590). The entire tympanomeatal flap is elevated with the entire annulus (Fig. 591). The elevation continues far anteriorly, and the malleus handle is cleared of the keratinized epithelium (Fig. 592).

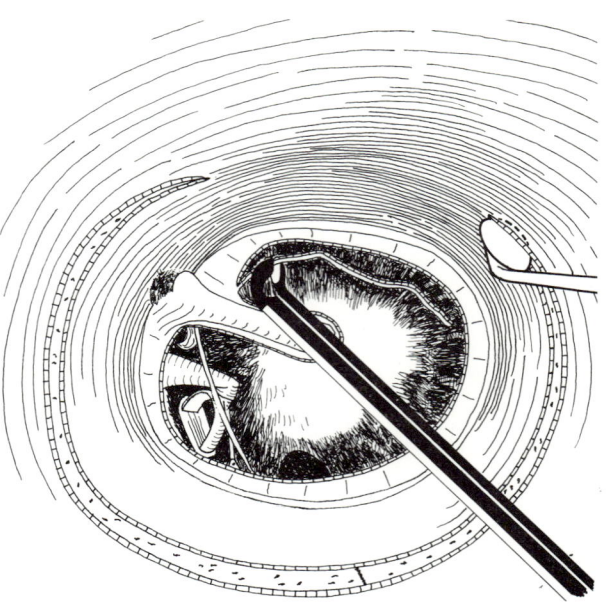

Fig. **590 Total elevation of the annulus in a total perforation.** The edge of the perforation is excised. An incision is made all the way round the ear-canal skin between the 2-o'clock and 5-o'clock positions

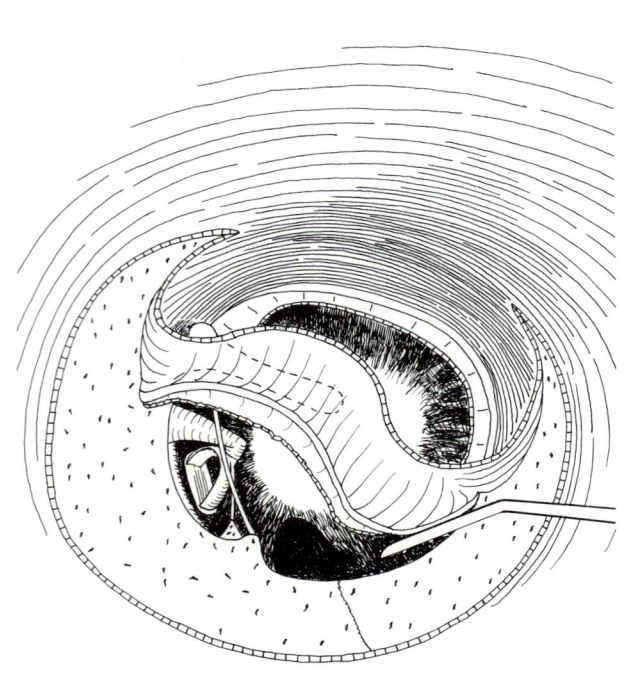

Fig. **591** The large tympanomeatal flap is elevated posteriorly

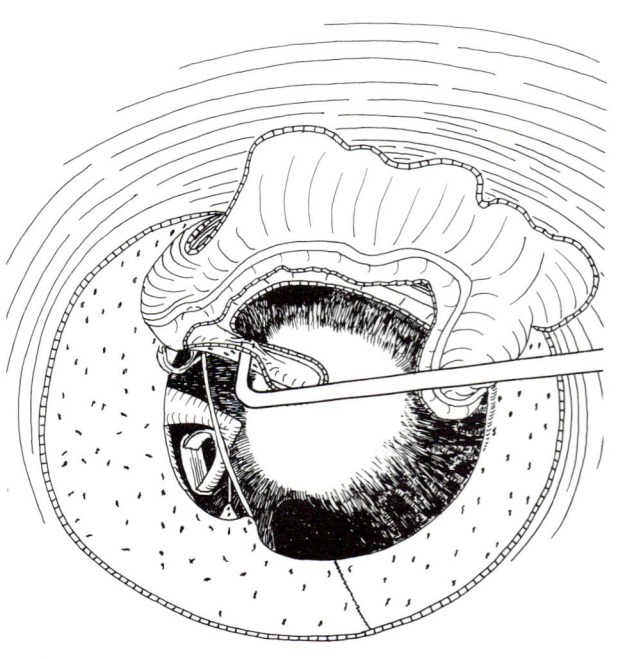

Fig. **592** The epithelium is elevated from the malleus, and a malleus flap is created

Total Elevation of the Fibrous Annulus 203

A small malleus flap is created. The annulus is further elevated all the way round and luxated out of the bony sulcus (Fig. **593** and **594**). The tympanic cavity is now free of pathology, and ready to be covered by an underlay fascia graft placed on the bone (Fig. **595**). The fascia is incised superiorly, and placed under the malleus handle. The anterior edge of the fascia is pulled posteriorly, covering Shrapnell's membrane (Fig. **596**), and then the posterior edge is pulled anteriorly, further covering the Shrapnell's membrane region and the short process of the malleus (Fig. **597**). The flaps are returned (Figs. **598, 599**).

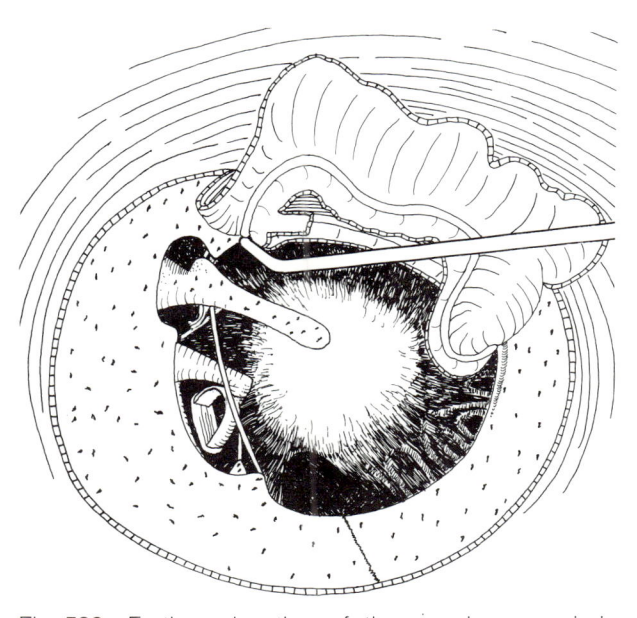

Fig. **593** Further elevation of the annulus superiorly and inferiorly

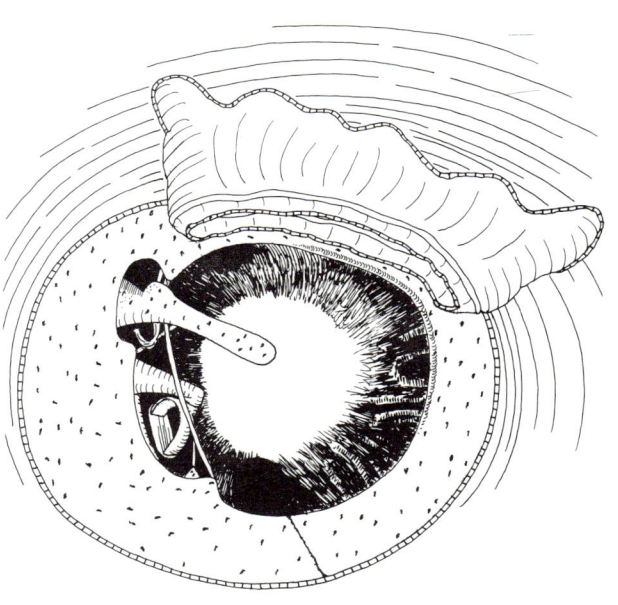

Fig. **594** Total elevation of the annulus

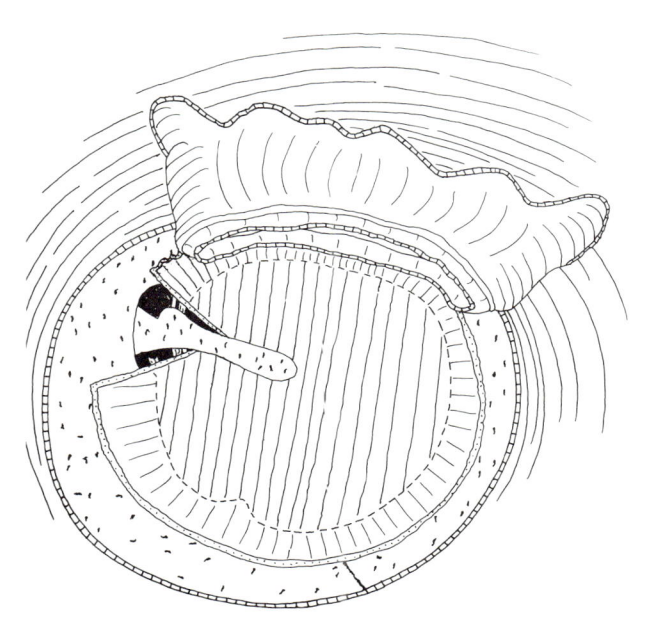

Fig. **595** Fascia with a superior slit is placed on top of the bony annulus and underneath the malleus handle

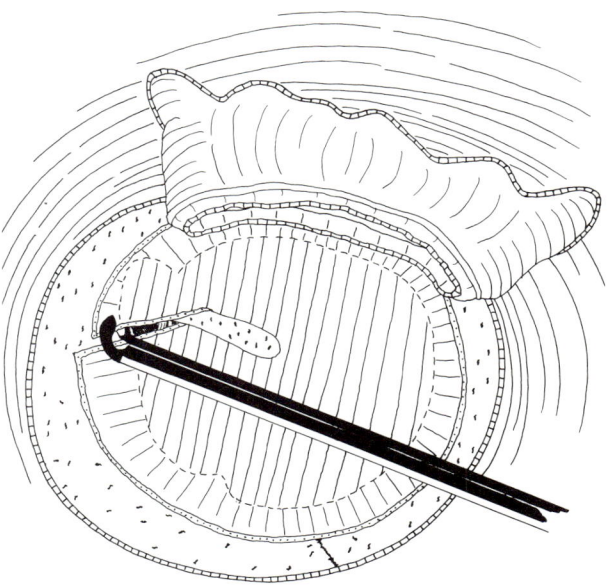

Fig. **596** The anterosuperior edge of the fascia is pulled posteriorly

11 Underlay Techniques

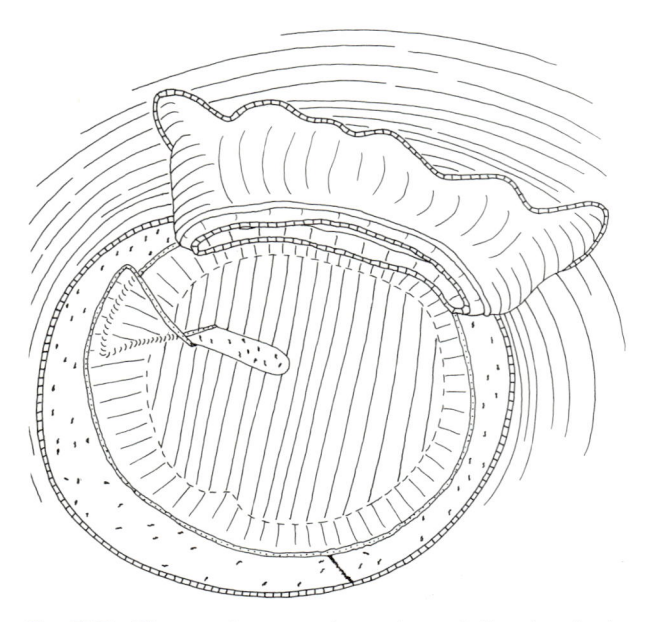

Fig. **597** The posterosuperior edge of the fascia is pulled anteriorly, closing the Shrapnell's membrane region

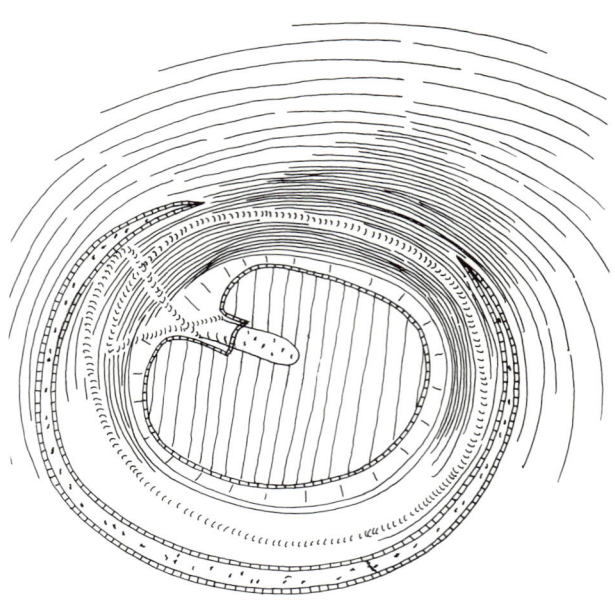

Fig. **598** The tympanomeatal flap is replaced

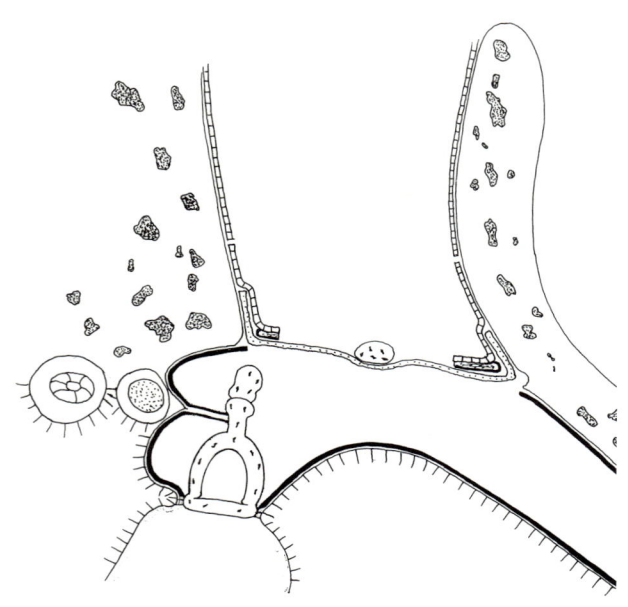

Fig. **599** Side view of the fascia placement under the malleus

The fascia can also be placed on the denuded malleus handle and the Shrapnell's membrane region. This method is easier to perform, and the fascia does not need to be cut (Figs. **600** and **601**). With a retracted malleus, placement on the malleus handle is an advantage, since it avoids the problem of graft adherence to the promontory.

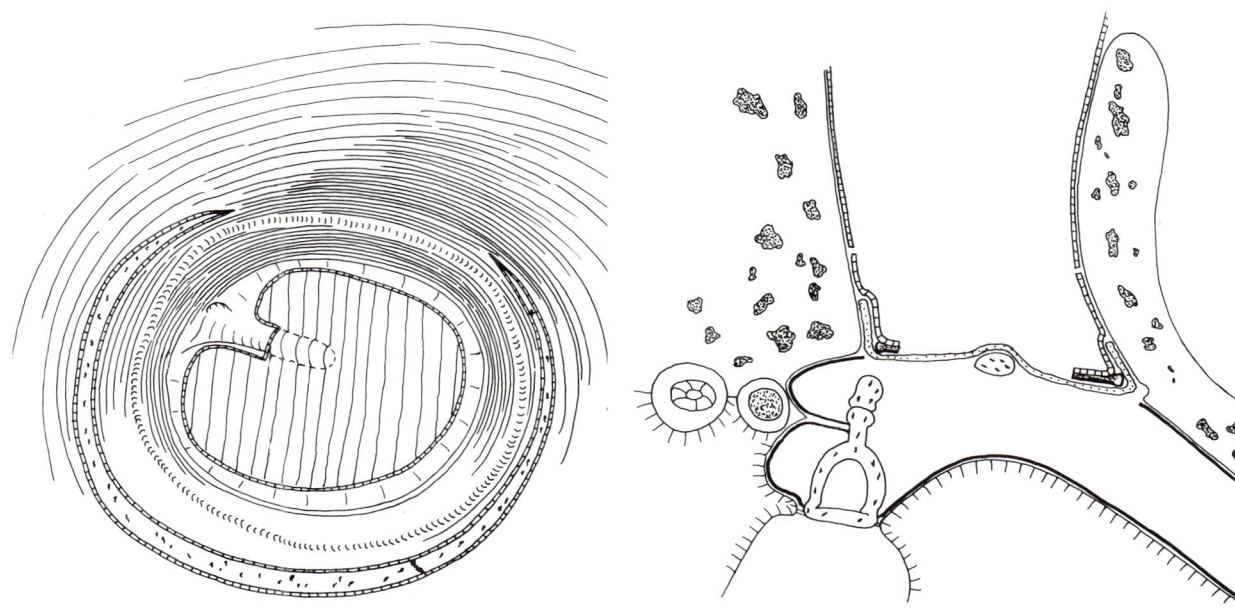

Fig. 600 The fascia is placed on the malleus handle

Fig. 601 Side view of the fascia in place on the malleus handle

Underlay Sandwich Techniques

The principle of this technique is that the fascia is placed under the annulus, while the previously removed canal skin is placed on top of the annulus. The method contrasts with Sheehy's onlay sandwich technique, which involves placement of the fascia on the annulus and covering the fascia with an ear-canal skin graft.

The concept of placing the graft under the drum remnant was in fact first introduced as a sandwich technique by Shea (1960) and Tabb (1960), who used vein as the graft material. In large and total perforations, they had to use two pieces of vein to cover the perforation. It was easier to place the two vein grafts under the annulus than on top of the annulus, especially because of the tendency of the vein to curl up. Also, the covering with skin was, in their opinion, easier if the mesodermal graft was placed under the annulus.

The methods of removing the canal skin for various approaches are described above (Figs. **47, 61–63, 152–157**), as is Sheehy's onlay sandwich technique (Figs. **526–531**).

The placement of the fascia in relation to the malleus handle and the annulus can be performed in different ways, but in all modifications, the mucosa under the fibrous annulus and under the drum remnant has to be carefully removed or elevated as far as the bony annulus. In addition, the malleus handle has to be cleared of keratinized epithelium, and the tympanic cavity has to be filled with Gelfoam.

The modifications of the fascia placement are:
1. Under the anterior and inferior annulus, and under the malleus handle (Keller 1976). To cover Shrapnell's membrane, the fascia is cut superiorly, and the anterior edge is pushed under the anterior superior annulus up to the Shrapnell's membrane region. The posterior edge also covers the Shrapnell's membrane region. Posteriorly, the fascia is placed on the annulus (Fig. **602**), with careful approximation to the inferior annulus. This means that the fascia has to cross from an underlay position anteriorly to an onlay position posteriorly. The canal skin covers part of the fascia, especially at the anterior and inferior tympanomeatal angle (Fig. **603**).
2. The posterior annulus is cut at the 9-o'clock position and elevated, allowing the fascia to be placed under the annulus anteriorly as well as posteriorly. After placement of the fascia, the posterior annulus is replaced on the fascia (Fig. **604**). The canal skin covers the Shrapnell's region, part of the fascia, and partly the denuded ear-canal bone (Fig. **605**).
3. The fascia is placed under the malleus handle, and under the entire annulus, but the annulus is not elevated. The size of the fascia has to be somewhat smaller. The fascia is first placed under the anterior and inferior annulus with an

11 Underlay Techniques

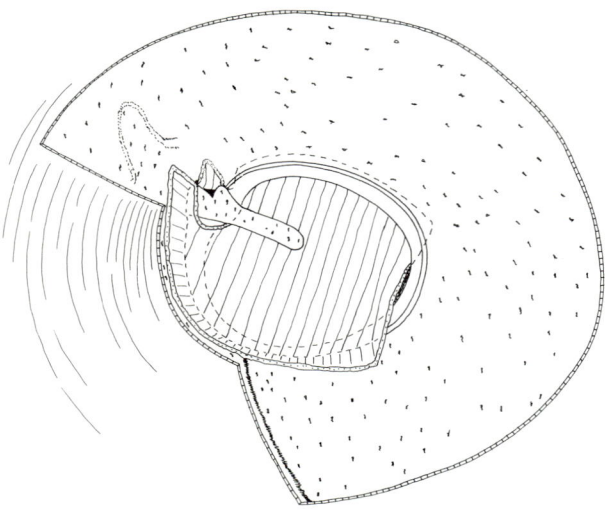

Fig. **602 Underlay sandwich technique.** After removal of the canal-wall skin and the drum-remnant epithelium, as in Sheehy's method, the fascia is placed under the anterior annulus and malleus handle. Inferiorly, the fascia crosses the annulus to be placed posteriorly on the drum remnant. Superiorly, a slit in the fascia is cut, and the anterior and posterior edges cover the Shrapnell's membrane region. Inferiorly, careful positioning of the fascia is necessary

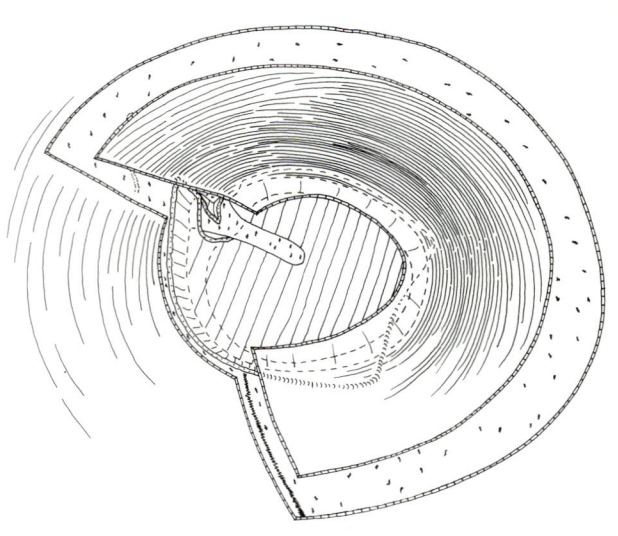

Fig. **603** The canal-wall skin partly covers the fascia, and partly the denuded bone

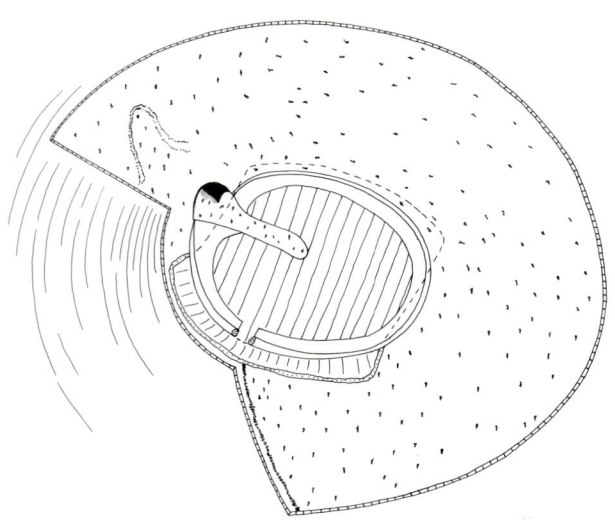

Fig. **604** The fascia is placed under the annulus, which has been resected at the 9-o'clock position and elevated

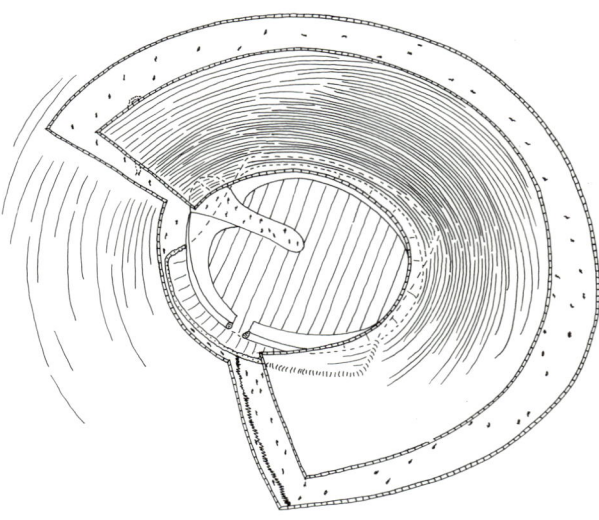

Fig. **605** The canal-wall skin covers the entire Shrapnell's membrane region and part of the fascia

angled rugine, and then under the posterior annulus (Fig. **606**). Shrapnell's membrane is covered by canal skin alone (Fig. **607**).

Underlay sandwich techniques can also be used in approaches other than Sheehy's. Various methods of removing the canal-wall skin while preserving the vascular strip are described: the anterior vascular strip (Wolfermann 1971); the inferior vascular strip (Farrior 1968, Fisch 1990); and the superior vascular strip (Fleury et al. 1974). With all these techniques, underlay sandwich methods of closing the perforations, as well as onlay methods, can be employed.

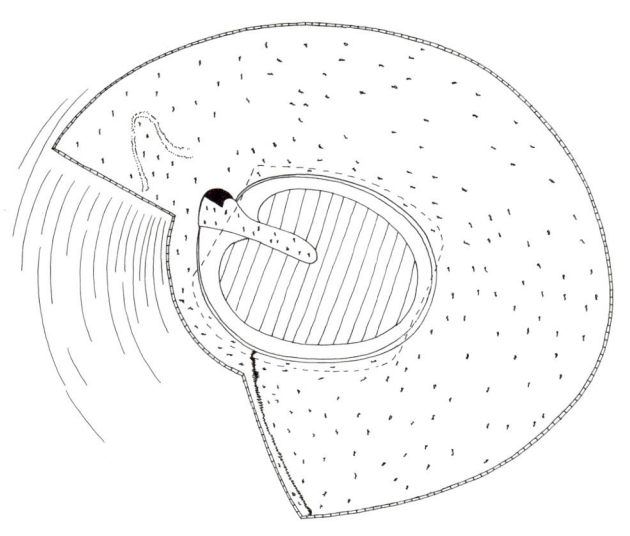

Fig. **606** The fascia is placed underneath the annulus

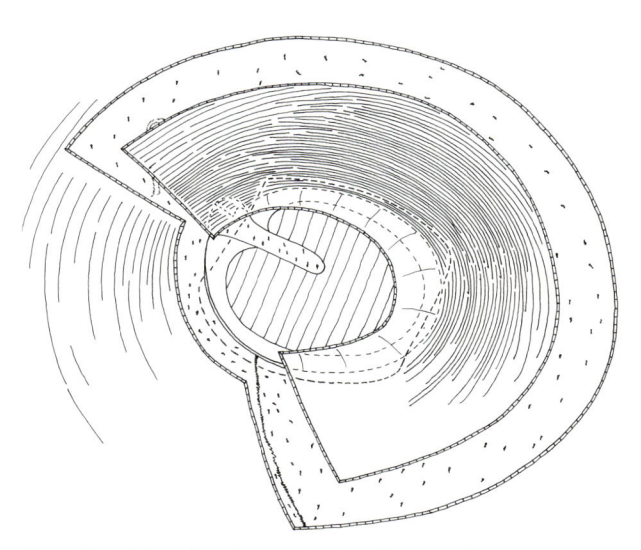

Fig. **607** The fascia and the Shrapnell's membrane region are covered by the canal-wall skin

12 Perichondrium and Cartilage in Myringoplasty

Utech (1959) was the first to introduce cartilage in tympanoplasty. Goodhill et al. (1964) introduced the use of tragal perichondrium together with tragal cartilage, Salen (1963) used septal cartilage and Heermann and Heermann (1964) used tragal and conchal cartilage in myringoplasty.

Perichondrium in Total Perforation

Perichondrium can, in principle, be used in the same way as fascia as an overlay, inlay, or underlay graft. In total perforations, Goodhill placed the perichondrium under the malleus handle, but over the deepithelialized fibrous annulus (Fig. **608**). The cartilage side of the perichondrium is turned toward the tympanic cavity (Fig. **609**). On the totally deepithelialized malleus handle, Goodhill placed another small piece of perichondrium (Fig. **610**).

Instead of removing of the epithelium, the author would recommend using the onlay three-flap method (Fig. **494**). Perichondrium is placed on top of the annulus but under the malleus handle (Fig. **611**). Another piece of perichondrium is placed on the malleus handle, (Fig. **612**), rolling the malleus handle up like a sandwich. The epithelium flaps are returned (Fig. **613**), and are fixed by Gelfoam balls. With this modification of the original Goodhill technique, closure of the perforation at its superior edge is more solid, and the epithelium flaps further secure the closure.

In closure of a total perforation, even the largest perichondrial graft from the tragus may be too small. Using perichondrium from both sides of the tragus as one piece, the perichondrium may be long enough, but its width may still be too small.

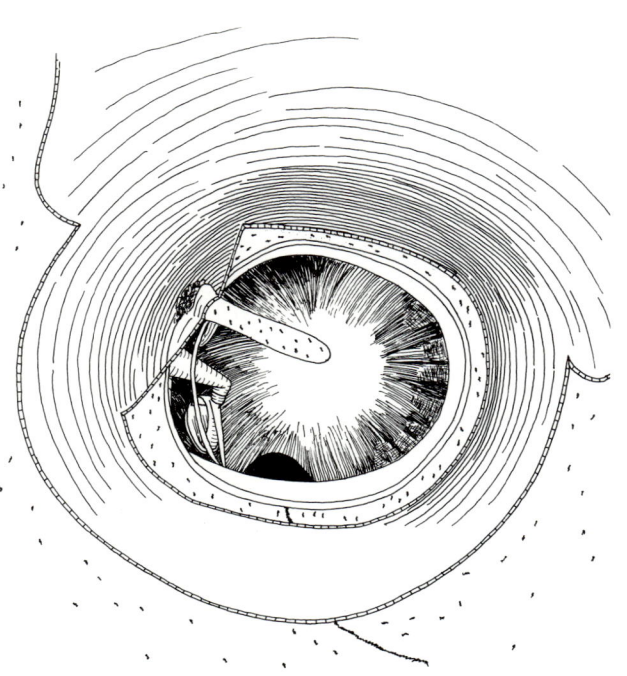

Fig. **608 Goodhill's method** of placing perichondrium on top of the annulus and underneath the malleus handle. The epithelium around the fibrous annulus is removed

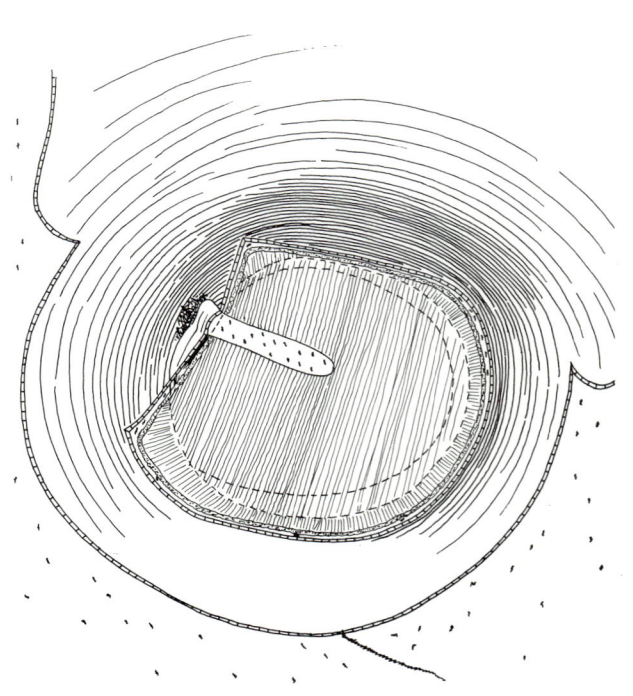

Fig. **609** The perichondrium is placed on top of the annulus and underneath the malleus handle

Perichondrium in Total Perforation 209

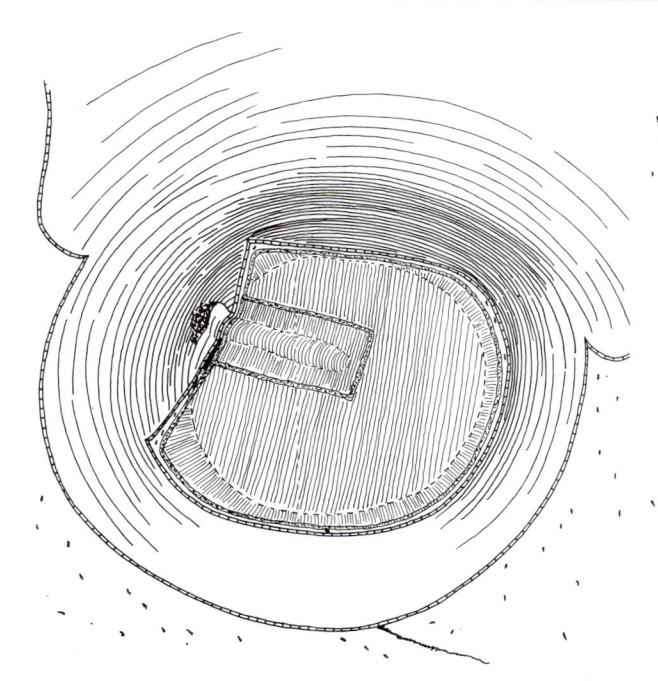

Fig. 610 Another piece of perichondrium is placed on the malleus handle

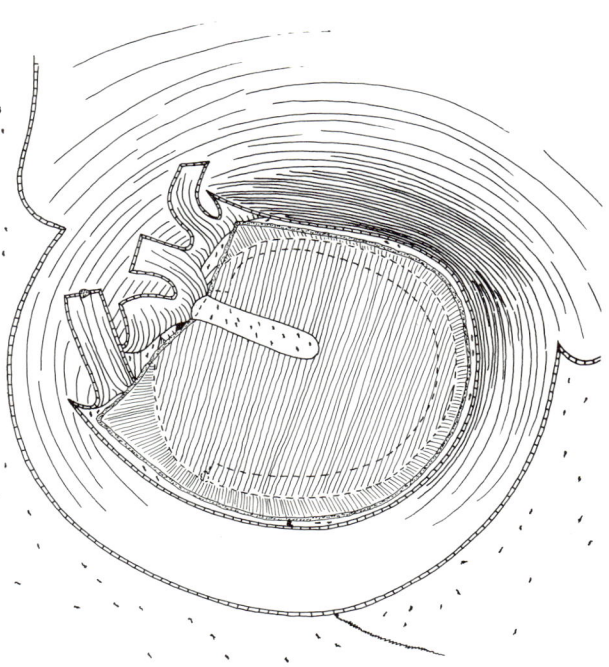

Fig. 611 **The three-flap onlay technique with perichondrium.** The epithelium from the fibrous annulus is removed all the way round, as shown in Figure **494**. The three superior epithelial flaps are elevated, and perichondrium is placed on top of the annulus and underneath the malleus handle

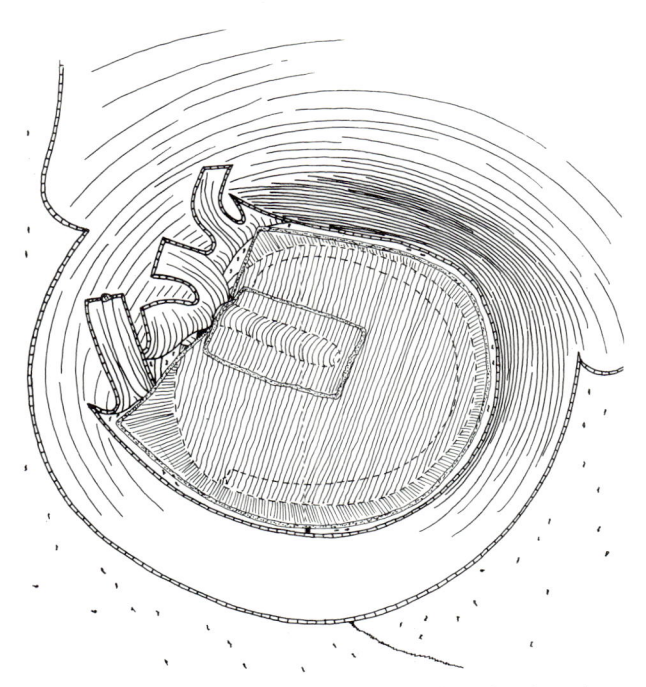

Fig. 612 Another piece of perichondrium is placed on the malleus handle

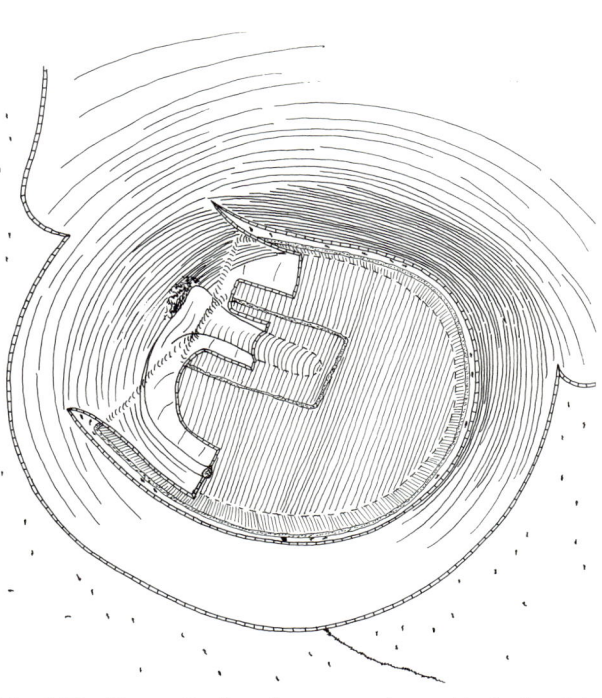

Fig. 613 The epithelium flaps are returned to their original positions.

Combined Perichondrium–Cartilage Grafts

Combined perichondrium cartilage grafts were also used by Goodhill in total perforation. The graft is tailored primarily from the tragal cartilage, and includes a horseshoe shaped cartilage (Fig. **614**). The cartilage is placed on the fibrous annulus, or in close contact with it (Figs. **615, 616**). Goodhill used this method especially in cases with an absent malleus.

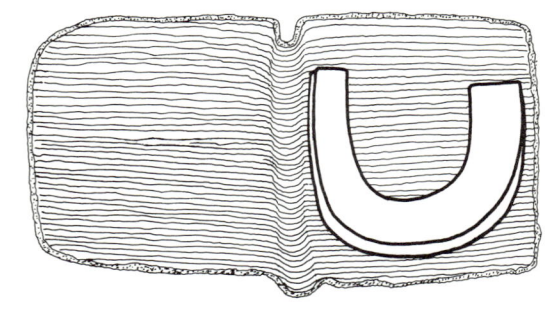

Fig. **614** Combined perichondrium–cartilage graft from the tragus, as used by Goodhill

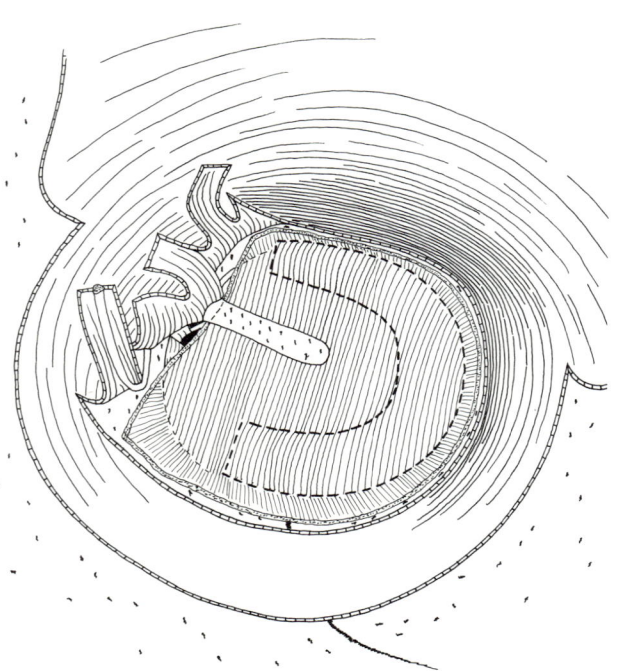

Fig. **615** The graft is placed in position in the three-flap onlay technique. The cartilage is at the level of the fibrous annulus. The perichondrium is placed on top of the fibrous annulus and underneath the malleus

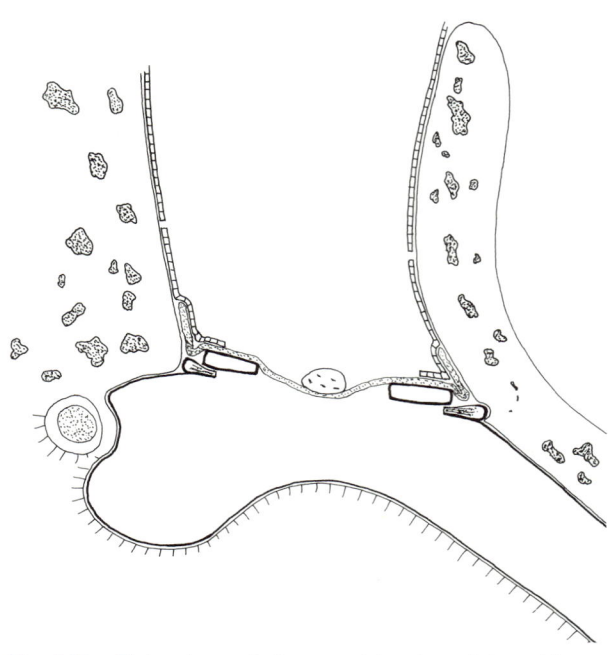

Fig. **616** Side view of the combined perichondrium–cartilage graft. Cartilage is placed on the edges of the annulus

Glasscock et al. (1982) use tragal perichondrium–cartilage graft in posterior perforations. In cases with posterosuperior retraction, adhesive otitis, and sinus cholesteatoma, cartilage of full thickness is used, and is trimmed exactly to the size of the posterior perforation. A piece of tragal cartilage is harvested, and the perichondrium is elevated from one side like a book cover (Fig. **617**). The exact size of the perforation is measured, and the remaining cartilage is removed from the perichondrium plate. The rest of the perichondrium is cut off. The perichondrium–cartilage graft is placed as an underlay graft. The anterior part of the perichondrium is pushed far anteriorly under the malleus handle (Fig. **618**). The cartilage with the middle part of the perichondrium fills out the perforation between the malleus handle and the posterior bony annulus, and the posterior part of the perichondrium lies on the posterior ear-canal bone. The size of the posterior part of the perichondrium depends on the approach used, or on the size of the tympanomeatal flap (Fig. **619**). In total perforation or total atelectasis, as well as in tensa-retraction cholesteatoma, a large piece of cartilage can be used.

Combined Perichondrium–Cartilage Grafts

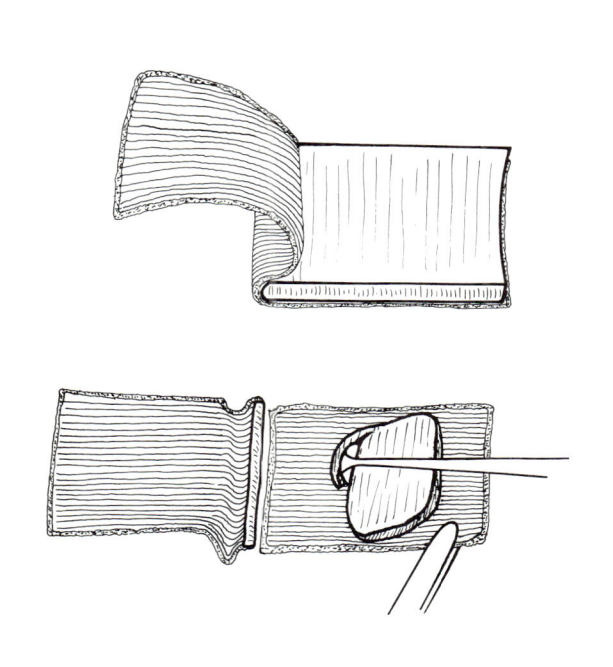

Fig. **617** **Glasscock's technique.** Dissection of a combined tragal perichondrium–cartilage graft for closure of the underlay posterior perforation

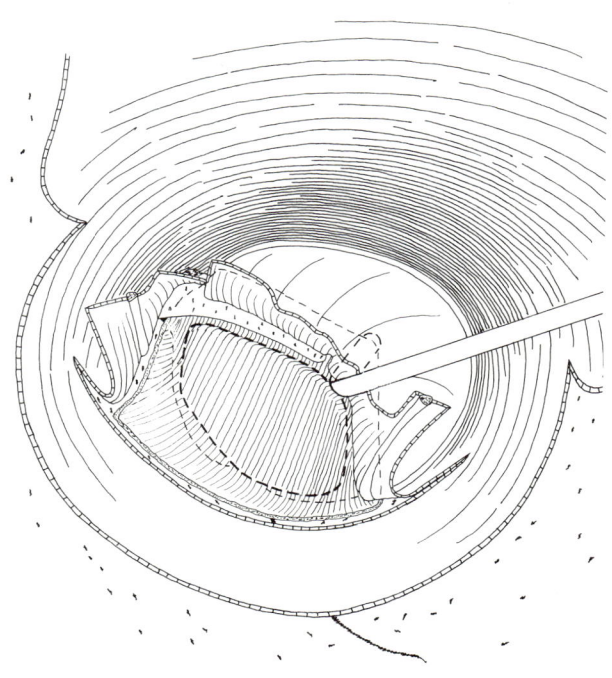

Fig. **618** The perichondrium is in a posterior perforation, placed under the malleus handle, and the cartilage is placed at the side of the perforation

Tragal perichondrium with cartilage has been used sometimes in ears with no ossicles after a canal wall–down technique for reconstruction of the drum. An interesting method is the "thumb touch" technique. The principle of this is a solid connection and concentration of a bony bridge connecting the head of the stapes (or the footplate) with the drum graft. A hole is created through the perichondrium–cartilage graft, which is trimmed in a way similar to that shown in Fig. **617**. A specially-shaped bony graft connecting the head of the stapes and the cartilage plate is placed in this hole (Fig. **620**). The cartilage plate is large, covering the total perforation. The perichondrium is placed on the annulus, with the cartilage in contact with the fibrous annulus, but superiorly the plate is placed on the facial-nerve prominence (Fig. **621**). The facial-nerve prominence can be elevated by some fibrous tissue or another piece of cartilage, but this is not always necessary.

There are no late results on this method as yet, but the principle of creating a hole to center and fix the prosthesis has been used in ossiculoplasty with a combined graft, and is described below (pp. 378–382).

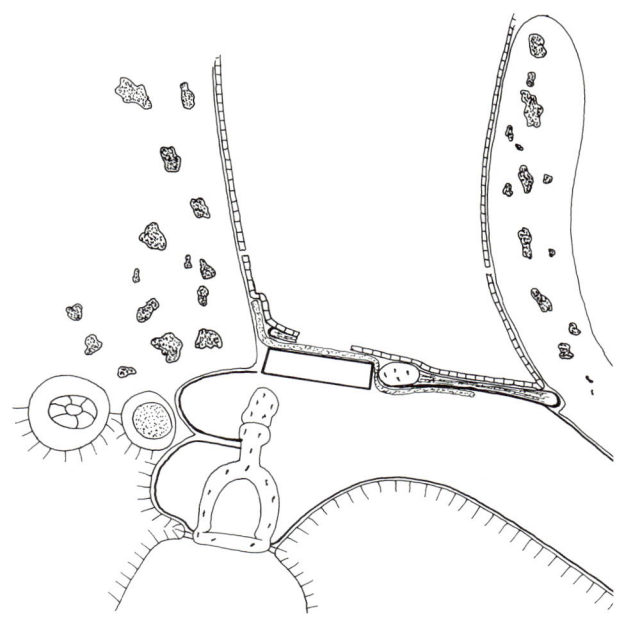

Fig. **619** Side view of the closure of a posterior perforation with an underlay perichondrium–cartilage graft. The cartilage is situated between the malleus handle and the bony annulus. The perichondrium is placed under the malleus handle

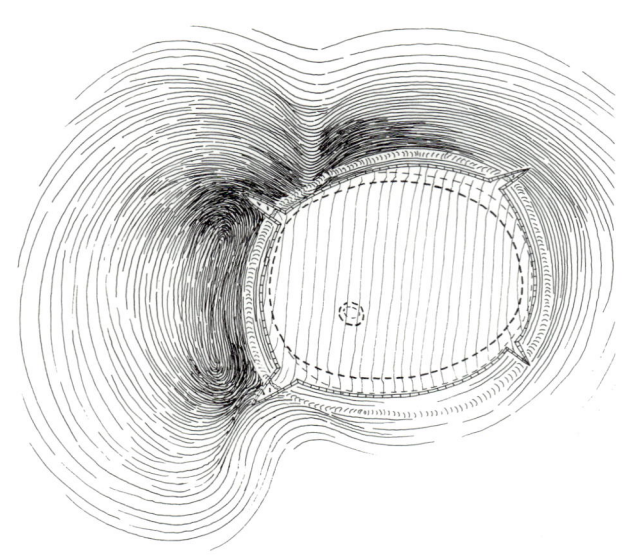

Fig. 620 **The thumb touch technique with a plate of cartilage.** A hole is made in the cartilage plate for a specially-shaped bony prosthesis to connect the head of the stapes and the cartilage plate. The cartilage plate covers the total perforation in a canal wall–down mastoidectomy. Perichondrium is placed on the cartilage

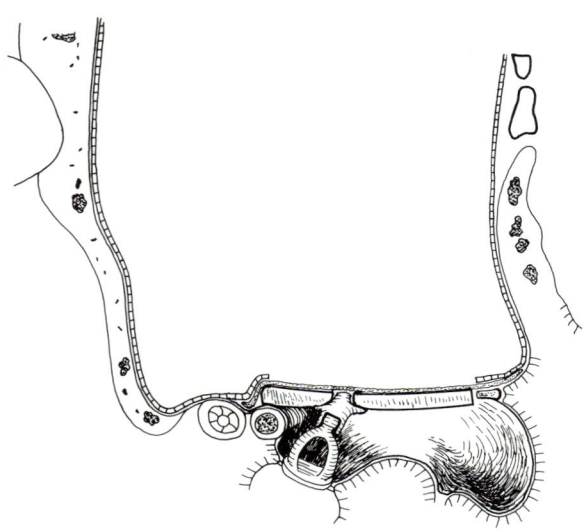

Fig. 621 Side view of the thumb touch technique, which is particularly appropriate after canal wall–down mastoidectomy. The cartilage plate is placed on the facial nerve prominence

Tragal and Conchal Cartilage Plates

Autogenous cartilage plates are widely used for reconstructing attic wall defects in canal wall–up mastoidectomy techniques, or for reconstructing the entire ear canal in canal wall–down mastoidectomy techniques. In addition, tragal cartilage is used in ossiculoplasty, both in type II as an interposition graft and in type III as a columella. These techniques are described in Chapters 16 and 21 below (pp. 279–281 and 360–368). To prevent extrusion of an artificial biocompatible prosthesis, autogenous cartilage plates of various thickness have been widely used.

In connection with fascia grafting of a perforation, cartilage plates can be placed for special purposes: to fortify part of the fascia and prevent retraction, usually posterosuperiorly, in a manner similar to that shown for perichondrium–cartilage grafts (Fig. **618**).

To fortify an atrophic retracted part of the drum which has been elevated by tympanoplasty, either in toto without perforation, or with a small perforation, a plate of tragal cartilage can be placed under the atrophic drum without fascia.

In elevated Shrapnell's-membrane retraction, further retraction can be prevented by placing a piece of cartilage under Shrapnell's membrane.

In myringoplasty, plates of the entire thickness of the tragal cartilage can be used, but usually thinner plates are cut in a special way (Fig. **622**).

Microsliced Septal Cartilage

Overbosch (1971) was the first to use microsliced septal cartilage in myringoplasty. Yamamoto et al. (1985) placed a large, 0.1–0.2 mm-thick allogenous septal cartilage plate under the fascia to prevent retraction. Allogenous septal cartilage is stored in 70% alcohol, and plates with thicknesses of 0.1, 0.2, 0.3, 0.4, and 0.5 mm are prepared before surgery using a dermatome. The cartilage is glued to the curved surface of the dermatome with an adhesive, and the required thickness is sliced with scalpel equipment. A wedge-shaped cut is made in the oval cartilage slide for the short process of the malleus (Fig. **623**). The slice is placed on the malleus handle and on the fibrous annulus (Fig. **624**), and an autogenous fascia onlay graft covers the cartilage (Fig. **625**). If an interposition has to be performed an opening in the wedge slide, the incision is enlarged, giving the prosthesis direct contact with the fascia (Fig. **626**).

Instead of allograft septal cartilage, autogenous tragal cartilage can be used, but the slices are not as regular as those made of septal cartilage.

Microsliced Septal Cartilage 213

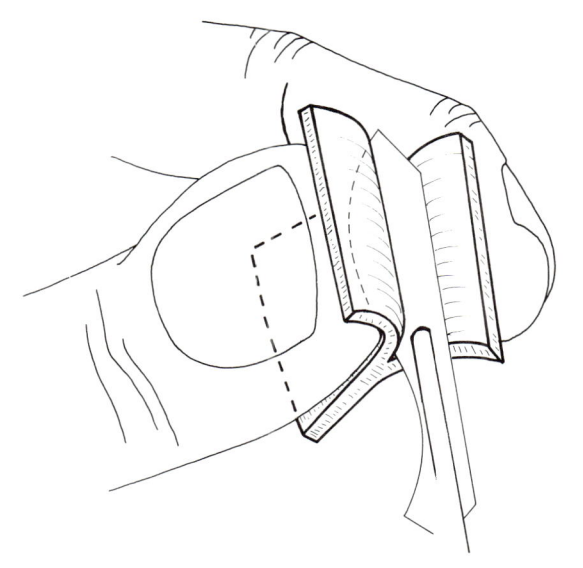

Fig. 622 **Cartilage slice technique.** Cutting a piece of tragal cartilage to create two cartilage slices

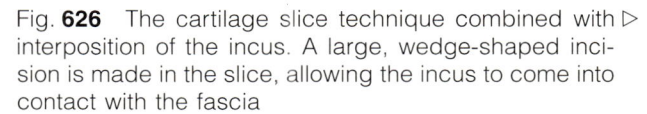

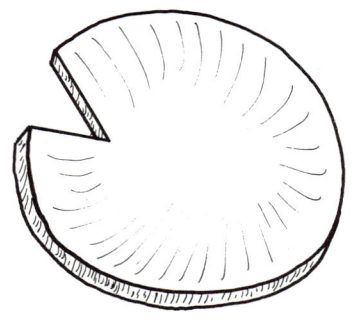

Fig. 623 A slice of homograft cartilage made by a dermatome (Yamamoto). The wedge-shaped cut is to fit the short process of the malleus

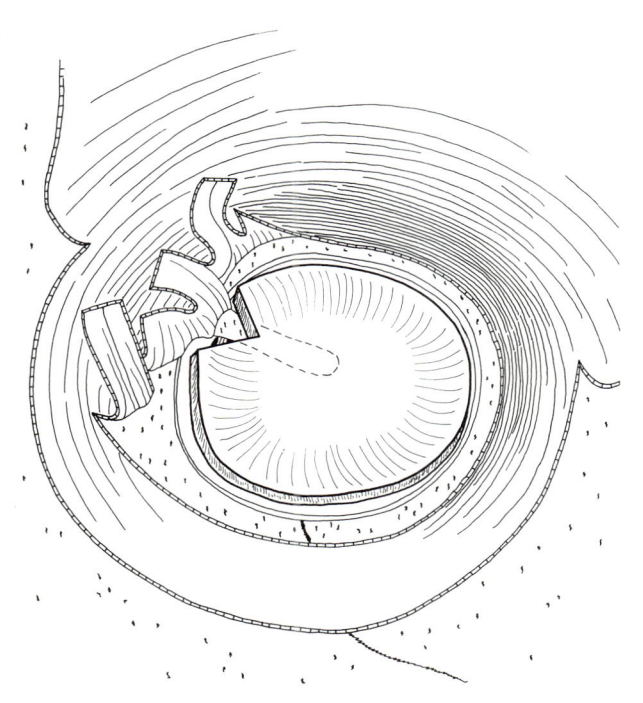

Fig. 624 The cartilage slice is placed on the annulus in a three-flap onlay technique, and will be covered with fascia

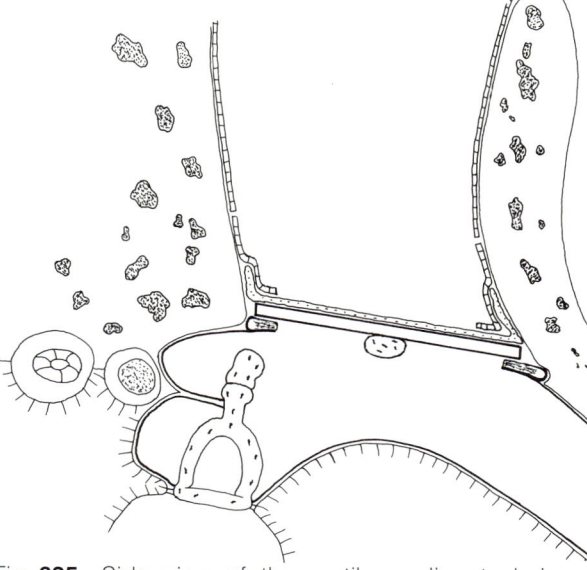

Fig. 625 Side view of the cartilage slice technique. The slice lies on the malleus handle, and is covered by fascia

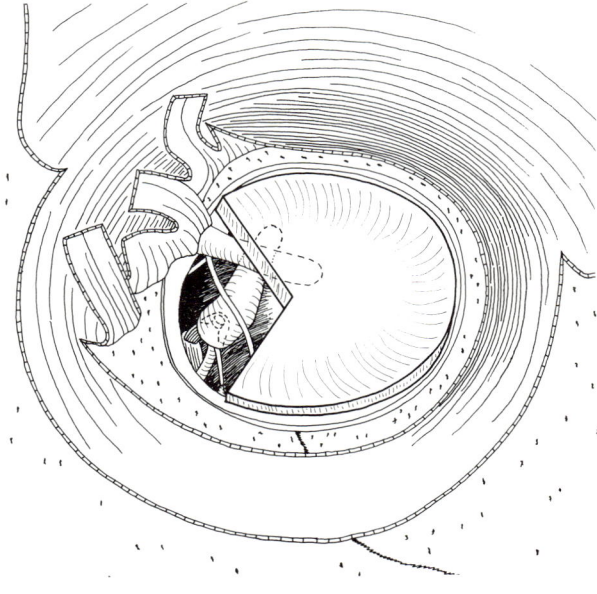

Fig. 626 The cartilage slice technique combined with ▷ interposition of the incus. A large, wedge-shaped incision is made in the slice, allowing the incus to come into contact with the fascia

Palisade Cartilage Tympanoplasty (Heermann)

Heermanns have used cartilage plates for myringoplasty since 1962, and has found that larger plates of cartilage may twist after some years. They therefore started to use palisades of conchal and tragal cartilage placed parallel to the malleus handle. Twisting of the cartilage is apparently avoided in this way (Heermann 1963, 1991, Heermann et al. 1970).

The palisades of tragal or conchal cartilage are about 1 mm broad, and contain perichondrium on one side. They are cut by scalpel blade no. 23 (Fig. **627**). The palisades from the concha can be quite long if the entire conchal cartilage is removed.

To close a total perforation, concha cartilage is preferable. It is harvested by a separate posterior incision, and has a curved shape, so that curved palisades can be obtained.

The approach necessary for palisade tympanoplasty is an extensive elevation of the tympanomeatal flap and the fibrous annulus (Fig. **628**), but the swing-door technique with elevation of the fibrous annulus inferiorly up to the 5-o'clock position can be applied (Fig. **629**). In total perforations, the first piece is placed far anterior in the tubal entrance, medial to the bony annulus (Fig. **628**). Superiorly, the palisade reaches the supratubal recess. This anterior palisade (Heermann's term is *semiring*) is an important part of the tunnelplasty at the tympanic orifice of the Eustachian tube. If the first palisade does not stay superiorly under the bony annulus, it can be supported by a 2.3-mm piece of cartilage (an architrave) resting on the prominence of the tensor tympani muscle (Fig. **629**). A similar architrave can be placed inferiorly to support the first palisade and hold it close to the undersurface of the bony annulus, keeping the tunnel open, especially in cases with granulating mucosa and atelectasis. The next palisade is also placed under the bony annulus. The third palisade

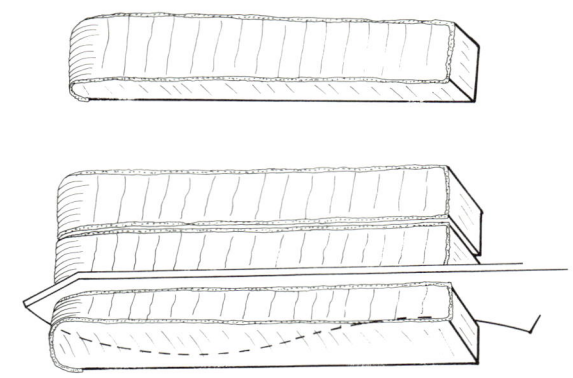

Fig. **627 Palisade cartilage tympanoplasty (Heermann).** Preparing palisades of tragal cartilage in palisade myringoplasty. The perichondrium is removed on one side of the cartilage. The slices can vary in width, but are usually 1 mm

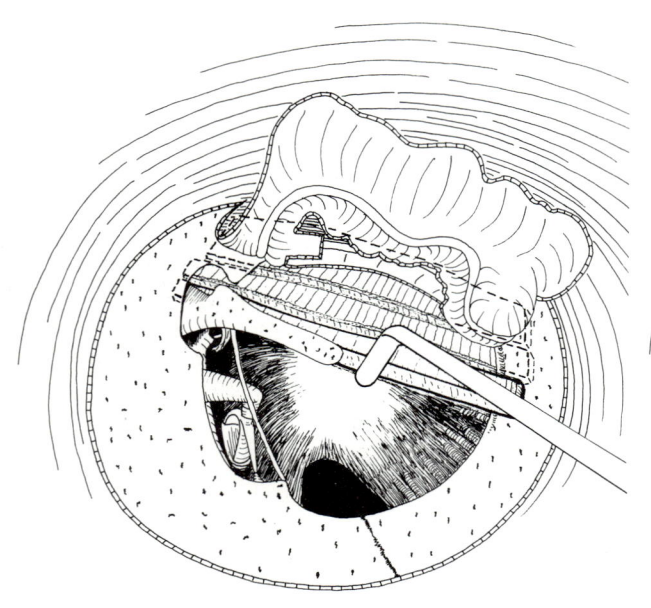

Fig. **628** The first two palisades are placed under the anterior bony annulus; the third is placed on the bony annulus

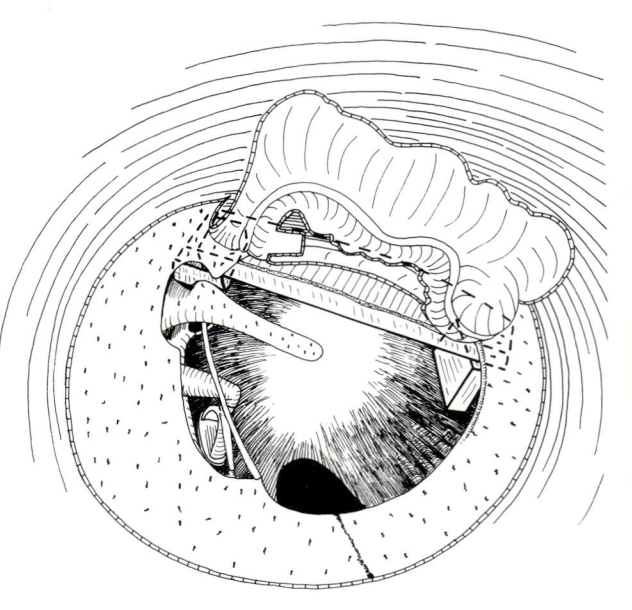

Fig. **629** Tunnelplasty. A piece of cartilage is placed superiorly on the tendon tympani muscle, and another is placed in the hypotympanum, supporting the first

has close contact with the malleus handle. Inferiorly, it is placed on top of the bony annulus, but beneath the fibrous annulus, which is elevated. The next palisades are placed posteriorly to the malleus handle but on top of the bony annulus. The most posterior piece of cartilage is placed with its posterior edge on top of the posterior bony annulus (Fig. **630**). The tympanomeatal flap is replaced, and the annulus is fixed all the way round, either by Gelfoam balls or some other fixation method (Fig. **631**). This method is used in total perforation with an intact ossicular chain and without mastoidectomy. Usually, the perichondrium is turned on the palisades toward the ear canal, but this is not necessary. In some palisades, it can also be turned towards the middle ear, and the palisades should be placed in such a way that there is no space between them. If there is a major space, the defect can be closed with a small piece of perichondrium, but the palisade method does not include general covering of the palisades by perichondrium or fascia.

In cases with a defective ossicular chain, but with the stapes present, Heermann uses a 3-mm wide annulus–stapes plate, placed inferiorly on the bony annulus at about the 5-o'clock position (Fig. **632**). It is placed under the malleus handle. Superiorly, it is placed on the head of the stapes. The other palisade, including the *"semiring"* is placed as shown in Figures **630** and **631**. The ossiculoplasty method is illustrated in the chapter on ossiculoplasty (p. 281).

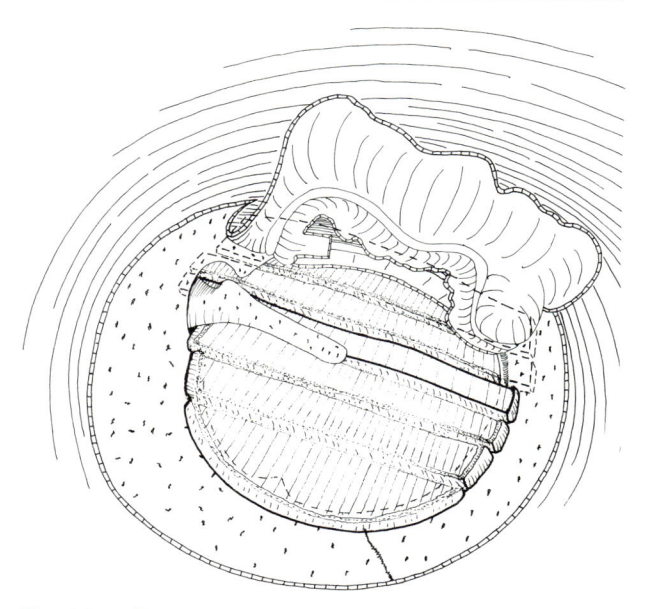

Fig. **630** Further palisades are placed anterior and posterior to the malleus, on top of the bony annulus but underneath the fibrous annulus. The most posterior plate is placed on the posterior bony annulus

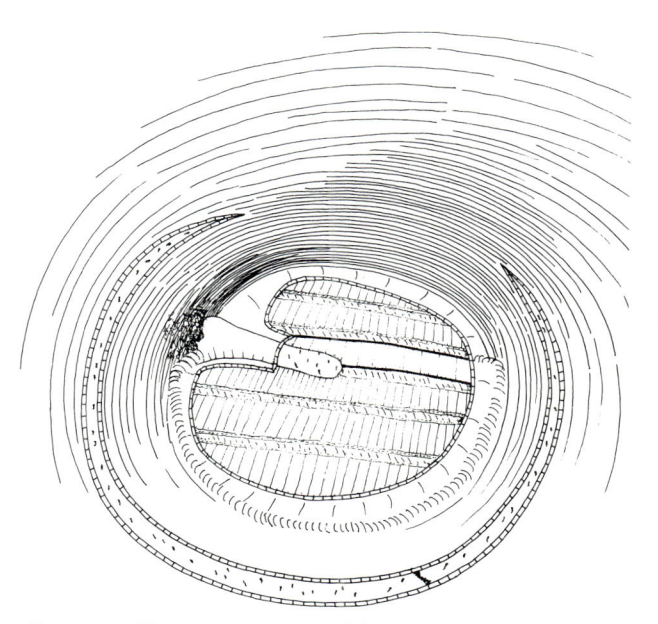

Fig. **631** The tympanomeatal flap is replaced

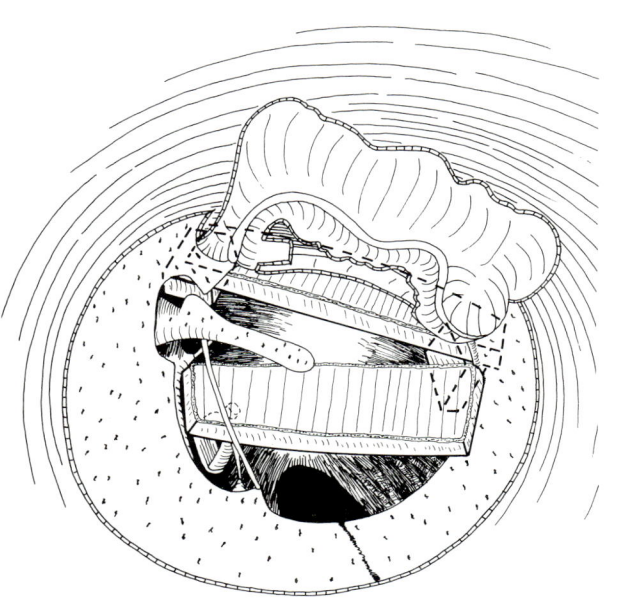

Fig. **632** The annulus–stapes plate placed on the bony annulus and the head of the stapes

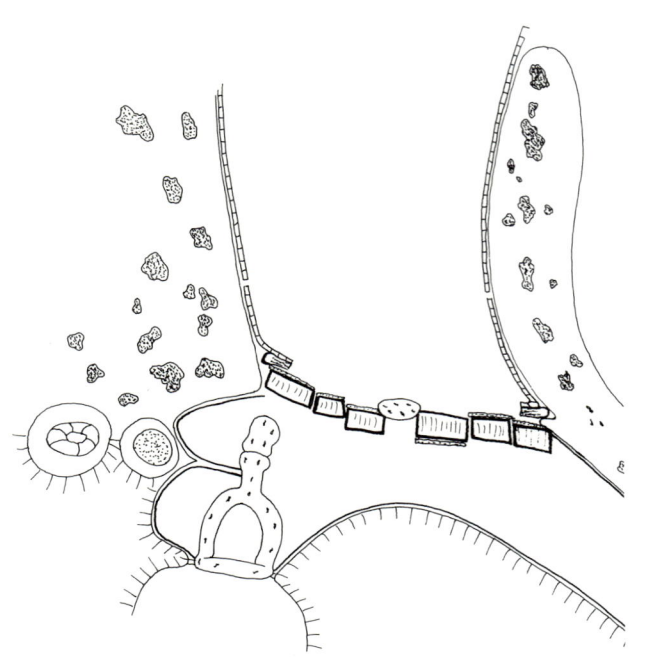

12 Perichondrium and Cartilage in Myringoplasty

Fig. **633** Side view of the palisade technique, illustrating the position of the first palisade and the most posterior palisade, as well as the palisades around the malleus handle

It is important to place the palisades under a certain amount of tension to achieve a relatively high tympanic cavity. Sometimes they can be placed as stairs, each in a more medial position than the other.

Although the cartilage plates or the palisade placed in the posterior part of the drum can prevent retractions, the method of covering the entire tympanic cavity with palisades looks extremely mysterious. Heermann claims excellent hearing results and almost no recurrent perforation, but he has never performed an reevaluation, and never published the results of his own technique. Some short-term results on small materials have recently been published with good results (Péré 1989, Amedee et al. 1989). Physiologically, the palisade cartilage cannot provide good hearing, simply because the drum is too thick (Fig. 633) and the cartilage has to be placed lower than the malleus handle in order to close tightly around the handle, resulting in a low tympanic cavity.

13 Myringoplasty in a Curved Ear Canal

A curved ear canal with a narrow anterior tympanomeatal angle seems to occur relatively more frequently in ears with chronic otitis media, especially cholesteatoma, than in normal ears. One of the explanations for the narrow anterior tympanomeatal angle may be the constricted and sclerotic mastoid process, as well as small and nonexistent pneumatization. These conditions are caused by infection or chronic tubal dysfunction, and by secretory otitis in early childhood, hampering the process of pneumatization and creating severe drum changes, which can later on progress to cholesteatoma or noncholesteatomatous chronic otitis. Even if there is no scientific documentation for the stated high incidence of the curved ear canal, otosurgeons feel that about 25% of ears with anterior, subtotal, or total perforations have such extensive bulging of the bony ear-canal wall and so narrow an anterior tympanomeatal angle that visualization with an ear-canal speculum of the anterior part of the perforation, including the anterior annulus, is hampered. This is especially true in revision operations, where poor visualization has significantly influenced the failure of the primary operation.

There are several options available to overcome these problems (Chandler 1976). All of these are valuable, and can be recommended in particular cases, but no single one is the best method in all cases. The problems differ between the different approaches.

Endaural Approach with an Ear Speculum

The author has performed tympanoplasty mainly through the ear speculum, with many reoperations when previous surgery has failed due to a prominent ear canal and poor visualization of the anterior tympanomeatal angle, since the late 1960s. He uses a transmeatal method, which definitively eliminates the prominence prior to the tympanoplasty, provides excellent visualization of the anterior annulus, allows short postoperative care, and promotes good postoperative epithelial migration without stagnation or crust formation in the ear canal. This method has been practised for more than 25 years in all cases with very pronounced prominences in total, subtotal, or anterior perforations in which the tympanomeatal angle, after maximal tilting of the patient's head, could not be clearly seen or instrumentally reached through the speculum. Since this method has not been published before, it will be described here in detail. The main principle involved is to preserve all ear-canal skin intact, with a broad superior connection allowing good vascularization of the canal skin immediately after it has been replaced. The myringoplasty can be performed as an onlay technique—which is preferable—or as an underlay technique.

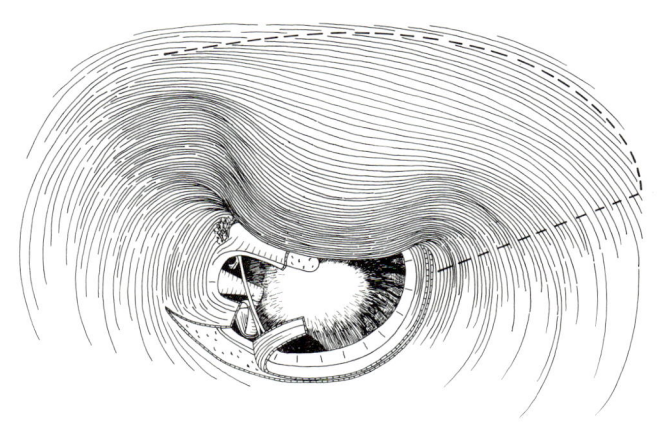

Fig. **634 Removal of the bony prominence.** A total perforation, with a prominent ear canal impairing visualization of the anterior part of the perforation. A radial incision at the 6-o'clock position and a lateral circumferential incision will be performed. Posterosuperiorly, an epithelial flap is elevated

The lateral anterior circumferential skin incision is performed far lateral to the prominence, usually at the bone–cartilage junction. The incision goes from the 1-o'clock to the 5-o'clock positions, or to the 6-o'clock or 7-o'clock position, depending on the extent of the prominence (Figs. **634, 635**). At the 6-o'clock or 5-o'clock position, a radial incision is performed, starting at the annulus and running outward.

Before this skin incision is started, the incision for the onlay myringoplasty procedure in the poste-

13 Myringoplasty in a Curved Ear Canal

rior part of the canal can be performed as described previously (Figs. **488–501**). A posteroinferior circumferential incision 1 mm lateral to the annulus is extended as far anteriorly as allowed by the ear canal protrusion. Posterosuperiorly, a skin flap is elevated, the keratinized epithelium from the umbo is removed (Fig. **634**), and the malleus epithelial flap (Fig. **636**) is elevated.

After completing work in the posterior part of the tympanic cavity, the radial skin incision is started at the annulus with a large sickle knife, running laterally. The anterior circumferential incision then starts at the 6-o'clock position, running anteriorly. Elevation of the epithelial flap (Fig. **637**) from the lateral part of the ear-canal prominence is easy to begin with, but it becomes more difficult medial to the bulge. After extensive drilling, the skin is gradually elevated medially to the bony prominence (Fig. **638**) using curved elevators. Continued drilling of the bony prominence (Fig. **639**) provides room for further elevation of the skin towards the anterior annulus (Fig. **640**), and when drilling continues medially more and more of the inferior annulus comes into view (Fig. **641**). After this, further elevation of the skin medial to the prominence (Fig. **642**) allows gradual removal of the bone (Fig. **643**). After exposure of the anteroinferior part of the annulus (Fig. **644**), drilling is continued superiorly to visualize its anterosuperior part (Fig. **645**). A small skin strip from the annulus and all keratinized epithelium from the drum remnant are removed, and an anterosuperior skin flap is elevated. Finally, all bone is removed as far as the mandibular fossa, without exposing the capsule of the

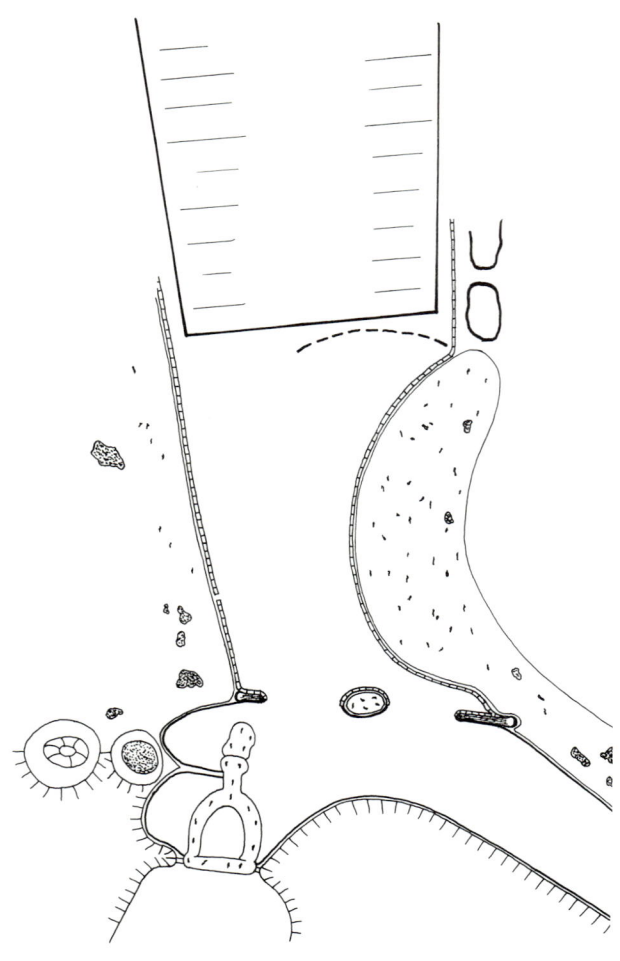

Fig. **635** Side view of the prominent anterior ear-canal wall in a total perforation, viewed through the ear speculum as a precondition for surgery

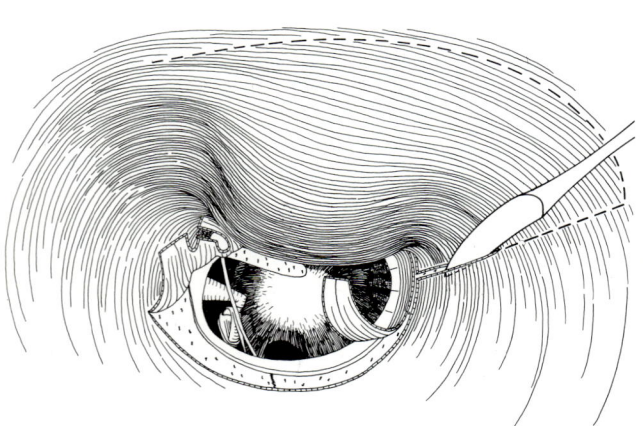

Fig. **636** Posteriorly, the malleus is cleaned, and the malleus flap is elevated. Epithelium from the posterior annulus is also removed. The radial incision is performed

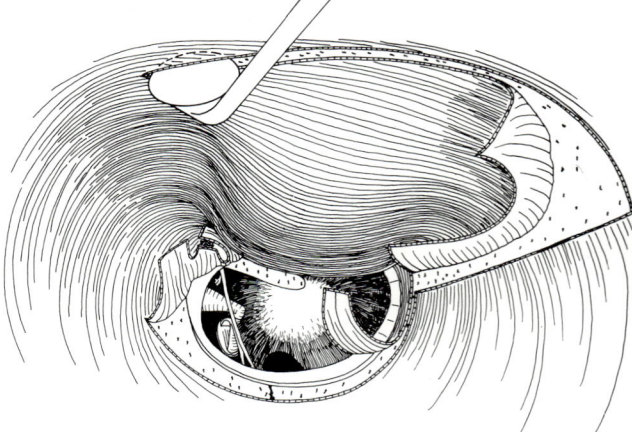

Fig. **637** The circumferential incision is finished, and the skin is elevated laterally

Endaural Approach with an Ear Speculum 219

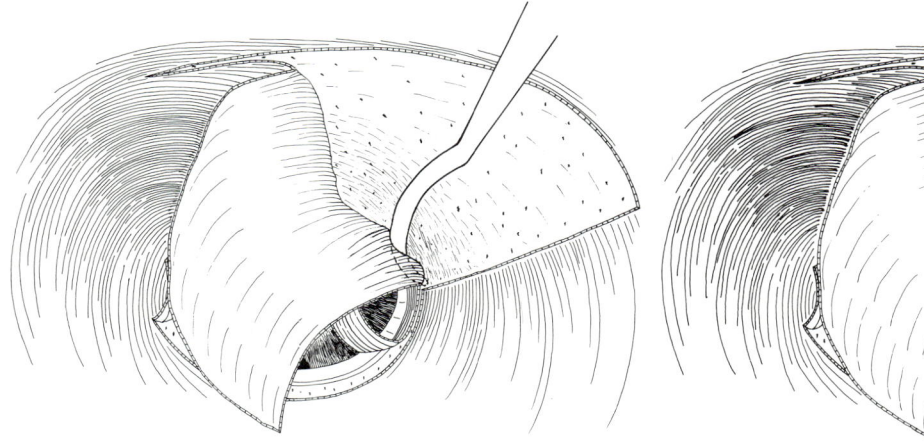

Fig. **638** Further elevation of the skin towards the prominence

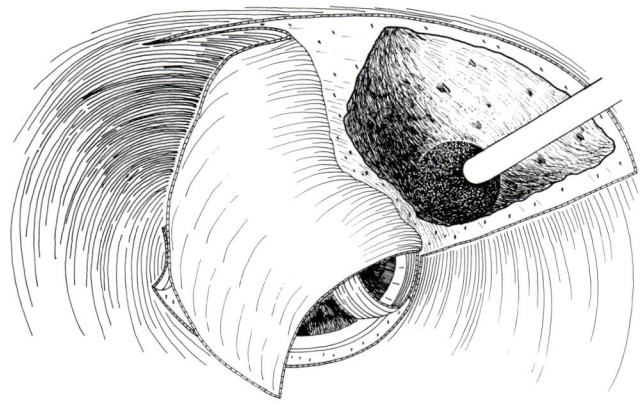

Fig. **639** Drilling of the anterior bony ear-canal wall with a diamond burr

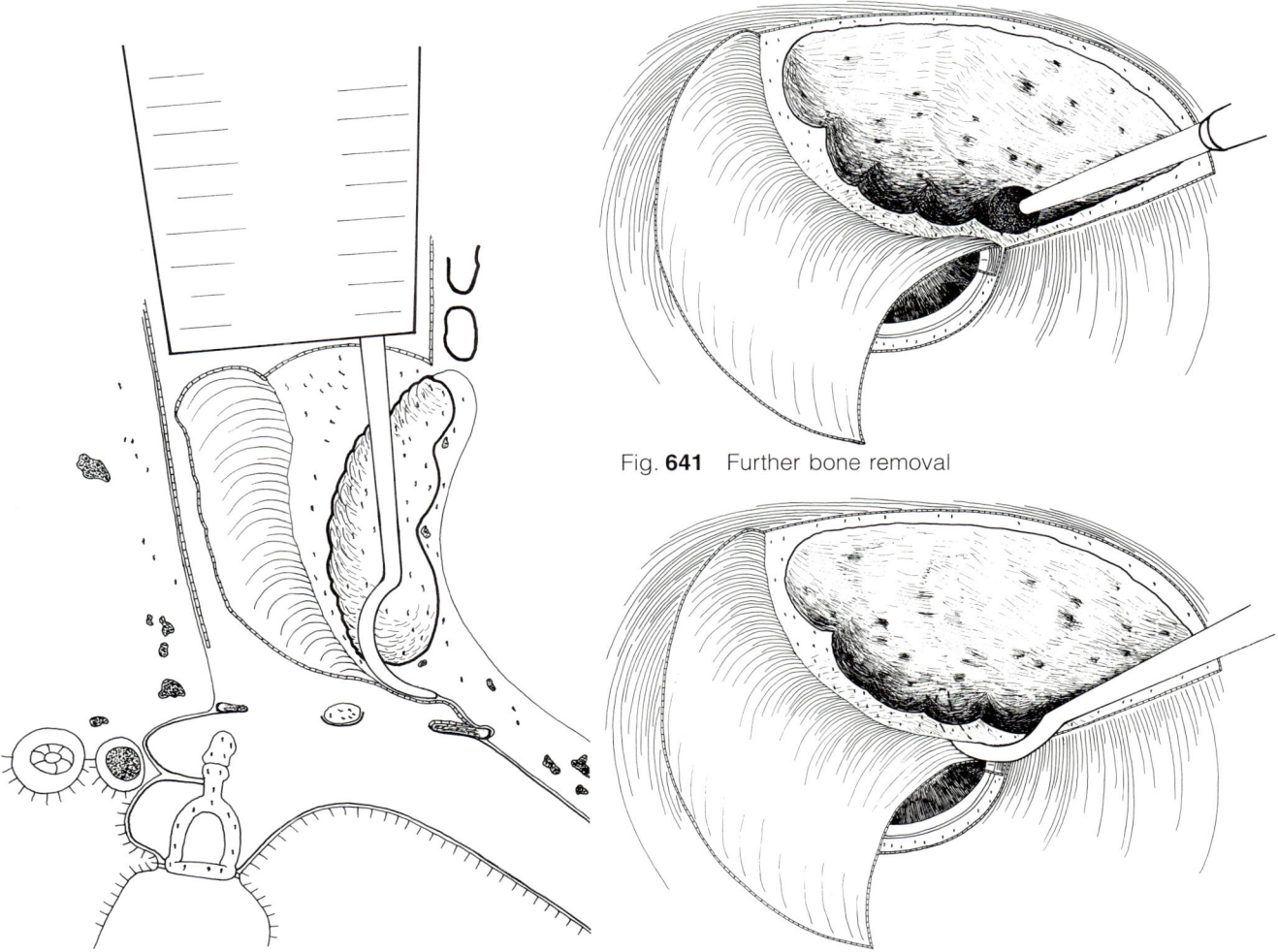

Fig. **641** Further bone removal

Fig. **640** Side view of bone removal at the anterior prominence and elevation of the skin under the prominence

Fig. **642** Further elevation of the skin medial to the prominence

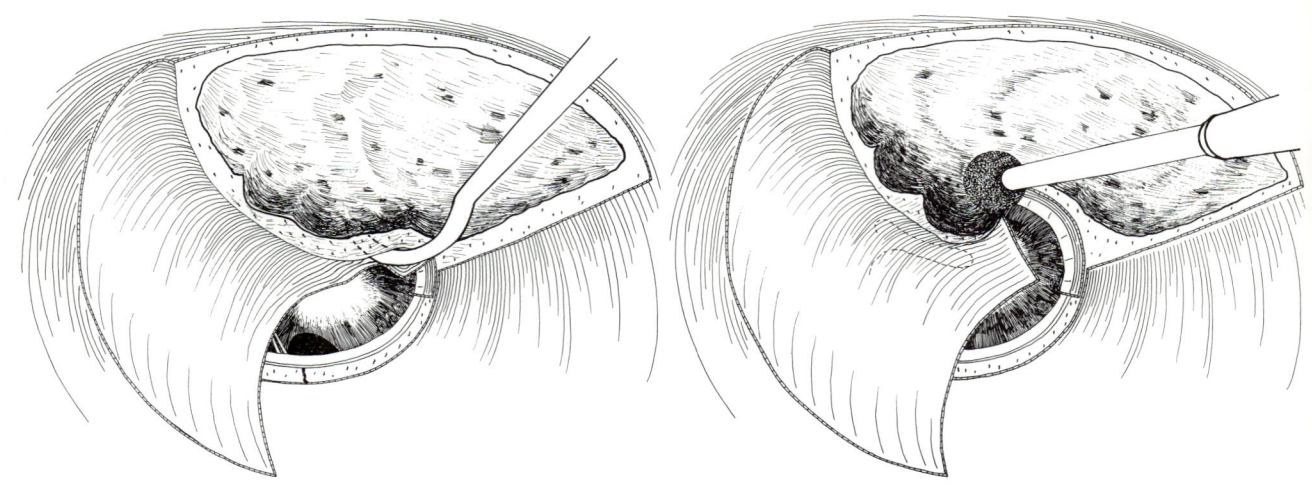

Fig. **643** More and more of the ear-canal prominence is removed, and the inferior annulus is visualized. Further elevation of the ear-canal skin

Fig. **644** The bone is removed, and the anterior annulus has become visible

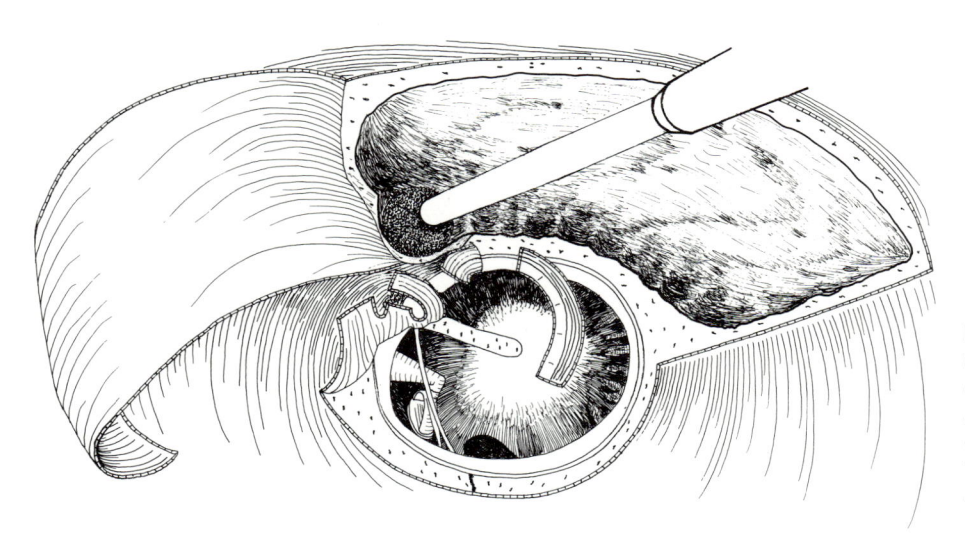

Fig. **645** The bony prominence has been almost completely removed. The annulus is visible in its entire circumference, and the superior epithelial flaps are elevated

mandibular joint (Fig. **646**), and all the bony irregularities lateral to the annulus, as well as at the superior and inferior edges of the previous prominence, are removed with a House curette, making the anterior wall smooth (Fig. **647**). After the fascia has been placed as an onlay graft, the entire anterior canal-wall skin is replaced, covering all the denuded bone, and even an edge of the fascia. The skin-canal flaps—i.e., the anterosuperior flap, the malleus flap, and the posterosuperior flap—are replaced, fixed by Gelfoam balls (Fig. **648**). Firm fixation of the fascia to the anterior annulus is provided by semidry Gelfoam balls (Fig. **649**) all the way round (Fig. **650**). The canal-wall skin is fixed by hydrocortisone–terramycin gauze strips placed in the ear canal and left for three weeks. Admittedly, the method is complicated and technically difficult, but it provides a permanent solution—widening the ear canal as far as physiologically possible.

Endaural Approach with an Ear Speculum 221

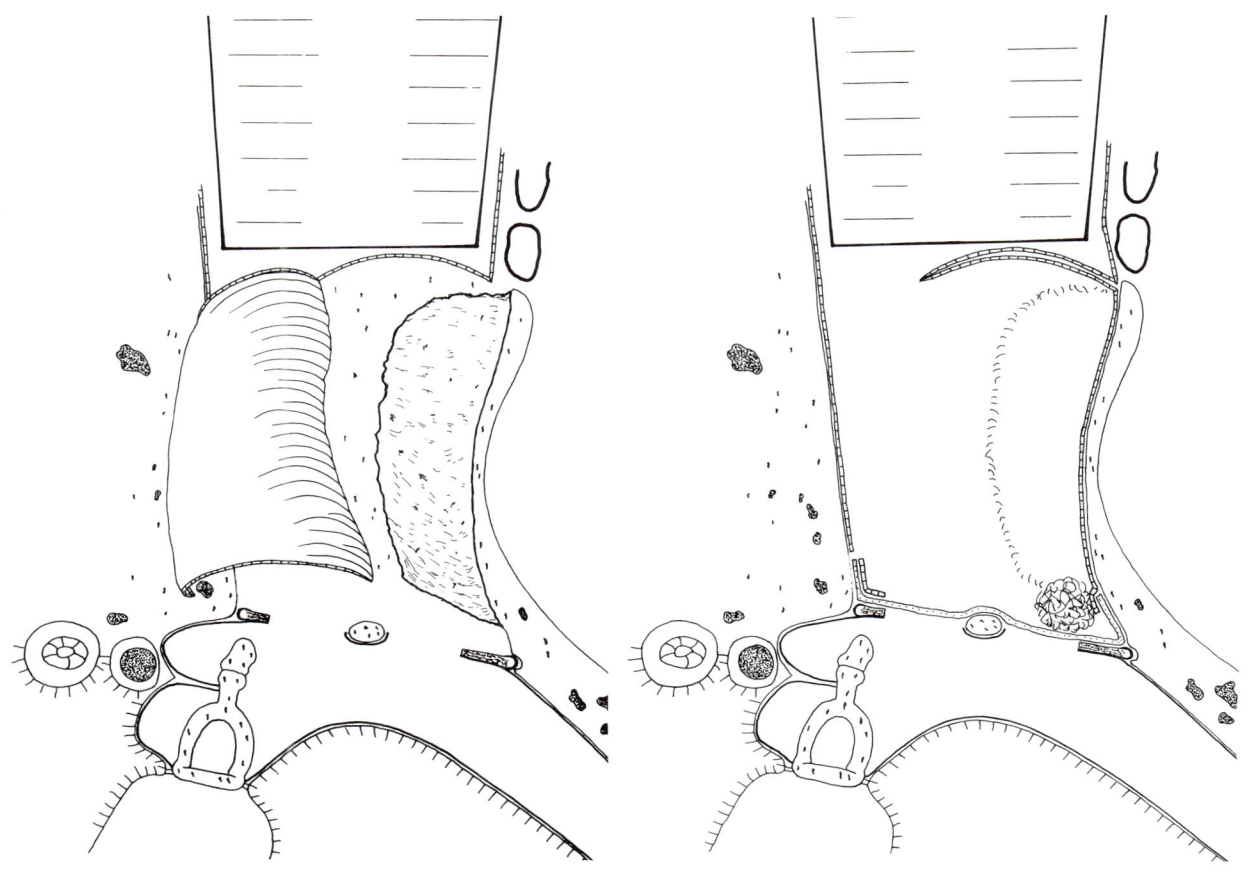

Fig. **646** Side view of the completed removal of the anterior bony prominence

Fig. **649** Side view in the final stage of the operation. Fascia is used as an onlay graft. The skin is replaced

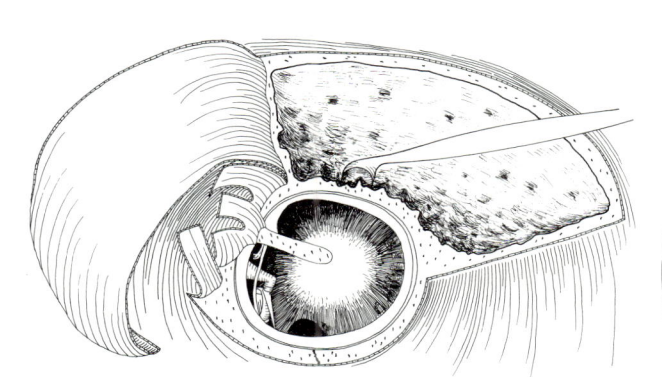

Fig. **647** Final removal of the bony margin using a House curette. The perforation is closed with a fascia onlay graft. The skin of the anterior ear canal is returned to its original position, and the epithelial flaps are replaced

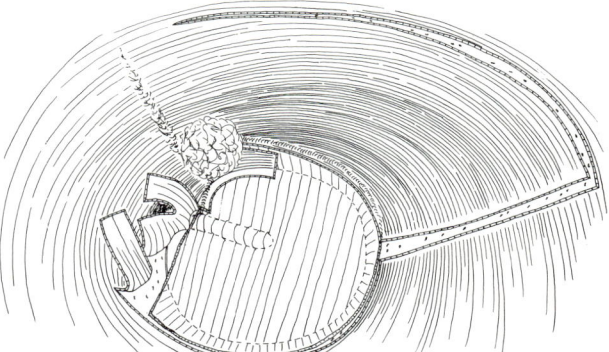

Fig. **648** The fascia is placed on the annulus, the anterior canal-wall skin and the anterosuperior skin flap are replaced, and fixation with Gelfoam is started

13 Myringoplasty in a Curved Ear Canal

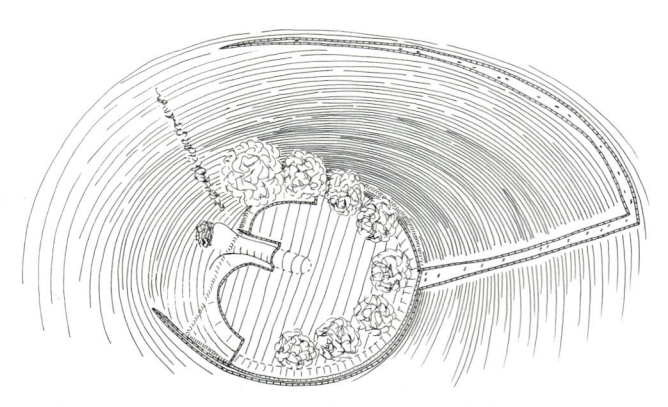

Fig. 650 Fixation of the fascia with Gelfoam balls all the way around. All three epithelial flaps are replaced

There are various modifications of the basic method described, using the same principle: maximal preservation of the canal skin:

1. An inferiorly-pedicled skin flap, achieved after a superior radial and lateral circumferential incision and an incision placed along the maximal prominence of the ear canal. In this way, a sufficiently large area of the bone is exposed, and it can be drilled away using a cutting burr until a thin bony shell is left. This shell is fractured forward by a House curette, exposing more skin medial to the prominence (Fig. **651**). When drilling of the bone is continued until a new, thin bone shell is created, which again can be broken down by a curette, gradual and safe removal of the bony prominence can be performed down to the annulus (Fig. **652**) without damaging the skin. Finally, the skin flap can be replaced, allowing good exposure for myringoplasty.
2. A similar procedure starts with a curved incision (Fig. **653**) anterior to the bony prominence, continuing over the top of the prominence, and outward to the inferior border of the prominence. A laterally-pedicled skin flap is elevated, and the bony prominence is removed in a way similar to that shown in Figures **651** and **652**.
3. A swing-door approach to the bony prominence starts with a laterally-placed anterior circumferential incision (Fig. **654**) at the bone–cartilage junction, and continues from there at the 3-o'clock position with a radial incision as far medially over the bone prominence as possible.

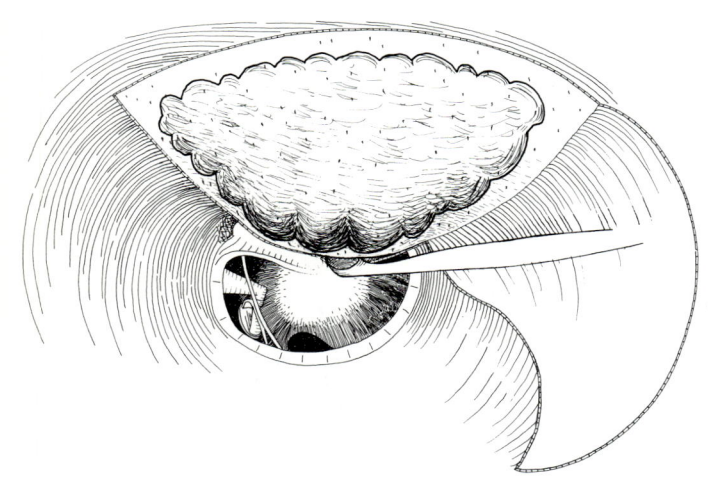

Fig. **651** **A modification of the removal method for the bony prominence.** A circumferential incision is performed laterally to the prominence, and a radial incision continues over the prominence. The skin is elevated, and the bony prominence is exposed and drilled away until a thin bony shell remains

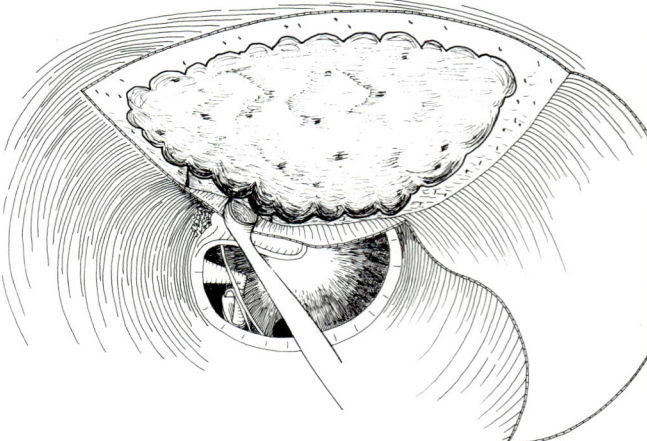

Fig. **652** The thin bony shell of the prominence is removed with a House curette, and the skin under the prominence is further elevated

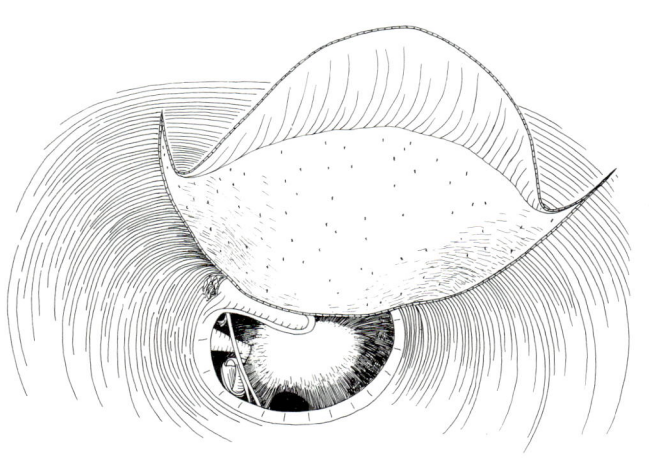

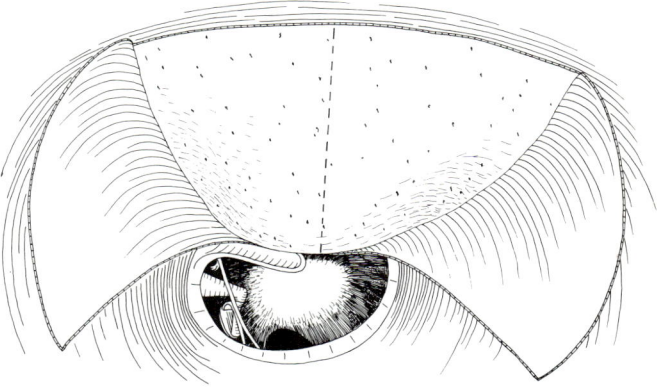

Fig. 653 **Another modification of the removal method for the ear-canal prominence.** Radial incisions are performed superiorly and inferiorly to the prominence, and a medial circumferential lincision connects the radial incisions. The skin is elevated, with the skin flap based laterally

Fig. 654 **A third modification of the removal method for the anterior ear-canal prominence.** The skin is incised lateral to the prominence with a circumferential incision, and at the 3-o'clock position, using a radial incision. Two skin flaps, based superiorly and inferiorly respectively, are elevated from the prominence

The skin is elevated, resulting in a superiorly-pedicled and inferiorly-pedicled skin flap, exposing the bone like a swing-door. The bone is drilled away, as indicated above (Fig. **652**), allowing exposure of some skin medial to the prominence. This piece of skin is cut at the 3-o'clock position, allowing further elevation of the two skin flaps from the medial surface of the bony prominence. By pressing a large sickle knife under the bony prominence and cutting the skin at the 3-o'clock position from the annulus outward (Fig. **655**), further elevation of the skin and complete removal of the bony prominence becomes possible.

4. A medially-pedicled skin flap, achieved by a lateral circumferential incision, two parallel radial incisions along the prominence, and elevation of the skin, is especially well situated for minor prominences, e.g., removing exostosis (Fig. **656**). By drilling the bone until a thin bony shell is left, removing this shell, further elevating the skin with a curved rugine (Fig. **657**), and repeating this sequence, skin elevation can be performed as far as the anterior tympanomeatal angle (Fig. **658**). After the skin flap has been replaced in its original position, the annulus becomes visible, and the tympanoplasty with underlay or overlay grafting can proceed.

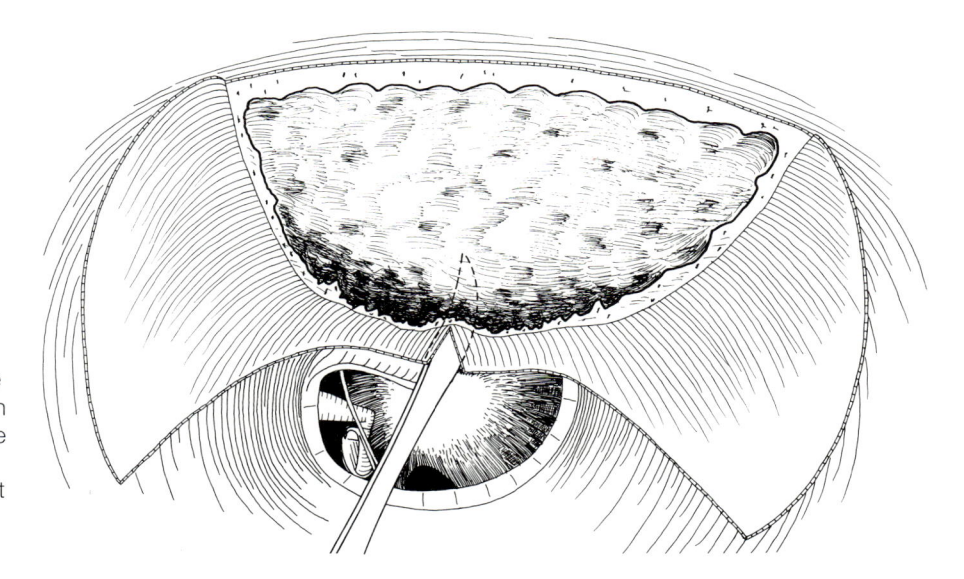

Fig. **655** After removal of the bone and elevation of the skin from the medial surface of the bony prominence, the ear-canal skin is further incised at the 3-o'clock position with a sickle knife

13 Myringoplasty in a Curved Ear Canal

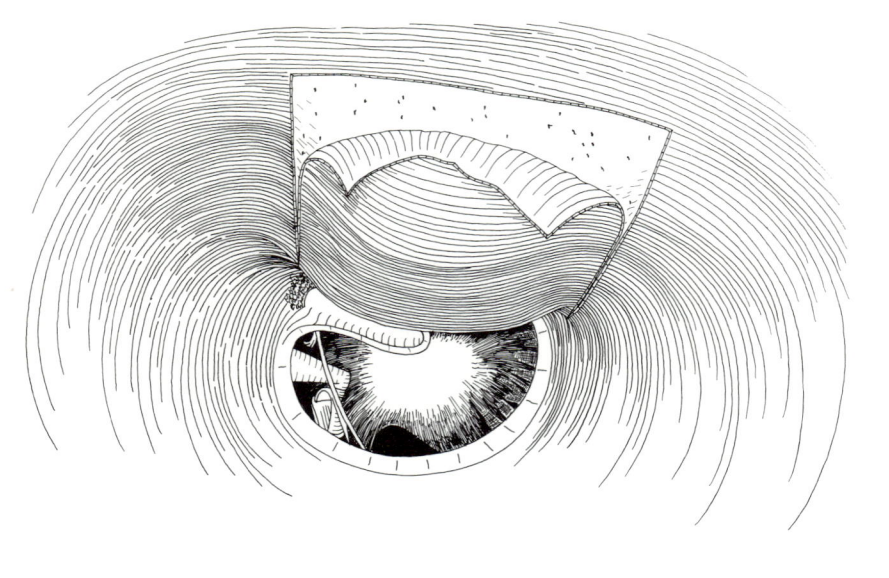

Fig. 656 **A fourth modification of the removal method for the bony prominence.** The elevated skin flap is based medially

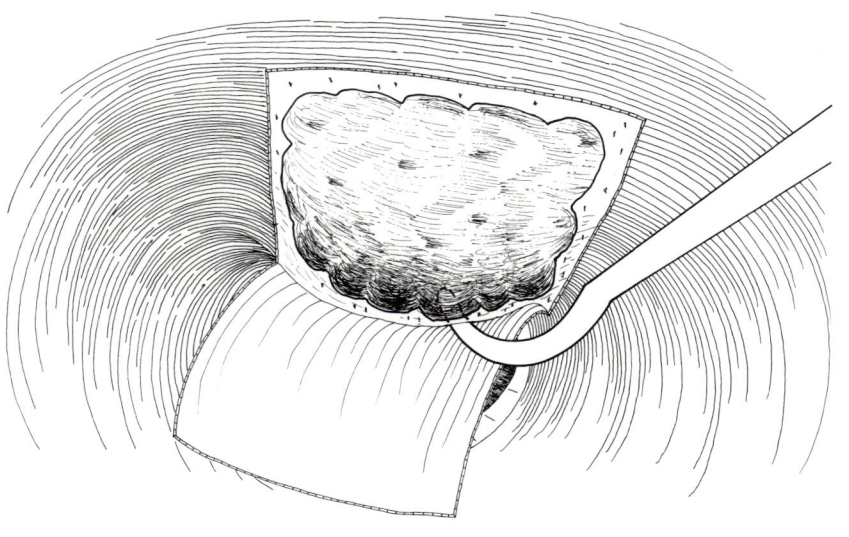

Fig. 657 The medially based skin flap is elevated, and the bone is drilled away

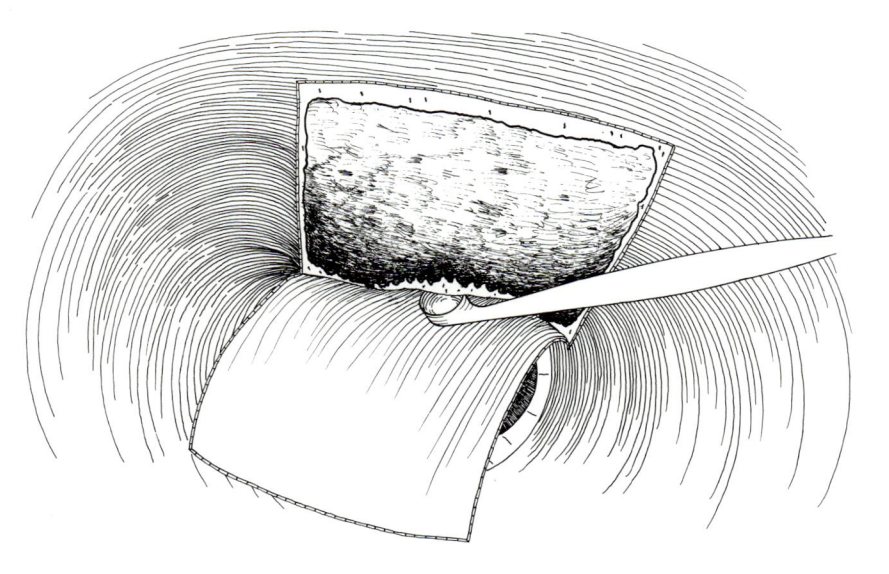

Fig. 658 Further drilling of the bone and elevation of the skin under the bony prominence

Retroauricular Approach

The retroauricular approach is a popular solution in an anterior perforation, giving optimal visualization of the anterior tympanomeatal angle. In subtotal and total perforations, the view of the anterior tympanum is also good with a retroauricular approach, but in cases with associated pathology in the tympanic sinus and in the deep regions of the posterior tympanum, the retroauricular approach has difficulties as far as adequate visualization of these regions is concerned. Both underlay and onlay methods can be performed with the retroauricular approach.

In cases in which removing the anterior prominence is desirable in order to improve the postoperative view to the anterior drum region through the ear-canal speculum, the bone should be removed by creating a laterally-pedicled skin flap with two radial incisions, at the 1-o'clock positions, respectively, and a medial circumferential incision connecting the two radial incisions just lateral to the annulus (Fig. **659**). The anterior canal skin is elevated far laterally, and the bone is drilled away by cutting or diamond burrs of various sizes. The most medial edges of the bone are usually best removed by a House curette (Fig. **660**). The laterally-pedicled skin flap is replaced, and the tympanoplasty can continue.

Fig. **659** **Removal of the bony prominence in the retroauricular approach.** The skin is incised using a radial incision just lateral to the annulus. After a circumferential incision, and after superior and inferior radial incisions, the laterally-based skin flap is elevated

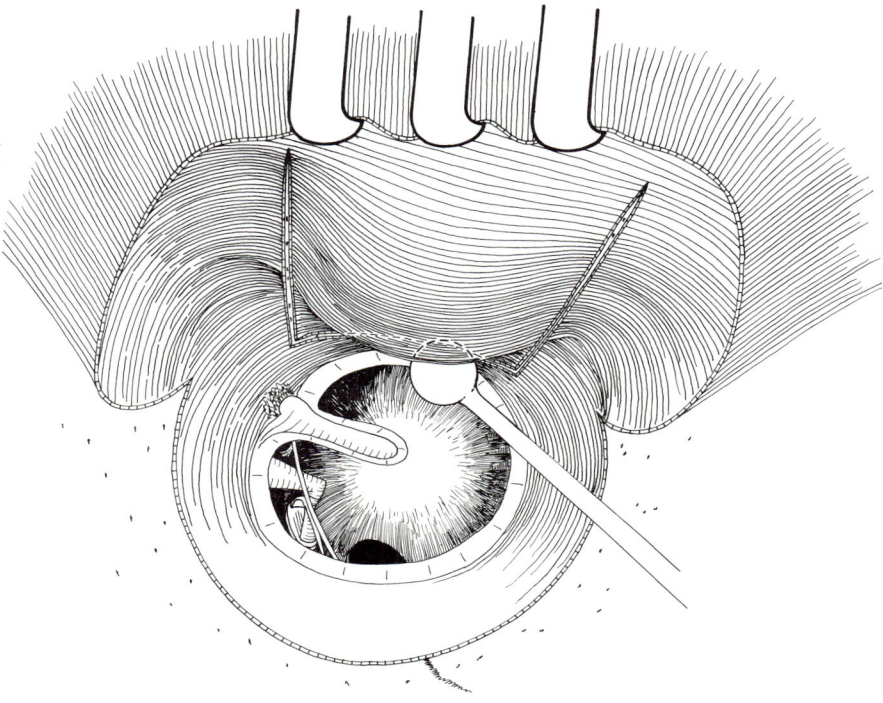

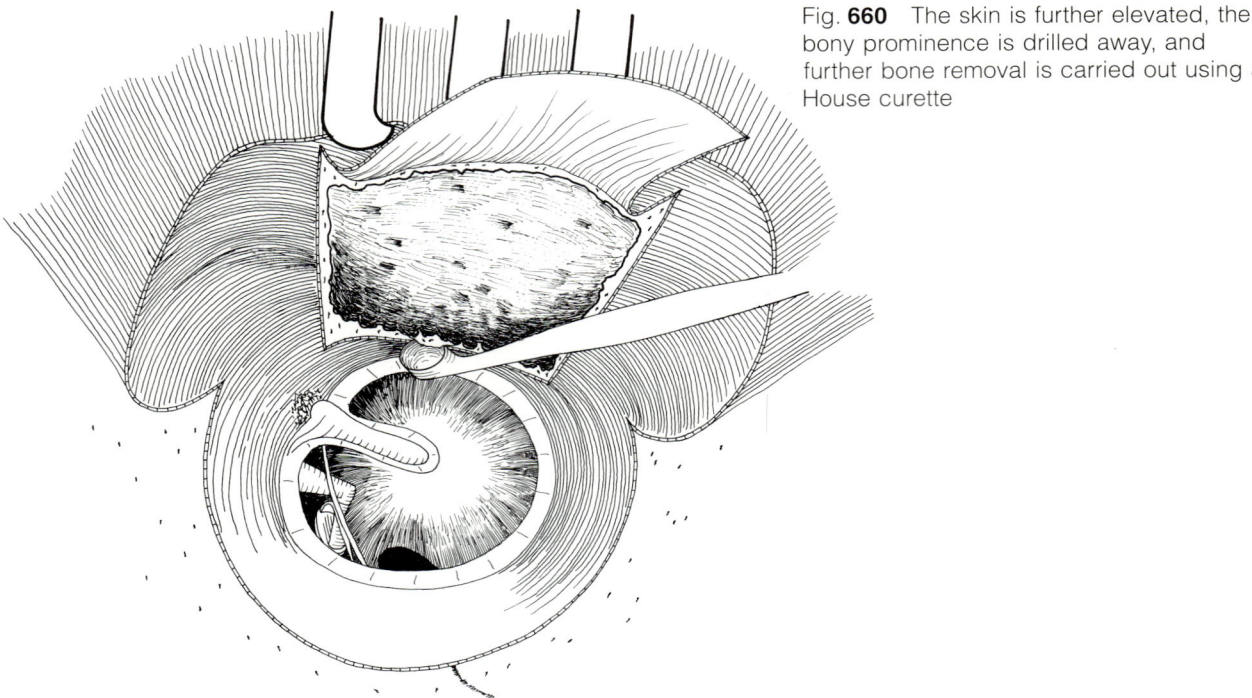

Fig. **660** The skin is further elevated, the bony prominence is drilled away, and further bone removal is carried out using a House curette

Endaural Approach

With the Heermann B incision, with a laterally-pedicled posterior skin flap, the posterior region is exposed, but a major anterior prominence of the ear canal has to be removed before myringoplasty. The intercartilaginous incision and a radial incision at the 12-o'clock position has already been performed as part of the Heermann B incision. From here, a circumferential incision can be performed (Fig. **666**) lateral to the anterior ear canal prominence, running from the 12-o'clock to the 6-o'clock position, and the skin can be elevated from the anterior bony canal wall. Because the prominence of the ear canal does not usually extend up to the 12-o'clock position, a separate radial incision just superior to the ear-canal prominence at approximately the 1-o'clock or 2-o'clock position is preferable. This leaves a strip of superior ear-canal skin intact between the 12-o'clock and 2-o'clock positions (Fig. **661**). The lateral circumferential incision goes to the 5-o'clock position. All skin is carefully elevated as far medially as possible, and the bone is exposed. The bony ear canal prominence is drilled off, starting laterally and superiorly (Fig. **662**), and continuing medially after careful elevation of the canal skin using a large curved elevator. Further drilling continues on the same principles (Fig. **663**): firstly, elevation of the skin, then drilling with a diamond burr until bone is removed and the anterior annulus is visualized. Finally, the edges of the bony wall are smoothed using a House curette. The canal skin is replaced, and myringoplasty with underlay or onlay grafting can be performed. Subsequently, the canal skin is attached medially along the annulus and inferiorly at the 6-o'clock position (Fig. **664**).

There are several other modifications of this technique, depending on the degree and localization of the prominence, as well as the tympanoplasty method used.

Endaural Approach 227

Fig. 661 **Removal of the bony prominence in the Heermann incision.** A circumferential incision and a radial incision are performed anterior and lateral to the bony prominence. The skin flap is elevated

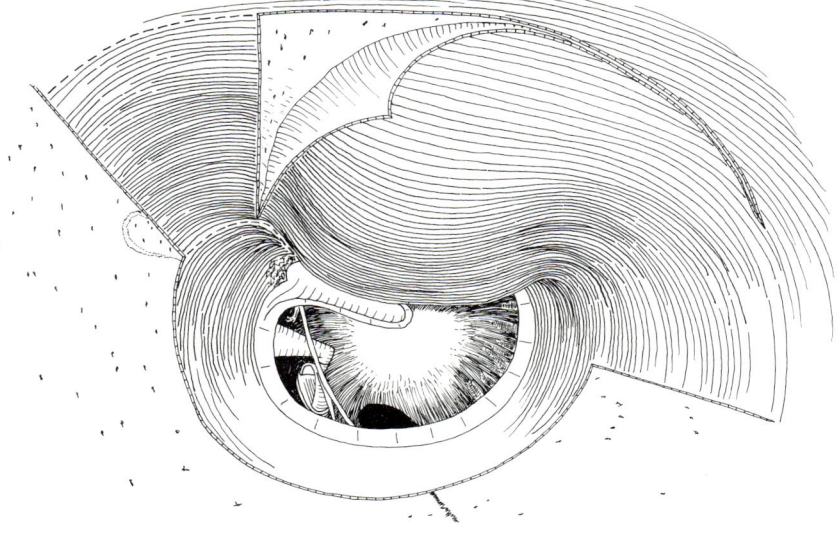

Fig. 662 Elevation of the skin flap and removal of the bony prominence. Further elevation of the skin under the prominence

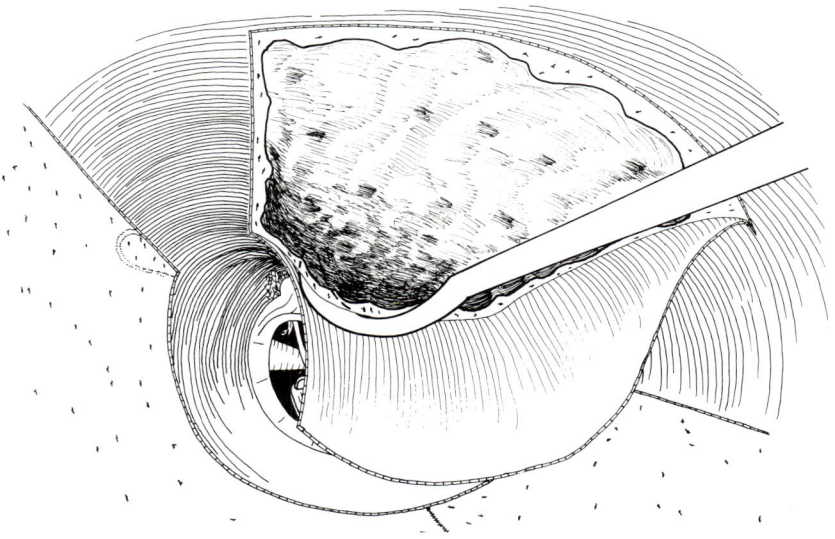

Fig. 663 Further removal of the bone, and elevation of the skin

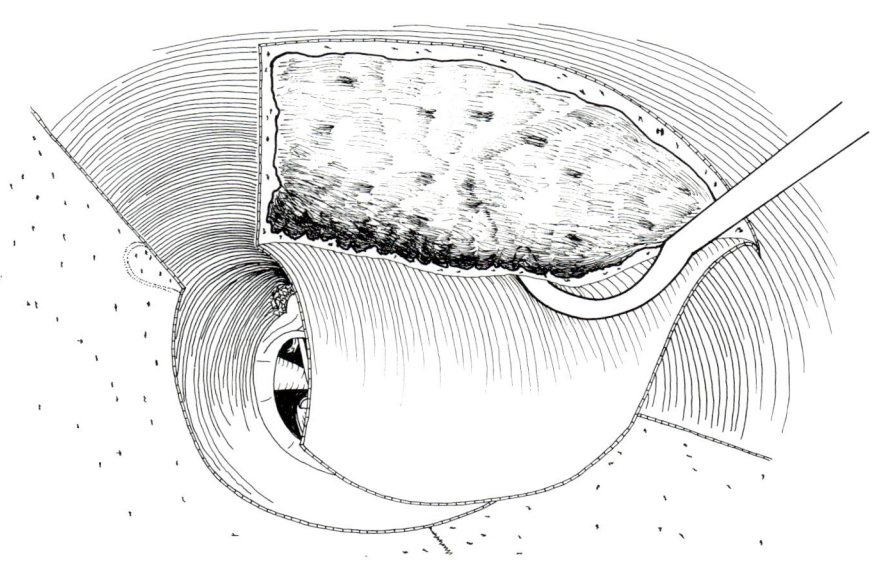

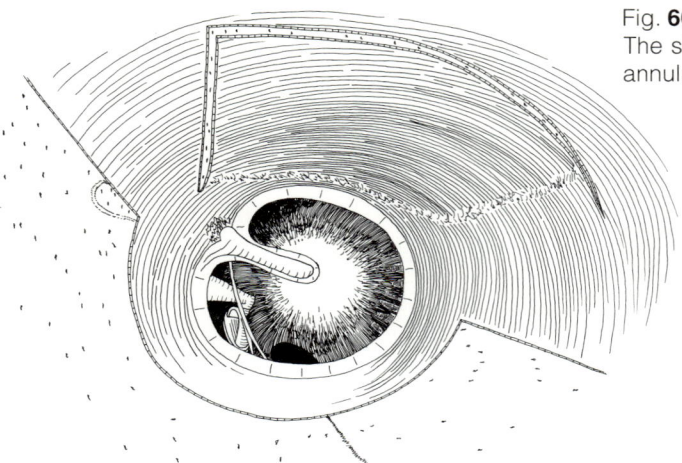

Fig. **664** Completed removal of the bone anteriorly. The skin flap is replaced in its original position, and the annulus is visible all the way round

The Shambaugh, Farrior and Fleury endaural incisions include methods with removal of the ear-canal skin. These methods were described above (pp. 25–30), and are used by some surgeons in cases with severe protrusions hampering the tympanoplasty. One of the purposes of skin removal has been to drill off overhangs on the anterior ear-canal wall, but in cases in which a tympanoplasty can be performed without bone removal, the ear-canal skin should be left intact.

Sheehy's Skin Removal Approach

Sheehy's sandwich technique of tympanoplasty is based on extensive skin removal, mainly to cover the fascia, and partly to be able to remove all irregularities and prominences of the ear canal. The Sheehy approach and the sandwich tympanoplasty techniques are described above (pp. 60–62 and 181–183). In cases with a prominent ear canal hampering visualization of the perforation, this technique can be performed. It is faster than the pedicled flap techniques we use, but in our opinion it is no better. In tympanoplasty and mastoidectomy surgery, the present author always prefers a flap technique to skin removal techniques. In flap techniques, the skin is replaced in exactly the same position as before. The vascularization and healing are rapid, and the migration process of the ear canal is not changed. After removal of the skin, exact replacement is seldom possible, especially if part of the skin is used as graft material in sandwich myringoplasty. The complicated mechanism of the migration process of the ear canal is disturbed, and in particular the outward orientation of the migration can be changed, as well as migration being slowed down, resulting in late accumulation of keratin and ear wax in the ear canal, and facilitating crust formation and infection—as is often seen in the cavities.

Removing the canal skin, in our view, is not optimal surgery. Using a diamond burr, any skin flap can be preserved after it has been elevated and pushed away during drilling.

14 Allogenous Ear Drum Transplantation

Allogenous eardrum has been used in several combinations:
1. simple closure of small perforations (Marquet 1972).
2. Replacement of the drum only.
3. Replacement of the drum and the malleus.
4. Replacement of the drum, malleus, and incus as a block, possibly together with the stapes.

Dissection of Allogenous Drum

Allografts are obtained from fresh cadavers within twelve hours of death. Two different methods, the transmeatal and transcranial routes, are used to collect the grafts. The *transmeatal route* permits removal of the drum together with the attached malleus, the annulus, and the deep meatal skin with periosteum. The other ossicles are removed separately. Circumferential incision is made all the way round through an ear speculum about 5 mm lateral to the annulus. The skin and periosteum are elevated, and the annulus is luxated from its bony sulcus all they way round (Fig. **665**). The malleus head is dislocated from the body of the incus, and the tensor tympani ligament, the chorda tympani, and the anterior and posterior ligaments of the malleus are cut with a relatively large forceps. The totally liberated drum–malleus allograft is displaced downwards by a forceps, the malleus head becomes visible in the tympanic cavity, and the graft can be removed (Fig. **666**). The tympanic membrane–malleus graft can be used with the attached tympanomeatal flap (Fig. **667**), or only with the fibrous annulus (Fig. **668**). The epithelial layer is removed from the tympanic membrane, from the fibrous annulus, and from the attached canal skin.

The tympanic membrane is separated from the donor malleus by slitting the fibrous sleeve on the medial side of the malleus handle by a hook (Fig. **669**). The fibrous sleeve is gradually elevated from the malleus handle until the free tympanic membrane is delivered (Fig. **670**).

The resected allogenous membrane can be stored in otimerate (Cialit), alcohol, or formaldehyde. Before use, the unbound fixative is removed by irrigation with Ringer's solution.

The *transcranial route* is performed on the temporal bone, which has been removed and kept frozen until dissection. To obtain the total block of the drum, including the malleus and incus, the trans-

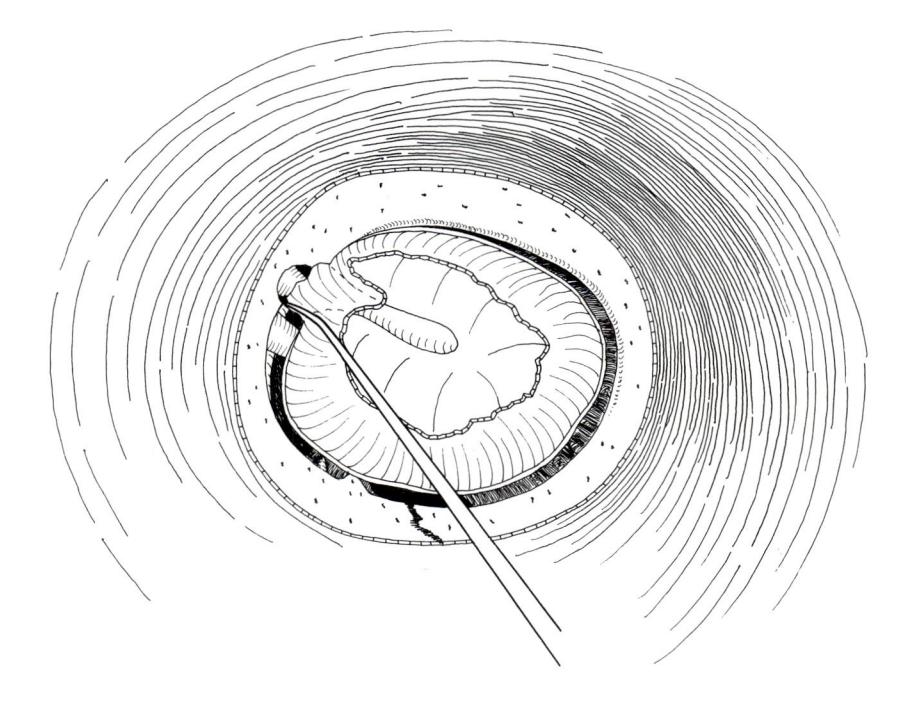

Fig. **665 Harvesting tympanic membrane–malleus allograft with the canal skin by a transmeatal route.** An attic incision is made in the canal skin, followed by elevation of the tympanomeatal flap and dislocation of the fibrous annulus. The canal skin is pushed onto the drum, and the malleus is dislocated from the incus

14 Allogenous Ear Drum Transplantation

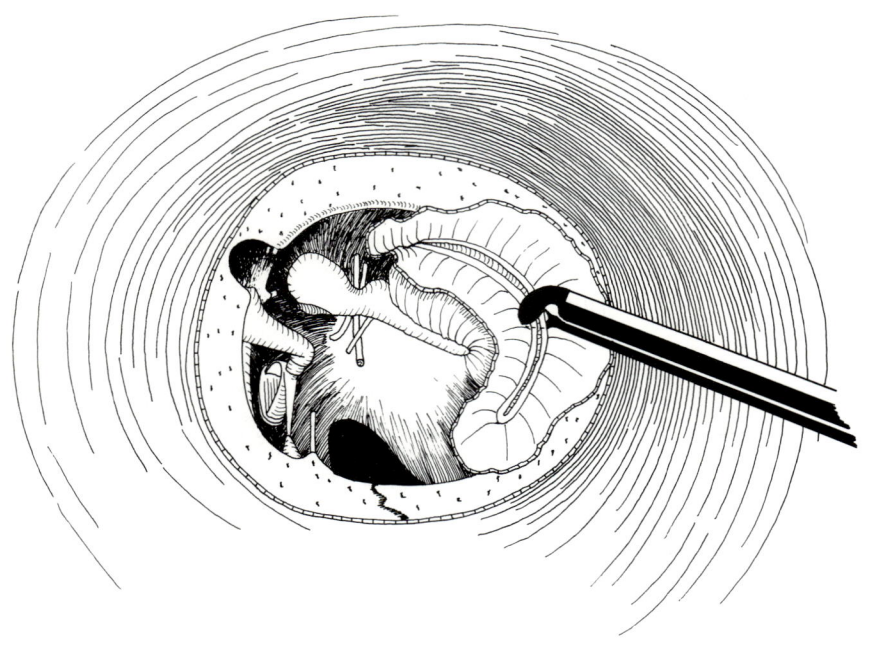

Fig. **666** The totally liberated drum–malleus allograft is displaced inferiorly in the tympanic cavity and will be removed by a forceps

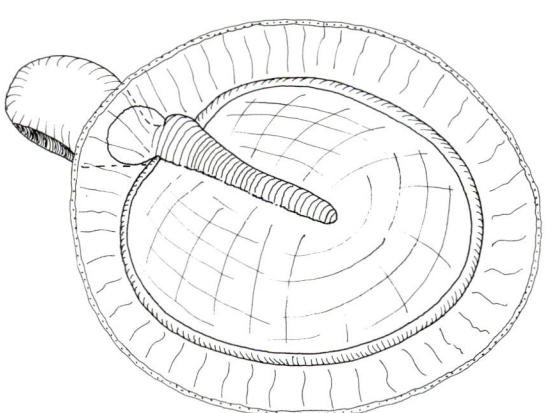

Fig. **667** The tympanic membrane–malleus graft with attached periosteum from the tympanomeatal flap, as used by Marquet

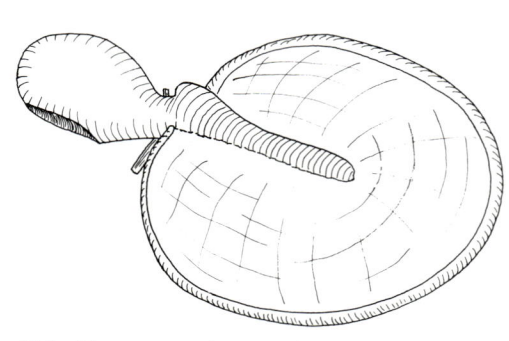

Fig. **668** The tympanic membrane–malleus graft with the fibrous annulus, as used by Perkins, Wehrs, and Brandow

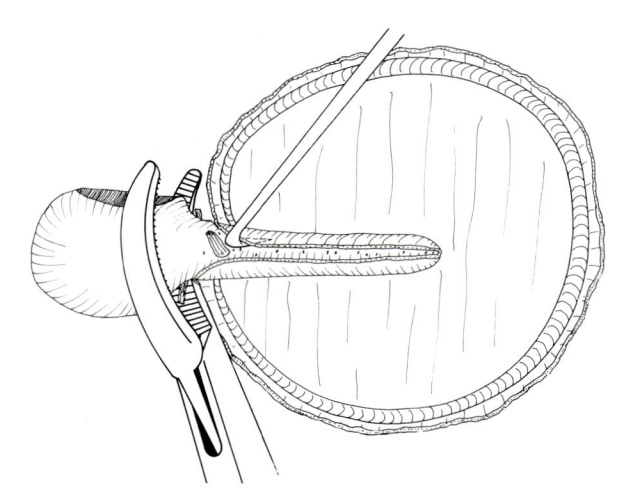

Fig. **669** Separation of a tympanic membrane from the malleus handle by section of the fibrous sleeve on its medial side

cranial route has to be employed. The technique of harvesting a total block is actually a complicated surgical procedure, and some experience is needed to avoid luxating the incudomalleus joint. The technique is especially difficult when the stapes is also included in the block. It is beyong the scope of this book to describe the techniques of removing the total drum–ossicular block.

Allograft Drum in Small and Middle-Sized Perforations

Marquet has used allogenous drum to close all types of perforations, even small ones. He cuts a piece of allogenous drum and covers the perforation as an onlay graft in a manner similar to the onlay technique with fascia or perichondrium. As far as I know, no-one other than Marquet (1966, 1971) has used allogenous drum in small perforations. In the 1970s in several places, drums with medium-sized perforations, even in noncholesteatomatous ears, were removed together with the annulus and the malleus, and replaced by an allogenous malleus–drum graft. We would definitely not recommended such procedure. It only produces failures and increases the percentage of reperforations.

Allogenous Drum in Total Perforation with Intact Malleus

In this pathology, replacement of the drum without the malleus has been used, and is still recommended. Two, in principle different, methods are used. The first method, *without removal* of the patient's annulus, involves placing the allogenous annulus onto the patient's annulus. The second method includes *total removal* of patient's annulus and replacement of it with a homograft annulus, which is palced in the bony sulcus. Both methods attempt to preserve as much of the drum-remnant epithelium and ear-canal skin epithelium as possible in order to cover the allogenous drum with skin. The first method was popularized by Brandow (1969, 1976). It is usually performed in an endaural approach with a speculum or in any endaural incision, but the retroauricular approach can also be used.

A circumferential skin incision is made between the 11-o'clock and 2-o'clock positions. Before or after the skin incision, an epithelial flap from the malleus handle is elevated (Fig. **671**). The ear-canal skin is elevated, together with the kera-

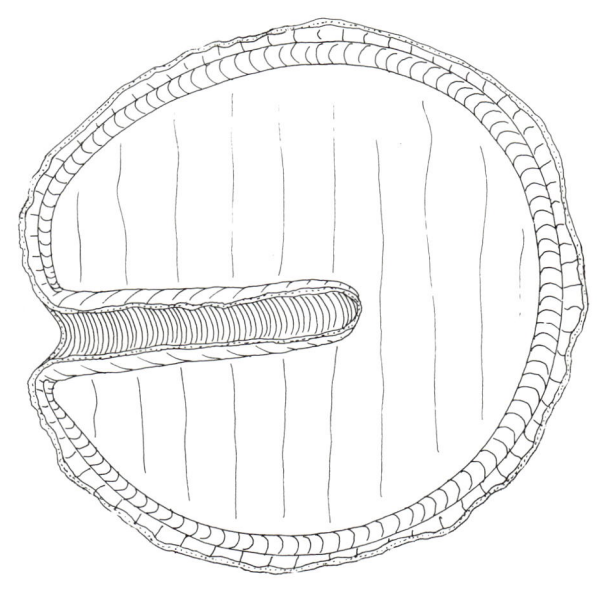

Fig. **670** The free tympanic membrane is totally separated from the malleus handle, and the fibrotic sleeve is illustrated

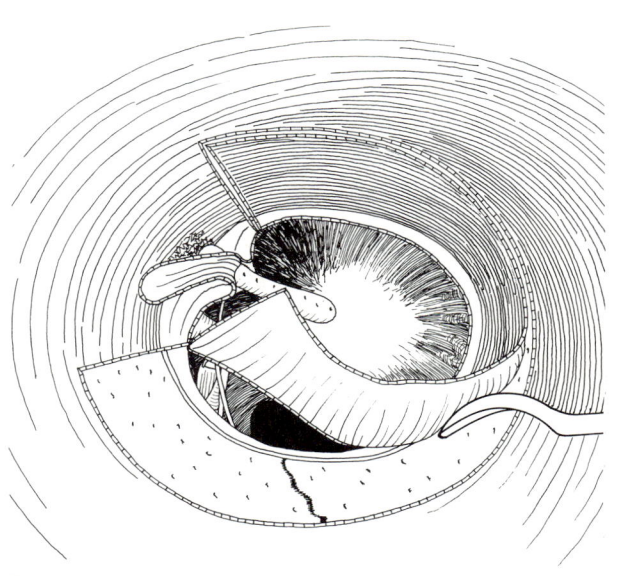

Fig. **671** **The Brandow method of allogenous drum transplantation.** A circumferential skin incision is made between the 11-o'clock and 2-o'clock position, and the malleus flap is elevated

tinized squamous epithelium of the drum remnant. After carefull elevation and removal of the large skin flap, it is stored in Ringer's solution during the operation. The superior tympanomeatal flap is elevated together with the malleus flap, exposing the Shrapnell's membrane region (Fig. **672**). The allogenous drum is carefully adapted and placed onto the patient's annulus. The fibrous sleeve of the allo-

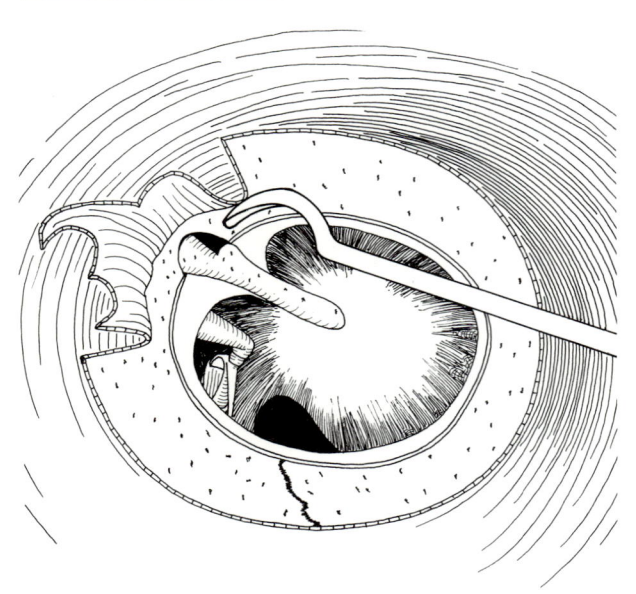

Fig. **672** The tympanomeatal flap and the keratinized drum remnant epithelium are removed. Elevation of the superior tympanomeatal flap together with the malleus flap

Fig. **673** The allogenous drum is placed on the patient's annulus, and the superior canal-skin flap is replaced

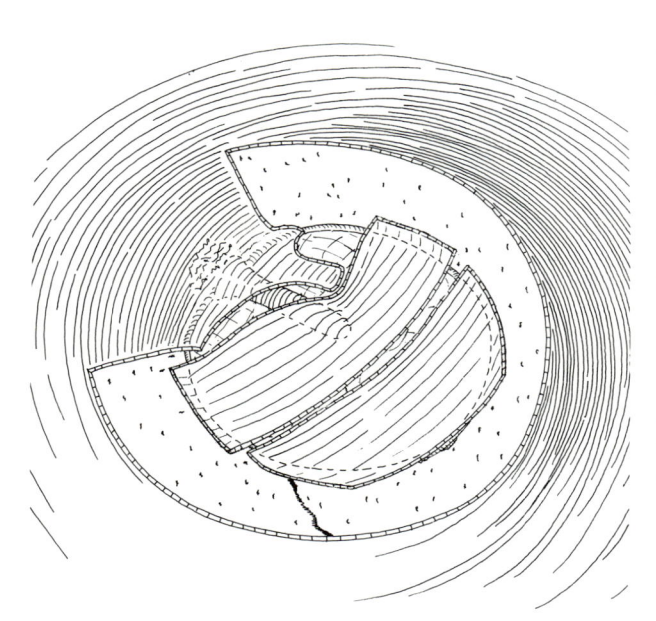

Fig. **674** The removed canal skin covers the allogenous drum area in two pieces

genous drum is carefully adapted to the malleus handle (Fig. **670**). The superior skin flap, including the malleus flap, is replaced. The malleus-handle skin flap is placed anterior to the malleus handle (Fig. **673**), allowing easier covering of the drum with canal skin. The removed ear-canal skin is cut into two pieces, which cover the majority of the allogenous drum area (Fig. **674**). The canal skin should be brought across the allograft to the anterior sulcus, but not up to the anterior meatal wall, to avoid blunting (Fig. **675**). The canal skin usually covers 75% of the allogenous graft surface. The ear canal is packed with Gelfoam. Wehrs (1982) used techniques similar to those of Brandow (1976), also mainly with an endaural approach.

The other method is to remove the annulus, mainly with a retroauricular approach (Perkins 1970, Marquet 1966, 1971).

Perkin's method is based on the creation of a posterior vascular strip flap, which is elevated retrograde (Fig. **676**) (Perkins 1970). An incision is performed at the 12-o'clock positions, and another at the 6-o'clock position, elevating a malleus handle flap. After a retroauricular incision, the posterior canal-skin flap is elevated and turned backwards, providing a good view of the anterior tympanomeatal angle and outward elevation of the anterior canal skin (Fig. **677**). Elevation of the squamous epithelium from the drum remnant takes

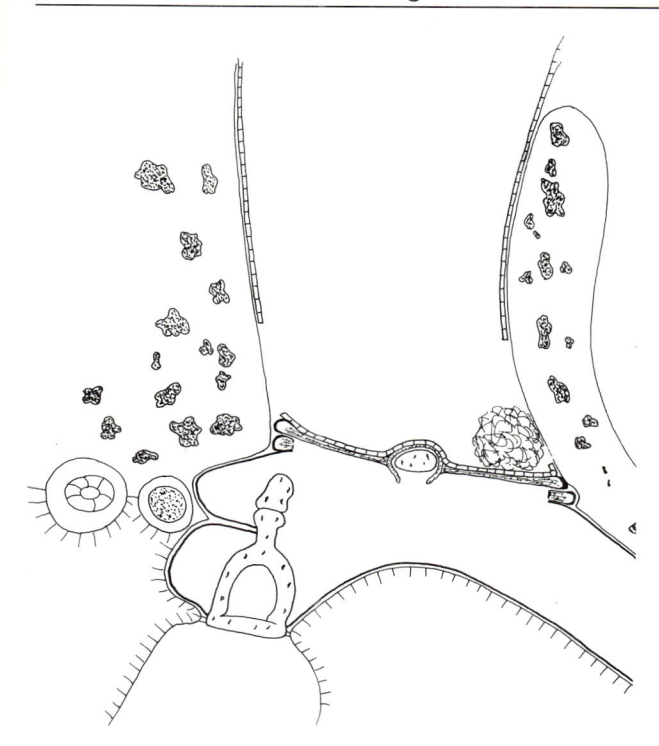

Fig. 675 Side view of the placement of the allogenous drum on the patient's fibrous annulus. The canal skin covers the allogenous drum

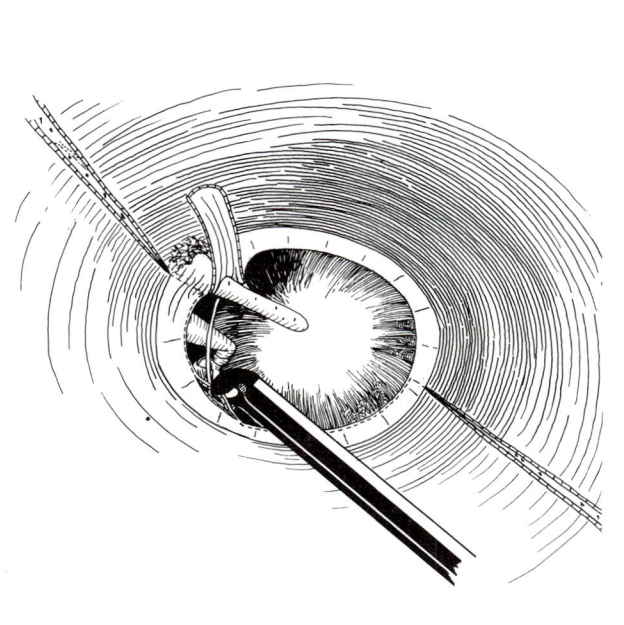

Fig. 676 **The Perkins method of allogenous drum transplantation.** Incisions are made at the 12-o'clock and 6-o'clock positions, and the malleus handle flap is elevated

place superiorly, exposing the Shrapnell's membrane region, and inferiorly, along the anterior annulus (Fig. **678**). Finally, all the annulus is luxated out of its bony sulcus (Fig. **679**) and removed (Fig. **680**). The allogenous ear drum with its annulus is placed in the empty bony sulcus and adapted to the malleus handle. Any space between the tympanic membrane and the bony sulcus is bridged with small pieces of autogenous fascia. The epithelial flaps are carefully replaced (Fig. **681**). The ear canal is packed with Gelfoam (Fig. **682**).

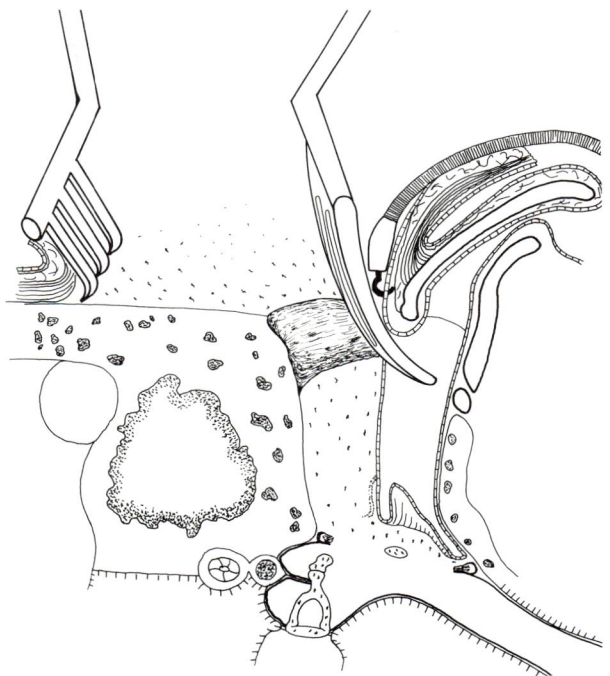

Fig. 677 In the retroauricular approach, the posterior meatal skin is elevated from the drum remnant together with the squamous epithelium and turned backward, providing a good view of the anterior tympanomeatal angle

234   14   Allogenous Ear Drum Transplantation

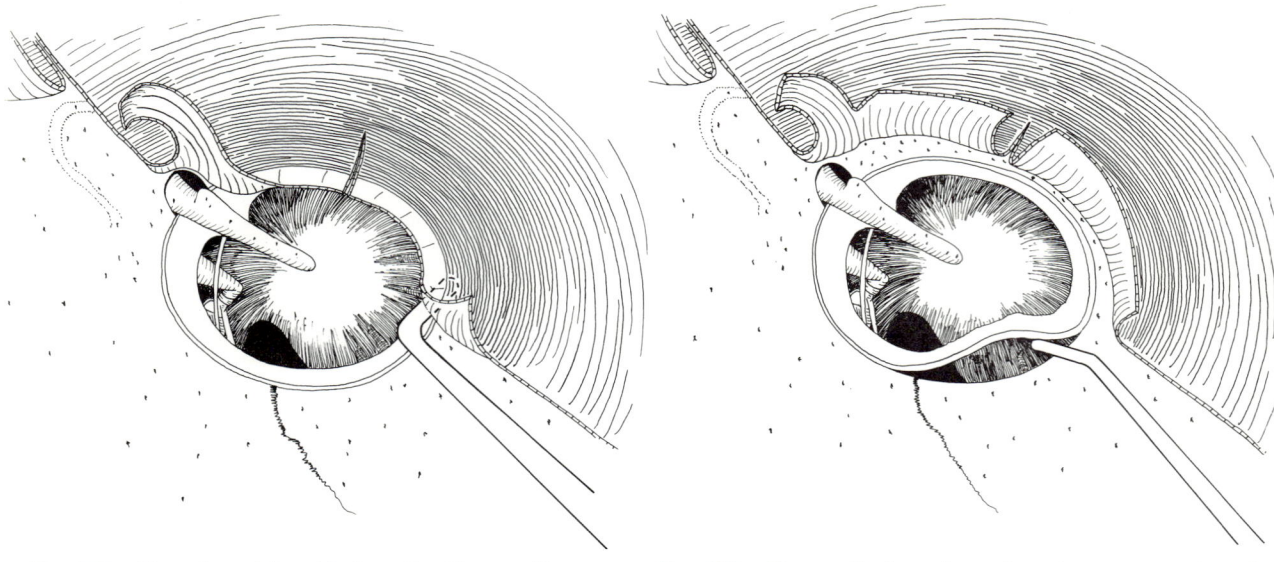

Fig. 678 Elevation of the skin from the Shrapnell's membrane region and inferior annulus

Fig. 679 The epithelium from the drum remnant and the-ear canal skin are elevated outward, and the posteroinferior part of the fibrous annulus is dislocated

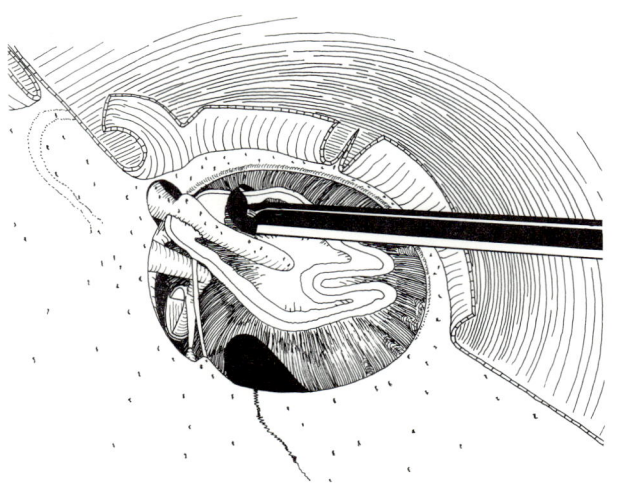

Fig. 680 The entire fibrous annulus is dislocated and is to be removed. The bony annulus is visible

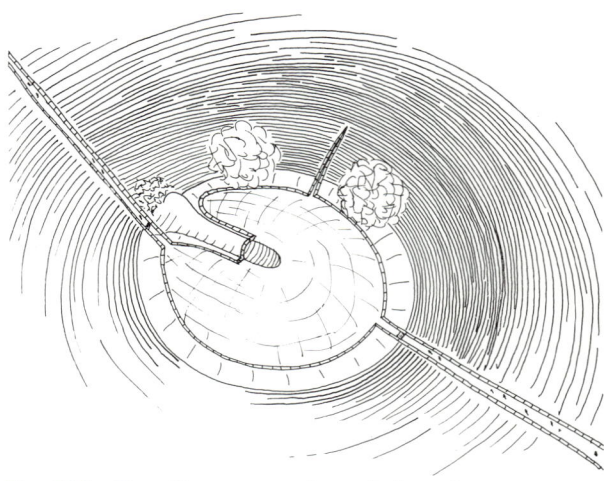

Fig. 681 The fibrous annulus of the allogenous ear drum is placed into the empty bony sulcus and adapted to the malleus handle. The epithelium flaps are replaced

Marquet (1971) uses allogenous drum together with neighboring periosteum (Fig. 667). The elevation of the ear-canal skin should therefore be much more extensive than with other methods. Elevation is started at the edge of the perforation, continuing outward along the bony meatal wall for about 1 centimeter from the annulus (Fig. 683). If the host annulus is absent, the allogenous annulus replaces it; if it is present, the allogenous annulus is placed on top of the host annulus. In this respect, Marquet's method is similar to that of Brandow. The graft periosteum is placed onto the bony meatal wall, and the host meatal and tympanic epithelium is gently replaced over the graft (Fig. 684).

Usually, Marquet's method of elevating the epithelium is performed transmeatally (Fig. 683) (Marquet 1971), but, on the other hand, a posterior atticotympanotomy is usually performed, and the approach is retroauricular, making elevation of the posterior meatal skin easier (Fig. 685).

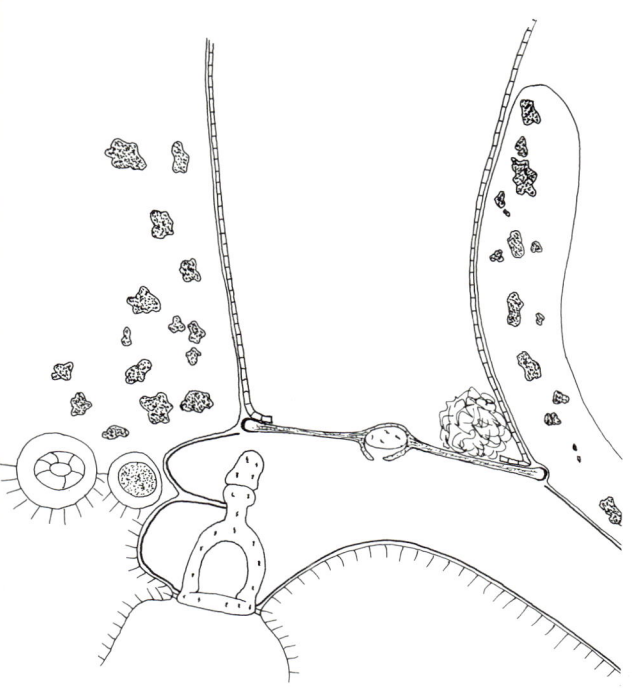

Allogenous Drum in Total Perforation with Intact Malleus 235

Fig. **682** Side view of the placement of the allogenous tympanic membrane after removal of the patient's fibrous annulus

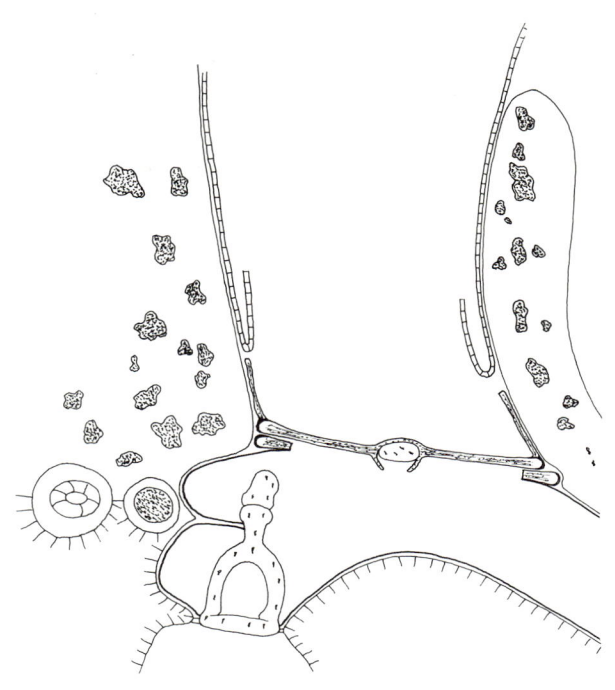

Fig. **683 The Marquet method of transcanal outward elevation of the drum-remnant epithelium and the ear-canal skin.** The allogenous tympanic membrane is placed on the patient's fibrous annulus, and the periosteum is placed on the denuded ear-canal bone

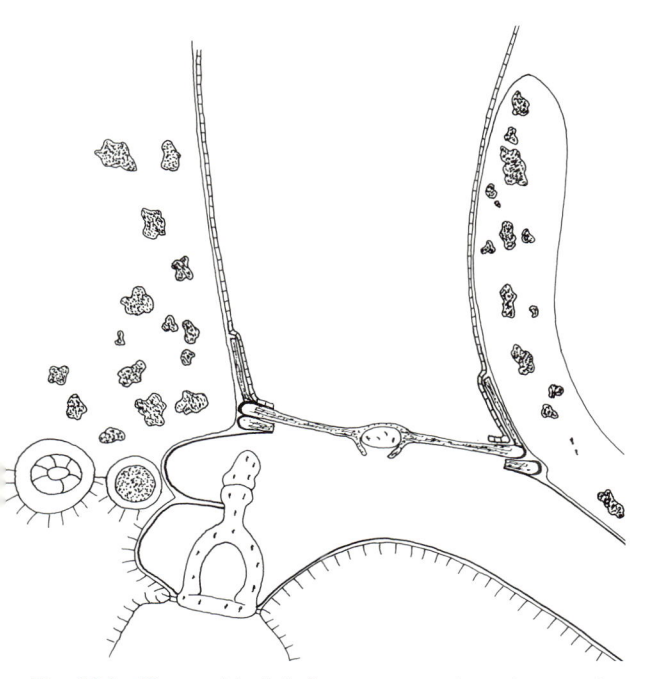

Fig. **684** The epithelial flaps are replaced, covering the allogenous periosteum

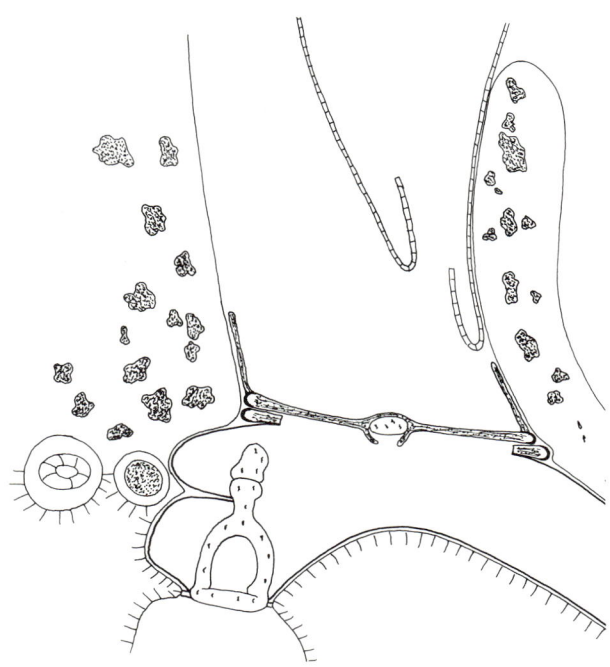

Fig. **685** Side view of elevation of the ear-canal skin in the retroauricular approach. The allogenous tympanic membrane with the periosteum is in position on the patient's fibrous annulus

In the late 1960s, the present author performed about 20 allograft tympanic membrane transplantations, but the results were definitely no better than those with autogenous fascia, and the method was soon abandoned. In cases with atelectatic and "too large" atrophic drums placement of an allogenous drum under the elevated atrophic membrane is quite satisfactory.

The problem of AIDS in relation to using allogenous drum (Glasscock et al. 1988) was mentioned above in connection with graft materials (p. 126–127).

Transplantation of the malleus should only be performed in cases in which it is absent. The technique is described below (pp. 229–235).

Part III
Ossiculoplasty and Tympanoplasty

15 Tympanoplasty—General

In chronic middle ear disease, the ossicular chain is often defective. It is reconstructed at the end of a tympanoplasty operation, just before reconstruction of the drum. Ossiculoplasty forms part of the tympanoplasty procedure, and means the reconstruction of a defective ossicular chain, either between the intact stapes or the footplate and the malleus handle or the drum only. The term "ossiculoplasty" therefore includes only some of the possible hearing-improvement procedures. It does not cover procedures in which the ossicles are not involved, e.g., the round-window protection technique and fenestration techniques. The term "ossiculoplasty" will be used here in connection with tympanoplasty, and the classifications presented refer to tympanoplasty in general.

Classification of Tympanoplasty

Over the years, several classifications of tympanoplasty have been proposed and used. The present author uses the following classification of tympanoplasty in daily practice and in clinical research:

Myringoplasty. Closure of the eardrum perforation in cases with a normal ossicular chain and without any other surgical procedures in the tympanic cavity or middle ear.

Tympanoplasty type 1. In cases with an intact ossicular chain at the end of the operation. This procedure can be nearly as straightforward as myringoplasty, and for instance simply involve removal of a retracted membrane in the tympanic cavity, or removal of adhesions around the ossicles; but it can also be an extensive and time-consuming procedure, for instance in cases of tensa-retraction cholesteatomas involving the entire tympanic cavity, but not the attic (Fig **686a**).

Tympanoplasty type 2. Ossiculoplasty in cases with a defective ossicular chain, but with the stapes present. Type 2 includes interposition techniques between the head of the stapes and the malleus handle or the grafted eardrum remnant (Fig. **686b**). Interpositions between the stapedial arch in cases with a missing head or neck of the stapes and the malleus handle or eardrum are also defined as tympanoplasty type 2.

Tympanoplasty type 3. Ossiculoplasty in cases with an absent, or severely defective, stapedial arch, if columella techniques are used. The columella goes from the footplate to the malleus handle or the grafted eardrum (Fig. **686c**).

Tympanoplasty type 4. This type does not involve ossiculoplasty as such, but is protection mechanism for the round window in cases with absent ossicles, including the stapedial arch, but with an intact and mobile footplate. The type 4 technique also includes the cavum minor technique or sound-protection techniques (Fig. **686d**).

Tympanoplasty type 5A. Fenestration of the lateral semicircular canal in cases with no ossicles and a fixed footplate. The stapedial arch may or may not be intact (Fig. **686e**).

Tympanoplasty type 5B. This means platinectomy in cases with a fixed footplate and no ossicles. Tympanoplasty type 5B has today almost totally replaced the fenestration procedure, which is very seldom performed (Fig. **686f**).

Fig. **686** The classification of tympanoplasty most commonly used
a Type 1. Intact chain
b Type 2. Defective long process of the incus. Interposition of an ossicle, or any other prosthesis, between the stapedial arch and the malleus handle or eardrum
c Type 3. Absent or severely defective stapedial arch. Placement of a columella between the footplate and the malleus handle or eardrum
d Type 4. Sound protection of the round window with a graft, and formation of an air space in the hypotympanum. The footpate is covered by keratinized epithelium
e Type 5A. Fenestration of the lateral semicircular canal (arrow) in cases with no ossicles and a fixed stapes footplate. In such cases the stapedial arch is usually missing. The round window is protected
f Type 5B. Platinectomy. The oval window niche is filled with fatty tissue or fibrous tissue

Classification of Tympanoplasty

a

b

c

d

e

f

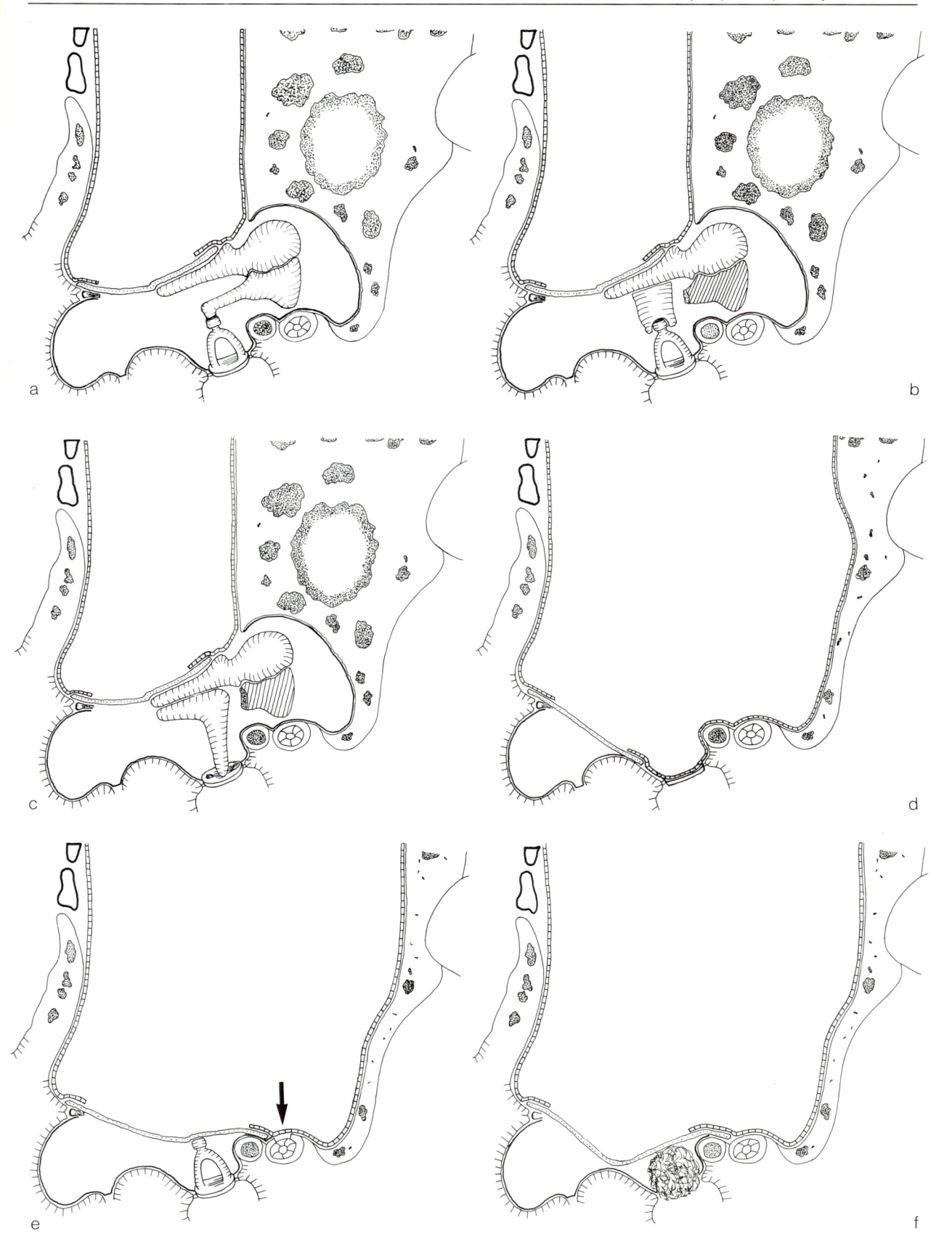

The author uses this tympanoplasty classification for procedures on the sound-conducting structures. If mastoidectomy, atticoantrotomy, or atticotomy is performed in addition to tympanoplasty, the same tympanoplasty classification is used, but the names of other procedures will be added, e.g., mastoidectomy and tympanoplasty type 1, or atticoantrotomy and tympanoplasty type 1, or mastoidectomy and tympanoplasty type 2, etc.

This classification is used currently by the majority of surgeons, and will be applied in this book. It deviates in some important points from the original Wullstein (1968) classification (Fig. **687a–e**): Tympanoplasty types 1, 4, and 5A are the same, but Wullstein assigns cases with a missing malleus handle but an otherwise intact ossicular chain to type 2. He places the graft on the intact incudostapedial joint—a myringoincudopexy. Very few surgeons today use the term "tympanoplasty type 2" for this situation alone. In fact, this type of situation is a rare condition. In our surgical material (Tos 1979), it appears in 3% of noncholesteatomatous cases, and 3% of cholesteatomatous cases. In patients with total perforation, a defective malleus handle was seen in 10%. Since the lenticular process is usually also resorbed in cases with resorption of the malleus handle, so that there is no connection between the stapes and the incus, and partly because the majority of surgeons disrupt the ossicular chain in cases with a defective malleus handle and perform interposition between the stapes and the drum, very few surgeons today perform Wullstein's original tympanoplasty type 2. It is therefore reasonable to use the term "tympanoplasty type 2" to cover all interpositions, as well as the few cases with an intact ossicular chain and resorbed malleus handle. Since the malleus is defective and the stapes are intact, Wullstein's original type 2—the myringoincudopexy—easily fits into our type 2 tympanoplasty. When Wullstein introduced his classification, the interposition techniques were in fact not in use. It is therefore reasonable for interposition techniques to be classified nowadays as tympanoplasty type 2.

Another problem with Wullstein's classification is with tympanoplasty type 3. According to Wullstein, type 3 denotes myringostapediopexy, and he did not include columellas in his classification. Myringostapediopexy is seldom performed today. The majority of surgeons today perform an interposition instead of a pexis, and place an ossicle or a prosthesis on the head of the stapes, mainly because myringostapediopexy usually requires a canal wall–down mastoidectomy and extensive removal of the posterosuperior bony wall. This is particularly apparent in cases with a low, posteriorly positioned stapes. The present author only performs myringostapediopexy in patients who have an established myringostapediopexy and good hearing, but if it is necessary to disrupt this connection due to other pathology, an interposition is performed instead of attempting a repeated myringostapediopexy. Since Wullstein's tympanoplasty type 3 is rarely used nowadays, there is a logical argument for type 3 to be used for columella techniques in cases in which the stapedial arch is absent.

Type 4 is the same in both classifications. It denotes protection of the round window. At the time the Wullstein classification was introduced, the 1950s, type 4 was the only method used in cases with an absent stapedial arch. This was, in connection with canal wall–down procedures, the method of choice at that time. Today, type 4 has been replaced by columellas and is seldom used.

Type 5 denotes fenestration of the lateral semicircular canal. Platinectomy was not used at that time.

Wullstein himself modified his own technique later, and the modification is similar to the classification used here (Wullstein and Wullstein 1990).

Farrior's classification, (1968) is as follows: a type 1 tympanoplasty denotes cases with an intact ossicular chain or myringoplasty. A type 2 tympanoplasty denotes reconstruction of a new eardrum, placed in contact with a normal, mobile incus in cases with a missing malleus handle, which is the same as Wullstein type 2—myringoincudopexy (Fig. **688**). Type 3 tympanoplasty denotes interposition of a bone graft between the intact stapes and the drum or the malleus handle, corresponding to our type 2 classification (Fig. **686b**). Type 4 tympanoplasty denotes cases with a missing stapedial arch, reconstructed by a columella, corresponding to our type 3 classification (Fig. **686c**). Type 5 tympanoplasty denotes fenestration of the lateral semicircular canal, which is the same as Wullstein's type 5 (Fig. **687e**). Type 6 tympanoplasty denotes myringoplasty in cases with no ossiculoplasty and no restoration of the hearing, for instance in scar tissue, tympanosclerosis around the windows, and disease of the Eustachian tube. This operation is termed myringoplasty here, since no other procedures are performed.

The difficulties in the use of the classic Wullstein classification with today's many different interposition techniques are clearly demonstrated by Kley's classification (1982). Kley still uses Wullstein's classification, but, recognizing that type 2 is today an extremely rare operation, includes the following situations in type 2:

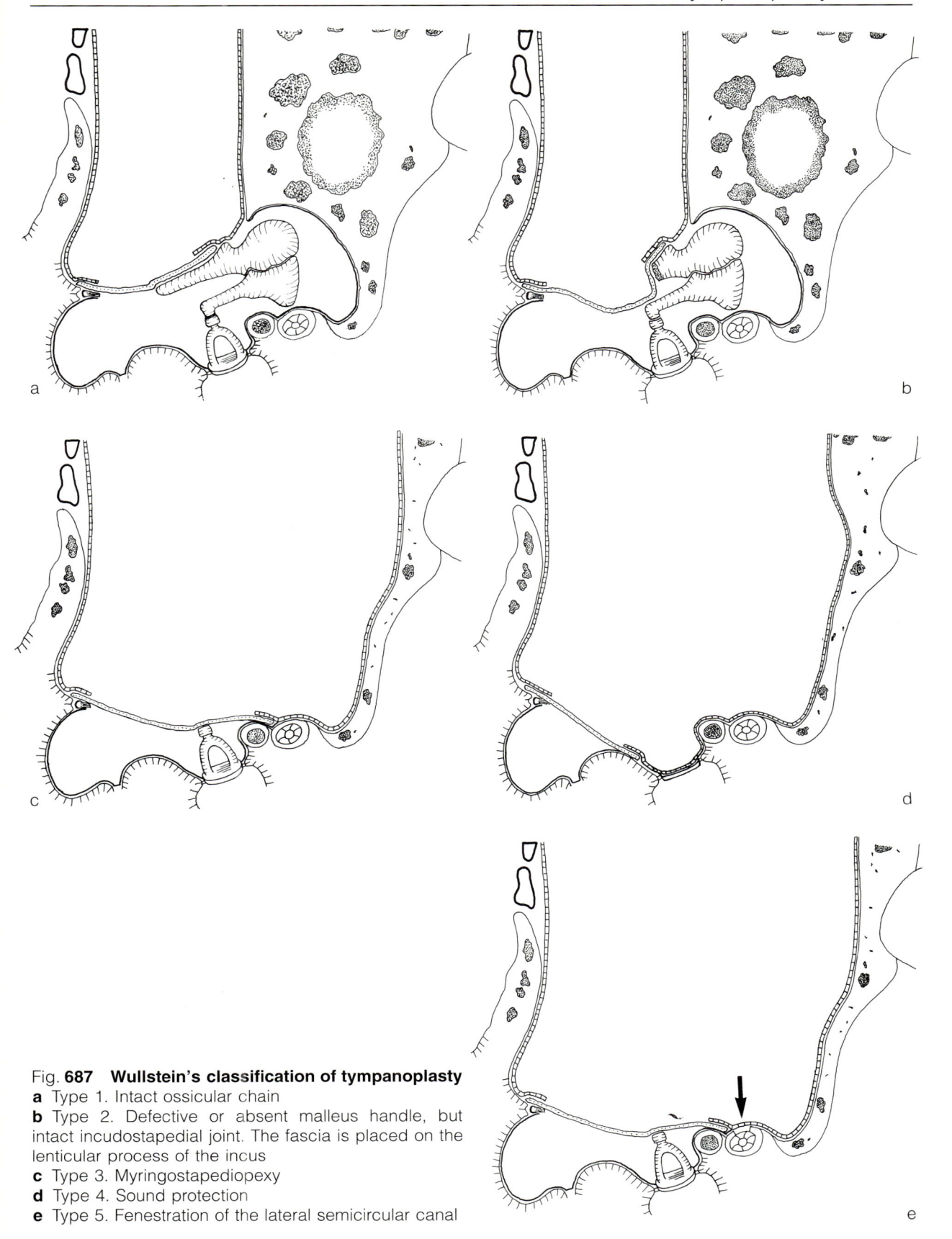

Classification of Tympanoplasty

Fig. 687 Wullstein's classification of tympanoplasty
a Type 1. Intact ossicular chain
b Type 2. Defective or absent malleus handle, but intact incudostapedial joint. The fascia is placed on the lenticular process of the incus
c Type 3. Myringostapediopexy
d Type 4. Sound protection
e Type 5. Fenestration of the lateral semicircular canal

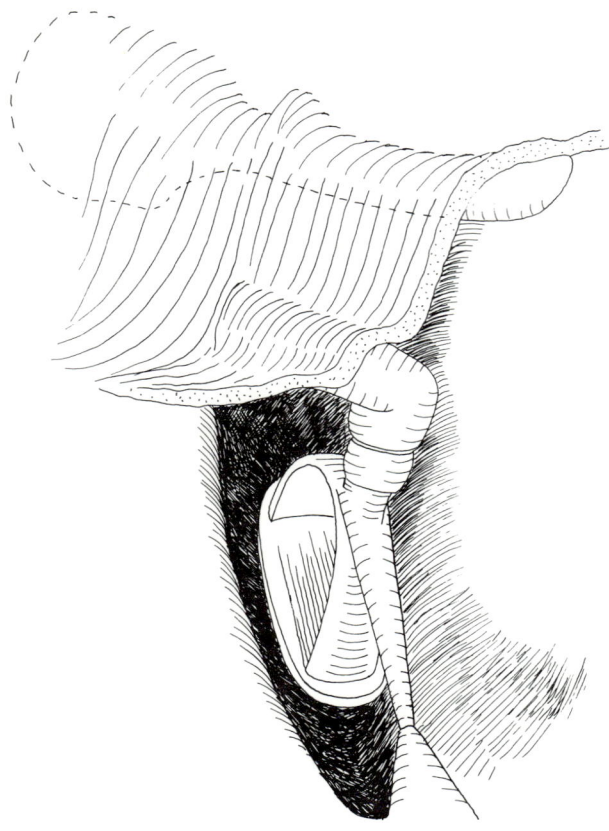

Fig. **688** Myringoincudopexy. The long process of the incus is cut from the body of the incus and covered with the fascia. This is a type 2 tympanoplasty in Kley's classification. The incudostapedial joint is intact

1. Minor defects of the long process of the incus with definite incudostapedial discontinuity, if such a discontinuity is restored by placing connective tissue between the stapes and the incus, or if the incus defect is bridged by a malleostapediopexy using a wire to connect the malleus to the head of the stapes.
2. Kley also classifies as type 2 a direct connection using steel wire between the malleus and the footplate, i.e., malleoplatinopexy. The majority of surgeons describe this as an incus replacement prosthesis (IRP) (Sheehy 1972).
3. A spontaneous type 2 tympanoplasty, if the tympanic membrane, or its remnant, covers the defective ossicular chain and provides good hearing. If the spontaneous bridging of the defect needs to be disrupted in order to remove the disease from the middle ear, then Kley's type 2 is transformed into type 3, even though the original pathology is present (intact stapes and missing long process of the incus).

In type 3 tympanoplasty, Kley uses the following subclassification: a) The classical Wullstein type 3, myringostapediopexy (Fig. **687c**). b) Type 3 plus building up of the stapes using the lenticular process (Fig. **688**). In these cases, the long process of the incus is cut off, and the fascia or drum remnant is brought into contact with the lenticular process—a myringoincudopexy. This type of myringoincudopexy can be performed either with the malleus intact, or in a canal wall–down procedure with total removal of the malleus. Also, all interpositions between an intact stapes and the malleus handle or drum are placed in this group, e.g., interposition of the incus or the malleus head, or a piece of cortical bone. c) Type 3 with replacement of the stapes by a columella, including all cases with the columella placed between the footplate and the malleus handle or drum.

It is evident that Kley's classification is the most confusing one, especially as interpositions with an intact stapedial arch, and columellas without a stapedial arch and a completely different prognosis, are mixed together in the same group as type 3 tympanoplasty. As indicated above, surgeons today clearly distinguish between interpositions with the stapes present, classified as type 2, and columellas with stapes crura absent, classified as type 3. The French school (Portmann, Wayoff, Charachon, Magnan, Deguine, and others) distinguishes clearly between type 2, with the stapes present, and type 3, with the stapes absent.

Bellucci (1969, 1973) incorporates all possible pathological variables into two broad groups, one representing the pathology of the conductive mechanism in the middle ear, and the other relating to middle-ear infection. The Bellucci dual classification classifies patients into four prognostic groups in relation to stabilized ear:

Group 1: Good prognosis; dry ear for a long period.
Group 2: Fair prognosis; ear stabilized but discharging during upper respiratory tract infection.
Group 3: Poor prognosis, persistent discharge.
Group 4: Very poor prognosis, with chronic discharge and nasopharyngeal malformations.

For the prognosis of hearing improvement, Bellucci includes a modified Wullstein classification:

Type 1: Intact ossicles.
Type 2: Minor ossicular defects.
Type 3: Severe ossicular defects but stapes arch intact.
Type 4: Cavum minor.

Incidence of Ossicular-Chain Pathology

In our study of 1100 consecutive primary cases of middle-ear surgery for chronic middle-ear diseases, consisting of 429 patients with chronic otitis sequelae, 165 with active granulating chronic otitis, 80 patients with adhesive otitis, and 426 patients with cholesteatoma, varying incidences of ossicular-chain defects were found in various middle-ear diseases (Table **2**). In attic cholesteatoma with retraction or perforation of Shrapnell's membrane, involvement of the incus body or the head of the malleus was much more common than resorption of the stapedial arch. Total resorption of the malleus handle did not occur in attic cholesteatomas.

In sinus cholesteatoma with posterosuperior retraction of the pars tensa, starting in the tympanic sinus around the stapes, a very high frequency of resorption of the long process of the incus and of the stapes was found.

In tensa-retraction cholesteatoma involving the entire pars tensa, in addition to a high incidence of stapes and incus pathology, resorption of the malleus handle was also common (Table **2**). This is logical, since tensa-retraction cholesteatoma is defined as retraction of the entire pars tensa, usually totally surrounding the malleus handle and continuing up under the anterior and posterior malleus folds and into the attic.

In a chronic otitis sequelae group with dry perforations without cholesteatoma, a very low incidence of stapes pathology was found; the incidence was somewhat higher in active granulating otitis (Table **3**).

There was a considerable difference in the ossicular-chain pathology between the anterior, inferior and posterior perforations. The incidence of a defective long process of the incus was highest with posterior perforations, and extremely low with anterior perforations (Table **3**). The ossicular pathology in cases of total perforation was similar to the pathology found in the posterior perforation group, the only exception being the malleus handle, which was relatively often resorbed in ears with total perforations. The frequency of ossicular-chain pathology was higher in active chronic otitis than in the sequelae group, but the distribution of pathology between the various perforation types was similar (Table **4**).

Austin (1971) distinguished tympanoplasty type 2, with the stapes present, into type 2A, with the malleus handle present, and type 2B, with an absent malleus handle. In tympanoplasty type 3, with the stapes crura absent, Austin also distinguished a type 3A, with the malleus handle present, and type 3B, with the malleus handle absent. Due to the immense importance of the malleus handle for the stability of the drum and for the hearing, this subdivision is logical, but as is seen from Tables **2-4**, the 2B and 3B types mainly occur in total perforations, as well as in tensa-retraction cholesteatomas.

Table **2** The frequency of ossicular defects in 1100 ears with chronic middle-ear disease

Missing part of ossicular chain	Cholesteatomas			Granulating otitis n = 165 (%)	Sequelae of otitis n = 429 (%)	Adhesive otitis n = 80 (%)	Total n = 1100 (%)
	Attic n = 152 (%)	Sinus n = 166 (%)	Tensa n = 108 (%)				
Intact	26	10	12	38	57	23	37
Malleus handle	–	1	15	10	10	8	7
Malleus head	24	4	7	–	–	–	5
Malleus total	1	2	10	–	–	1	2
Long process of incus	39	75	73	56	39	75	53
Incus body	35	13	14	2	1	3	9
Stapedial arch, partial	5	7	10	6	3	5	5
Stapedial arch, total	16	40	35	15	5	24	18

Table 3 The frequency of ossicular defects with different perforations in 165 cases of chronic granulating otitis without cholesteatoma

Missing part of ossicular chain	Total n = 72 (%)	Anterior n = 13 (%)	Inferior n = 14 (%)	Posterior n = 66 (%)	All perforations n = 165 (%)
None (intact)	35	54	57	33	38
Malleus handle	18	–	14	2	10
Long process of incus	56	46	36	64	56
Incus body	3	–	–	3	2
Stapedial arch, partial	4	15	–	8	6
Stapedial arch, total	14	15	–	20	15

Table 4 Pathology of the ossicular chain in sequelae to otitis group

Missing part of ossicular chain	Total n = 429 (%)	Perforation				No perforation n = 32 (%)	Tympanosclerosis n = 58 (%)
		Total n = 137 (%)	Anterior n = 36 (%)	Inferior n = 42 (%)	Posterior n = 124 (%)		
None (intact)	57	58	92	81	52	25	45
Malleus handle	10	18	–	5	2	–	19
Long process of incus	39	34	8	17	48	63	52
Incus head	1	1	–	–	–	13	–
Stapedial arch, partial	3	2	–	2	2	6	3
Stapedial arch, total	5	7	–	2	5	6	9

16 Type 2 Tympanoplasty, Stapes Present

Ossicles, Bone, Cartilage, Tooth

From Table 2 (p. 243), it is evident that the incidence of resorption of the long process of the incus is the most common ossicular-chain pathology. It is three times more common than absence of the stapedial arch. Consequently, type 2 ossiculoplasty is the most common procedure in middle-ear surgery.

Type 2 tympanoplasty can be divided into:
1. interposition,
2. transposition, and
3. pexis

Interposition means placing an ossicle, a bony or cartilaginous graft, or any other prosthesis, between the stapes or stapedial arch and the malleus handle or drum.
   Transposition refers to procedures in which an ossicle is still partly attached to its origin, e.g., the drum, but is transposed onto the stapes. Transpositions of the ossicles are seldom used. They consist of transposition of the incus, transposition of the neck of the malleus or of the umbo, or transposition of the entire malleus onto the head of the stapes.
   The various types of pexis are myringoincudopexy, myringostapediopexy, and various kinds of ossicular wiring.

Interpositions

The most common interposition we use is interposition of autogenous incus, followed by other prostheses, in the following order: 1) cortical bone, 2) allogenous incus, 3) allogenous malleus head, 4) tragal cartilage, 5) conchal cartilage, 6) autogenous malleus head, and 7) biocompatible materials, e.g., partial ossicular replacement prostheses. Every surgeon has his own preference, but the majority prefer autogenous materials.

Use of Autogenous Incus

Some surgeons do not use incus if it has been in contact with the cholesteatoma membrane. Plester et al. (1989) found histological signs of cholesteatoma in the Haversian channel of one incus, and recommended not to use incus at all in cholesteatoma ears. The present author does not use autogenous incus if there is major erosion of the incus body, simply because there is no sound bone left, but in all other cases does use the incus, in spite of possible contact with the cholesteatoma membrane. In cholesteatoma cases, the incus is cleaned after extraction under the operating microscope, and it is easy to remove the cholesteatoma membrane from the incus body. Usually, there is mucosa under the matrix, still covering the incus. If there is any doubt as to whether the cholesteatoma has been removed or not, cleaning can be continued at a higher magnification, and any suspicious region of the incus can be drilled off. During the many years that we have systematically examined for possible cholesteatomas arising from the interposed incus at reoperations, we have not found any such cases. The risk of iatrogenic cholesteatoma when using autogenous materials is much lower than the risk of bone resorption when using allograft material, or extrusion when using artificial materials.

Extraction of the Incus

Extraction of the incus is in fact the most difficult procedure in type 2 tympanoplasty, with a risk of damaging the chorda and of causing trauma to the inner ear, leading to high-tone hearing loss, and even luxation of the stapes.
For safe extraction of the incus remnant, the following details are important:

1) The incus should initially be dislocated from the head of the malleus and rotated out of the attic. During the dislocation, the malleus head is pushed anteriorly. In cases with bony fixation of the malleus head, this movement is not possible, and dislocation and rotation of the incus are difficult.
2) Before starting the extraction, exposure of the posterosuperior part of the bony annulus should be sufficient, and the bony annulus should be drilled off in order to allow rotation of the incus. Even in ears with a small distance between the stapes and the malleus, so-called "otosclerosis" drilling is necessary (Fig. **689**), particularly in ears with a pronounced remnant of the long process of the incus. Even in cases with total

16 Type 2 Tympanoplasty, Stapes Present

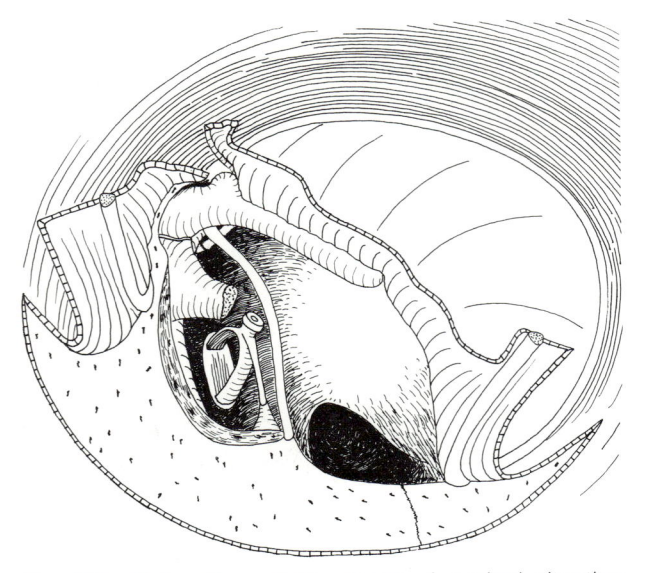

Fig. **689** **Extraction of the incus.** A typical situation prior to extraction of the incus, with an absent long process in a posterior perforation. The bony annulus is drilled away, the stapes is intact and mobile, and the joint between the malleus and incus is visible

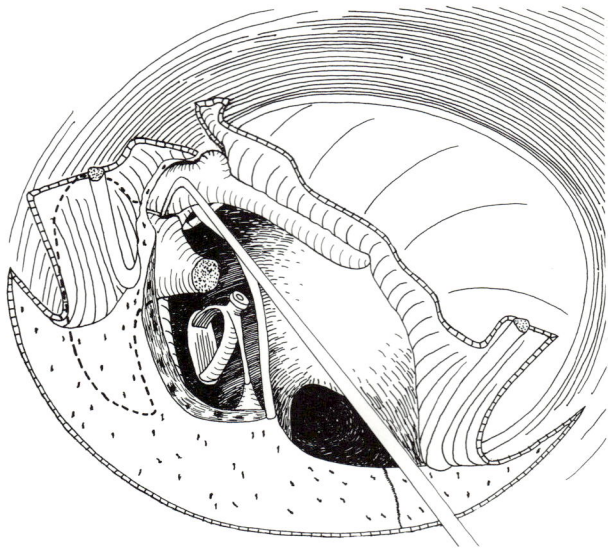

Fig. **690** The mobility of the malleus head is tested by palpation, and the incus is dislocated posteriorly with a hook

resorption of the long process, the final action in rotating the incus can be impossible due to insufficient drilling of the bony annulus.
3) The rotation is clockwise in the right ear and counterclockwise in the left ear.
4) The rotation takes place lateral to the stapes in one of two ways, either: a) medial to the chorda, i.e., between the chorda and the head of the stapes, or b) lateral to the chorda, i.e., between the bony annulus and the head of the stapes. In the latter type, removal of the bony annulus should be more extensive, and in addition to the clockwise rotation, a movement in the anteroposterior direction also takes place.

Before starting to extract the incus, the lower edge of the joint between the malleus head and the incus body should be exposed by elevating the posterosuperior skin flap (Fig. **689**). The bony annulus is removed by drilling with a diamond burr or by curettage, exposing the entire stapes, the sinus tympani, and the pyramidal process. The extent and location of the bone drilling is similar to that used in otosclerosis surgery, and we therefore call it "otosclerosis drilling." The chorda tympani should also be mobilized (Fig. **689**). The drilling should extend superiorly towards Shrapnell's membrane. Sometimes the bony annulus is prominent here, and rotation is not possible, even if enough bone is removed further inferiorly. The malleus head is palpated with a hook. If it is mobile, then dislocation between the incus body and the malleus head is performed with the same hook (Fig. **690**). With the hook, the dislocation is continued by pulling gently on the incus in a posterior direction. The body is luxated and rotated (Fig. **691**). This initial procedure can be performed with a curved double-cup forceps instead of a hook (Fig. **692**).

The forceps are introduced *medial to the chorda,* carefully catching the edge of the incus and pulling it in a posteroinferior direction with small jerking movements. Care should be taken not to luxate the incus into the antrum. It has happened that the forceps have slipped and the incus has shot like a projectile into the antrum. Further attempts to catch it are fruitless, and extensive drilling towards the attic only creates unnecessary weakness in the attic wall. An allograft can be used in such cases.

Further extraction and rotation of the incus takes place between the chorda and the head of the stapes (Fig. **691, 693**). Pulling the incus outward is not possible in this phase. The incus should be carefully rotated under the malleus handle (Fig. **694**) to frees it from the chorda, and finally, when the incus is freed from the chorda tympani and the stapes, it can be softly rotated outwards into the ear canal and

Interpositions

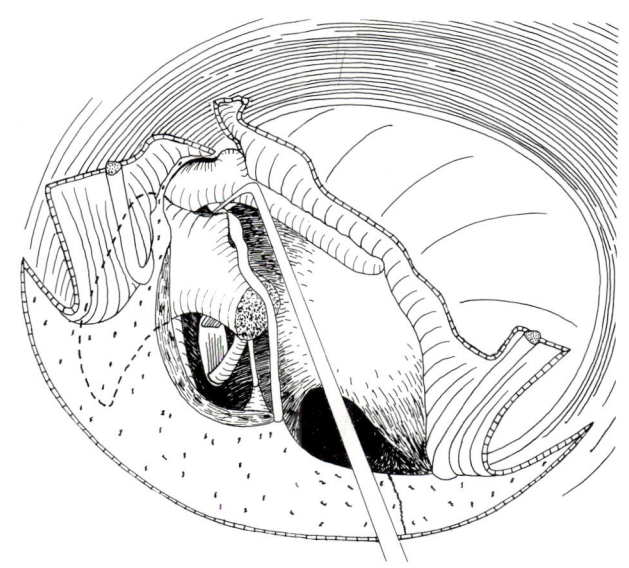

Fig. **691** Clockwise rotation of the incus with a hook medial to the chorda tympani

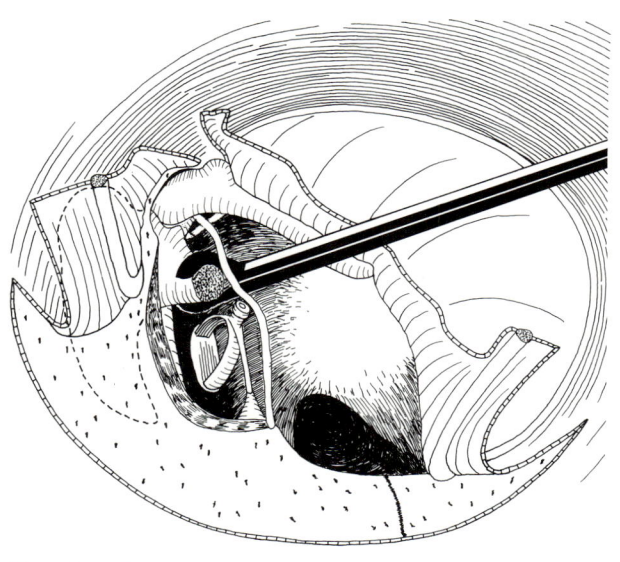

Fig. **692** Rotation of the incus with a curved double-cup forceps

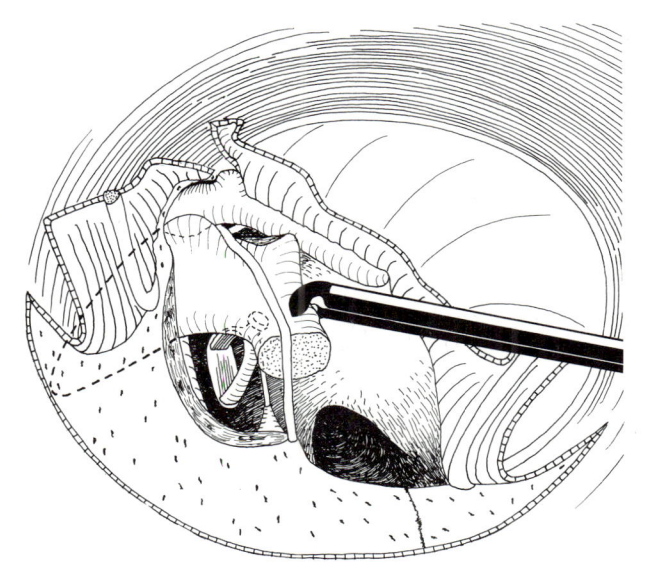

Fig. **693** Further rotation of the incus between the chorda and the stapes

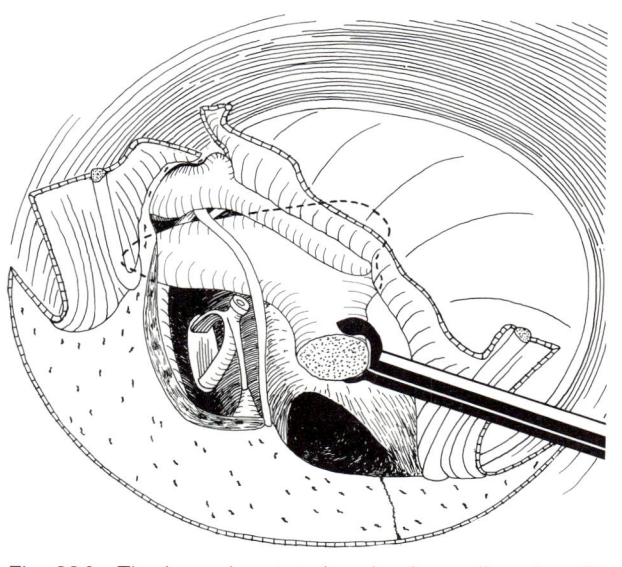

Fig. **694** The incus is rotated under the malleus handle

removed (Fig. **695**). The rotation of the incus between the stapes and the chorda is clear: first, the short process of the incus points posteriorly (Fig. **691**), then superiorly (Figs. **693**, **694**), and finally anteriorly (Fig. **695**). While this is being done, the chorda should be kept lateral to the incus. Sometimes the chorda has to be carefully stretched during the incus rotation in order to gain space between the stapes and the chorda. After the chorda has been stretched and placed over the incus body (Fig. **693**), further rotation is not difficult, and there is no further risk to the chorda or the stapes (Fig. **695**).

16 Type 2 Tympanoplasty, Stapes Present

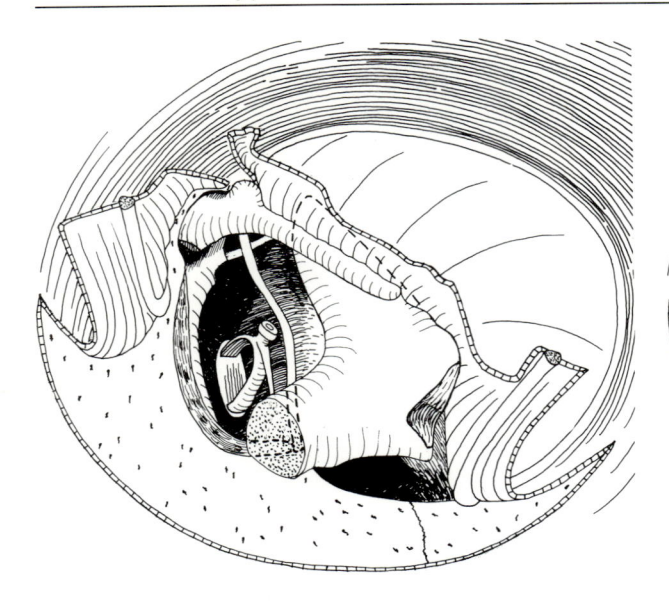

Fig. **695** Finally, the incus is rotated lateral to the chorda tympani, out of the tympanic cavity

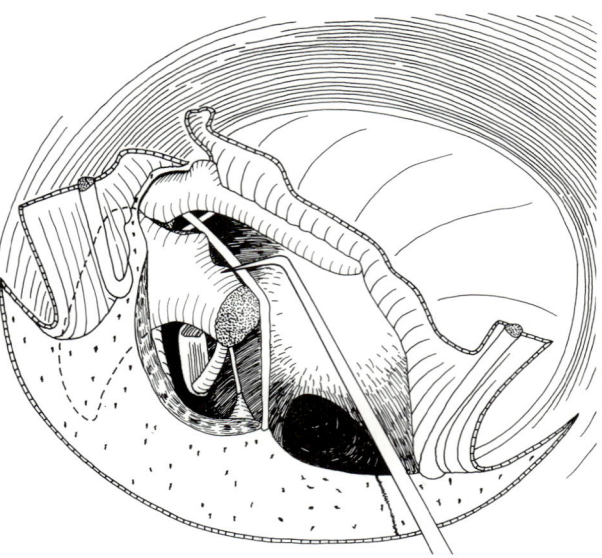

Fig. **696** Extrusion of the incus lateral to the chorda tympani. The incus is luxated out and rotated postero-inferiorly, and the chorda is pushed underneath it

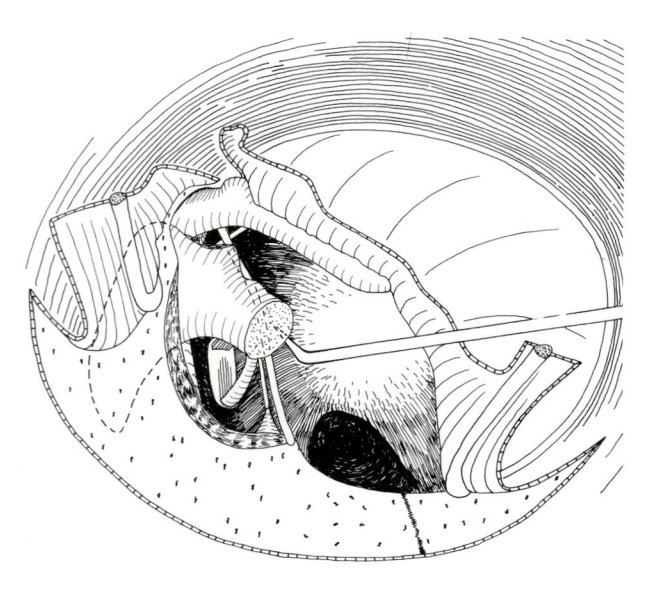

Fig. **697** The incus is rotated toward the posterior bony annulus, while the chorda is placed under the incus

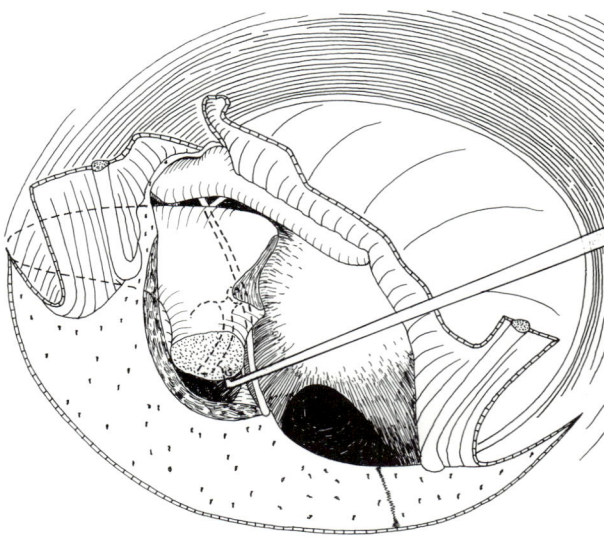

Fig. **698** At the posterior bony annulus, the long process of the incus is elevated into the ear canal

Before extraction of the incus *lateral to the chorda,*, i.e., between the bony annulus and the chorda, the incus is rotated lateral to the stapes, stretching the chorda (Fig. **696**), which is elevated with a hook and pushed under the incus (Fig. **697**). Further rotation of the incus is now possible, but the critical point of rotation can be the postero-superior bony annulus (Fig. **698**) in cases with long remnant of the long process of the incus and insufficient drilling of the superior bony annulus close to the Shrapnell's membrane. By gentle elevation of the remnant of the long process laterally with a hook or a forceps, the long process can be placed lateral to the bony annulus and softly rotated out (Fig. **699**).

Interpositions

Disruption of the Incudostapedial Joint

As seen from Table 3 (p. 244), erosion of the long process of the incus, including the lenticular process, is the most common ossicular defect in chronic otitis, with or without cholesteatoma. The degree of resorption of the long process of the incus is extremely variable, ranging from just slight resorption of the surface of the long process—usually caused by retraction of the posterosuperior part of the pars tensa onto the long process of the incus (myringoincudopexy)—to total resorption of the long process.

In some cases, the connection of the long process of the incus and its lenticular process is maintained by fibrous tissue, with good preoperative hearing. When an attempt is made to remove the epithelial membrane and the fibrous tissue under the membrane, the previously intact connection can be partly disrupted, resulting in decreased transmission (Figs. **700, 701**). In such cases, it is necessary to totally disrupt the connection between

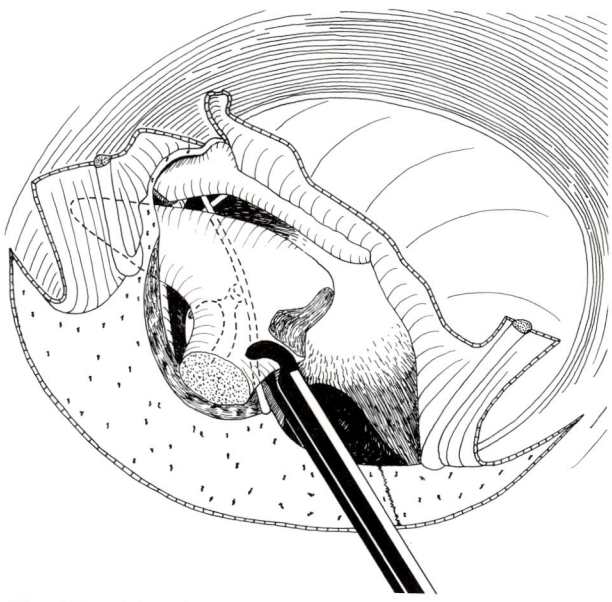

Fig. **699** After further rotation laterally, the incus can be safely removed

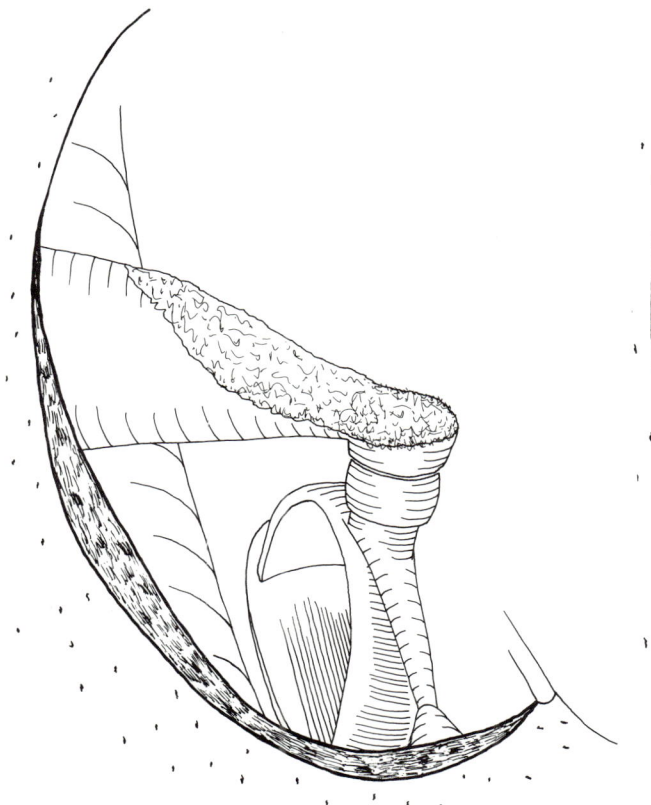

Fig. **700** **Disruption of the incudostapedial joint.** A small defect in the lenticular process and the long process of the incus, with relatively good function since fibrous tissue bridges the gap. A myringoincudostapediopexy is established

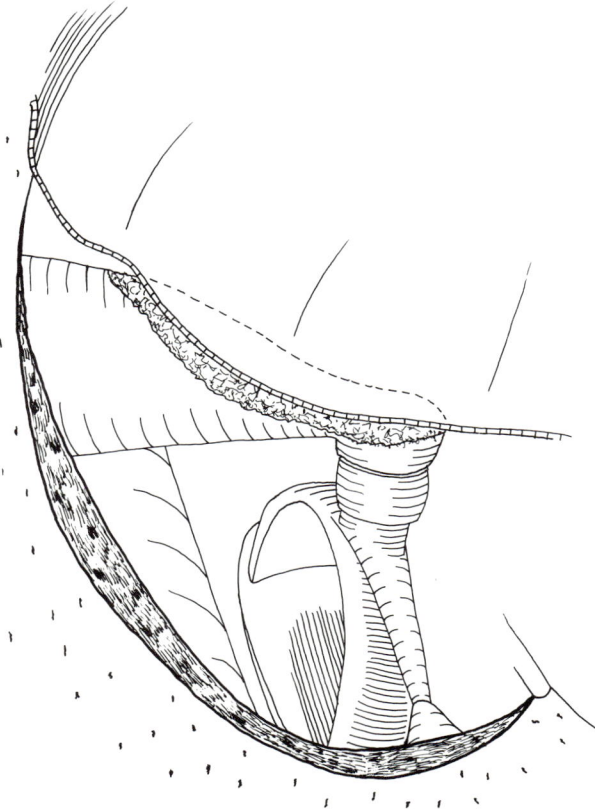

Fig. **701** Poorer connection after removal of the epithelium

16 Type 2 Tympanoplasty, Stapes Present

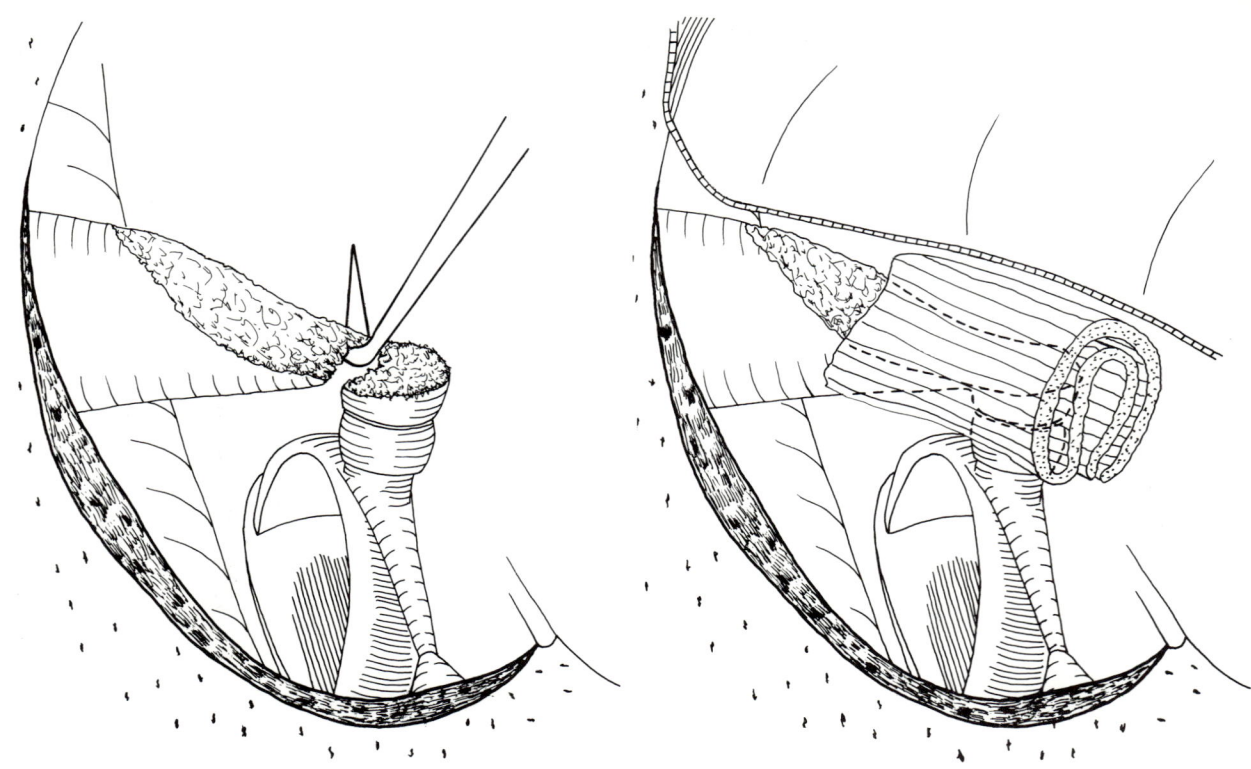

Fig. **702** After removal of the fibrous tissue, the incus is disconnected from the stapes

Fig. **703** Strengthening a partly resorbed long process of the incus using fascia or fibrous tissue, also to avoid contact between the squamous epithelium and the bone

the long process and the remnant of the lenticular process (Fig. **702**) and interpose the incus. The interposition of the incus or any other form of prosthesis prolongs the operation. Before removal of the fibrous tissue around the incudostapedial joint, it is therefore important to check the intergrity of the bony connection and decide whether this connection will provide sufficient function in the long term, or if it is necessary to disrupt it totally and perform a type 2 tympanoplasty, which generally has a poorer prognosis than type 1. In these cases with good preoperative hearing, we often leave the fibrous tissue around the long process of the incus intact, and may even fortify it with fascia (Fig. **703**).

In patients with a low stapes or a high tympanic cavity, the lenticular process can be left attached to the head of the stapes and the incus can be interposed onto it. The lenticular process is cleaned of fibrous tissue, exposing the bone and thus facilitating good contact between the stapes and the interposed incus (Fig. **704**).

Sometimes it is better to remove the remnant of the lenticular process together with the fibrous tissue. This is achieved by introducing a small hook under high magnification, posteriorly into the joint between the stapes and the lenticular process (Fig. **705**). By carefully moving the hook in the direction of the tendon of the stapes, the gap is enlarged, and the lenticular process is dislocated anteriorly and removed with the forceps in the same phase (Fig. **706**).

Because of chronic infection, ossification of the incudostapedial joint can occur. In such cases, removal of the lenticular process is impossible, and even dangerous (Fig. **707**). The stapes, which is usually mobile in chronic ears in contrast to otosclerotic cases, is exposed to excessive movement, risking a sensorineural high-tone hearing loss. In these cases it is therefore definitely better not to attempt to remove the lenticular process (Fig. **707**). The remnant of the lenticular process is cleaned of fibrous tissue, and the incus is interposed.

Interpositions 251

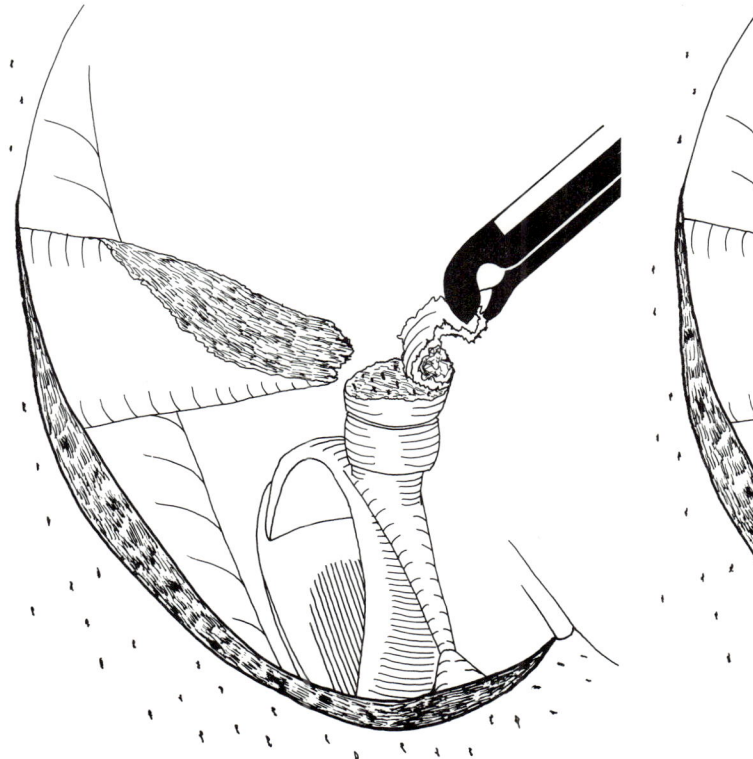

Fig. 704 The fibrous tissue is removed from the lenticular process, which is not disrupted from the stapes. After the incus is extracted, it is placed on the stapes

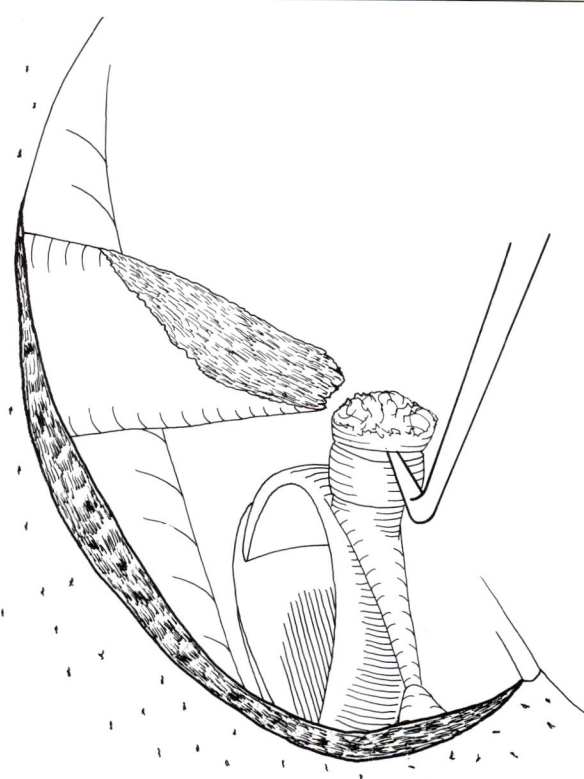

Fig. 705 Disarticulation of the lenticular process using a small, sharp hook placed at the level of the incudostapedial joint, just above the stapes tendon

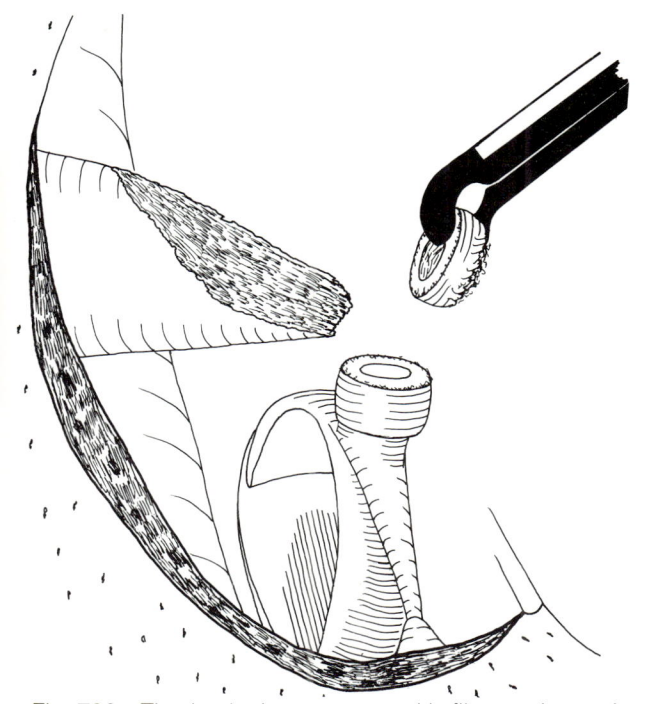

Fig. 706 The lenticular process, with fibrous tissue, is removed

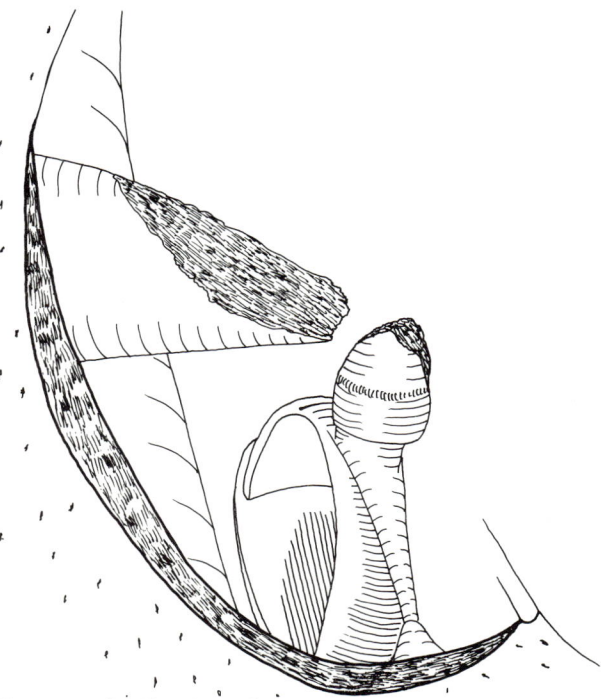

Fig. 707 Ossification of the incudostapedial joint, and a defective long process of the incus. The lenticular process cannot be removed, and the interposed incus is placed on the defect

Disruption of the Intact Ossicular Chain

Disruption of the incudostapedial joint with an intact incus has been a common procedure in large-fenestration stapedectomy. In otosclerosis this type of disruption is much easier, due to the fixation of the stapes, and there is no risk of sensorineural hearing loss during this procedure. In chronic otitis the stapes is mobile, and the capsule of the incudostapedial joint is usually fibrotic and thickened. In such cases, disruption is a difficult procedure, as the stapes tends to follow the movements of the instrument when it is introduced into the incudostapedial joint (Fig. **708**). A small hook is inserted posteriorly into the incudostapedial joint just above the stapedius tendon, disrupting the capsule and enlarging the joint. When the gap between the lenticular process and the head of the stapes is sufficiently large, an incudostapedial knife can be introduced and pushed in an anterior direction, dividing the fibers (Fig. **709**) and totally separating the joint (Fig. **710**).

Separation of an intact incudostapedial joint has been used in attic cholesteatoma cases to ensure

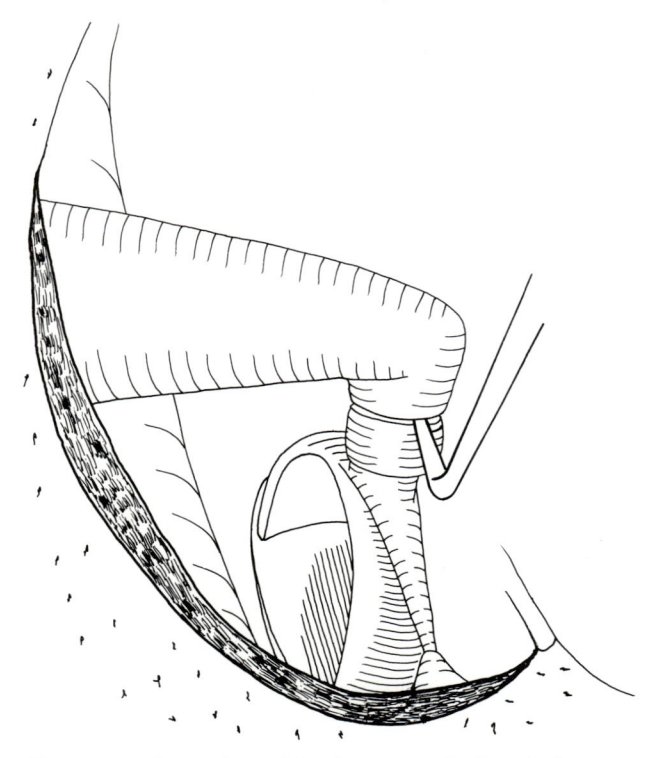

Fig. **708** **Disruption of the intact ossicular chain.** Disruption of an intact incudostapedial joint, using a hook introduced into the joint just above the stapes tendon

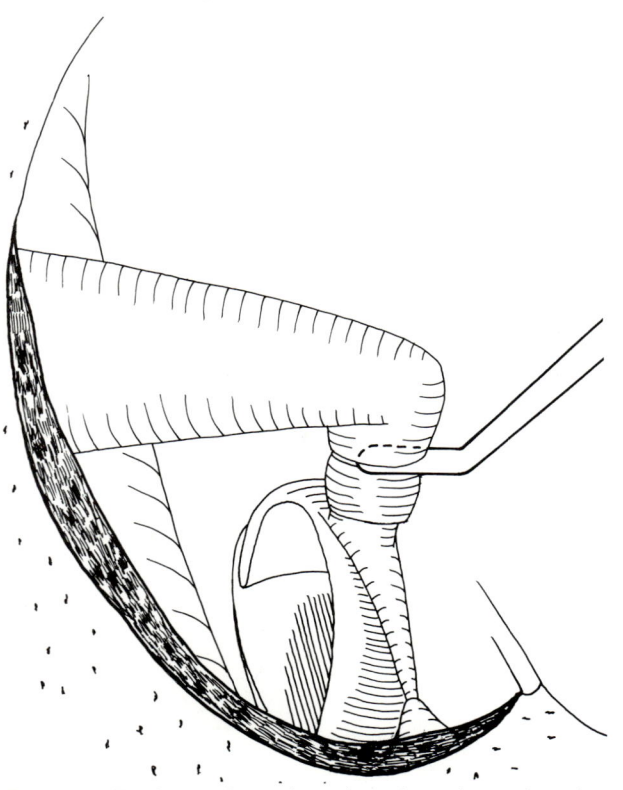

Fig. **709** Further disruption by inserting the incudostapedial knife into the incudostapedial joint

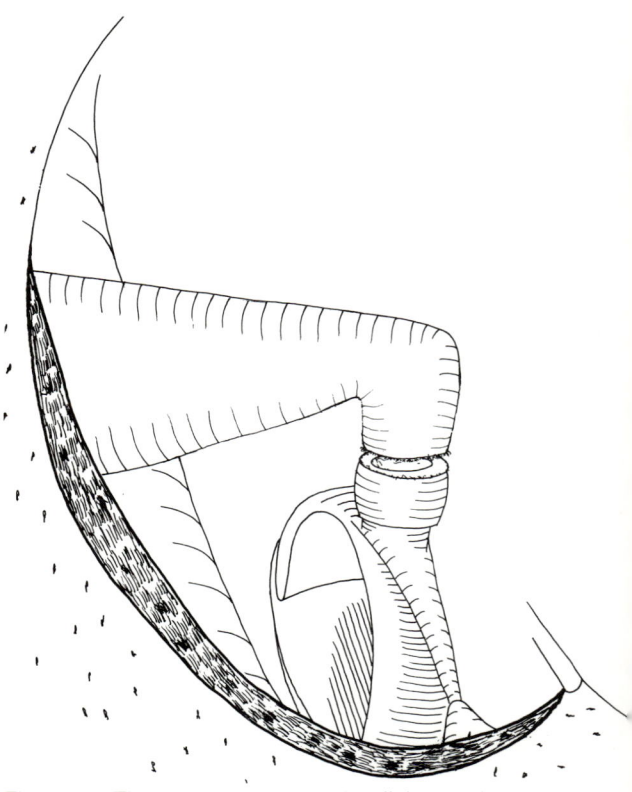

Fig. **710** The incus is now totally dislocated

safe cleaning of the cholesteatoma membrane from the incus body or malleus head. A few surgeons have separated the joint in cases of posterior atticotympanotomy (Smyth 1980) or anterior atticotympanotomy in combination with intact canal wall tympanoplasty. In cases with bony fixation of the incus or malleus, requiring drilling of the bony bridge through an anterior atticotomy, the incudostapedial joint is separated before drilling. The purpose of this separation is to avoid trauma to the inner ear from manipulation of the incus and malleus. After this operation, the incudostapedial joint can be glued together with fibrin glue or ionomer cement. Unfortunately, in such circumstances the majority of surgeons today extract the incus and perform an interposition, which gives poorer results and has a poorer prognosis in the long term than the intact ossicular chain.

The present author tries to preserve the ossicular chain whenever possible, and our series has shown that the long-term hearing results are much better and more stable if the chain is left intact, as opposed to type 2 tympanoplasty (Tos and Lau 1991). This is especially true in cholesteatoma (Fig. **711**), tympanosclerosis, and bony fixation within the attic. Disruption of an intact ossicular chain is a rare procedure in our hands in ears with chronic otitis and its sequelae.

After an intact ossicular chain has been disrupted, and before interposition with the incus, is performed, the incus has to be extracted. However, it is almost impossible to extract in incus with an intact long process by rotation without a significant amount of drilling of the posterosuperior wall. It is therefore necessary to cut the long process before rotating of the incus. Cutting is performed by introducing the guillotine-like punch under the long process of the incus. Even the smallest punch is of considerable size (Fig. **712**), and introducing it is not always easy. The bony annulus should at least be drilled away to the same extent as for stapedectomy. The punch can sometimes also be introduced between the malleus handle and the long process of the incus (Fig. **713**). Other methods of cutting the long process of the incus include using crura scissors, as for resection of the crura in small-fenestration stapedotomy techniques, or drilling with a diamond burr or using the laser if it is easily available. Sometimes it is necessary to rotate the incus out into the ear canal and then resect the long process (Fig. **714**).

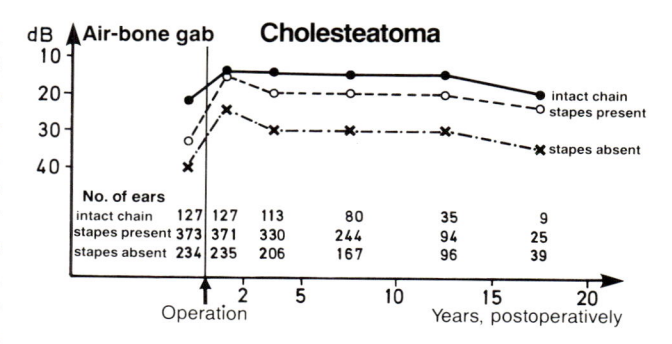

Fig. **711** Mean air–bone gap closure (frequency range 500–2000 Hz) in cholesteatoma, before, and at various times after surgery in intact ossicular chain tympanoplasty type 2, with the stapes present, and type 3, with the stapes absent (Tos and Lau 1991)

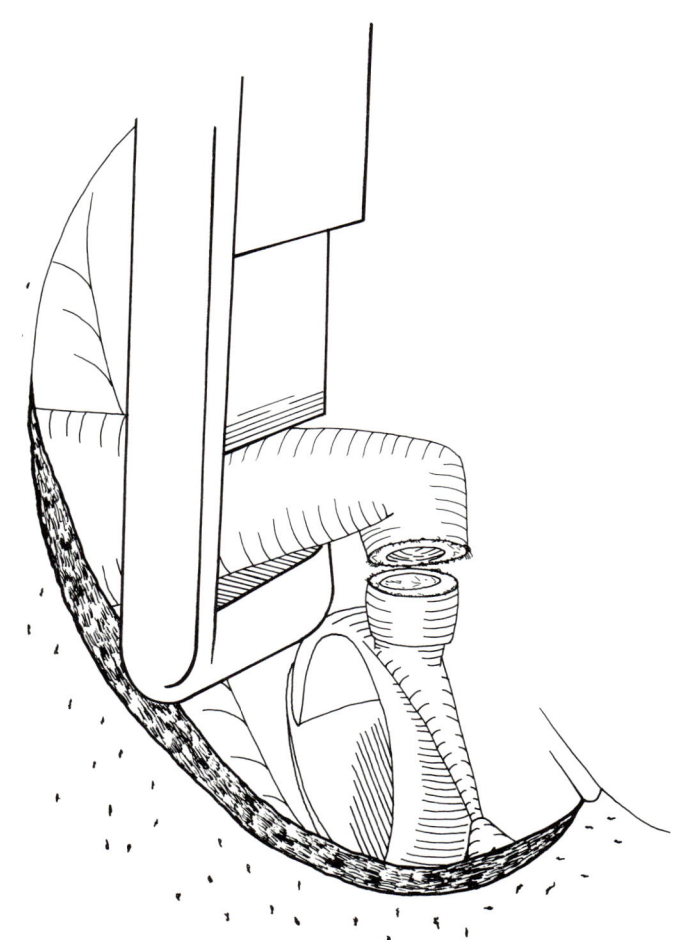

Fig. **712** Resection of an intact long process of the incus using a punch placed between the long process and the bony annulus to allow the incus to be extracted

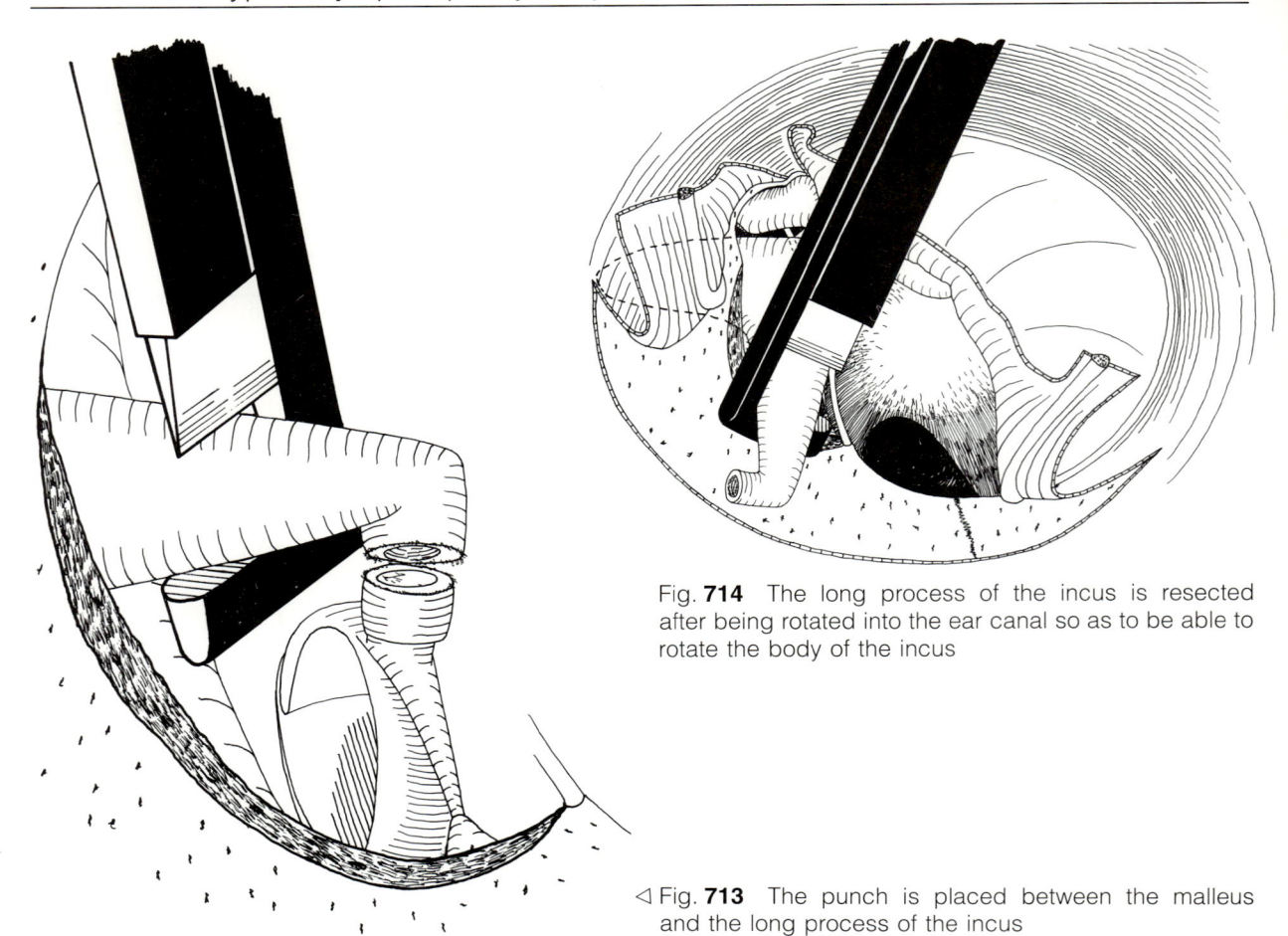

16 Type 2 Tympanoplasty, Stapes Present

Fig. 714 The long process of the incus is resected after being rotated into the ear canal so as to be able to rotate the body of the incus

◁ Fig. 713 The punch is placed between the malleus and the long process of the incus

Interposition of the Incus

As mentioned above, this procedure is by far the most common type of ossiculoplasty. There are no significant differences in technique whether an autogenous or allogenous incus is used, but an autogenous incus may have more extensive resorption of the long process than an allogenous one, which is usually complete. The autogenous incus is usually covered with mucosa, especially in noncholesteatoma cases. The appearance of the allogenous incus will depend on the method of storage and sterilization employed. We always prefer autogenous incus as the first choice if it is available, but allogenous incus is used as the second choice in endaural procedures and as the third choice in retroauricular procedures.

The situation after extraction of the autogenous incus in a posterior perforation is seen in Figure 715. Some small pieces of Gelfoam are placed in the mesotympanum to hold the short process of the incus in place, and some on the prom-

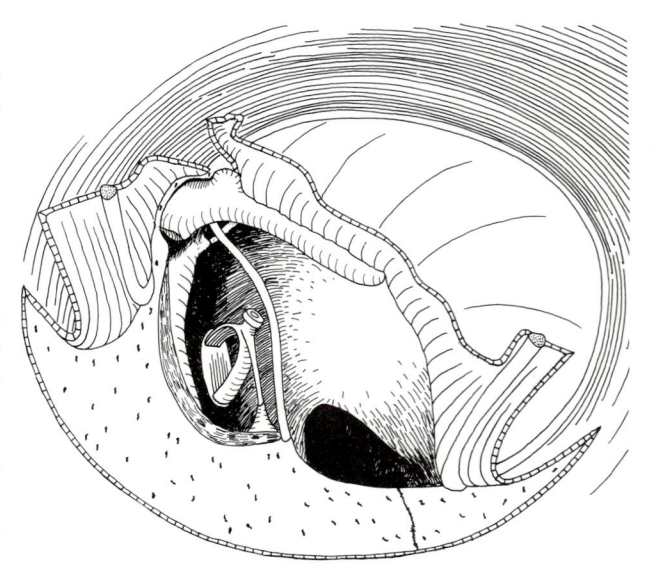

Fig. 715 **Interposition of the incus.** The typical situation after extraction of the incus and just before interposition of the incus

ontory to support an underlay graft. In general, the author does not place Gelfoam in the posterior tympanum, except in cases where it is felt that the incus is not stable.

Incus interposition was first described by Hall and Rytzner (1957), the Swedish otologists, but American surgeons soon popularized the method, especially Guilford (1965). Wullstein favored myringostapediopexy without interposition, and Zöllner (1951) showed that excellent hearing could be obtained in a radical operation with myringostapediopexy. The German school therefore adopted incus interposition relatively late.

The incus can be interposed in many ways, depending on the many different situations pertaining within the tympanic cavity and the attic, and in particular on the relation between the malleus handle and the stapes. Variations in the height of the stapes and in the distances to the posterior bony annulus, to the facial nerve, and to the malleus handle, are important, as well as the size of the tympanic cavity, the position of the malleus handle, the drum retraction, the thickness of the middle-ear mucosa, and the presence of adhesions, all of which can influence the placement of the incus. In many situations, the interposed incus will prevent a new adhesion of the drum, and the placement will depend on whether a canal wall–up or canal wall–down procedure is performed.

In the classic incus interposition, described and popularized by Guilford, the incus body is placed directly on the head of the stapes, the remnant of the long process is directed inferiorly, parallel to the malleus handle, and the short process towards the tympanic orifice of the Eustachian tube under the malleus (Fig. **716**). There should be a gap between the interposed incus and the posterior bony annulus, in order to prevent bony fixation of the incus. Bony fixation between the facial prominence and the incus body should also be avoided. The classic incus interposition is therefore used mainly in patients with a high stapes. In classic incus interposition, the incus occupies most of the posterosuperior quadrant of the tympanic cavity, and hence tends to prevent retraction in this region. The prevention of retraction is an extremely important factor, which explains why incus interposition in the classic manner is still a very popular interposition method, despite the many techniques available for shaping the incus and ossicles, as well as the many forms of artifical graft that are commercially available.

Before final placement of the incus, the chorda should be placed superior to the incus. Using a fine hook, the chorda is elevated (Fig. **716**) and gently

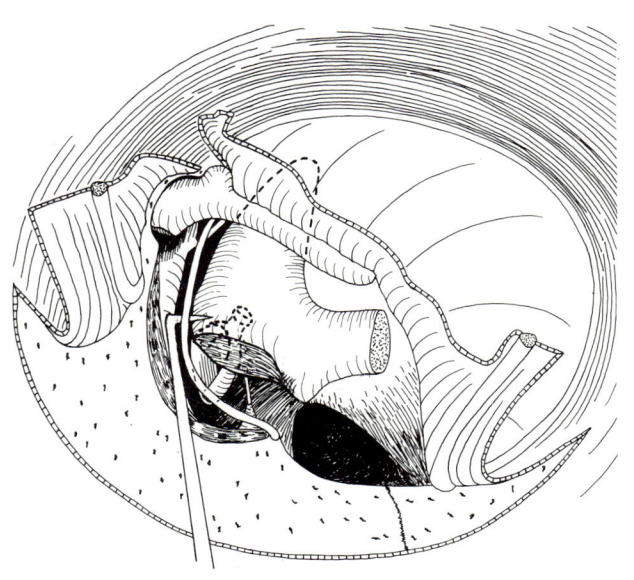

Fig. **716** The classical placement of the incus as advocated by Guilford, with the short process pointing anteriorly under the malleus, and the remnant of the long process pointing inferiorly almost parallel to the malleus handle

pulled onto the incus body, thereby fixing the incus to the head of the stapes (Fig. **717**). There is no need to use any glue to fit the incus to the stapes or malleus handle.

The fascia in a posterior perforation can be placed on the posterior side of the malleus handle (Figs. **718, 719**), or under the malleus handle, i.e., between the short process of the incus and the malleus handle (Fig. **720**). Placement of the fascia after ossiculoplasty is, in fact, a very delicate phase of tympanoplasty, and can spoil the efforts made in the ossiculoplasty by dislocating or tilting the incus or other graft. This is especially the case in underlay grafting of a posterior perforation, so that several surgeons prefer ot place the fascia under the malleus handle before placing in incus graft on the stapes. The problem is similar when grafting a total perforation with the fascia placed under the malleus handle. In onlay myringoplasty techniques, and in underlay techniques with the fascia placed on the malleus handle, interference with the ossiculoplasty is less of a problem. Several surgeons and, unfortunately, an increasing number of institutions specializing in otology, use the popular argument in favor of a second-stage procedure that "the ossiculoplasty is easier in the second operation, and therefore the ossiculoplasty is not performed in the first stage." The present author finds it completely unacceptable not to attempt an ossiculoplasty at the first

16 Type 2 Tympanoplasty, Stapes Present

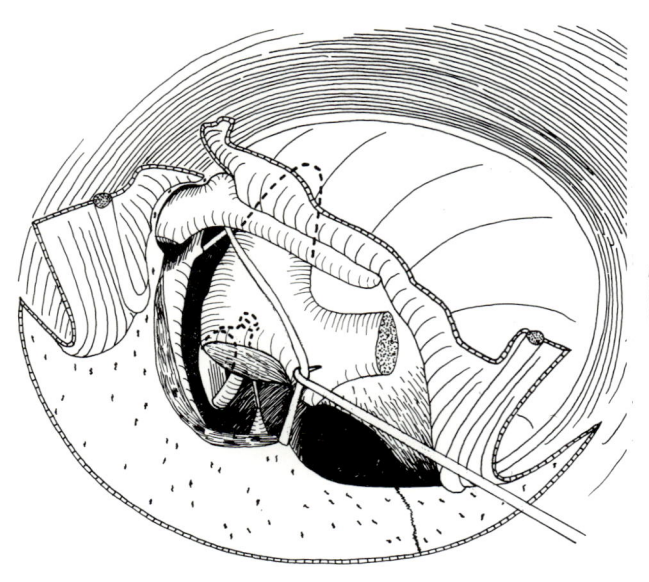

Fig. 717 The chorda is pulled over the body of the incus, providing fixation

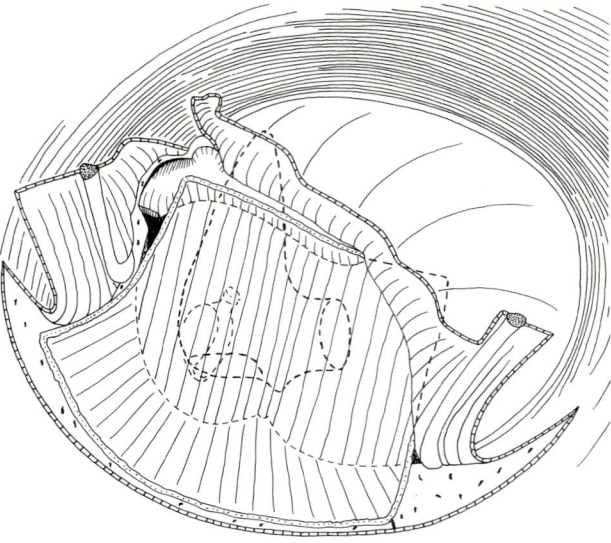

Fig. 718 The incus and posterior perforation are covered by fascia placed posteriorly on top of the malleus handle and underneath the umbo

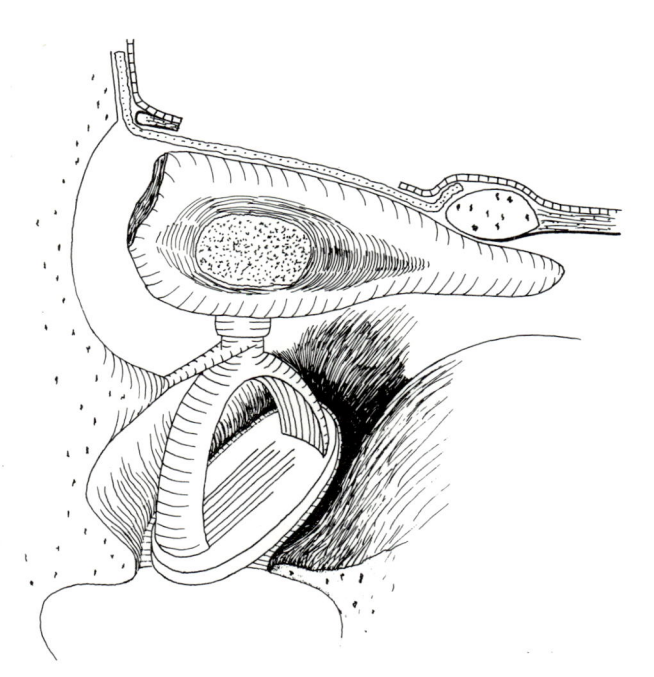

Fig. 719 Side view of the interposed incus, with the long process pointing inferiorly and the short process under the malleus handle. The fascia is placed on the lateral and posterior aspects of the malleus handle. The hole has not yet been drilled in the incus body

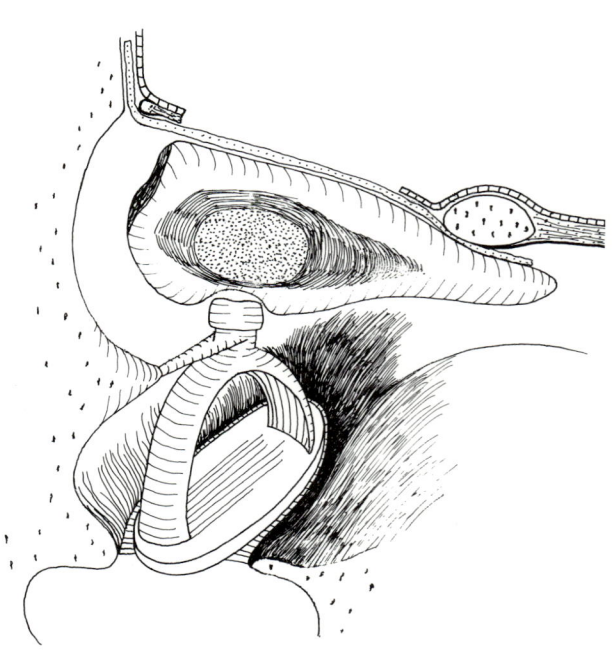

Fig. 720 The hole has been drilled in the incus body. The incus is placed with the short process under the malleus handle. The fascia is placed under the malleus handle and under the drum

stage, since this can provide hearing improvement without the need to wait for a second procedure. A slight alteration in the grafting methods, e.g., from underlay to onlay grafting, or placing the fascia on, instead of under, the malleus handle, help to avoid a second stage by facilitating "primary" ossiculoplasty. Opening of the inner ear in a second stage, after the eardrum perforation has been closed, is, of course, an exception to these statements.

A hole can be drilled on the medial side on the incus body for the head of the stapes (Fig. **720**), although the need for such a hole (Fig. **719**) depends on the surgeon's judgment of the circumstances. Sometimes, a hole seems to be a logical and good solution, and should definitely be performed. Sometimes, the incus body with a hole placed on the head of the stapes is too low, with a risk of subsequent fixation to the facial prominence. In such cases, it is advisable to avoid making a hole, so as to keep the incus in a slightly lateral position. Similarly, when a second hole is required to achieve a better position, there is a risk of the incus medially, in contact with the facial nerve prominence. Because of these problems, the author rarely tries to make a hole in the classic incus interposition, and prefers simply to place the incus on the head of the stapes, without any drilling of the incus body, as indicated in Figure **719**.

After the skin flaps have been replaced (Fig. **721**), the position of the incus should be maintained by a probe. The incus should not be placed too close to the posterior bony annulus. This can sometimes happen during the replacement of the skin flaps.

Assessment of the position and of any movement of the interposed incus can be detected at any time after the operation under the operating microscope using the Siegles pneumatic otoscope, or with a probe. Bony fixation, fibrous fixation, or lateralization of the incus can easily be detected.

In some situations, partcularly in cases where there has been extensive spontaneous resorption of the posterosuperior bony annulus, or after extensive drilling, the long process of the incus can be rotated so that it is pointing in a superior, instead of an inferior, direction (Fig. **722**). This method is used to prevent retraction when there is a superior bony defect, or in cases where the incus simply fits better into the tympanic cavity. The short process of the incus is still placed under the malleus handle (Fig. **722**). Fixation with the chorda is easier, and the risk of bony fixation of the long process of the incus to the facial prominence seems to be lower using this variation. The fascia is placed under the malleus handle (Figs. **723**, **724**), or it can be placed on the

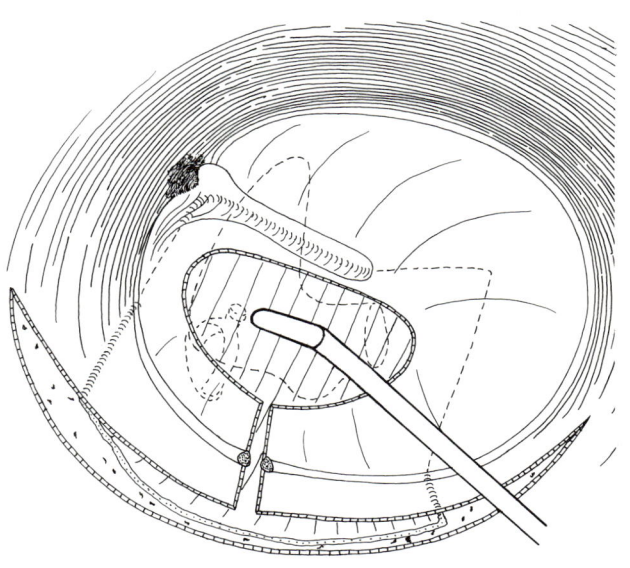

Fig. **721** The skin flaps are replaced, and the position of the incus is checked with a probe

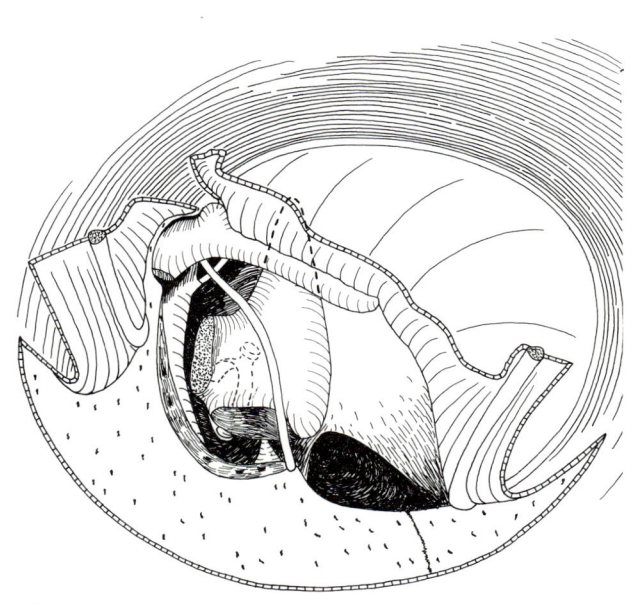

Fig. **722** Placement of the incus with the short process under the malleus, but with the long process pointing superiorly

posterior side of the malleus handle, as illustrated previously (Figs. **718, 719**). A hole can be drilled in the body of the incus (Fig. **724**), or the hole may be avoided, depending on the circumstances, as discussed above.

In some canal wall–down mastoidectomy techniques, or atticoantrotomies with partial obliteration of the cavity and repneumatization of the attic, a superior extended incus may be an advantage to include the drum of the attic region in the new drum, particularly in cases with low mobility of the inferior part of the drum.

Another modification of incus interposition is placement of the short process of the incus on the neck of the malleus, pointing anterosuperiorly towards the anterior attic (Fig. **725**). The remnant of the long process will be in contact with the lower part of the malleus handle and the malleus neck. In cases with type 4 attic retraction (Tos and Paulsen 1979), with considerable spontaneous erosion of the lateral attic wall, there is enough space to place the short process of the incus onto the malleus neck. Retraction of the posterosuperior region can be prevented. In this type of situation, the fascia is usually placed onto the posterior side of the malleus handle, and covers the attic retraction region (Fig. **726**) after careful elevation of the keratinized epithelium. The fascia is carefully pushed under the drum only at the umbo region, without displacing the assembly between the malleus handle and the remnant of the long process of the incus (Fig. **726, 727**). Similarly in this technique, a hole can be drilled in the incus body, stabilizing the malleus assembly (Fig. **727**).

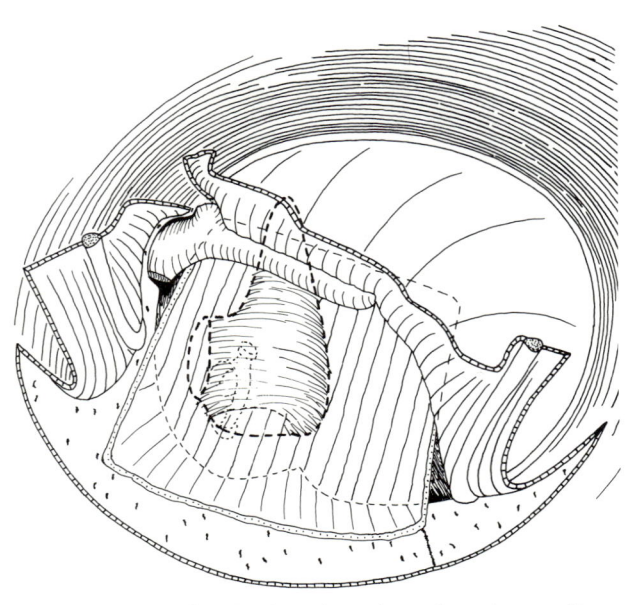

Fig. **723** The fascia is placed under the malleus handle and under the drum in a posterior perforation

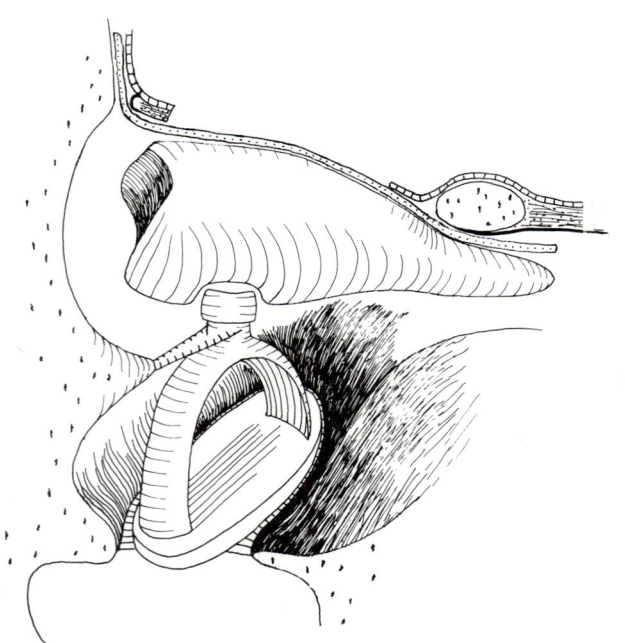

Fig. **724** Side view of the interposition of the incus with a hole drilled in the incus body. The short process points anteriorly, and the long process superiorly. The fascia is placed under the malleus handle

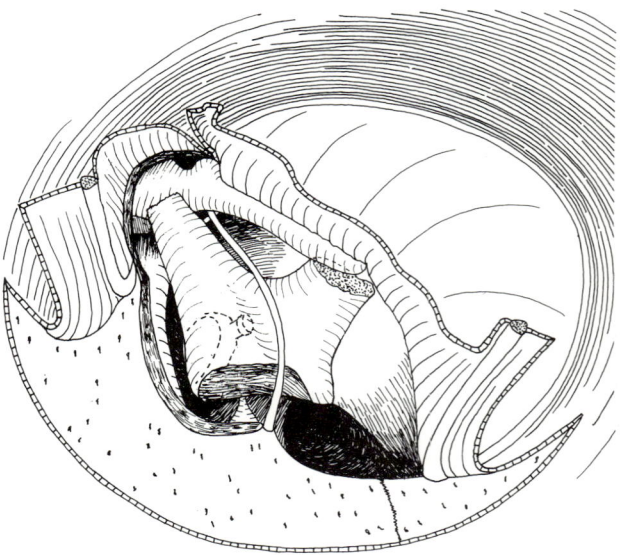

Fig. **725** Placement of the short process of the incus superiorly on the neck of the malleus in cases with attic retraction and with bone resorption of the lateral attic wall. The remnant of the long process is placed as an assembly towards the umbo

Interposition of the Incus

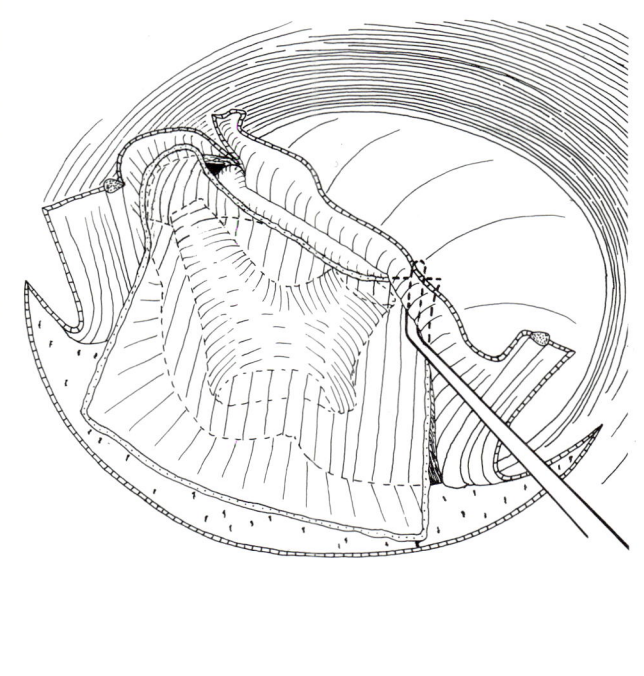

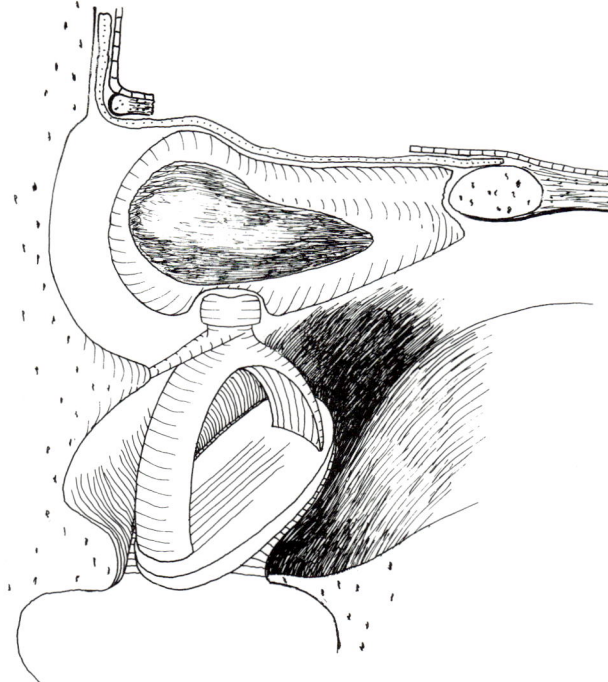

Fig. 726 The fascia is placed lateral to the malleus and under the umbo

Fig. 727 Side view of an incus interposition, illustrating an assembly between the stapes and the malleus handle. The short process of the incus is placed on the neck of the malleus

In certain circumstances, the short process of the incus is placed under the umbo (Fig. 728) pointing towards the anterior hypotympanum. The remnant of the long process of the incus is in contact with the upper part of the malleus handle, and the incus body is placed on the head of the stapes, preventing retraction. The fascia can be placed on the lateral aspect of the malleus handle and on its short process, following the same principles illustrated above (Figs. 718, 719, 726). In this situation, the fascia is usually placed under the malleus handle. Firstly, the fascia is placed under the superior part of the malleus handle and carefully adapted so as not to dislocate the remnant of the long process of the incus (Fig. 729). Finally, the fascia is placed under the umbo, and on the short process of the incus (Fig. 730). With a perpendicular rugine, the fascia is carefully pushed anteriorly along the short process of the incus, and adapted to the undersurface of the drum. In such cases, a 3×3-mm piece of the thinnest Silastic sheeting is usually placed under the umbo region (Fig. 728), preventing later fixation of the short process to the promontory. This type of incus interposition is sometimes used after extensive elevation of the retracted malleus.

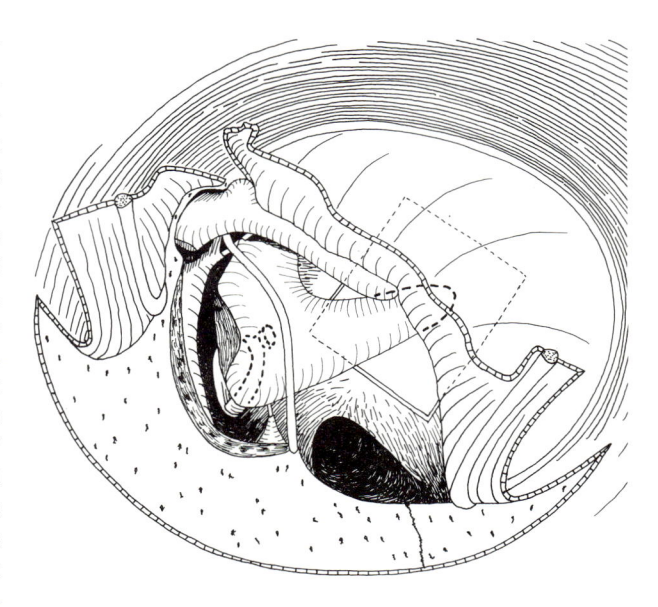

Fig. 728 Interposition of the incus, with the short process placed under the umbo. The remnant of the long process is pointing anteriorly towards the mesotympanum. The retracted malleus handle has been pulled laterally, and a 3×3-mm Silastic sheet is placed on the promontory

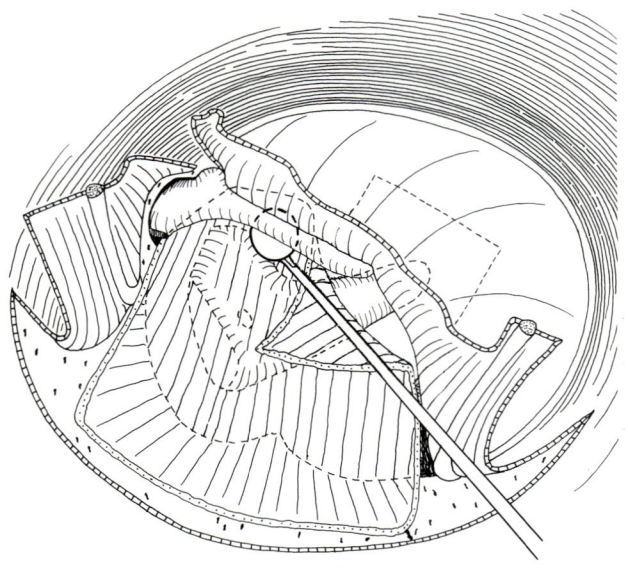

Fig. **729** The fascia is placed under the malleus handle

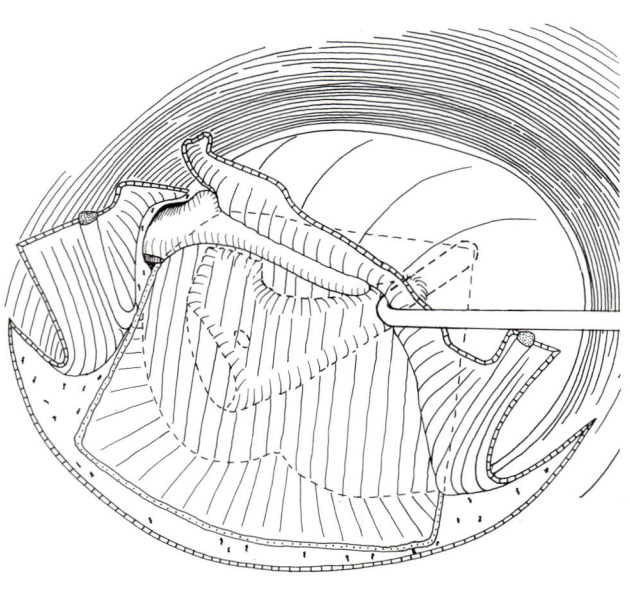

Fig. **730** Final placement of the fascia under the umbo and under the drum remnant

Incus Interpositions in Patients with a Retracted Malleus

Retracted malleus is a consequence of long-lasting retraction and atrophy of the eardrum, which is caused by long-term tubal dysfunction or secretory otitis in childhood, or both. Epidemiological studies of children have demonstrated a highly significant correlation between alterations in the drum, particularly atrophy and retraction, and the duration or severity of tubal dysfunction and secretory otitis (Tos et al. 1984). Atrophy of the eardrum is most often diffuse, but may be restricted to the posterior and inferior parts of the pars tensa. Tympanosclerosis of the drum is not associated with the retracted malleus, simply because the drum is stiff and does not allow any major retraction. The condition of retraction and atrophy of the drum with a retracted malleus is classified as atelectasis of various degrees. If the drum adheres to the medial wall of the tympanic cavity, the condition is desribed as adhesive otitis (Sadé and Berco 1976, Tos and Paulsen 1979). In these cases, the umbo usually adheres to the medial wall of the tympanic cavity. In posterior atrophy and retraction, the following consecutive conditions are often observed: 1) Posterosuperior or diffuse atrophy and retraction, 2) myringoincudopexy, 3) resorption of the long process of the incus, and 4) myringostapediopexy. Later on, 5) perforation of the atrophic part of the drum can occur, which stabilizes the condition, or 6) further retraction can occur, with adhesion to the medial wall—adhesive otitis—or 7) sinus cholesteatoma, or 8) tensa-retraction cholesteatoma. This last condition is usually associated either with a retracted malleus (75%) or a missing malleus handle (25%) (Table **3**, p. 244). Retracted malleus handle and adherent umbo is therefore a commonly encountered pathology in type 2 tympanoplasty.

A number of options are available in these circumstances.

1) Division of the adhesions between the promontory and the umbo (Fig. **731**), *elevating* the malleus handle laterally using a strong perpendicular rugine (Fig. **732**). The elevation has to be performed a few millimeters more laterally than its normal position. During this procedure, the tendon of the tensor tympani muscle is stretched, and the malleus handle remains in this position, mobile, but without natural elasticity. Cutting the tendon of the tensor tympani muscle is also used by some surgeons.

Sometimes in such cases, after placing a 3×3-mm thin Silastic sheet over the promontory, incus interposition is performed with the short

Interposition of the Incus

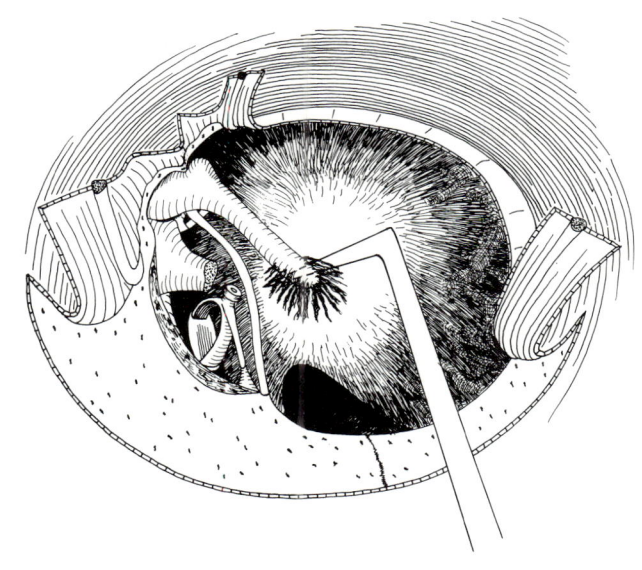

Fig. **731** Total perforation, with the malleus handle retracted and adherent to the promontory. The adhesions are separated with a hook. The Palva swing-door technique for underlay grafting is performed

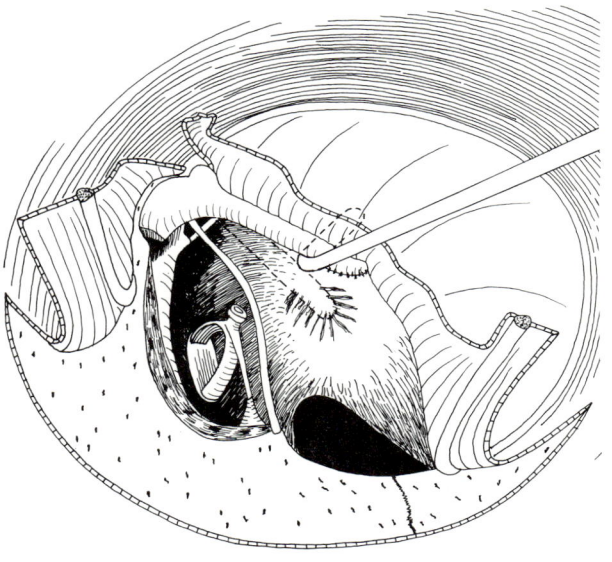

Fig. **732** Retracted malleus and umbo adherent to the promontory (dotted line). The adhesions are separated, and the malleus is pulled laterally with a perpendicular elevator or hook

process placed under the umbo (Fig. **728**). Placement of the underlay fascia is not difficult, since the malleus handle is hypermobile (Figs. **729**, **730**). If the umbo and fascia are in a stable position, it is preferable not to support them with Gelfoam balls within the tympanic cavity, but to place semidry Gelfoam balls in the ear canal at the junction between the edge of the perforation and the fascia, in order to fixate the fascia from outside. This method of fixing an underlay graft is described in the Chapter on myringoplasty (pp. 144–150).

The classic interposition of the incus is commonly used in these situations (Fig. **717**). Sound transmission is mainly direct, via the incus body to the stapes, so that having, a large area of the incus body in contact with the drum is the best solution. It also prevents, fascia graft retraction in the posterosuperior region.

2) Division of the adhesions between the umbo and the promontory (Fig. **732**) *without elevating* the malleus handle, if it is mobile. After placing a 3×3-mm piece of thin sheet of Silastic sheeting under the umbo, the short process of the incus is sometimes placed on the retracted malleus handle (Fig. **733**). The body of the incus, either with or without a hole for the stapes, is placed on the head of the stapes. The long-process remnant of the incus points in an inferior direction, without being too close to the posterior bony annulus. The short process crosses the lower half of the retracted mal-

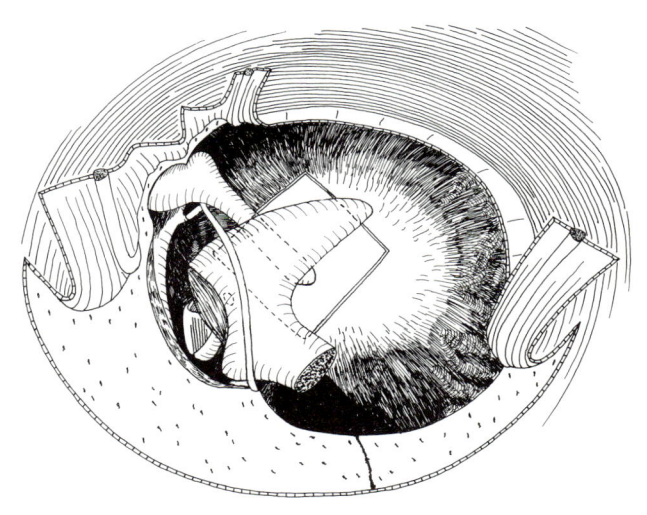

Fig. **733** After extraction, the incus body is placed on the head of the stapes and the short process is placed on the retracted malleus. A 3×3-mm piece of Silastic is placed on the promontory

leus, pointing anteroinferiorly (Fig. **734**). The fascia is placed on the incus–malleus assembly, keeping the tympanic cavity at a sufficient height. We only use this method when closing a total perforation, as in Figure **735**, showing the underlay swing-door technique. Anteriorly, the fascia has to be

16 Type 2 Tympanoplasty, Stapes Present

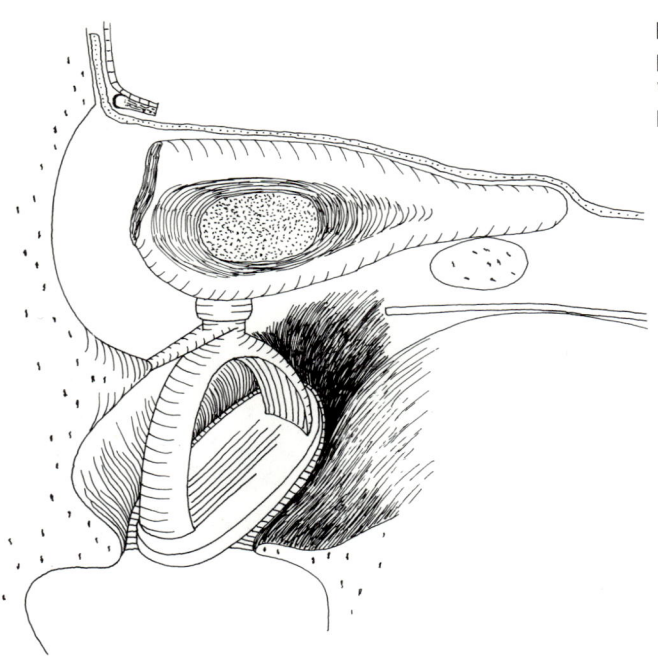

Fig. **734** Side view of the short process of the incus placed on the retracted malleus handle and covered with fascia. Silastic is placed between the umbo and the promontory

fixed to the bone by elevating and removing the mucosa under the fibrous annulus, hence avoiding too much Gelfoam in an adhesive ear.

3) In the adhesive ear, we prefer to use the onlay technique with three superior flaps (Fig. **736**), described in detail above (Figs. **488–504**). An incus is shaped and placed with its hole on the on the head of the stapes. The short process is tilted towards and along the malleus handle (Fig. **736**). Since the fascia is supported on the annulus all round the circumference, and by the short process of the incus in the center of the middle-ear cavity (Figs. **737, 738**), as well as in the center of the incus body in the posterosuperior region, Gelfoam is unnecessary in the tympanic cavity in these cases.

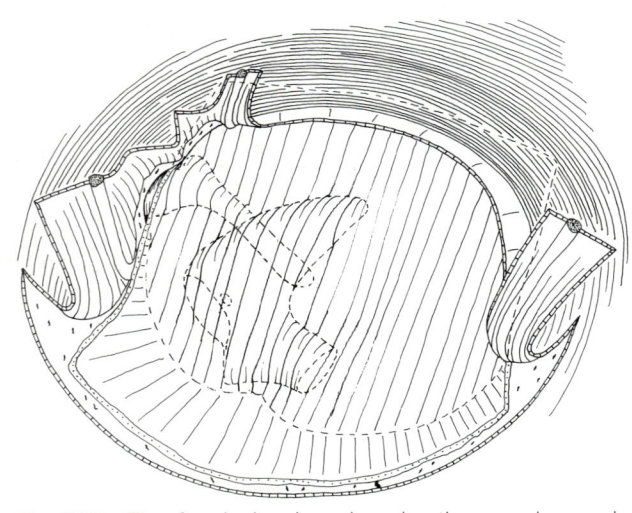

Fig. **735** The fascia is placed under the annulus and over the incus

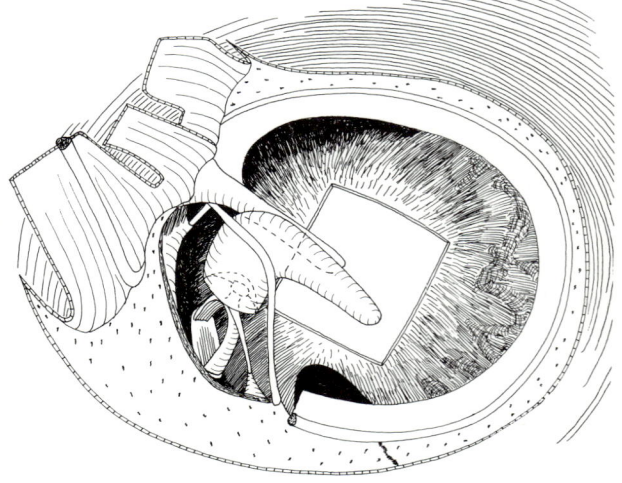

Fig. **736** Total perforation, with a retracted and adherent malleus handle. The adhesions have been loosened, the piece of Silastic is placed under the umbo, and a specially-shaped incus prosthesis is placed with its hole on the head of the stapes, tilted towards and along the malleus handle. The myringoplasty will be carried out as an onlay technique

Interposition of the Incus

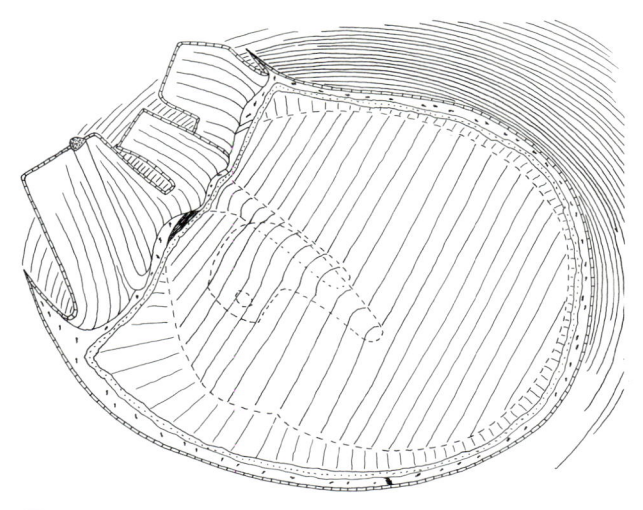

Fig. **737** The fascia is placed on the umbo and brought into contact with the incus and the retracted malleus

Fig. **738** Side view at the level of the umbo, showing ▷ the incus prosthesis in contact with the malleus handle and the fascia placed quite medially, in contact with both ossicles

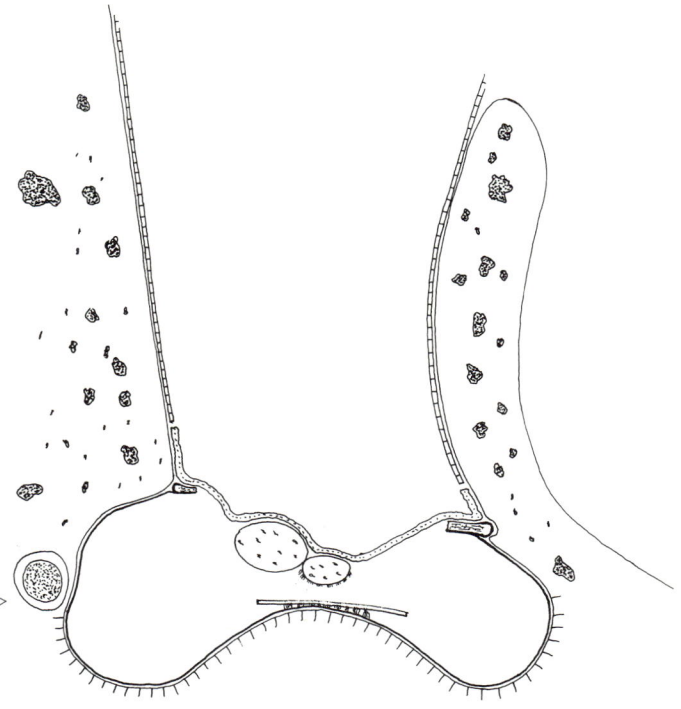

4) Some surgeons cut off and remove the adherent umbo, and place the fascia under the remnant of the malleus handle. Firstly, the adhesions between the promontory and the umbo should be cut with a sickle knife or a hook (Fig. **739**). The malleus handle is then elevated in order to get the punch underneath it (Fig. **740**). The umbo is removed, and the incus is interposed before the fascia is placed under the shortened malleus handle and over the interposed incus (Figs. **741, 742**). The rationale for this unphysiological procedure is to avoid lateralization of the drum in relation to the malleus when using an onlay technique (Fig. **743**), or for fixation of the drum when using underlay technique. We do not recommend removal of the umbo, since it is very important for maintaining the conical shape of the drum. When using an underlay technique, a 3×3-mm piece of thin Silastic sheeting will prevent adhesions, and the fascia can be placed under the umbo (Fig. **744**). If the umbo is cut, the new drum is already lateralized, and its function is not optimal. This is also the case in the onlay technique (Fig. **745**).

In patients with a retracted malleus handle, using the onlay technique, or at least placing the fascia on the retracted malleus handle, is in our opinion better than the underlay technique.

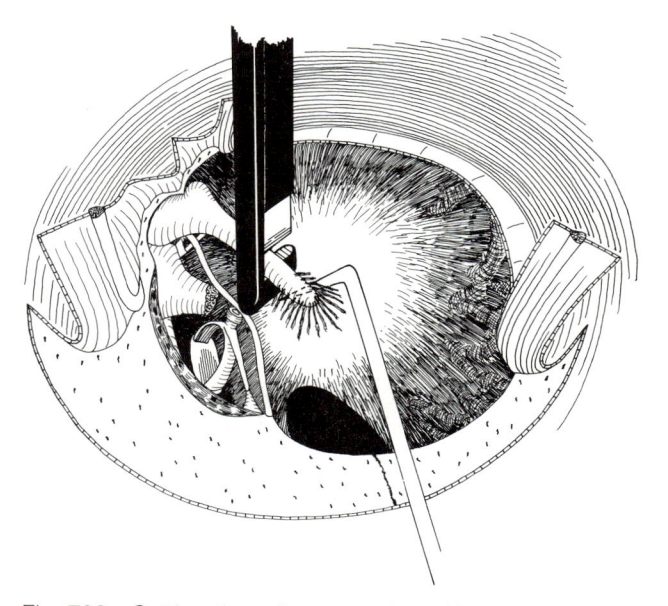

Fig. **739** Cutting the adherent umbo with a punch after disruption of the adhesions

16 Type 2 Tympanoplasty, Stapes Present

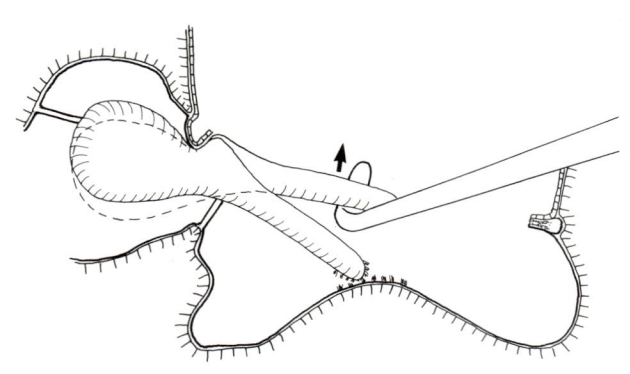

Fig. 740 Side view, showing the elevation of the retracted malleus handle

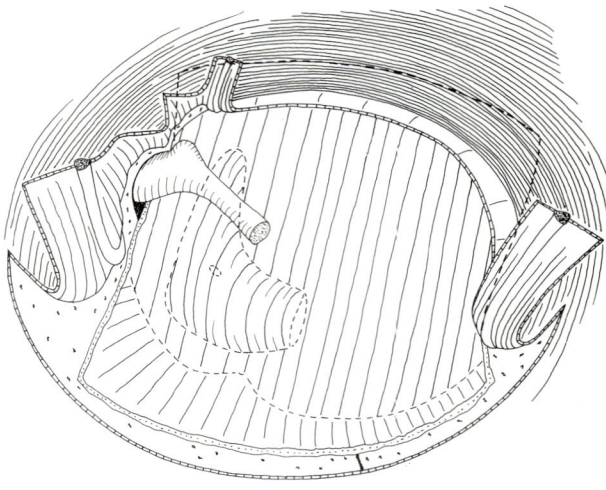

Fig. 741 Underlay fascia grafting after cutting of the umbo and interposition of the incus. The fascia is placed under the remnant of the malleus handle as an underlay graft

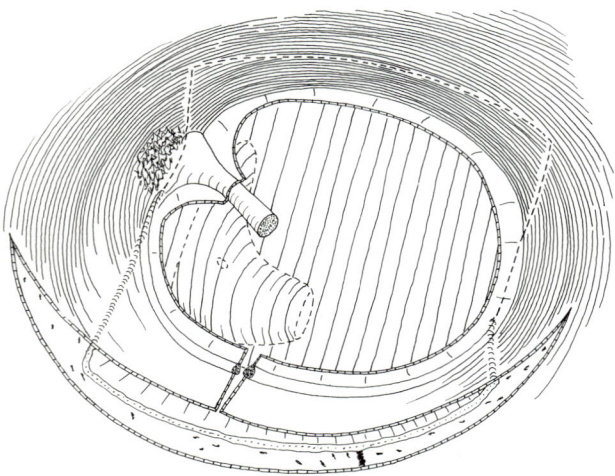

Fig. 742 The epithelial flaps are returned. The malleus handle is not covered

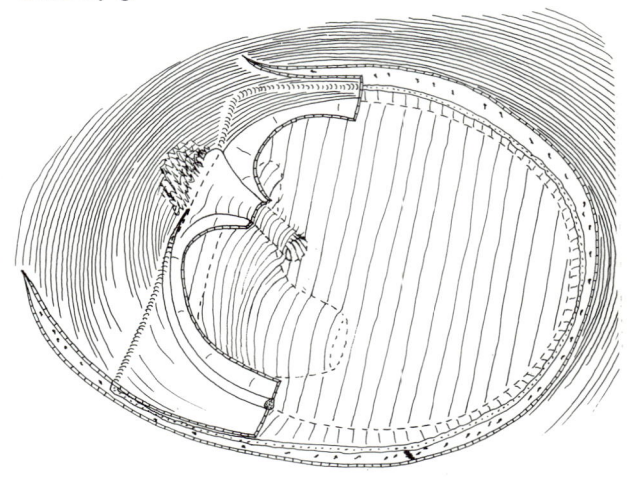

Fig. 743 Onlay grafting. The fascia is placed *on top of* the malleus handle

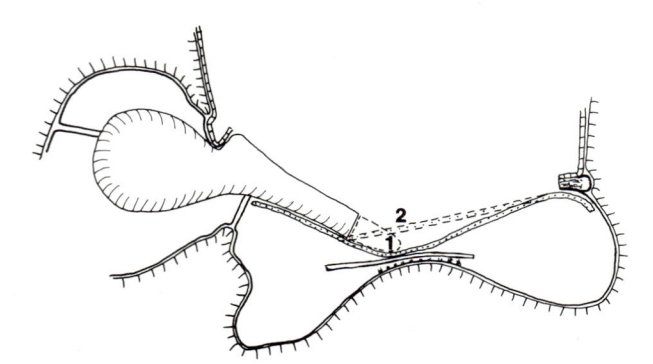

Fig. 744 Side view of the underlay grafting under the retracted malleus handle. The fascia is pushed under the intact umbo (1), or under the remnant of the malleus handle after the umbo has been removed (2). Silastic is placed on the promontory

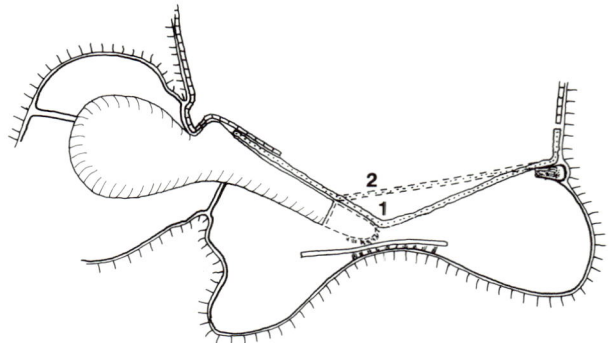

Fig. 745 Side view of onlay technique in retracted malleus handle. The fascia is placed on the umbo (1). After resection of the umbo, the fascia is lateralized (2)

Shaping the Incus

Up to now, the use of whole, unshaped incus has been described and discussed, but autogenous or allogenous incus can be shaped in such way that it fits exactly into the defect between the head of the stapes and the malleus handle (Pennington 1973). Shaping is sometimes a necessity, because of anatomic variations in the relationship between the head of the stapes and the malleus handle. In addition, the position of the bony annulus and the position of the tympanic membrane when healed is important for ossiculoplasty (Pulec and Sheehy 1973). The bony annulus can be drilled away if its position is too close to an interposed incus, but the relationship with regard to the distance between the malleus and the stapes cannot be changed, so that the ossicles have to be shaped (Fig. **746**). When there is a small distance between the head of the stapes and the malleus handle, and a small angle between the bony annulus and the malleus handle, the ossiculoplasty is straightforward and stable. The prosthesis has to be short, and quite a lot of the incus body and the short process of the incus therefore has to be drilled away (Fig. **747**). When there is a larger distance between the head of the stapes and the malleus, the prosthesis is long, and the entire length of the short process and the body of the incus has to be used in order to bridge the distance (Figs. **748–750**). Sound transmission from the malleus handle to the stapes is not as good, and is mainly maintained via the posterosuperior part of the drum. When there is a low stapes and a large tympanic cavity, the entire incus has to be used, with very little shaping (Fig. **751**).

While the shaping is being done, the incus should be stabilized during the drilling process. This can be performed in several ways:

1) With the Sheehy ossicle-holding forceps (Figs. **752, 753**). A screw holds the ossicle securely during drilling, but the disadvantage of this holder is the time-consuming change of position of the ossicle in relation to the forceps, which often occurs during drilling.

2) Holding the ossicles with ungloved fingers, as Marquet practiced. He claimed to have no contamination when operating without gloves. Recent research in our hospital has in fact shown that the amount of bacteria on the surface of the surgeon's hand is extremely low when compared with other possible sources of contamination during the operation. Gloves are recommended mainly to protect the surgeon and for aesthetic reasons. When shaping an allograft ossicle for storage in a bank of ossicles,

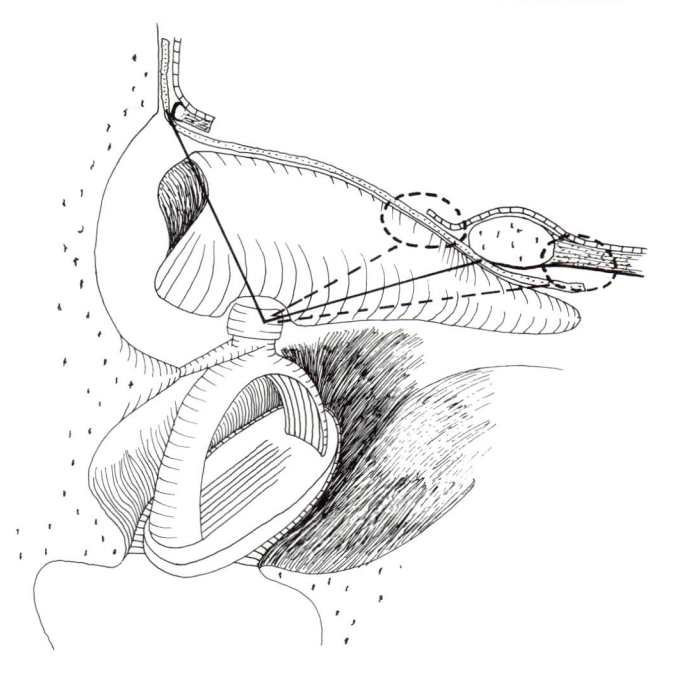

Fig. **746 Shaping the incus.** Various distances between the malleus handle and the head of the stapes, the posterior bony annulus and the malleus handle

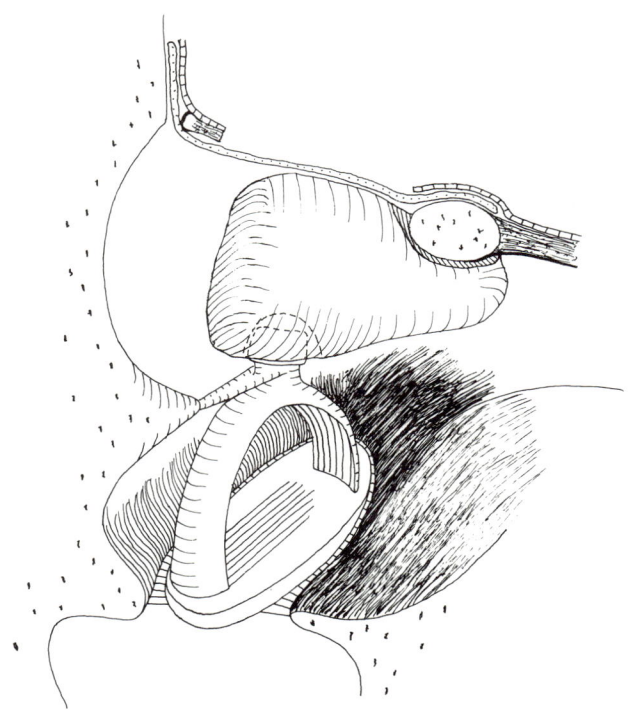

Fig. **747** Shaped incus in a patient with a small distance between the malleus handle and the head of the stapes. A hole is made for the head of the stapes and a groove is made for the malleus handle

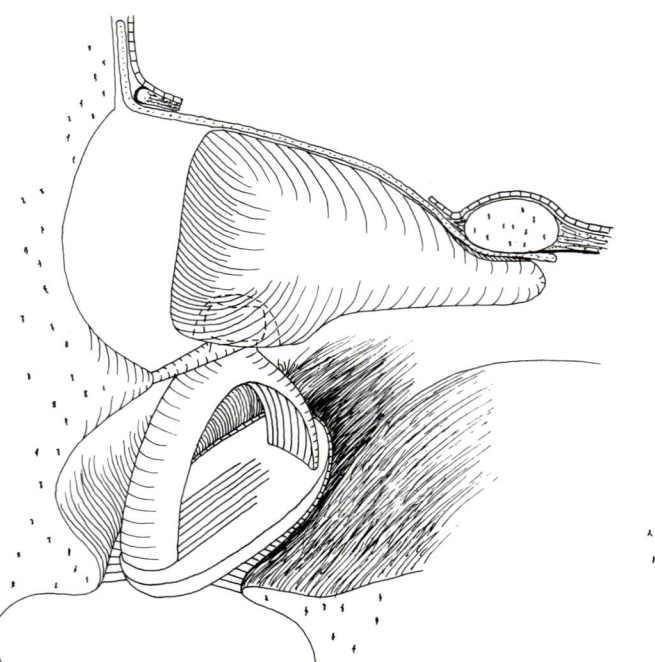

Fig. 748 Shaped incus with a hole at the long process end, solid contact between the incus body and the drum and between the groove in the short process and the malleus handle

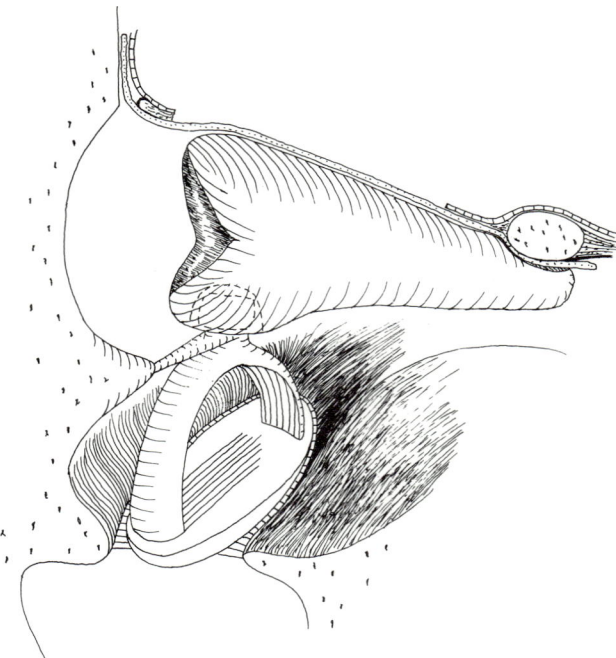

Fig. 749 Shaped incus in a patient with a wide distance between the malleus handle and the head of the stapes. There is solid contact between the prosthesis and the drum

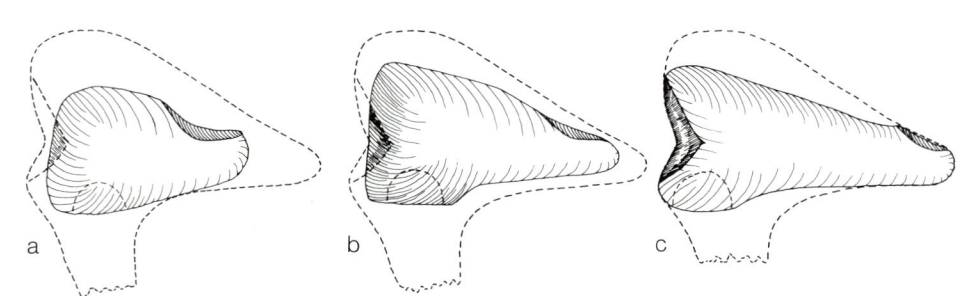

Fig. 750 Shaping the incus with various distances between the malleus handle and the head of the stapes. **a** Distance is small and much of the incus have to be drilled off. **b, c** The distance is large and relatively little of the incus has to be removed

including the malleus, incus, or stapes, we never use gloves, but the ossicles are later boiled or autoclaved. The most precise drilling can be performed when holding the ossicles with the fingers.

3) For shaping ossicles, we use a simple surgical clamp (Fig. 754), the advantage of which is that changing of the position of the ossicle during drilling is easy. However, there is a risk of the ossicle slipping during drilling.

Only the incus, cortical bone, or malleus can be held by forceps or clamps during drilling. The allogenous stapes is too fragile for instruments, and should be held with the fingers and shaped before surgery. Some surgeons claim that a clamp or holders cause microfractures of the ossicles, but microfractures have no influence on the movement and sound transmission of the ossicles. When a piece of cortical bone is harvested with a chisel, many microfractures occur, and the cortical bone can also be used as an interposition graft or a columella.

Before starting to shape the incus, the surgeon should measure the distance between the head of the stapes and the malleus handle. This can be done with a perpendicularly-curved instrument, e.g., a long hook, a curved elevator, or the incudostapedial

Shaping the Incus

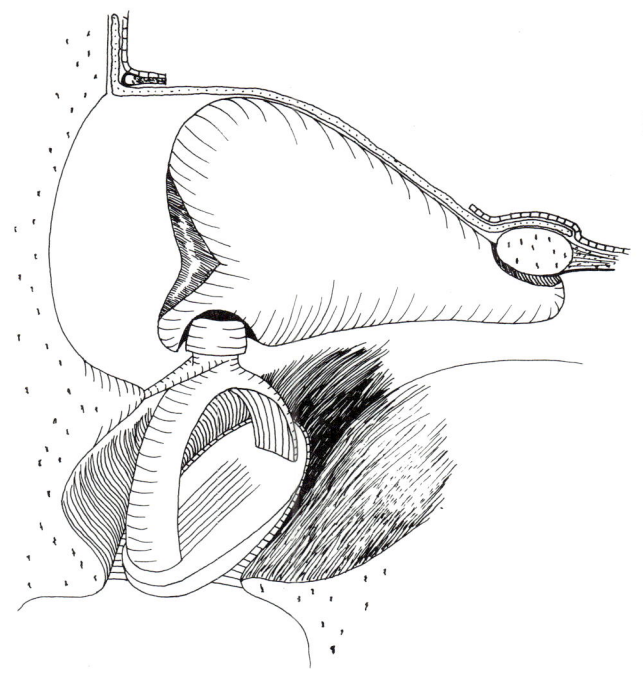

Fig. 751 The entire incus remnant is used. A groove is made in the long process end, and the short process is in contact with the malleus. Contact with the drum is solid

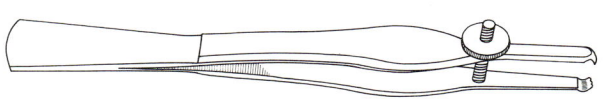

Fig. 752 The Sheehy ossicle-holding forceps

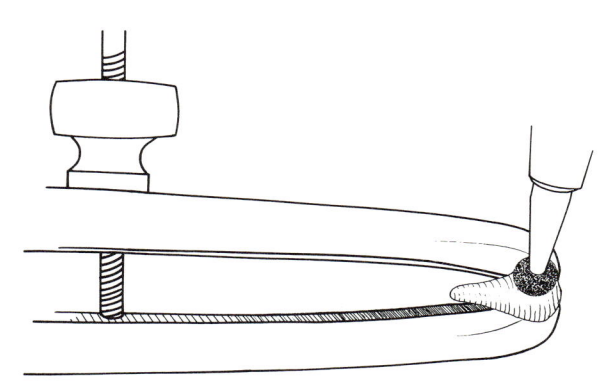

Fig. 753 The incus is securely fixed with a screw during the drilling

knife. The measurements should be compared to the incus. The surgeon must have an idea of how the new graft should look:

1) Should it have an acetabulum — a hole or a groove for the head of the stapes?
2) Should the graft be in contact with the malleus handle only, or both the malleus and the drum?
3) Should the graft be of the maximum or minimum possible size?

Answering these three questions provides at least 27 variant grafts. The varying distance between the head of the stapes and the malleus handle, the variation in the degree of malleus-handle retraction, and differences in the height of the stapes, increase the number of possibilities for shaping the graft even more.

The position of the surgical clamp has to be changed several times during drilling. The size of the prosthesis should be checked during drilling, and diminishes gradually. It is a frustrating fact that the prosthesis, despite measurements, is often still too large even after repeated attempts at shaping.

Severed principles should be followed when shaping the incus:

1) Minium shaping, e.g., by drilling away the irregularities of the articular surface of the incus

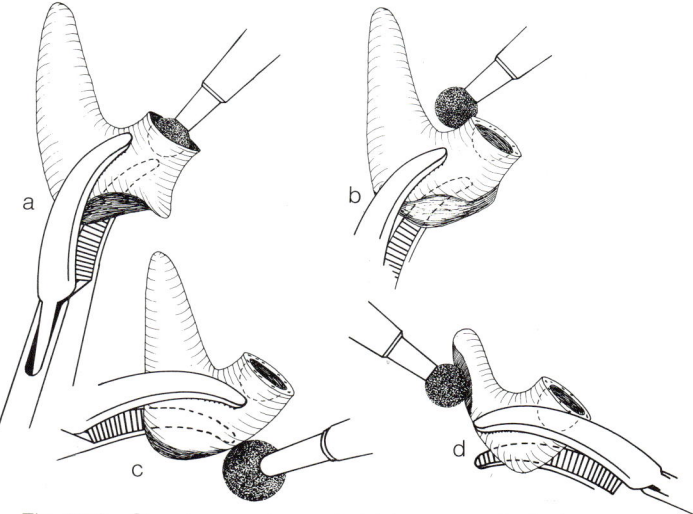

Fig. 754 Shaping an incus held by a surgical clamp. Its position should be changed several times during the drilling

body to enlarge the distance to the posterior bony annulus in the classic incus interposition (Fig. 716) and its variations (Figs. 722, 725, 728, 733). Drilling an acetabulum or a hole in the incus body is also minimal shaping (Fig. 746).

16 Type 2 Tympanoplasty, Stapes Present

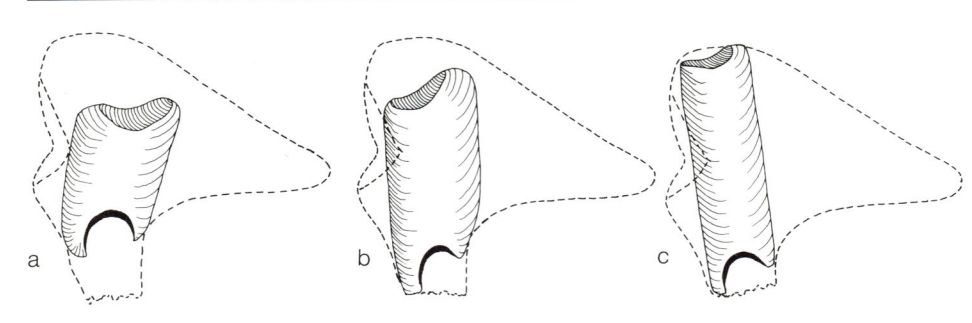

Fig. **755a, b** Shaping bony bridges between the malleus handle and the head of the stapes without major contact to the drum. **c** The Goodhill semi-incus prosthesis

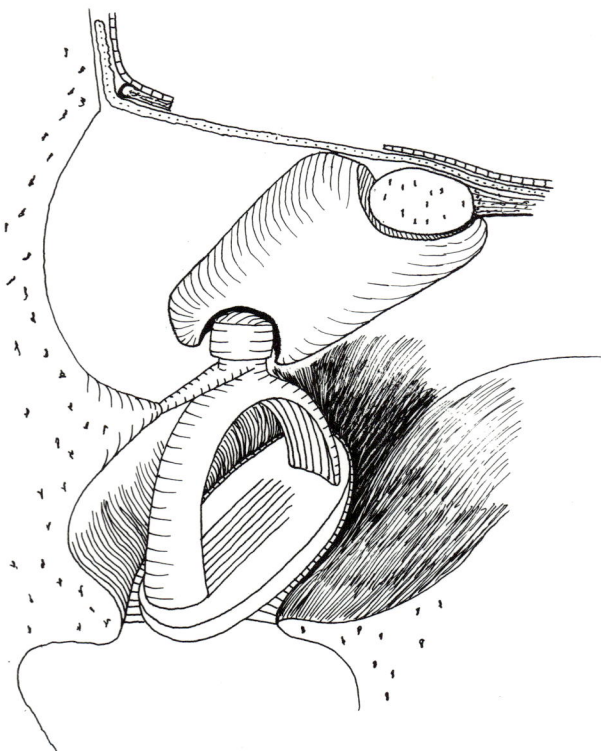

Fig. **756** A small bridge providing contact between the stapes and the malleus handle

2) Shaping an incus graft with a hole in the remnant of the long process, and with extensive contact between the superior surface of the incus body and the drum. The superior edge of the short process is in contact with the malleus handle in a groove shown (Figs. **747–750**). In ears with a low stapes and a high tympanic cavity, with a large distance between the head of the stapes and the malleus handle, the entire incus can be placed with its long-process remnant lying on the head of the stapes, providing maximum contact with the drum (Fig. **751**). This is especially important in well-ventilated ears, e.g., after traumatic incus luxation (Elbrønd 1970). Lateralization of the drum in relation to the incus graft is prevented.

3) Bridging the gap between the head of the stapes and the malleus handle with a bony bridge that has no contact with the drum. A large part of the incus has to be drilled away in this type of prostheses (Fig. **755**). The Goodhill (1967) semi-incus columella prosthesis is similar to the long interposition graft, shown in Figure **755c**. In cases with a small distance between the stapes and the malleus, there will be a good connection, and even some contact with the drum surface (Fig. **756**). In cases with a long distance between the stapes and the malleus, the position of the prosthesis is quite oblique, and sound transmission is, poor (Figs. **757, 758**).

4) Shaping a small incus prosthesis, with some contact with the drum and the malleus handle (Fig. **759**). Most of the incus is drilled away (Fig. **754d**). The fascia grafting is easy to perform, both in underlay techniques (Fig. **760**) and in onlay techniques, but there is a risk of retraction around, and especially posterior to the prosthesis.

Prostheses that are in contact both with the drum and with the malleus handle are preferable (Figs. **747–750**). The risk of retraction of the posterosuperior part of the drum is also smaller. Bridging techniques are popular in second-stage opera-

Shaping the Incus

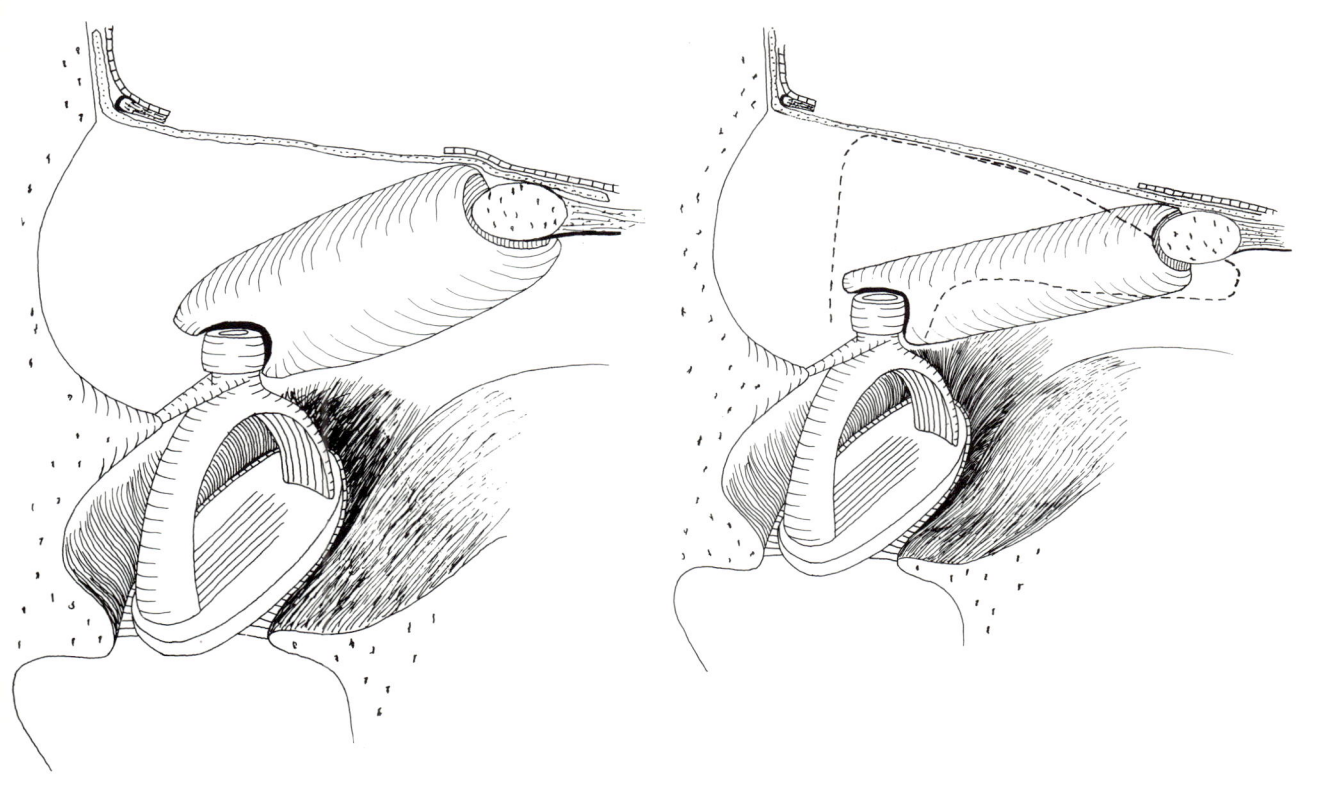

Fig. **757** Oblique position of a bony bridge, shaped from the incus with a groove for the head of the stapes and a groove for the malleus handle

Fig. **758** The semi-incus prosthesis, with a groove for the head of the stapes and a groove for the malleus handle, is positioned very obliquely to bridge the large distance between the stapes and the malleus handle. The dotted line indicates the incus prostesis with solid contact to the drum

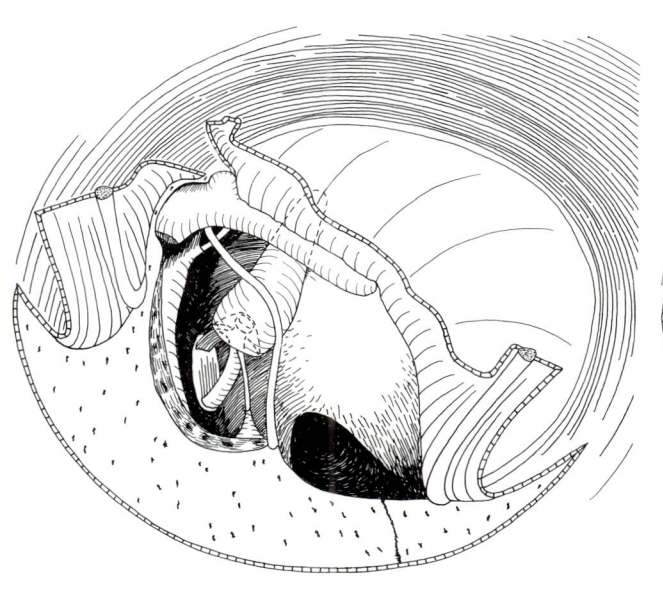

Fig. **759** The classic way to place a shaped incus with a thin short process under the malleus handle, with a hole drilled in the body of the incus for the head of the stapes. The tympanic chorda secures the prosthesis

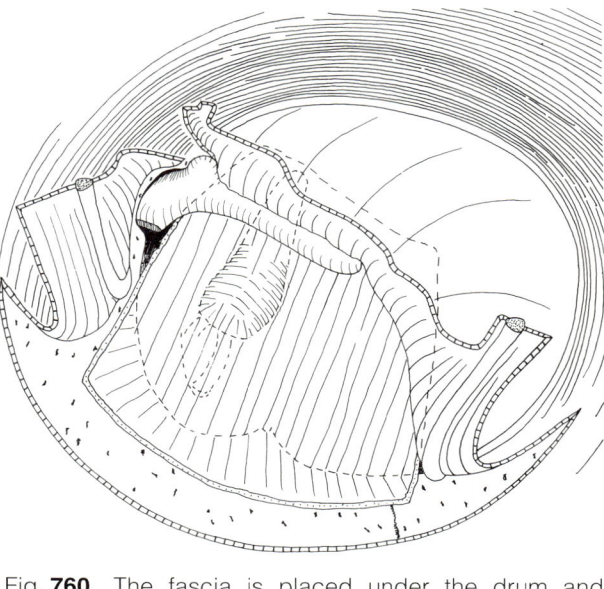

Fig. **760** The fascia is placed under the drum and under the malleus handle, and between the prosthesis and the malleus handle

16 Type 2 Tympanoplasty, Stapes Present

tions, because the drum has already healed in its original position, and if the malleus handle is present, it is easy to fit a bridge between the malleus and the stapes.

Sometimes it is not wise, nor even possible, to place the short process of the incus under the malleus handle. In these cases, placing a shaped prosthesis parallel to the malleus handle (Fig. **761**) provides firm fibrous contact both to the drum and the malleus (Fig. **762**). Placing a small, L-shaped graft between the drum and the stapes is also a popular method (Fig. **763**).

There are no scientific data comparing long-term hearing results in classic interposition techniques with shaping, and similarly there are no data comparing shaping of the incus that provides contact with the drum with shaping for bridging alone. There are not even any data comparing shaping of the incus performed in a one-stage procedure with that performed in two stages. English et al. (1971) found little difference in the hearing results obtained with autogenous and allogenous incus. At 1–3 years after surgery, 47% of patients with autogenous grafts had social hearing (0–30 dB) compared with 44% of those with allogenous grafts.

Finally, shaping of the allogenous incus with an intact long process of the incus is interesting: cutting the short process of the incus, drilling a small hole for the stapes head, facing the articular surface toward the drum, and placing the slender long process under the malleus handle (Fig. **764**).

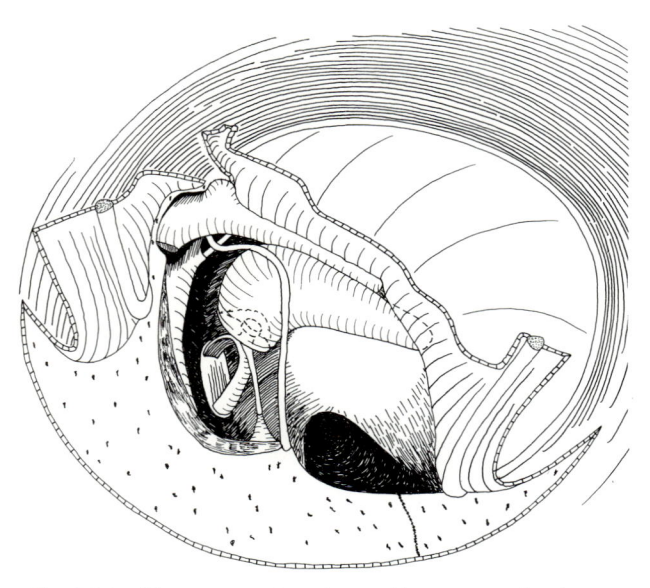

Fig. **761** Placement of a shaped incus prosthesis parallel to the malleus handle

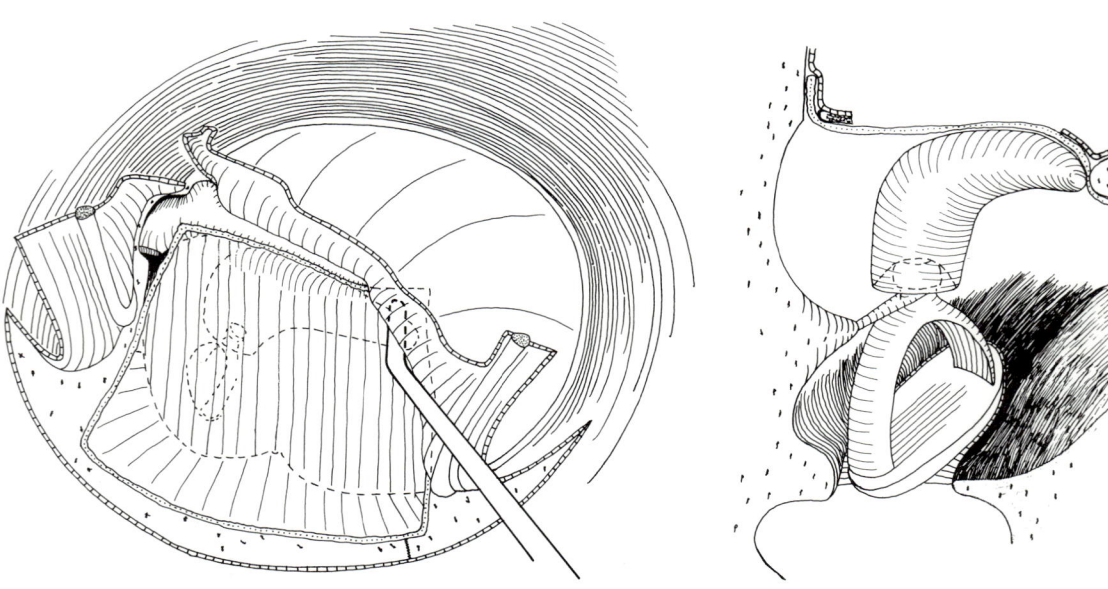

Fig. **762** The fascia is placed on the posterior aspect of the malleus handle and under the drum remnant inferiorly

Fig. **763** A small, shaped prosthesis of the incus, in contact both with the drum and the malleus handle. Fascia is placed under the malleus handle

Shaping the Malleus Head

Fig. 764 Shaping the incus by cutting the short process of the incus and placing the long process under the malleus handle

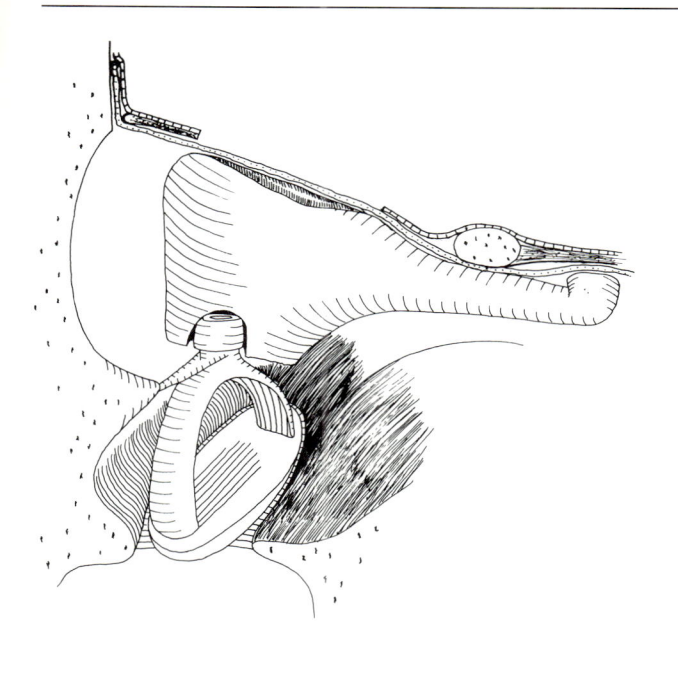

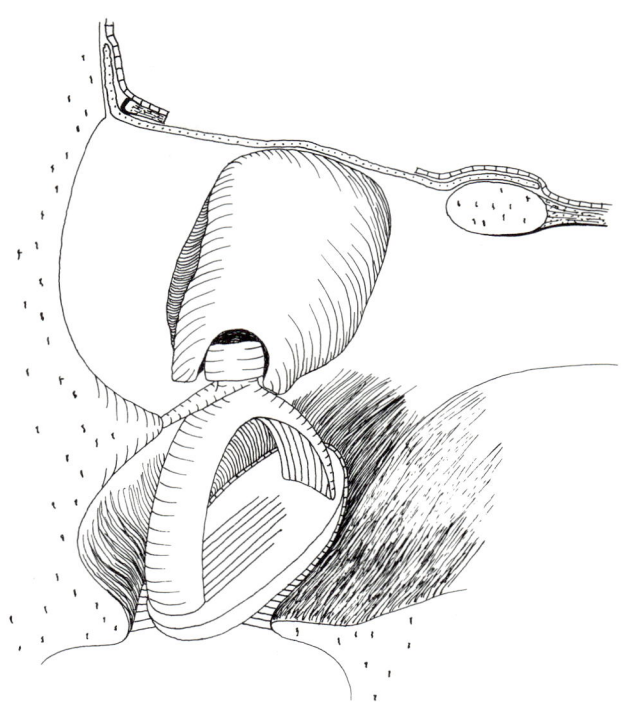

Fig. 765 **Shaping the malleus head.** The classsic use of the malleus head, with a groove drilled in the neck of the malleus and the top of the head in contact with the drum

Shaping the Malleus Head

An autogenous malleus head is seldom the only ossicle available, since the incus body is usually also available. In cholesteatoma cases with resorption of the incus body, the malleus body will also be resorbed. In cholesteatoma cases requiring mastoidectomy, cortical bone is easier to harvest than resection of the malleus head for use in ossiculoplasty. In tympanoplasty with an endaural approach, the allogenous malleus head is used.

The malleus head, with its neck, provides the length required to bridge the gap between the drum and the head of the stapes, and major shaping (apart from making a hole or a groove) is not necessary (Fig. 765). An unshaped malleus head can also be brought into contact with the malleus handle (Fig. 766).

Shaping of the malleus head usually includes a groove or a hole in its neck—an acetabulum—for the head of the stapes. For contact with the malleus handle, a groove is created (Fig. 767). Usually, the malleus head is in contact with the drum as well as the malleus handle (Fig. 768). Sometimes a bridge is established between the malleus handle and the head of the stapes, without drum contact (Fig. 769).

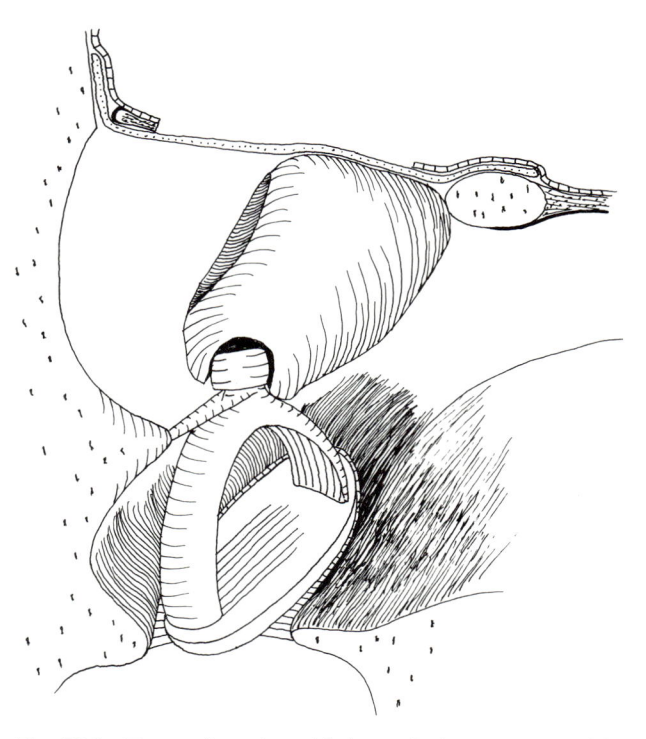

Fig. 766 The malleus head is brought into contact with the drum and malleus handle. A groove is created for the head of the stapes

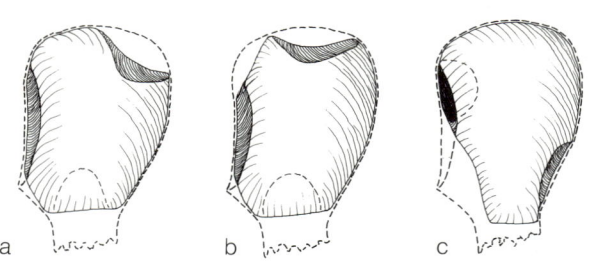

Fig. 767 Examples of how the malleus head can be shaped. **a, b** The classic method, with a hole or groove in the malleus neck region. **c** A hole drilled in the region of the joint surface, and a groove for the malleus handle

The malleus head can be placed on the stapes head with a hole drilled in its articular surface for the stapes. The neck region, with a groove, will be in contact with the malleus handle, and a major part of the malleus head will be in contact with the drum (Figs. **767c, 770**).

In general, the malleus head is suitable in cases with a short distance between the stapes and the malleus handle, but it is too small to bridge a longer distance, or for shaping an L-prosthesis, where contact both with the drum and the malleus handle is desirable.

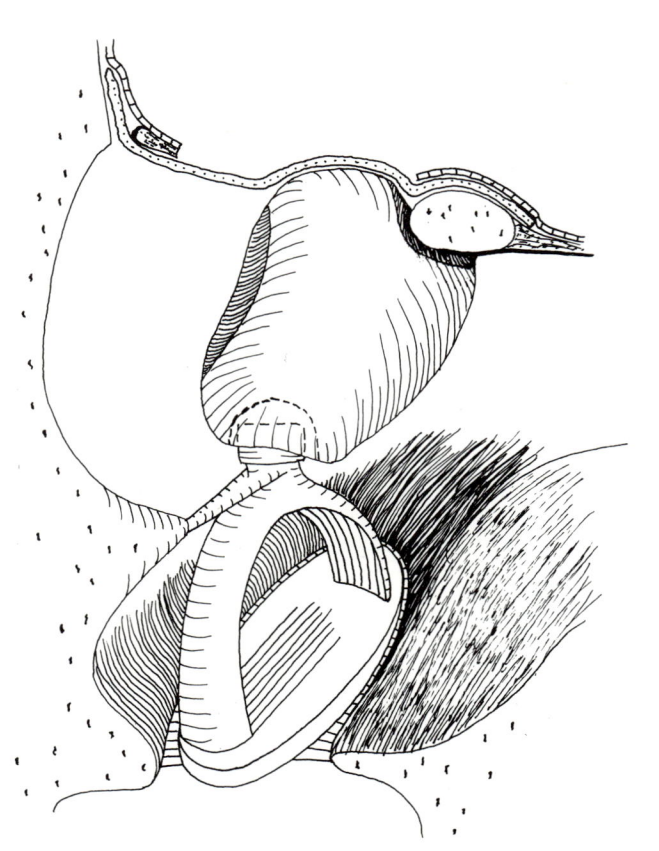

Fig. 768 Placement of the shaped malleus head. There is a hole in the neck region and groove in the head for the malleus handle

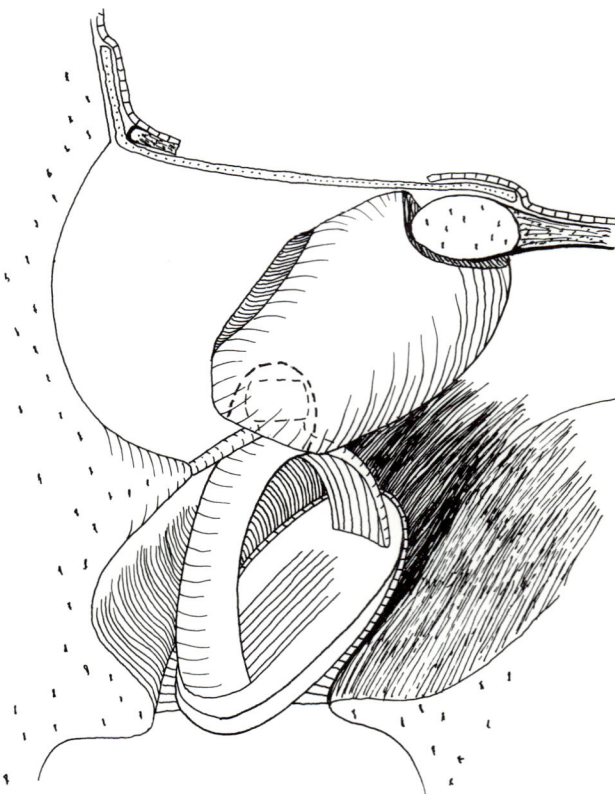

Fig. 769 Oblique placement of the malleus head when there is a greater distance between the stapes head and the malleus handle. A groove is drilled on top of the malleus head to achieve maximum contact with the malleus handle

Shaping Cortical Bone 273

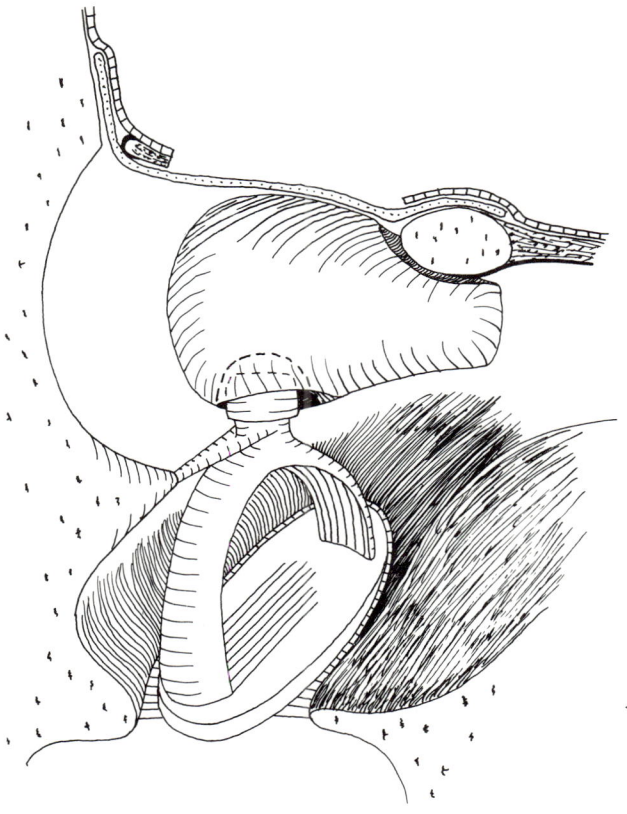

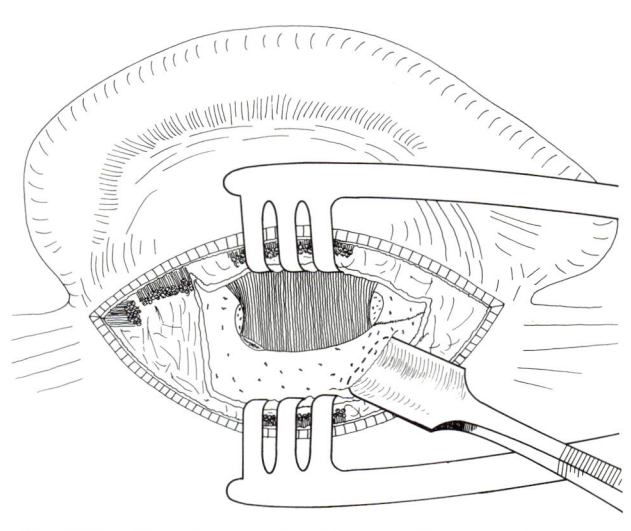

Fig. 771 **Shaping cortical bone.** Chiseling the cortical bone using a large chisel in a retroauricular approach

◁ Fig. 770 A hole or a groove is drilled on the head of the malleus, which is brought into contact with the head of the stapes and the malleus handle

Shaping Cortical Bone

The use of cortical bone as a shaped graft between the stapes and the malleus handle or tympanic membrane was first described by Zöllner (1960) and Andersen et al. (1962). Zöllner called this prosthesis a columella, and described the technique of harvesting the optimal bone shape.

Retroauricular cortical mastoidectomy begins by chiseling off the cortical bone that is to be used for ossiculoplasty, reconstruction of the ear canal, or for cavity obliteration in the form of bone chips (Figs. **771, 772**). By using a large curved chisel, inserting it into the posteroinferior part of the mastoid process, and directing it tangentially into the cortex anterosuperiorly, a piece of bone 1–2 mm thick is fractured off. There is no reason to fear a lesion of the sigmoid sinus. Several large pieces of cortical bone can be obtained in this way.

A suitable piece of bone is fixed into the surgical clamp and shaped for the prosthesis (Fig. **773**). During shaping, the fractured edge of the bone is drilled away with a cutting burr, making the bone fragment smaller.

During the 1960s, unshaped pieces of cortical bone, 2×3-mm in size, were often used in interpositions (Bauer 1966). The thicker end of a 2×3-mm piece was placed on the head of the stapes, and the thinner end under the malleus handle (Fig. **774**).

In contrast to incus grafts, those shaped from cortical bone are thin (Fig. **775**) with relatively sharp edges, and it takes some time to make them smooth. An L-shaped prosthesis with a groove or a hole for the head of the stapes and a groove for the malleus handle can be interposed in the same way as a shaped incus. A simple piece of bone with a groove for the head of the stapes can be placed under the drum along the malleus handle (Fig. **776**). Several other grafts can be shaped from cortical bone, e.g., grafts with significant contact with the drum (Fig. **775c**), or contact with the malleus handle alone (Fig. **777**).

The classic malleus–stapes assembly described by Austin (1971) is usually shaped from cortical bone (Fig. **778**). The prosthesis is in firm contact with the posterior aspect of the malleus handle, and its groove is placed on the head of the stapes. The prosthesis is somewhat thicker posteriorly, and is also in firm contact with the drum

16 Type 2 Tympanoplasty, Stapes Present

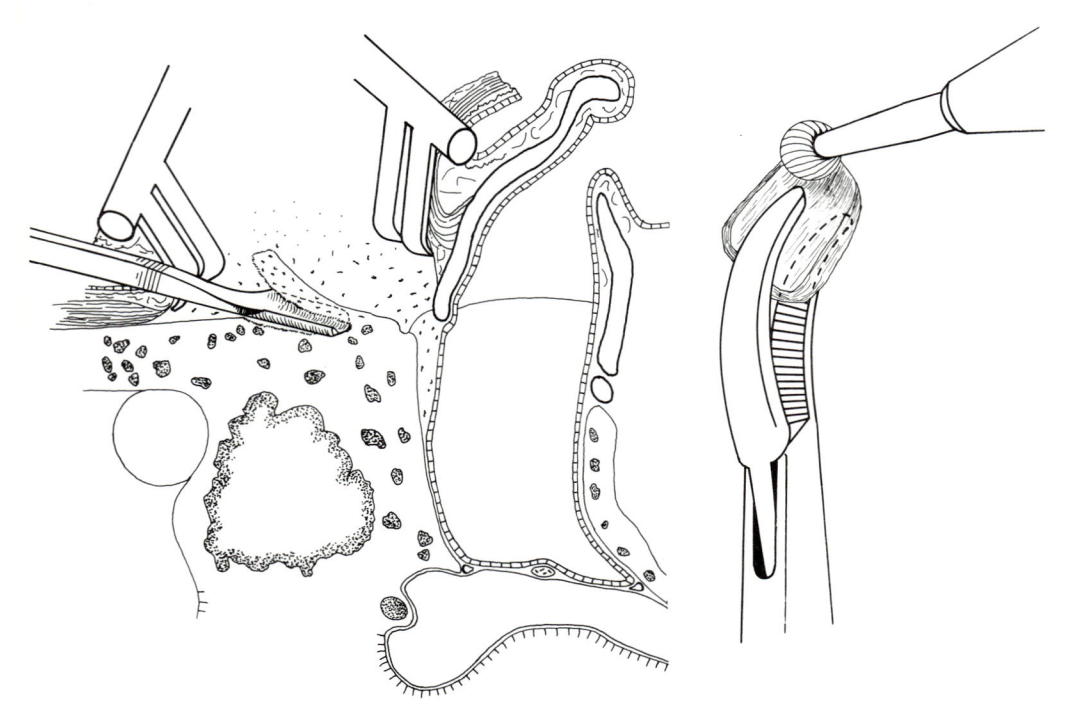

Fig. 772 Side view of chiseling of the cortical bone in a retroauricular approach, showing the tangential placement of the chisel

Fig. 773 Fixing the bone with a surgical clamp and shaping it as a graft

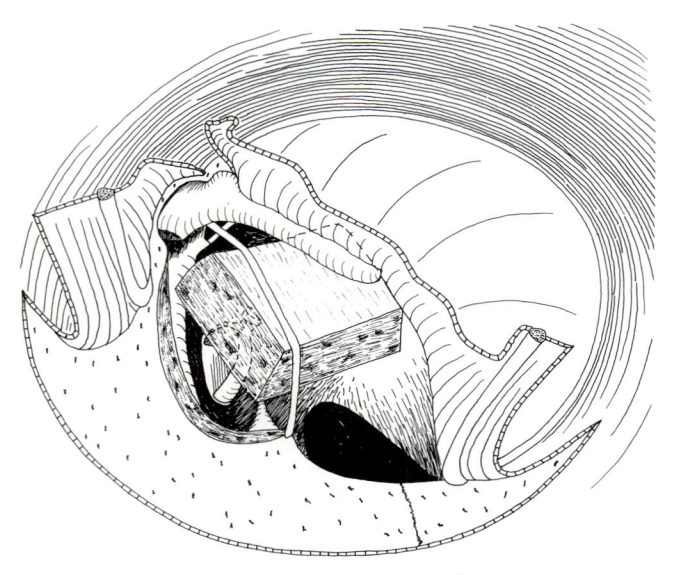

Fig. 774 A relatively large piece of cortical bone is placed on the head of the stapes and under the malleus handle. It is fixed by the tympanic chorda

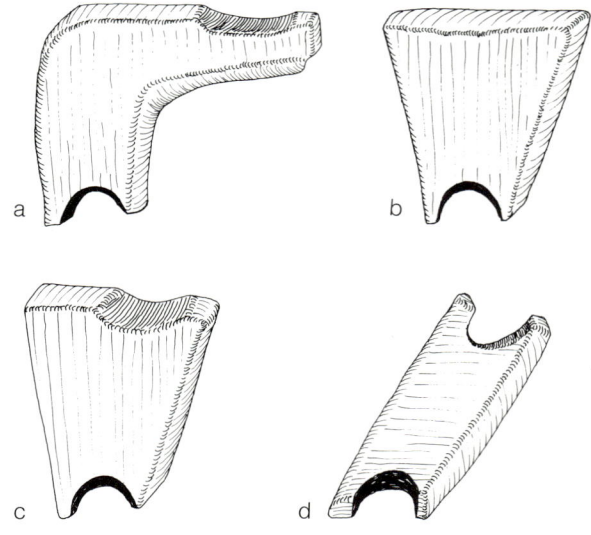

Fig. 775 Shaping of the cortical bone. **a** An L-prosthesis with grooves for the head of the stapes and for the malleus handle. **b** A shaped triangular piece of bone, with a groove for the malleus head. **c** A shaped triangular piece of cortical bone, with grooves for the head of the stapes and malleus handle. **d** A shaped bony bridge between the malleus handle and the stapes, with grooves at both ends

Shaping Cortical Bone

(Fig. **779**). A long, thin, L-shaped prosthesis is placed on the retracted malleus handle, bridging it almost perpendicularly (Fig. **780**). A hole is drilled for the head of the stapes (Fig. **781**).

Vizkelety et al. (1989), in cases with intact stapes, used a shaft of cortical bone—a columella—placed on the footplate between the stapedial arch and the facial prominence (Figs. **782, 783**). In the

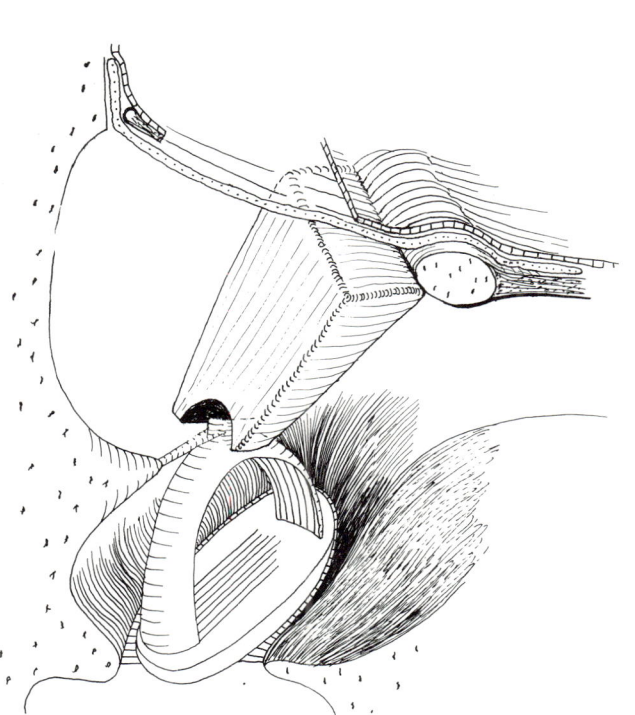

Fig. **776** A triangular cortical bone prosthesis placed parallel to the malleus handle

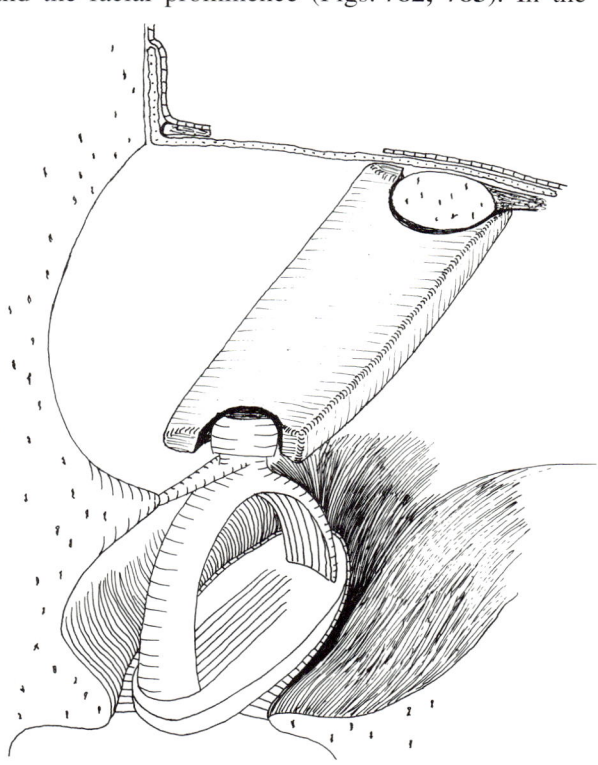

Fig. **777** A bridge of cortical bone placed with its groove between the stapes and the malleus handle

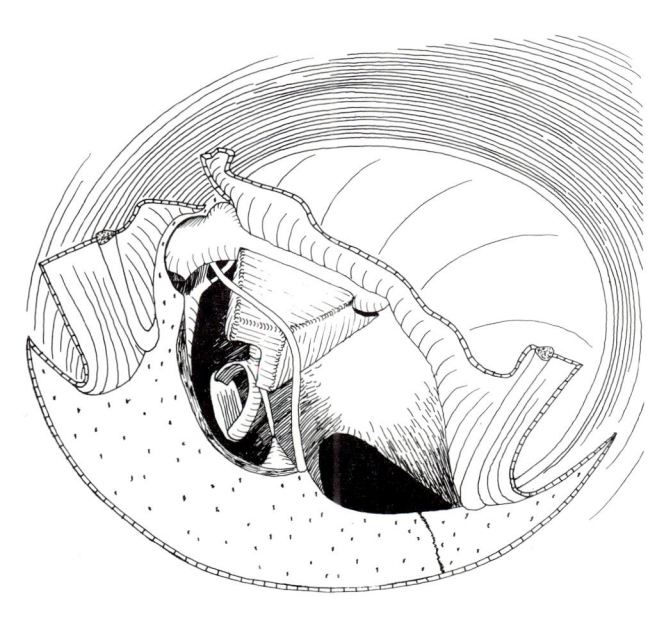

Fig. **778 Austin's malleus–stapes assembly,** with solid contact to the posterior aspect of the malleus handle and with a groove to the head of the stapes

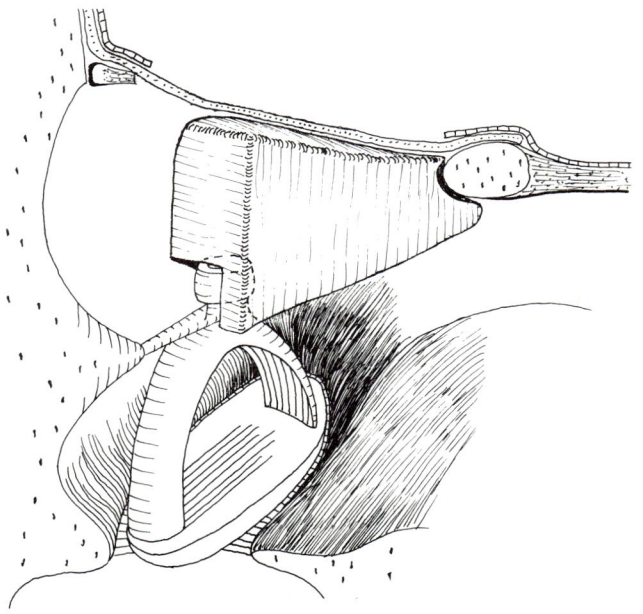

Fig. **779** Side view on the malleus–stapes assembly, showing good contact between the prosthesis and the drum

16 Type 2 Tympanoplasty, Stapes Present

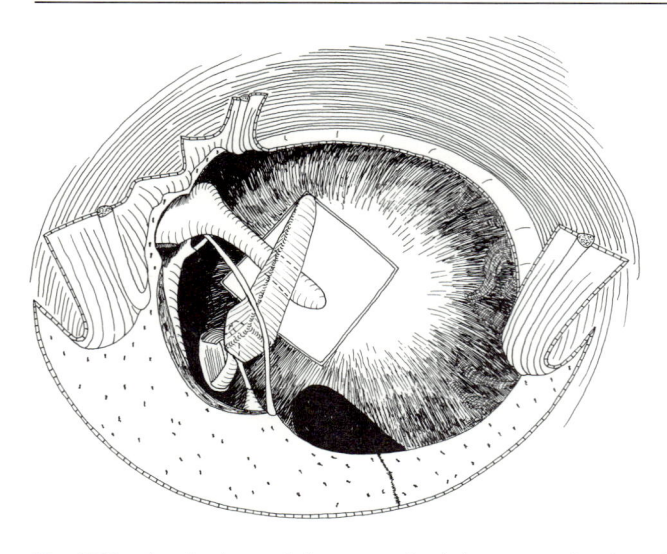

Fig. **780** An L-shaped long cortical bone prothesis, placed on the retracted malleus handle. A piece of Silastic is placed under the umbo

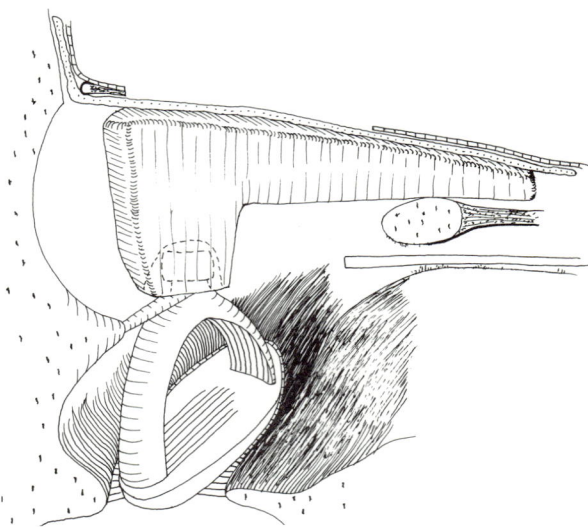

Fig. **781** Side view on the long L-shaped prosthesis in the retracted malleus handle with a hole for the head of the stapes. There is Silastic under the malleus handle

lateral part of the shaft, a groove is drilled, and the shaft is placed under the malleus handle. They claim better results with this technique than with interposition of the cortical bone between the head of the stapes and the malleus handle. To place a

columella between the facial prominence and the stapedial arch must, in long term, cause bony fixation of the prosthesis. On the other hand, Hüttenbrink (1992a) recently showed that a straight columella from the malleus handle to the footplate

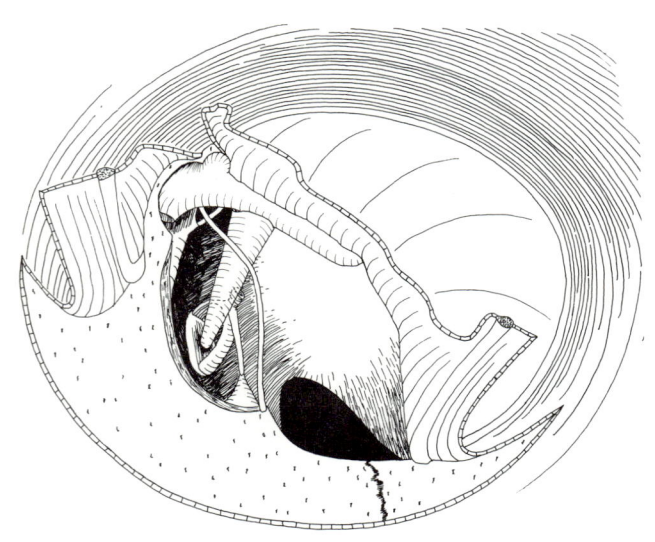

Fig. **782** A long shaft of cortical bone is placed between the malleus handle and the footplate in cases with intact stapes

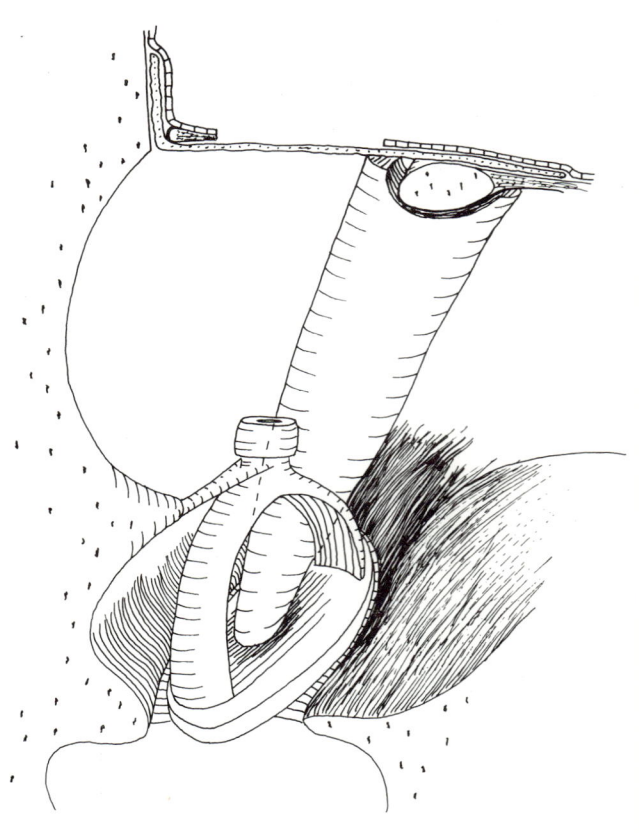

Fig. **783** Side view of the cortical bone columella ▷

experimentally produces better hearing than an oblique prosthesis going from the malleus handle to the head of the stapes.

Allogenous cortical bone has been harvested 12 hours after death from the tibia of a young adult (Gersdorff et al. 1986) and shaped as an incus replacement prosthesis or a total replacement prosthesis. The grafts are defatted in a 1:1 solution of chloroform–methanol. The cellular membranes are destroyed, and the lipids and lipoproteins are dissolved. After rinsing, the implants are freeze-dried and subsequently sterilized. The results obtained were better than with Ceravital.

Allogenous Stapes

Allogenous stapes can be interposed between the stapes and the drum. A hole is drilled in the middle of the allogenous footplate, and the stapes is placed on the autogenous arch and the stapedial tendon (Fig. **784**). The fascia is in contact with the head of the allograft stapes (Fig. **785**).

This method is seldom used, and it is hard to see any advantage in interposing all allogenous stapes instead of an incus body, malleus head, cartilage, or any other prosthesis; however, in type 3 tympanoplasty an allogenous stapes is often used as a columella in our hospital.

Cartilage

Autogenous and allogenous cartilage is relatively commonly used in tympanoplasty. It is easy to harvest and cut. Its disadvantage is that it may be too thin in one layer to bridge the gap between the head of stapes and the drum. In addition, the cartilage graft may become fibrotic after some years, with a progressive reduction in sound transmission. The great advantage of cartilage is that there is very little fibrotic fixation of the prosthesis to the surroundings, and, in contrast to bony prostheses or incus prostheses, there is no bony fixation with a cartilaginous prosthesis. A piece of cartilage can be placed close to the posterior bony annulus, pyramidal process, and facial prominence without fear of firm fixation. The cartilage is soon covered with mucosa (Glasscock and Shea 1967). Tragal cartilage, conchal cartilage and cartilage from the spine of the helix, septal cartilage, and rib cartilage can all be used.

Autogenous septal cartilage has seldom been used in tympanoplasty, despite the fact that harvesting a 5×6-mm piece of septal cartilage by

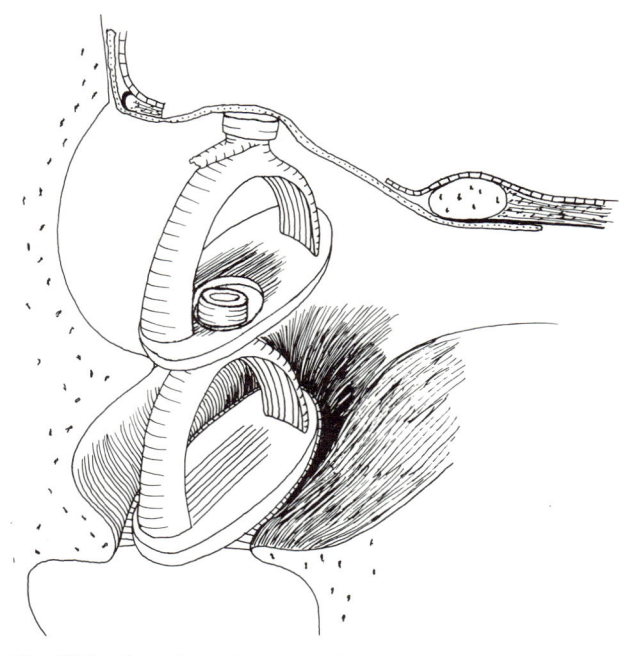

Fig. **784** An allograft stapes is placed on the stapes, riding on the stapedial tendon and stapedial arch

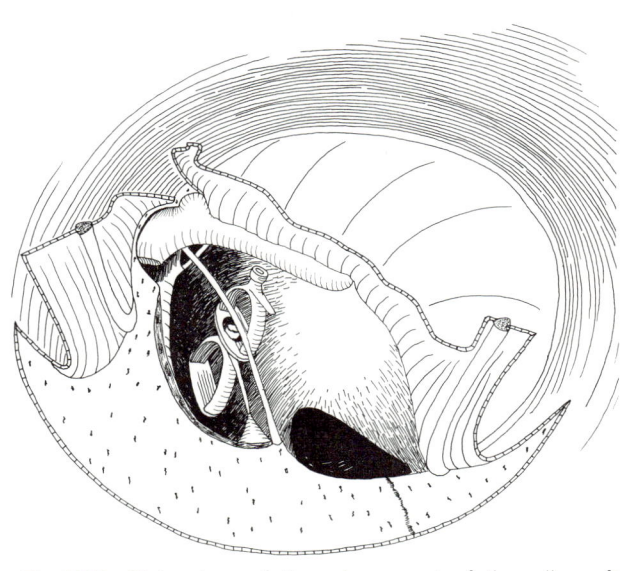

Fig. **785** Side view of the placement of the allograft stapes

an incision a few millimeters behind the columella is a simple, easy, and fast procedure. Allogenous septal cartilage has been used more often in tympanoplasty. As early as the late 1950s, Jansen (1963) used allogenous septal cartilage in type 2 tympanoplasty in cases with the stapes present, as a short T-prosthesis (Fig. **786**). He claimed that the septal cartilage has greater stability when compared

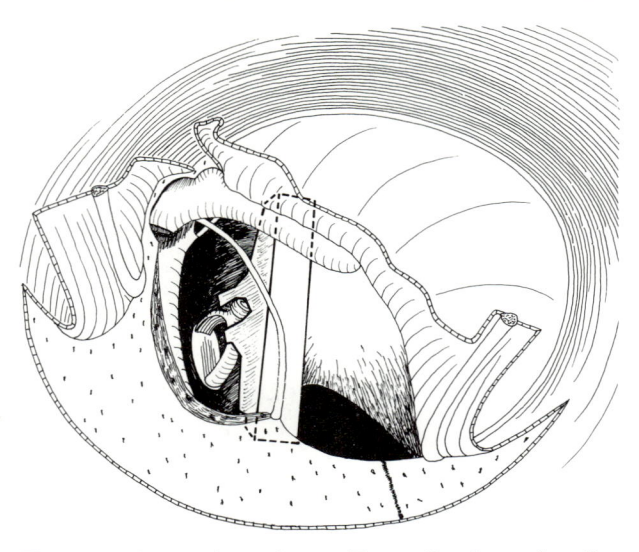

Fig. **786 Jansen's short T-prosthesis of allogeneous septal cartilage**, with a groove on the cartilage for the head of the stapes

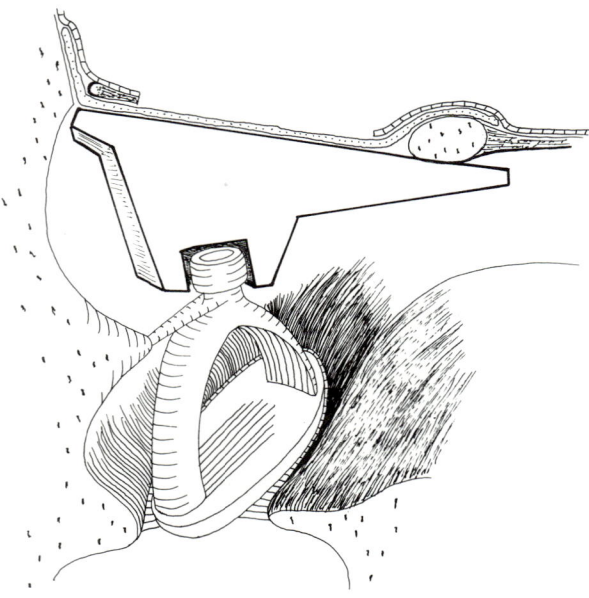

Fig. **787** Side view of the septal cartilage T-prosthesis, showing good contact with the drum

with conchal cartilage. There is no invasion of the cartilage by fibrous tissue, and the cartilage is soon covered with mucosa. The long horizontal portion of the T-prosthesis lies against the tympanic membrane and the malleus handle, and the prosthesis is fixed to the head of the stapes by a groove (Fig. **787**). Allogenous cartilage from the meniscus has also been used.

The author uses autogenous tragal cartilage for ossiculoplasty as the third choice of material, after autogenous and homogenous incus when using an endaural approach with the ear speculum, or after autogenous incus and cortical bone in the retroauricular approach.

Harvesting tragal cartilage was described above (Figs. **255–263**). The entire tragal cartilage can be harvested (Fig. **260**) and as well as a piece of cartilage for ossiculoplasty, its perichondrium can be used for myringoplasty. For an interposition graft, a 4×5-mm rectangular piece of cartilage is sufficient. A piece of this size can be excised from the lateral edge of the tragal cartilage, which is its thickest part. After exposing both sides of the lateral part of the tragal cartilage (Fig. **255**), two parallel incisions in the tragal cartilage are performed, and a rectangular piece is pulled in an anterior direction by a forceps (Fig. **788**) and excised using a scalpel.

The first surgeon to use tragal cartilage was Utech (1959, 1961), in the later 1950s. He placed a rectangular piece of the tragal cartilage on the stapes tendon. The piece of cartilage is brought into contact with the drum (Fig. **789**), and the prosthesis "rides" on the stapes tendon. Suzuki (1988) nowadays still uses this so-called "horse-rider" prosthesis, with good results. In a similar manner, Utech made a groove on the tragal cartilage plate for the head of the stapes (Fig. **790**). The plate is brought into contact with the drum or the fascia adjacent and parallel to the malleus handle. A more stable "horse-rider" tragal cartilage prosthesis is used by Glasscock and Shea (1967). The prosthesis is in contact with the stapes, anterior crus, malleus handle, and drum (Fig. **791**).

The most common tragal cartilage prosthesis is a 3×4-mm piece of cartilage placed on the head of the stapes, occupying the space between the malleus handle and the posterior bony annulus (Fig. **792**) (Spencer 1976). This type of prosthesis is sufficient in cases with a high stapes and a low tympanic cavity. In cases with a low stapes and a high tympanic cavity, two pieces of tragal cartilage have to be used. Only placing one piece of cartilage on the head of the stapes will cause the drum to be too low, and it may later lateralize (Fig. **793**), losing

Cartilage 279

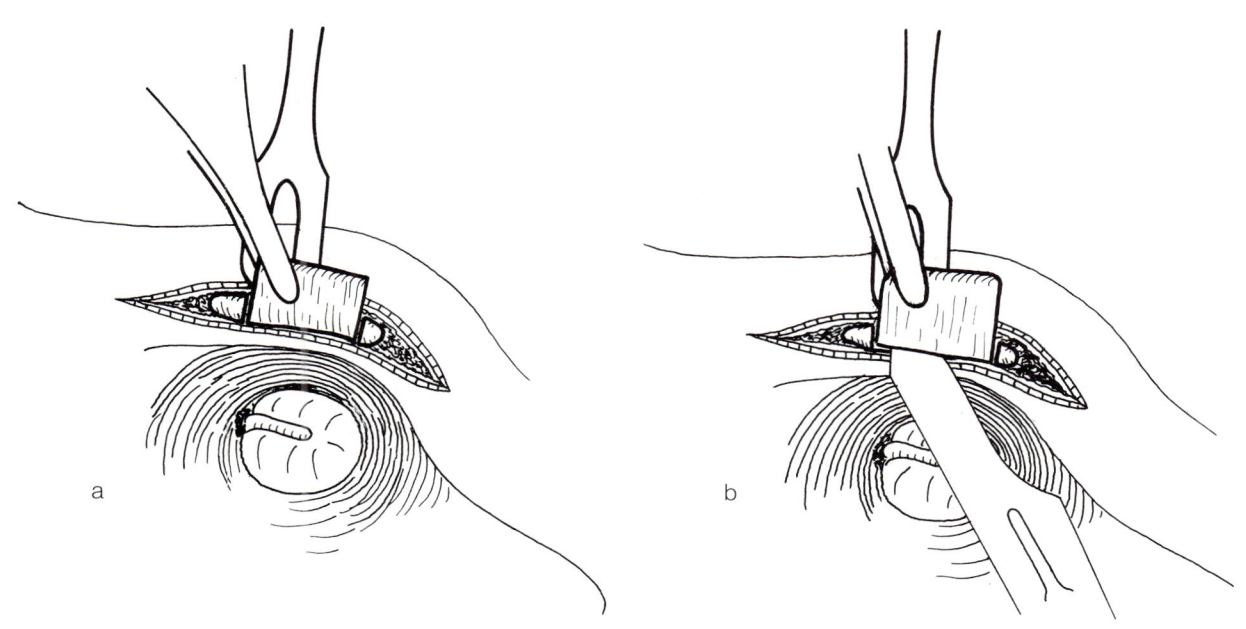

Fig. 788 Harvesting a small lateral piece of tragal cartilage. **a** After two incisions, the piece is pulled out and **b** excised with a scalpel

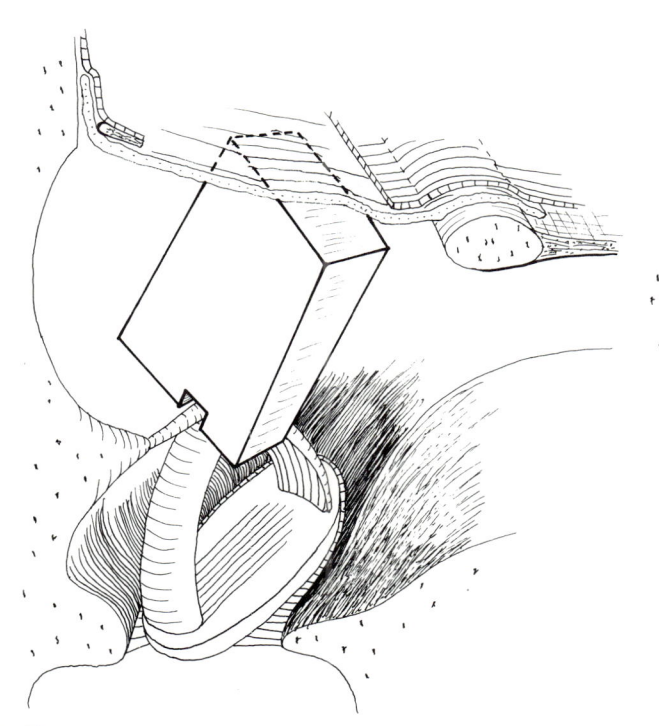

Fig. 789 The tragal cartilage prosthesis used by Utech, with a groove for the tendon of the stapes—the horse-rider prosthesis

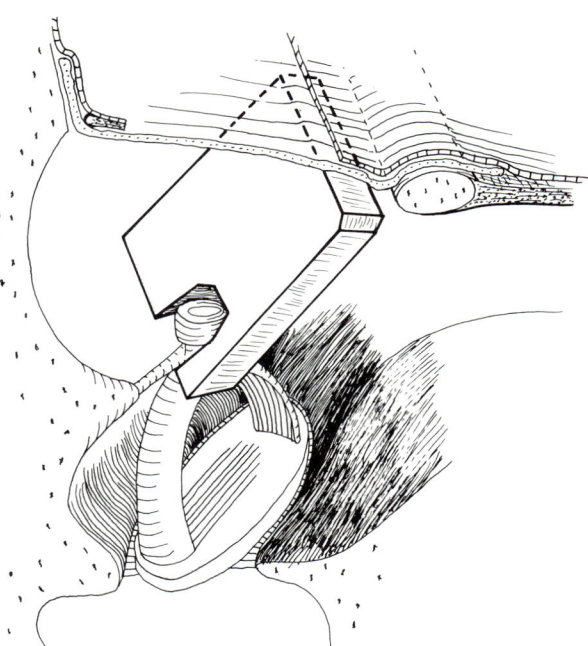

Fig. 790 Tragal cartilage, with a groove placed on the head of the stapes and parallel to the malleus handle

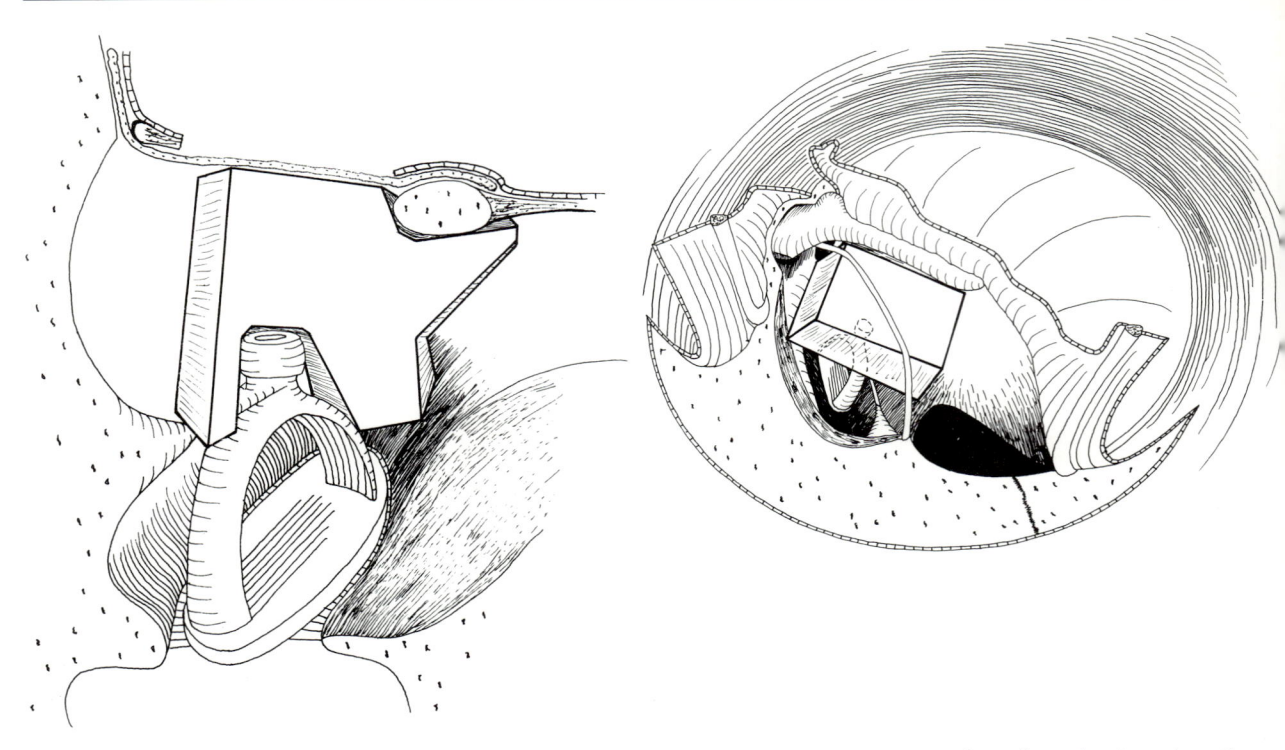

Fig. **791 Glasscock's tragal cartilage prosthesis,** with a groove for the head of the stapes and contact with the tendon of the stapes and the anterior crus

Fig. **792** A 3x4-mm piece of cartilage is placed on the head of the stapes

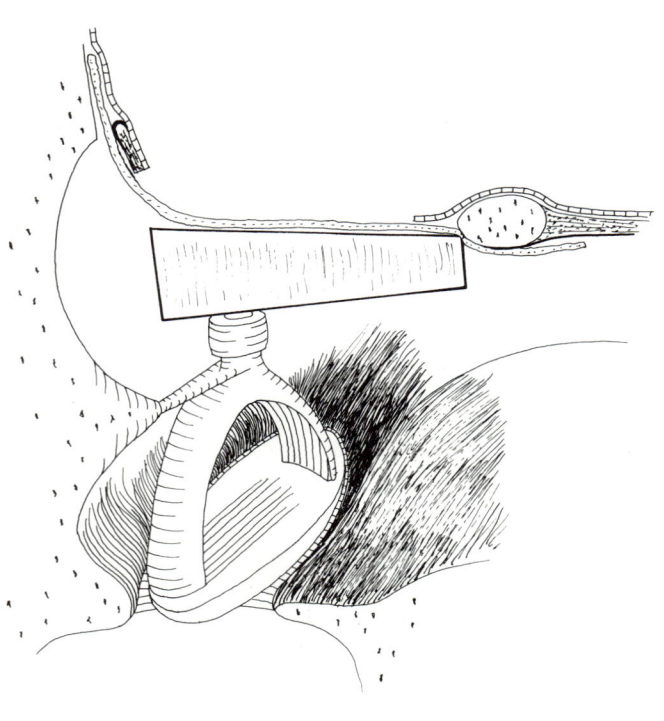

Fig. **793** Side view of the tragal cartilage, which may be positioned too low in cases with low stapes

contact with the graft. When two pieces of cartilage are placed, one piece can be placed on the head of the stapes and under the malleus handle, and the other, smaller, piece is placed on top of the larger one (Fig. **794**). In this way, the drum remains in its original position, and contact from the drum to the stapes is maintained (Fig. **795**).

A hole for the head of the stapes can be drilled using a small diamond burr, stabilizing the prosthesis, but this type of acetabulum may again cause the tragal prosthesis to lie in a lower position.

Heermann et al. (1970) and Heermann (1991) recommend an annulus–stapes cartilage plate of tragal or conchal cartilage, placed on the bony annulus at the 5-o'clock and 6-o'clock positions and on the head of the stapes (Fig. **796**). The prosthesis is positioned under the umbo. The perichondrium is attached to the cartilage on one side. This construction may be used as a part of Heermann's palisade myringoplasty.

Suzuki (1988) uses, and recommends the use of, cartilage from the spine of the helix as an interposition graft. Harvesting the spine of the helix is easy in an endaural approach with the Heermann, Lempert, Shambaugh, and other incisions, because the spine of the helix is easy to expose. The

Cartilage 281

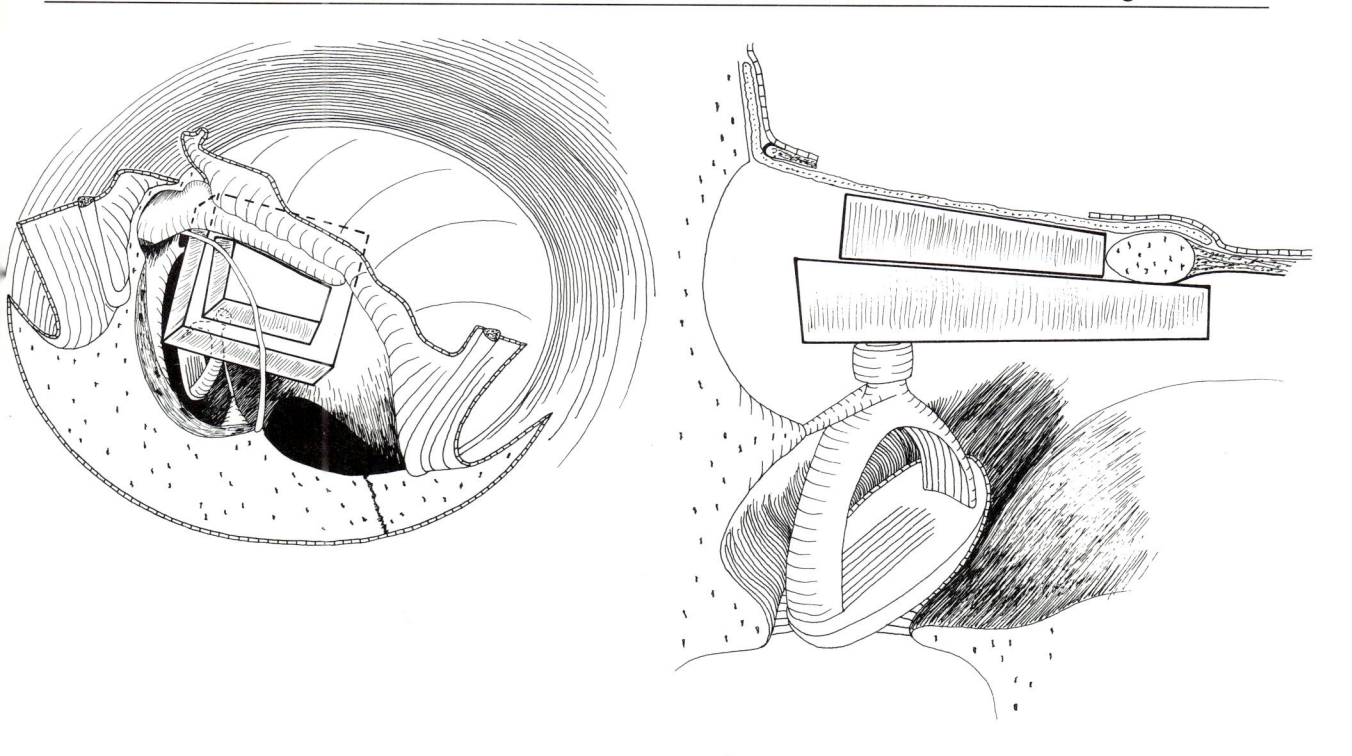

Fig. 794 Placement of two pieces of tragal cartilage, one on the head of the stapes, and the other, smaller one, on top of the larger one

Fig. 795 Side view of two pieces of the tragal cartilage prosthesis, with good contact both to the malleus handle and to the drum

exposed spine is excised with a scalpel, preserving the continuity of the helix. The cartilage of the spine of the helix is large enough for interposition (Fig. 797). Using the spine of the helix is recommended. In an endaural approach with the ear speculum, the spine of the helix can easily be exposed with a small separate skin incision. A hole is drilled for the head of the stapes, and the convexity of the spine is brought into contact with the drum (Figs. 798, 799).

The main problem associated with using cartilage in ossiculoplasty is its unpredictable degradation and loss of stability. The prosthesis will lose its stiffness and become softer after some years, mainly due to fibrous degeneration or resorption of the cartilage (Steinbach et al. 1992). In contrast to cartilage grafts, ossicular grafts have good long-term stability (Hildmann et al. 1992).

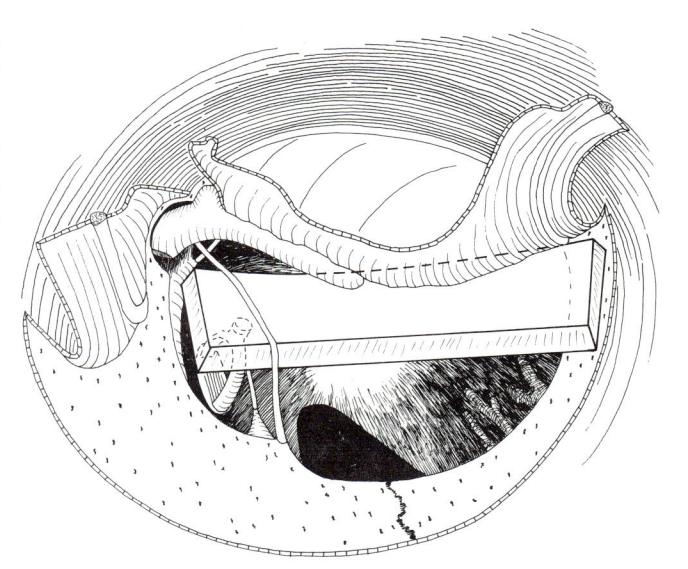

Fig. 796 **The Heermann annulus–stapes cartilage plate.** A large tragal or conchal cartilage plate is placed on the bony annulus at the 5–6-o'clock position and on the stapes head

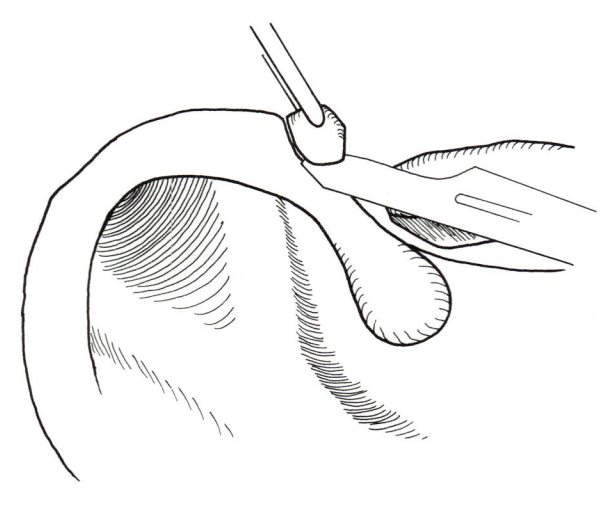

Fig. 797 Excision of the helix spine

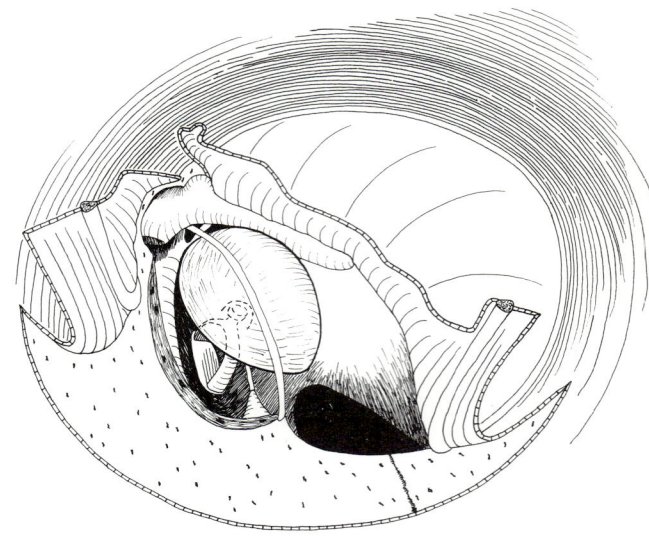

Fig. 798 The helix spine is placed on the head of the stapes

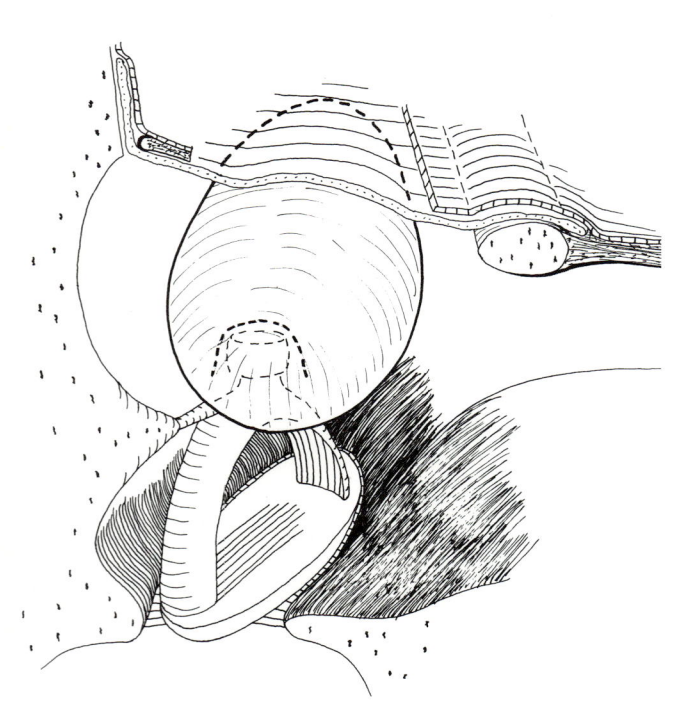

Fig. 799 Side view of the helix spine prosthesis, with a hole drilled for the head of the stapes. The cartilage prosthesis is placed parallel to the malleus handle

Allogenous Costal Cartilage Prostheses

Costal cartilage is stiffer than tragal or conchal cartilage, and is therefore more suitable for ossiculoplasty. Cole (1992) created a prosthesis from allogenous rib cartilage and found that this had several advantages:

1) Rib cartilage is easily obtainable from cadaver donors and up to 50 prostheses can be made from one cadaver.
2) The struts can be fashioned prior to surgery.
3) Preformed struts can be stored indefinitely in 70% alcohol.
4) The use of alloplastic material is avoided.
5) Allogenous cartilage is well tolerated in the human middle ear.
6) The strut made from the costal cartilage has a self-stabilizing shape, and is not as prone to displacement as the L-shaped cartilage struts.
7) Fixation of cartilage to the adjacent bony annulus does not seem to affect the resultant hearing in the way that fixation of allogenous bone does.
8) Extrusion of allograft cartilage from the human middle ear is a rare event.

The Cole technique for producing the struts is as follows. Rib cartilage is obtained from a cadaver, preferably a young person between 1-7 years of age. The cartilage is cut transversally into 8-mm long segments. Using a dermal punch 4-mm in diameter, a uniform 4-mm thick cylinder is made (Fig. **800a, b**). Using a 2-mm dermal punch pushed into the center of the 4-mm cartilage cylinder, and advanced to within 1-mm of the opposite round surface (Fig. **800c**), a new 2-mm cylinder is created. With a scalpel, the platform of the strut is excised (Fig. **800d**). The platform is exactly 1-mm thick, with a diameter of 4-mm, and the strut is 7-mm long (Fig. **800d**). After the distance between the stapes head and the drum has been measured, the strut is shortened to the size of a partial ossicular replacement prosthesis (PORP), and a hole is drilled into the costal cartilage (Fig. **801**). The strut is inserted on the head of the stapes (Fig. **802**). It is in broad contact with the drum, and has some contact with the malleus handle (Fig. **803**).

The preformed cartilage strut is sterilized by irradiation with cobalt 60, and then stored in 70% alcohol. Before use, the strut is washed in Ringer's solution for one hour in the operating room, and shaped to fit the individual distance between the head of the stapes and the tympanic membrane (Figs. **802, 803**). Since 50 prostheses can be made out of one person's rib, it is possible to eliminate the risk of HIV infection, especially as struts can be sterilized by irradiation.

Zini (1992) uses allogenous costal cartilage for most ossiculoplasties. The Zini PORP-C prosthesis is T-shaped, and has contact with the posterior bony annulus. The prosthesis is fibrotic, but has no osseous fixation to the posterior bony annulus (Fig. **804**). By moving the malleus handle or the drum, excellent sound transmission is achieved. This prosthesis is especially suitable in intact canal-wall mastoidectomies, and tympanoplasties with preserved bony wall. In canal-wall techniques, the effect of the fibrotic fixation of the prosthesis to the posterior bony wall is not produced.

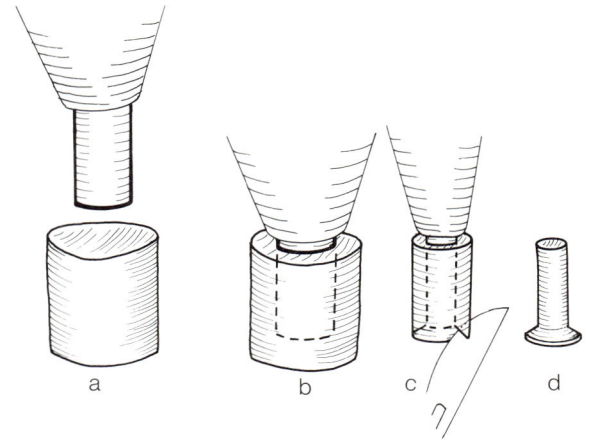

Fig. **800** **Cole's technique of preparing a costal strut. a** An 8-mm piece of costal cartilage is cut. **b** Using a 4-mm dermal punch, a 4-mm uniform cylinder of cartilage is cut out. **c** Using a 2-mm dermal punch, a small strut is cut out. Cutting stops 1-mm before the punch comes through, and the last millimeter provides the platform of the strut. The platform is cut with a scalpel. **d** The platform is 1-mm thick, and has a diameter of 4-mm

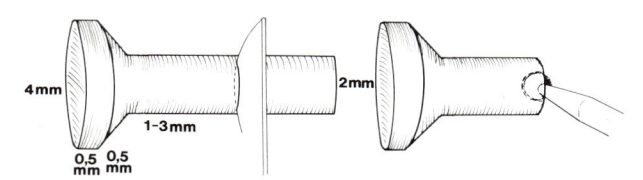

Fig. **801** Measurement and cutting of the allogenous concha strut to a PORP, and drilling a hole with a diamond drill for the head of the stapes

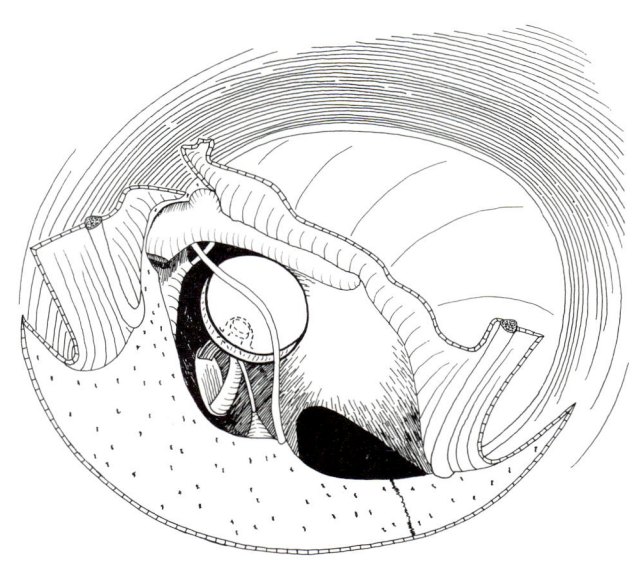

Fig. **802** The allogenous concha PORP is inserted onto the head of the stapes

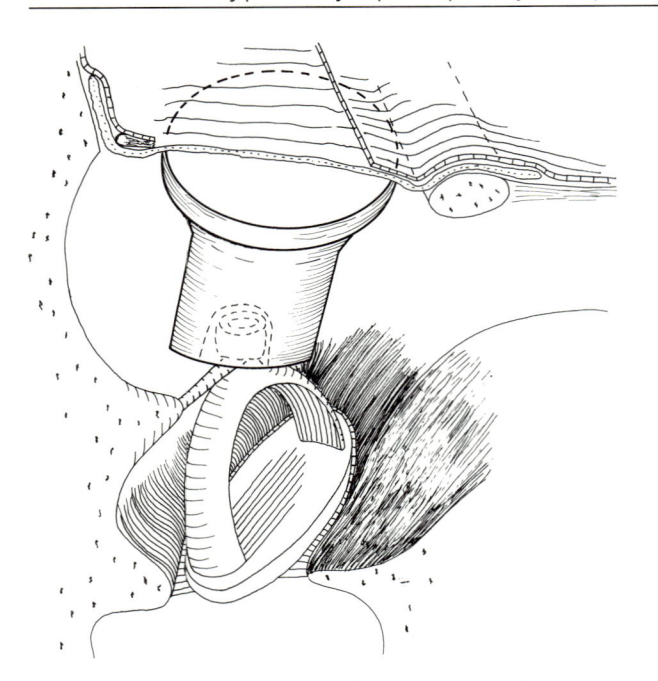

Fig. 803 Side view of the allogenous costal cartilage PORP, with broad contact to the drum and some contact to the malleus handle

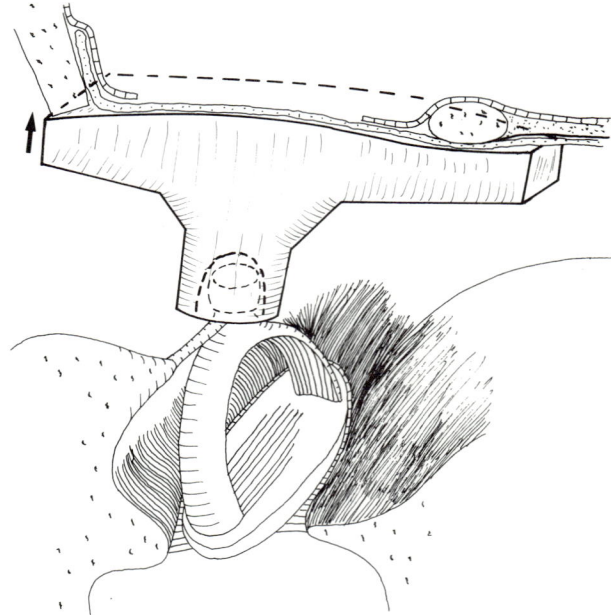

Fig. 804 **The Zini T-shaped allogenous costa cartilage prosthesis** (PORP-C), placed on the head of the stapes and under the posterior bony annulus (arrow), offering good stability and sound transmission

Allogenous Dentin Prostheses

Dentin was introduced into ossiculoplasty by Zini (1970), and independently by Gibb and Steward (1972). Dentin, with 20% organic material, lies between bone and enamel in its mineral content and hardness. Its inorganic component consists mainly of calcium apatite. Prostheses from dental roots can be easily shaped using a diamond drill, and the shaping is in principle the same as it that described below for ceramic and cement prostheses. Teeth have some potential advantages in ossiculoplasty: a) they are readily available, even from heterogenous sources; b) they are easy to shape; and c) they have little bioactivity and produce no bone formation. Degradation and resorption probably take place (Gibb and Steward 1972), and this may be the reason why teeth are not used in ossiculoplasty more often.

17 Type 2 Tympanoplasty with Biocompatible Materials

Since the origin of ossiculoplasty at the beginning of the 1960s, several synthetic biocompatible materials have been introduced as incus replacement prostheses. A short review of the first published prostheses illustrates that the shaft shape of the prosthesis used 30 years ago was basically the same as that used today. There have been improvements in the newer materials in the shape of the prosthesis platform, resulting in better contact with the drum.

Synthetic Biomaterials: Polyethylene, Teflon

Synthetic biomaterials such as polyethylene or compact Teflon were the first prostheses used. Shea (1958) used polyethylene prostheses as a replacement for stapes crura in stapedectomy.

As an incus replacement prosthesis, polyethylene was used by Harrison (1960, 1969), Portmann (1963), Guilford (1964), Sheehy (1965), Siedentop and Brown (1966), and others. The prostheses were tube-shaped, with (Fig. **805a**) or without (Fig. **805b**) a platform, with a sunflower-type platform (Fig. **805c**), or a mushroom type (Fig. **806**), or as a groove for the head of the malleus.

Several polyethylene tube prostheses were in use during the 1960s (Fig. **807**). The incudostapedial joint prosthesis for small defects of the long process of the incus (Fig. **807a**) is a polyethylene tube inserted onto the remnant of the long process. A hole was made on the side of the tube for the head of the stapes. In another modification (Fig. **807d**), the polyethylene tube was partly cut, and its lower end rotated perpendicularly and brought into contact with the head of the stapes. The stapes–malleus prosthesis (Fig. **807b**) was fixed to the undersurface of the neck of the malleus, or the malleus handle, and to the stapes. A prosthesis with a small platform facing the undersurface of the drum, or placed between the two ossicles, was used in cases of dislocated incus (Fig. **807c**). The long process of the luxated incus was pushed up laterally under the drum by a small strut inserted between the head of stapes and the lenticular process, resulting in a myringoincudopexy.

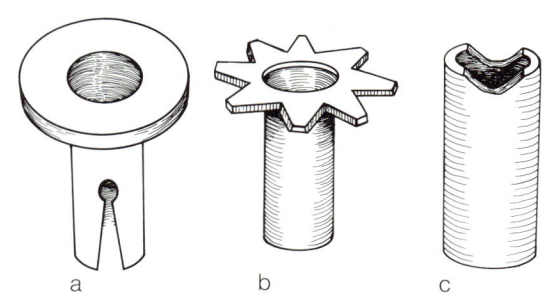

Fig. **805** Polyethylene prostheses used in the early 1960s, as incus replacement prosthesies between the head of the stapes and the drum or malleus handle. **a** A tube with a round platform and a slit for the stapes, **b** A tube with a sunflower-shaped platform, to be placed under the drum. **c** A tube with a groove, to be placed between the head of the stapes and the malleus handle

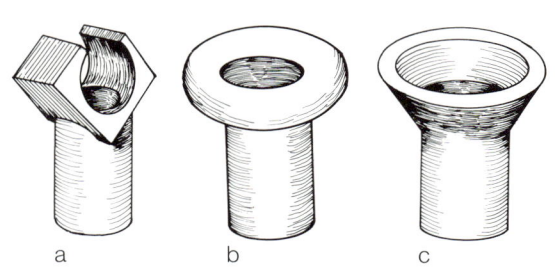

Fig. **806 a** Stapes–malleus prosthesis, with the head of the prosthesis to be fixed under the neck of the malleus. **b, c** Polyethylene tubes with mushroom-type platforms

The extrusion rate was extremely high with polyethylene prostheses—30–50% within the first year and 70% within the first three years—and they were therefore abandoned. Polyethylene shafts have, for some years, been used in composite prostheses, i.e., together with incus or cortical bone.

The author only used polyethylene in a few cases in the early 1960s, mainly in cases of traumatic incus dislocation. The prostheses were placed between the two ossicles (Fig. **807b, c**) with excellent initial results, but even in these cases the long-term results were not reliable. Due to the stiffness of the polyethylene, the head of the stapes or the anterior crus of the stapes became resorbed after long-term contact with the polyethylene.

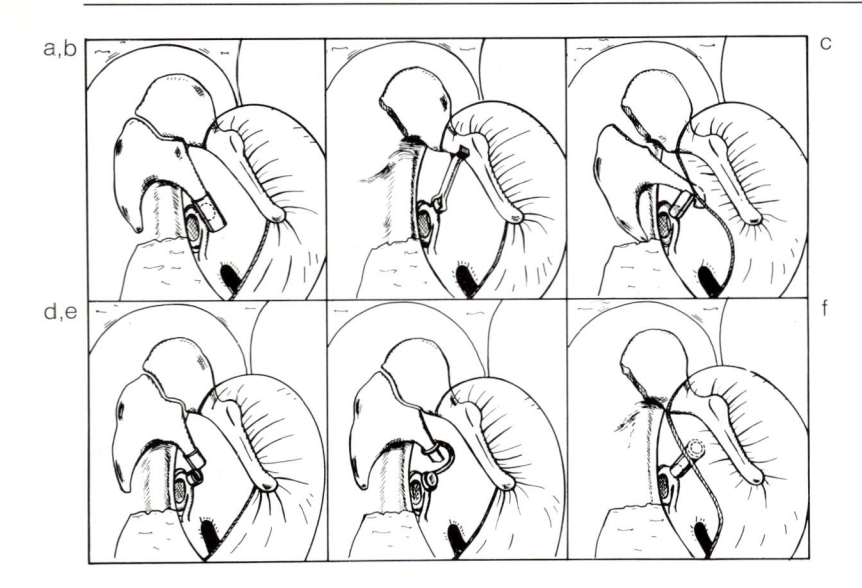

Fig. 807 Sketches from the mid-1960s, of some polyethylene tube prostheses. **a, d** Incudostapedial joint prostheses. **b** The malleostapediopexy prosthesis. **c** A polyethylene tube between the head of the stapes and a luxated incus, pushing the lenticular process laterally and making contact with the drum. **e** An incudostapediopexy prosthesis with a wire. **f** A tube with a small platform, placed between the head of the stapes and the drum

Porous Plastic

Porous plastics include porous polyethylene, Proplast (Vitek Inc., Houston), Teflon plus vitrified carbon, Plasti-Pore (Smith and Nephew, Richards Medical Company, Memphis), pure polyethylene, and Polycel Xomed-Treace Company, Memphis). The essential property of these materials is their porous structure, which enables them in principle to be infiltrated by living tissue, leading to effective integration and biocompatibility.

Proplast was introduced into otology by Shea (Shea and Homsy 1974). In 1978, he abandoned Proplast in favor of Plasti-Pore, a high-density polyethylene sponge (Shea and Emmet 1978). Partial ossicular replacement prostheses (PORPS) have been produced in several shapes. The shaft is tubular (Figs. **808, 809**), and the platform can be either thick or thin. Usually, sharp edges on the platform are avoided. There are combinations of a polyethylene or Teflon tube and a Plasti-Pore platform, or a fluoroplastic tube and a hydroxyapatite platform (Fig. **810**).

Porous plastic also tended to extrude, even when covered with cartilage slices. For a time, porous plastic was used in direct contact with the drum, but today placement of porous plastic in contact with the drum has been largely abandoned by most surgeons. Nearly all surgeons recommend cartilage covering of Polycel prostheses, because of their high extrusion rate, which is about 10%, but Shea still uses it without cartilage covering. He believes that cartilage interferes with tissue ingrowth into the Plasti-Pore prostheses.

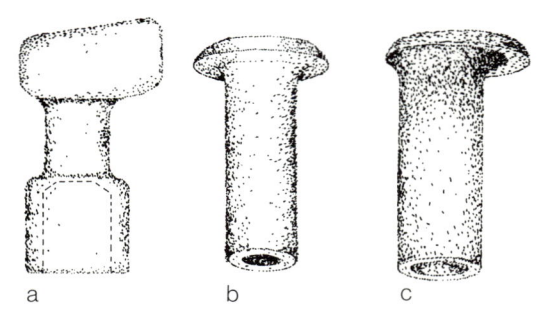

Fig. **808** Some Polycel prostheses. **a** Malleus to stapes strut, as endorsed by. Shea. **b** Sheehy's PORP prosthesis. **c** Austin prosthesis, with the head off-center from the shaft

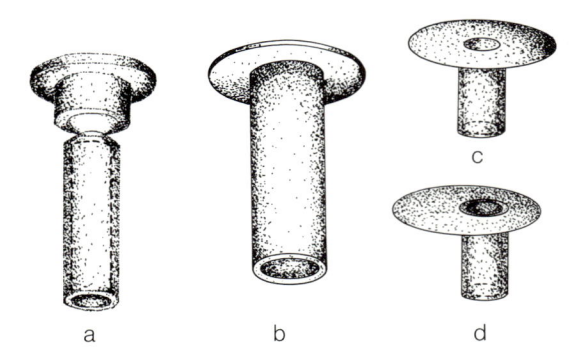

Fig. **809** Plasti-Pore prostheses. **a** Multi-PORP prosthesis. **b, c** Sheehy's PORP prosthesis, with a thin head. **d** Sheehy's prosthesis, with the head off-center from the shaft

Porous Plastic

Sheehy uses a Plasti-Pore PORP routinely, but covers it with a thin slice of cartilage. When a piece of tragal cartilage is put on a plate and held with a finger, it can be cut into thin slices with a concave shape (Fig. 811). A PORP with an angulated and asymmetrically placed platform (Smith and Nephew, Richards Medical Company) is placed on the head of the stapes (Fig. 812) and covered with a slice of cartilage. The convex side of the slice is in contact with the drum or fascia (Fig. 813).

In a special Polycel prosthesis (Xomed-Treace Company), the platform consists of a groove for the malleus handle. The prosthesis is placed on the head of the stapes and the groove under the malleus handle, so that any contact with the drum is completely avoided (Fig. 814).

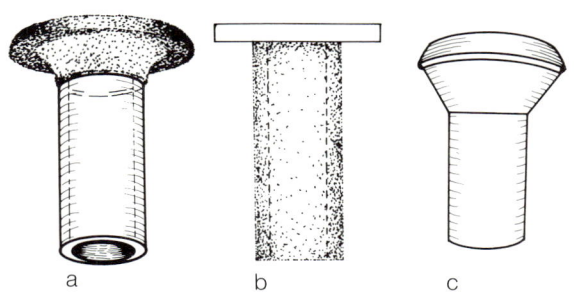

Fig. **810** PORP prostheses with combined materials. **a** Teflon shaft and Polycel head. **b** Plasti-Pore shaft and hydroxyapatite head. **c** Fluoroplastic and hydroxyapatite (Shea)

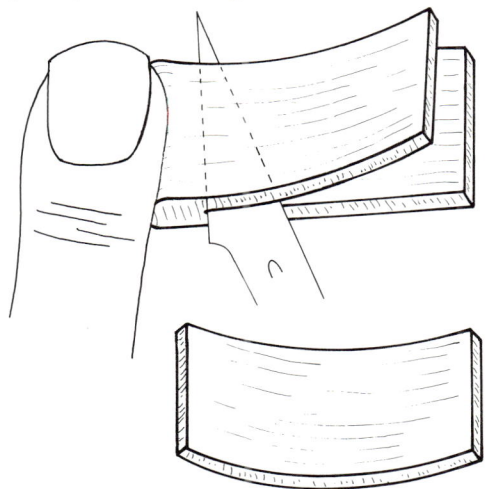

Fig. **811** **Sheehy's method of slicing tragal cartilage**

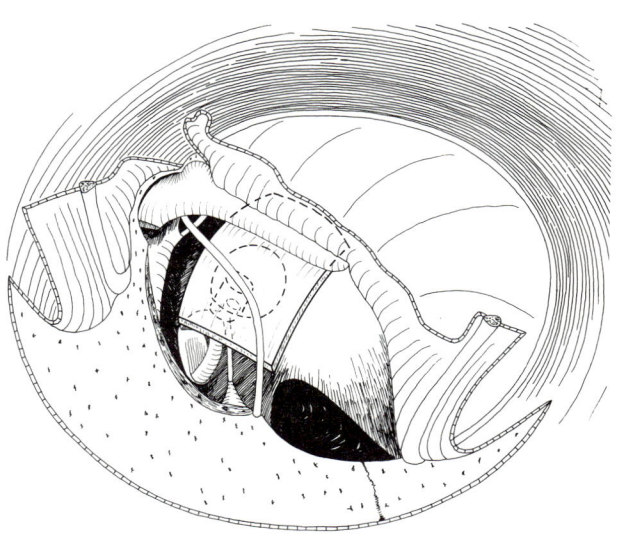

Fig. **812** A Plasti-Pore PORP with an angulated and asymmetrically placed platform covered with cartilage slice (Sheehy)

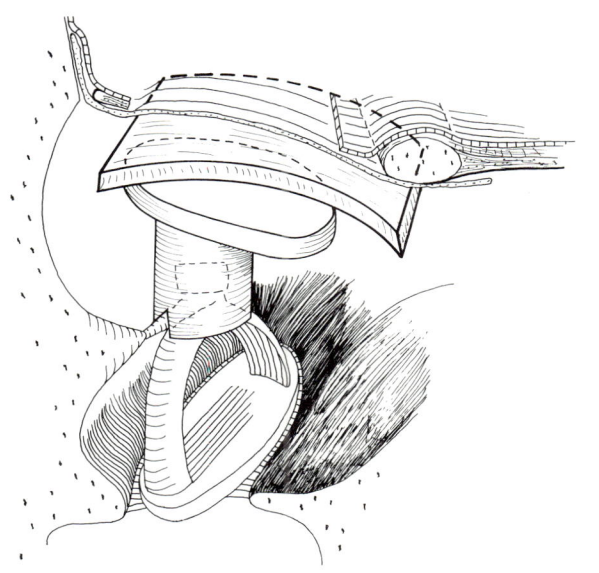

Fig. **813** Side view of the PORP, showing the connection between the cartilage and the drum

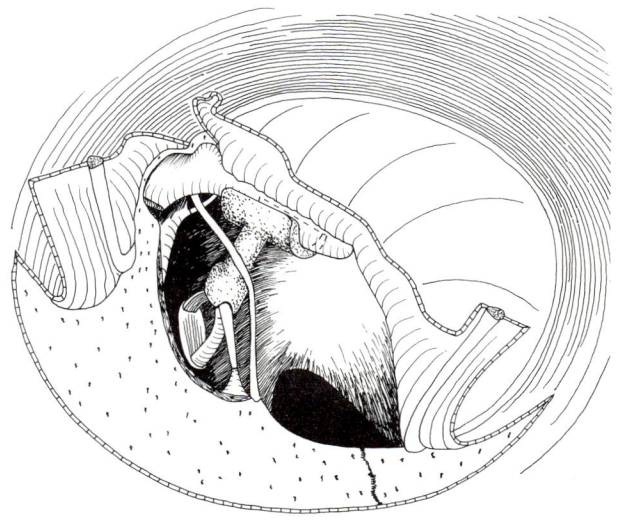

Fig. **814** Polycel prostheses placed between the head of the stapes and the malleus handle

Jackson and Glasscock (Jackson et al. 1983) recommend suturing the tragal cartilage to the platform of a total ossicular replacement prosthesis (TORP) or partial ossicular replacement prosthesis (PORP) as follows (Fig. 815). A curved needle with a 6-0 silk suture is stitched through the Plasti-Pore platform on one side of the shaft (Fig. 815a). The needle goes through the tragal cartilage plate (Fig. 815b) and returns again through the cartilage plate and through the platform on the other side of the shaft (Fig. 815c). The ends of the silk thread are sutured along the shaft and under the platform. The remaining cartilage is cut off with a scalpel (Fig. 815d). Sometimes fixing the prothesis and the cartilage with forceps can damage the cartilage or the prosthesis, and the following modification of the method just described can therefore be used. The cartilage and the prosthesis are placed on the edge of the plate and fixed gently with forceps. A needle is introduced on the right side of the shaft from above, through the platform and the cartilage (Fig. 816a). The needle then goes back from below, along the edge of the supporting plate, up through the cartilage and the platform (Fig. 816b) After the cartilage has been sutured to the platform, the remaining cartilage can easily be cut with a scalpel without damaging the prosthesis (Figs. 816c, d, 817).

Sanna et al. (1982) found that, at 6–24 months after surgery, there was a 15% extrusion rate in the group without cartilage covering, against 2% for those with covering. The same extrusion rate occurred with PORPS as with TORPS. Late results of Plasti-Pore are generally unavailable, but the impression is that few reports will stand the test of time. Smyth (1982) found an 11% extrusion rate in the long term (five years) and a 56% failure rate (air–bone gap closure within 10dB) with PORP and 78% with TORP).

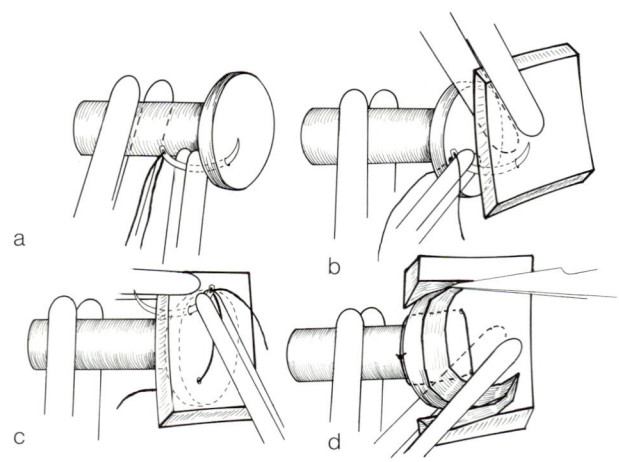

Fig. 815 **The Jackson and Glasscock method of fixing the cartilage slice to the PORP. a** A needle with the silk goes through the platform and the PORP, **b** through the cartilage plate, **c** returns on the other side of the shaft through the cartilage and platform, and is sutured. **d** The remaining part of the cartilage is cut off

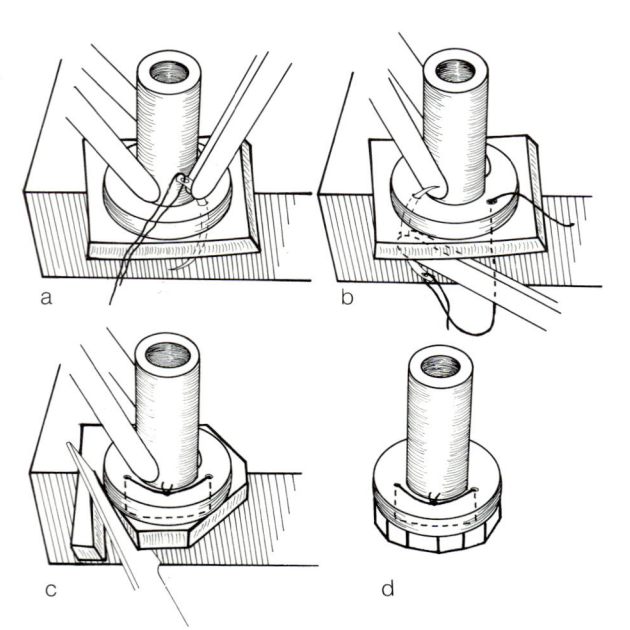

Fig. 816 An alternative way of fixing the cartilage plate to the platform of a PORP. **a** The cartilage and the prosthesis are placed on the edge of a plate. **b** A needle is brought through and returned. **c** The silk is sutured, and **d** the remaining cartilage is cut off with a knife (D)

Ceramics

During the 1980s, ceramics, which were by then widely used in dental surgery, became popular and are now extensively used in otosurgery as well. Ceramics are nonorganic crystalline materials. Initially, the powder is compressed under high-pressure and high-temperature conditions (1000 to 1300 °C). Ceramics are good thermal insulators, but they are fragile, and have to be shaped carefully with a diamond drill under constant irrigation. Their other main properties are:

They have good biocompatibility, with no toxic or inflammatory reactions.

Their porosity varies from 5–600 µm. If the pores have a diameter of at least 100 µm, living tissue, especially bone tissue, can invade the ceramics.

Their biodegradability varies from nil for aluminum oxides to total for certain calcium phosphates, which are absorbed in a few months.

Their bioactivity depends on the type of ceramic. Some are very active, with intense osteogenesis around the implant (bioactive ceramics), while others are totally bioinert. In ossiculoplasty, both bioinert and bioactive ceramics are used.

Bioinert Ceramics

In ossiculoplasty, bioinert ceramics such as Frialit (Friedrichsfeld Company, Germany), made of aluminum dioxide (Al_2O_3) have been introduced and used by Jahnke et al. (1979) and Jahnke and Plester (1980). Another example is Bioceram (Kyocera Company, Japan), which was introduced by Yamamoto (1982, 1985).

The shaft of the Frialit ceramic is a tube (Fig. **817**). It should be shortened to the proper length with a diamond drill under constant irrigation. It is best to hold the implant with two fingers without gloves during drilling (Fig. **818**). Fixation can also be carried out using a forceps covered with plastic, but the graft should not come into direct contact with the metal. The drilling should be gentle, without pressure on the ceramics material.

The implant should always be shaped by drilling to the required dimensions in order to achieve exact position, good stability, and optimal physiological conditions. On the platform, one groove can be deepened and broadened in order to prevent slipping of the malleus handle (Figs. **818, 819**). In the groove, the blood vessels are located. By drilling small holes into the platform, the attachment of the prosthesis to the tympanic membrane can be improved through the subsequent ingrowth

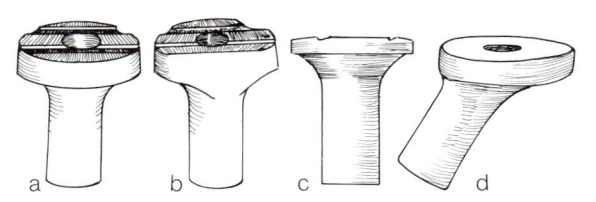

Fig. **817** The first generation of bioinert aluminum oxide ceramic PORPs. Straight hollow-shafted PORPs with round heads (**a, c**) or an oval head (**b**). **d** The prosthesis with an angulated shaft

Fig. **818** Shaping the platform of a PORP by drilling a large groove for it to fit under the malleus handle. The prosthesis is held by two fingers without gloves, and drilled

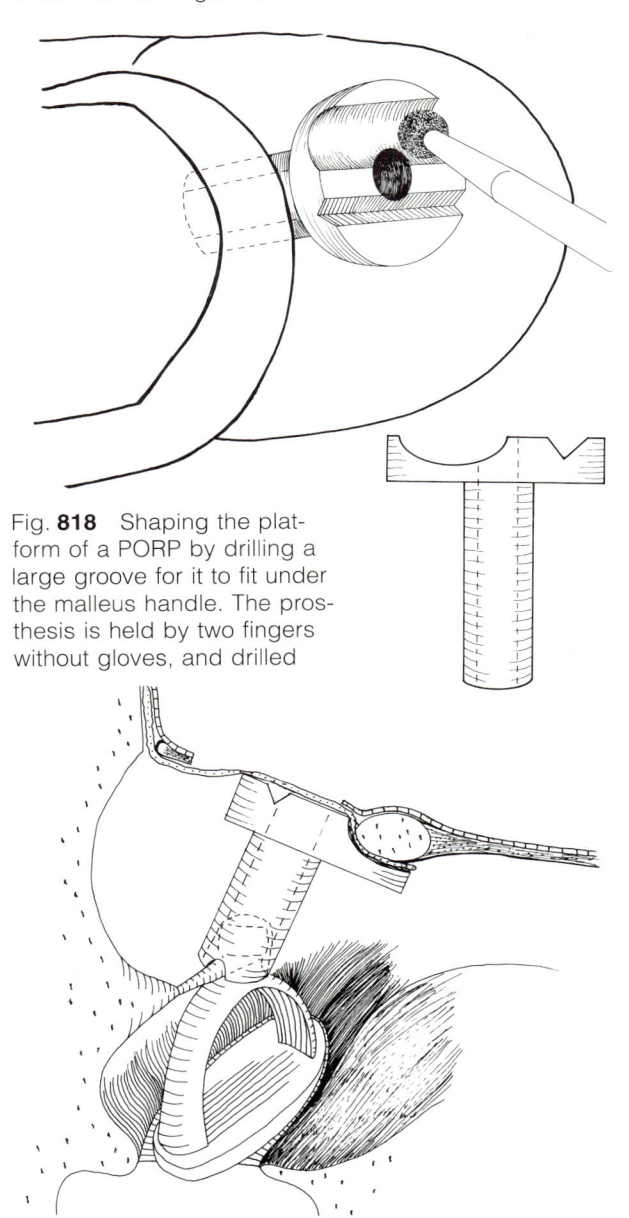

Fig. **819** A Frialit ceramic prosthesis with a hollow shaft is placed on the head of the stapes, and one groove of the platform is widened to be adapted to the malleus handle. A groove is made for the stapedial muscle tendon

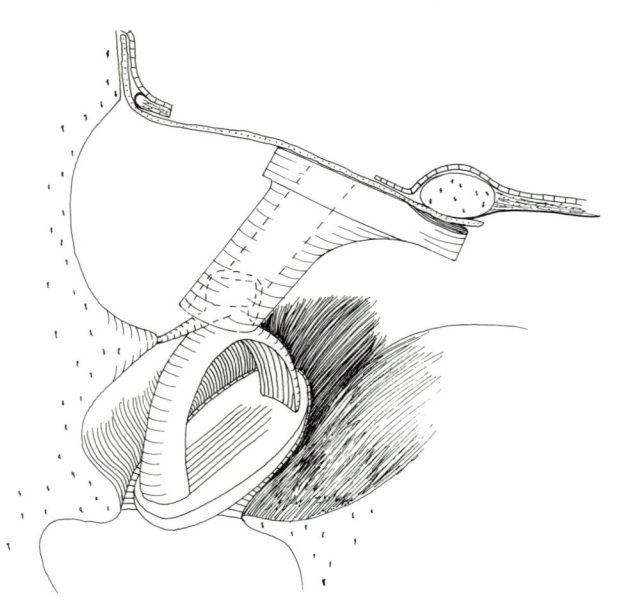

Fig. 820 An angled Frialit ceramic PORP prosthesis, for use when there is a large distance between the malleus handle and the head of the stapes

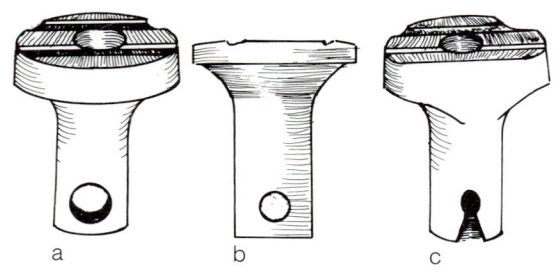

Fig. 822a, b The second generation of Frialit ceramic prostheses, with grooves on the oval-shaped platforms and small holes in the side of the hollow shaft. **c** The CORP-P Bioceram prosthesis, with an oval-shaped head

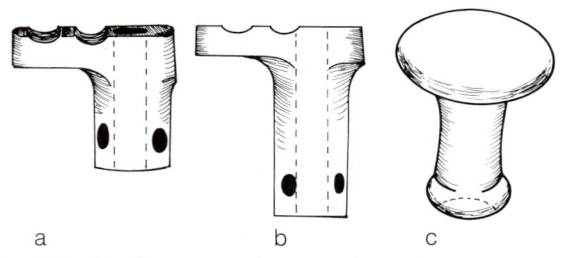

Fig. 822a, b The second generation of Frialit ceramic prostheses, with grooves on the oval-shaped platforms and small holes in the side of the hollow shaft. **c** The CORP-P Bioceram prosthesis, with an oval-shaped head

of fibrous tissue into the holes. In cases with an atrophic drum, the prosthesis should be covered with cartilage.

The connection between the rigid prosthesis and the head of the stapes results in a joint-like linkage (Jahnke and Plester 1981). The attachment to the head of the stapes can be improved by drilling a groove into the shaft in such a way that the implant can be placed on the tendon of the stapedius muscle (Fig. **819**). In cases with a long distance between the malleus handle and the head of the stapes, a prosthesis with an angled shaft can be used (Fig. **820**), or a large piece of cartilage can be placed on the platform of the ceramic prosthesis. The prosthesis is covered by a thin layer of epithelium within three weeks, and healing is completed after four weeks. No foreign body reaction has been seen.

With a retracted malleus, cutting the tendon of the tensor tympani muscle and elevating the handle with interposition of the prosthesis is recommended. Jahnke and Plester reported better primary results with ceramics than with porous plastic prostheses.

Recognizing that there are problems with the stability of the connection between the head of the stapes and the stiff ceramic prosthesis, as well as with the medial anchorage of the implant in general, Jahnke (1988) proposed drilling large holes in the end of the shaft (Fig. **821**), to facilitate ingrowth of fibrous tissue from outside the shaft to the head of the stapes. A keyhole-like notch made in the end of the shaft is considered to improve the fitting of prostheses to the tendon of the stapedial muscle. Jahnke recommends filling all of the hollow shaft with fibrous tissue.

In the second generation of Frialit ceramics (Jahnke 1992), the manufacturer provides various small holes, produced by an industrial laser beam. The holes are placed distally in the hollow shaft at various levels, allowing shortening of the shaft without removing all the holes (Fig. **822**). During the operation, the shaft is filled with fibrous tissue partly through the large hole, and partly through the small holes on the side of the shaft (Fig. **823**). This is performed with a small hook or a thin needle (Fig. **824**). The prosthesis is shaped to fit underneath the malleus handle. It is recommended to drill off all sharp edges of the prosthesis that might have possible contact with the drum.

Jahnke (1992) uses ceramics in 40% of tympanoplasties, but covers the majority of the prostheses with cartilage. Long-term results for major series are still lacking. Jahnke and Swan (1991) reported good hearing improvement in 99 ears 1–6 years postoperatively.

Ceramics

Yamamoto uses CORP-P (ceramic ossicular replacement prosthesis—partial) (Bioceram, Kyocera Company, Japan). The prosthesis permits smooth contact with the fascia graft and prevents extrusion. The base, which contacts the stapes, is disk-shaped, with a longer diameter than the shaft (Fig. **822c**). The base has a depression which fits easily and exactly onto the stapes head. The CORP-P has various shaft lengths—3, 4, and 5 mm. Yamamoto uses ceramics in combination with microslices of allogenous septal cartilage in open canal wall–down mastoidectomy (Figs. **623–626**). In cases with the stapes present but with a missing malleus handle, a CORP-P is fitted to the head of the stapes (Fig. **825**). A large piece of allogenous cartilage slice with a slit, placed under the annulus, covers the whole tympanic cavity, the attic, and the aditus and antrum. The head of the prosthesis protrudes through the slit (Fig. **826**). The cartilage and the prosthesis is covered with a large piece of fascia extending to the bony walls of the cavity (Figs. **827, 828**).

Yamamoto (1987) achieved good results with these techniques, with air–bone gap closure within 10 dB one year postoperatively in 45%, and 3–4 years postoperatively in 42%. The CORP-P was extruded in 8% of the ears. During repeat surgery for patients with unsatisfactory hearing, displacement of the prostheses was found. Yamamoto claims the following advantages with the prostheses: the convex head allows smooth contact with the fascia graft; the graft can be seen on X-rays, and the position of the prosthesis evaluated; no bony fixation on the graft occurs; and initial and long-term results are stable. Shinkawa and Sakai (1992) reported similar results.

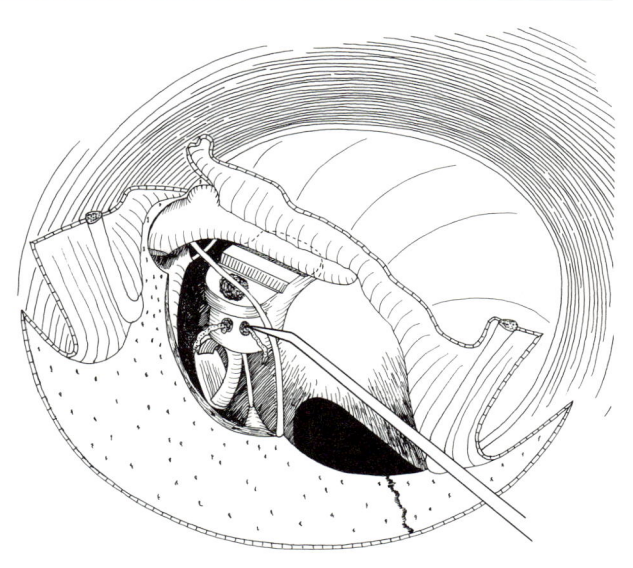

Fig. **823** Placement of a PORP Frialit ceramic on the head of the stapes. with a needle, fibrous tissue is pushed into the small holes. The large hole is filled with fibrous tissue

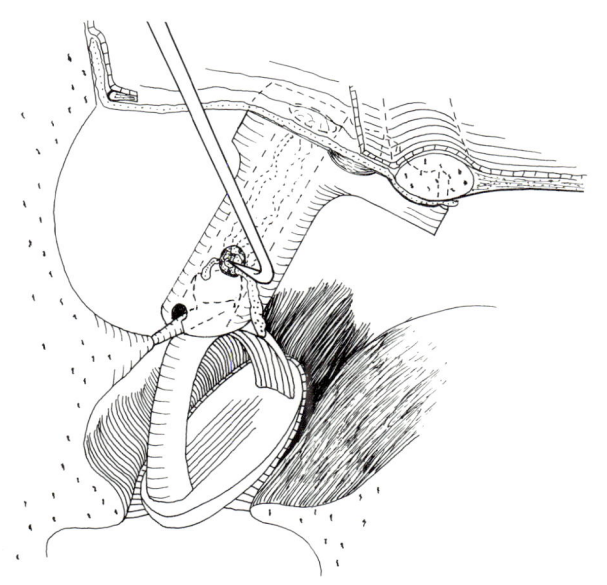

Fig. **824** Side view, showing the fibrous tissue in the hollow shaft

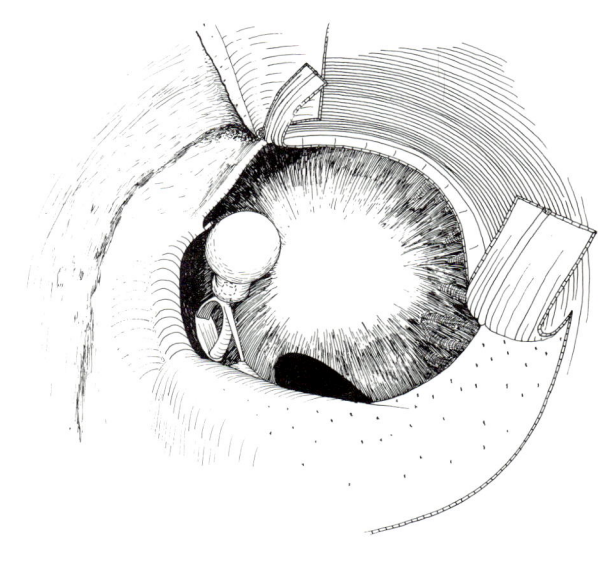

Fig. **825 Yamamoto's method.** A situation in a canal wall–down mastoidectomy, with the stapes present and an absent malleus handle. The CORP-P ceramic prosthesis (Yamamoto) is placed on the head of stapes

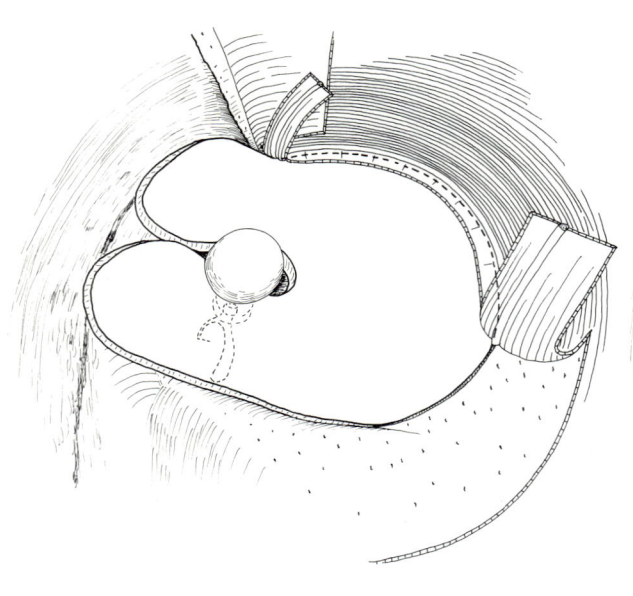

Fig. 826 The total perforation, the attic, and the aditus and antrum are covered with a slice of homogeneous septal cartilage, with the prosthesis protruding through a superiorly positioned slit

Fig. 827 The cartilage slice is covered with a large fascia, placed as an underlay graft, and extended over the walls of the cavity

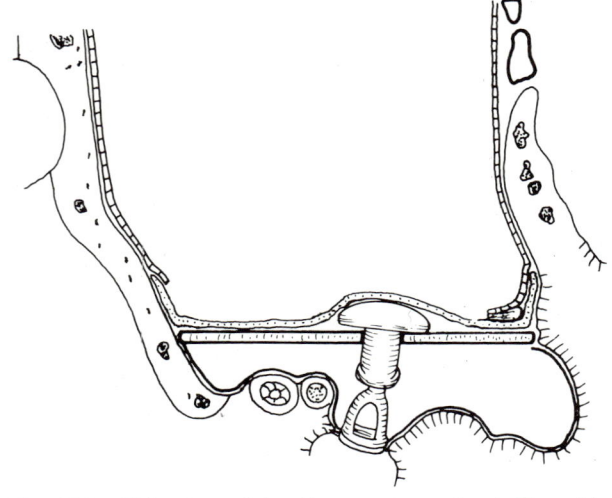

Fig. 828 Side view of the Yamamoto method. The attic and tympanic cavity are covered with cartilage. The head of the prosthesis protrudes through the slit. The cartilage is covered with fascia

Bioactive Ceramics

Bioactive ceramics are capable of establishing an ionic balance with the surrounding tissue, stimulating growth of bone that is in contact with them. This group consists of glass ceramics and calcium-phosphate ceramics.

Glass ceramics contain silicon dioxide (SiO_2) and are very similar to glass. In this category, products available are Macor (Smith and Nephew, Richards Company), Bioglass (USA) and Ceravital (Xomed Company, Jacksonville, USA).

Ceravital was introduced by Reck (1984) and has been used in 1300 cases. It has also been, and still is, used elsewhere. Ceravital develops an osteogenic surface reaction favorable to fixation. Interposition of cartilage is not only unnecessary, but contraindicated, since it prevents the osteogenic surface reaction that promotes fixation of the implant to the tympanic membrane. To activate the reaction, Reck used bone paste to cover the platform of the ceramic implant facing the drum. Gersdorff interposed a thin layer of bone powder–fibrin adhesive sheet (Gersdorff et al. 1986). The sheet is made as follows. The bone powder is obtained from drilling, either of the mastoid process in the retroauricular approach, or of the ear canal or bony annulus in the endaural approach. A bone collector can be used.

The bone paste is rinsed in a saline solution and dried. A small quantity of two components of fibrin glue (Tissucol or Tissel, Immuno Company, Vienna) is mixed, and, with a press, this homogenous agglomerate is pressed into a thin sheet that can be cut by a scalpel or a pair of scissors into the required shape. The bone paste–Tissucol sheet is inserted between the drum and the Ceravital prosthesis.

The anatomical results with this method are better than with Plasti-Pore (Gersdorff et al. 1986). Reck (1989) found the following long-term effects with Ceravital: a) in an aerated and uninfected ear cavity, no noticeable degradation of the graft surface was observed, but long-lasting inflammatory processes regularly destroy the implanted material. This degradation takes place if the ceramic is covered by an infected mucosa. b) Perforation of the tympanic membrane in contact with the prosthesis has never been found. c) Extrusion phenomena different from those known from allogenous ossicles did not occur. d) In contact with the overlying tympanic membrane in atelectic ears, the implant surfaces are stable.

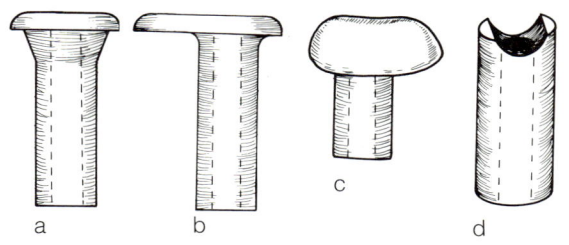

Fig. **829** Dense hydroxyapatite incus replacement prostheses. **a** The Shea PORP. **b** The Shea off-center PORP. **c** The Black prosthesis, with an egg-shaped head and a fluoroplastic shaft. **d** Kartush prosthesis, made of hydroxyapatite

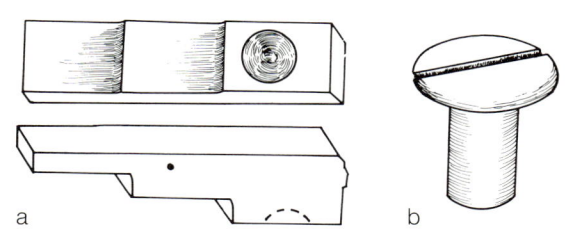

Fig. **830a** The Grote prosthesis. **b** The Yanagihara prosthesis, made of Apoceram-P

Calciumphosphate ceramics. There are several types of calcium phosphate. *Calcium phosphate* is, in fact, plaster of Paris, which has been used for obliteration of the cavity (Högset and Bredberg 1986). *Tricalcium phosphates* (Ca_3PO_4) are also used to fill cavities. They have a slow degradation rate, and after 12–18 months are replaced by new-formed bone. *Hydroxyapatite* has direct osteogenic effects, is only slightly degradable, and integrates perfectly with the surrounding bone. Hydroxyapatite is, in fact, the mineral matrix of bone, and is therefore ideal for middle-ear reconstruction. Hydroxyapatite can be made in a dense form, without macropores, for ossicles, which provides good integration. It is like bone, and produces no resorption, with or without infection. The other form contains macropores, and can be granulated. It becomes filled with fibrous tissue, and over three months is replaced by bone (van Bitterswijk and Grote 1989). This material is used for obliteration.

Dense hydroxyapatite has become very popular, and several simple and complex PORP prostheses have been developed during recent years. The simple prostheses do not differ from polyethylene, Polycel, and Plasti-Pore prosthesis. The Shea prostheses (Fig. **829a, b**) with the shaft and head made of hydroxyapatite, is similar to the Plasti-Pore prosthesis. The Black prosthesis (Fig. **829c**) (Black 1987, 1990) has an overall egg-shaped head, made of hydroxyapatite, with no sharp edges. The shaft is made of fluoroplastic. The Kartush (1989) prosthesis is a hydroxyapatite tube that is placed between the head of the stapes and the malleus handle (Fig. **829d**).

Grote (1989) designed an incus prosthesis (Fig. **830a**), which can be used for any distance between the stapes head and the malleus handle. The prosthesis is based on an assembly method, in which the interposed prosthesis is placed between the remnants of the ossicular chain. It is 6 mm long, 1.5 mm wide, and 1.5 mm in height. In cases with a large distance between the malleus handle and the head of the stapes, the prosthesis can be placed on the malleus handle (Fig. **831**). The periosteum and drum remnant is elevated from the outer surface of the malleus handle with a sickle knife, creating a pocket, and the thin end of the hydroxyapatite implant is pushed into this pocket (Fig. **832**). The cap of the prosthesis is placed on the head of the stapes. There is no need for an interposition betweeen the drum and the hydroxyapatite prosthesis.

The Yanagihara hydroxyapatite prosthesis (Apoceram-P–type prosthesis) has a hollow shaft and a smoothly curved platform (Fig. **830b**). The groove across the platform may help to fit the prosthesis between the malleus handle and the stapes. Yanagihara cuts the prosthesis with a special fine-disk diamond burr (Yanagihara et al. 1988).

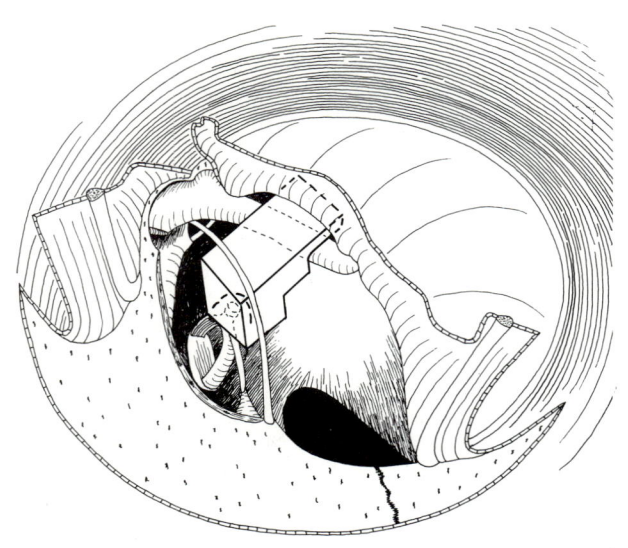

Fig. 831 The Grote prosthesis is placed on the head of the stapes and in a pocket on the malleus handle

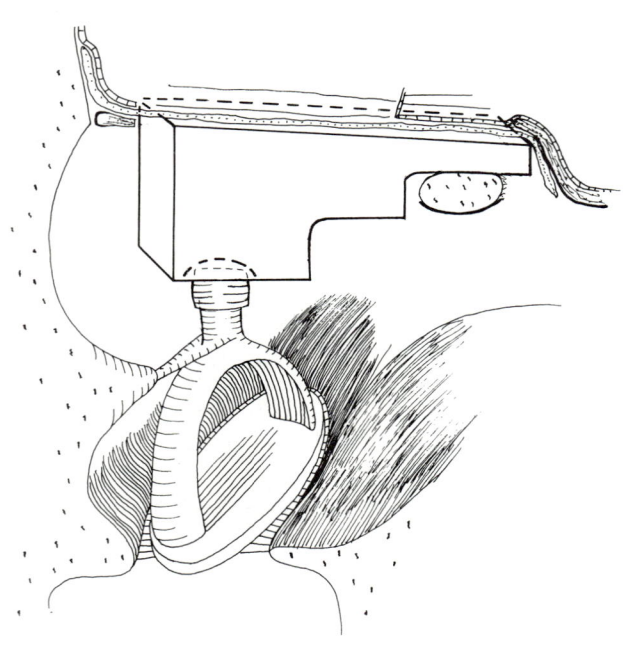

Fig. 832 The Grote prosthesis in position in side view

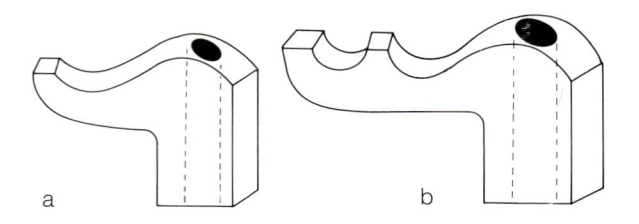

Fig. 833 The Wehr hydroxyapatite prosthesis, **a** with one notch and **b** with two notches

The Wehr incus prosthesis (Smith and Nephew, Richards Company) is well sculptured, and has a cannulated shaft also made of hydroxyapatite (Wehrs 1987). As an incus prosthesis, it is made either with a single notch (Fig. 833) for a short distance, or with a double-notch prosthesis for long anterior distances between the malleus handle and the stapes head. Before placement of the prosthesis, the anterior distance to the malleus handle should be measured by an angulated instrument. This is the horizontal distance from the malleus handle to a vertical line going through the head of the stapes. If the anterior distance is between 2 and 3 mm, a single-notch prosthesis should be used; if the distance is longer, a double-notch prosthesis is recommended. The prosthesis can be adapted by drilling with a diamond burr to the appropriate size and shape. The prosthesis should be placed on the head of the stapes first (Fig. 834). The malleus handle is elevated with a hook, and the prosthesis is gently pushed under the malleus with a small rugine in a cranial direction. Properly adapted, the prosthesis has good stability when the malleus handle is present (Fig. 835).

Goldenberg (1990) developed a hybrid prosthesis system, with a hydroxyapatite head and a Plasti-Pore shaft. The advantage of Plasti-Pore is its easy trimming and shaping, in contrast to hydroxyapatite. The Plasti-Pore shaft is directed medially, and is applied to the bone of the remaining ossicles. The Goldenberg hydroxyapatite–Plasti-Pore prostheses (1990, 1992) have various shapes. The small malleus-to-stapes prosthesis has a centering hole on the head, with a hollowed Plasti-Pore shaft (Fig. 836). The head of the prosthesis may be angled inferiorly or superiorly along the malleus handle (Figs. 837, 838). The large, wedge-shaped Goldenberg prosthesis has a relatively large hydroxyapatite platform, facing either the malleus handle or the undersurface of the drum. The hydroxyapatite head can be cannulated (Fig. 839) for visualization of the head of the stapes. The relatively large platform can face the drum and the malleus handle (Fig. 840). The Plasti-Pore shaft is malleable for proper angulation against the drum or malleus handle (Figs. 841, 842). Goldenberg (1992) published good hearing results with this prosthesis, with an extrusion rate of 3–4%. The mean follow-up time was about one year.

The Black spanner prosthesis (Smith and Nephew, Richards Company) consists of a hydroxyapatite head for the malleus handle (Fig. 836b) and a fluoroplastic shaft, with crural notches for alignment on the stapes (Fig. 843). The hydroxyapatite head is attached to the trimmed shaft after proper

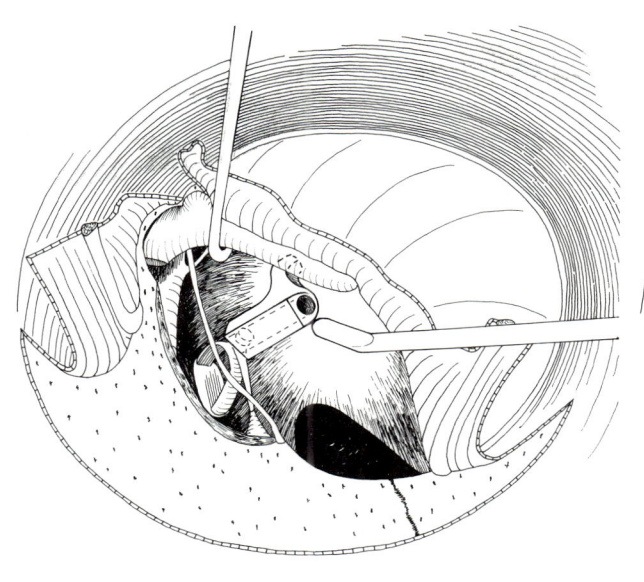

Ceramics 295

Fig. **834** The Wehr prosthesis placed on the head of the stapes. The malleus is elevated, and the prosthesis is pushed underneath it

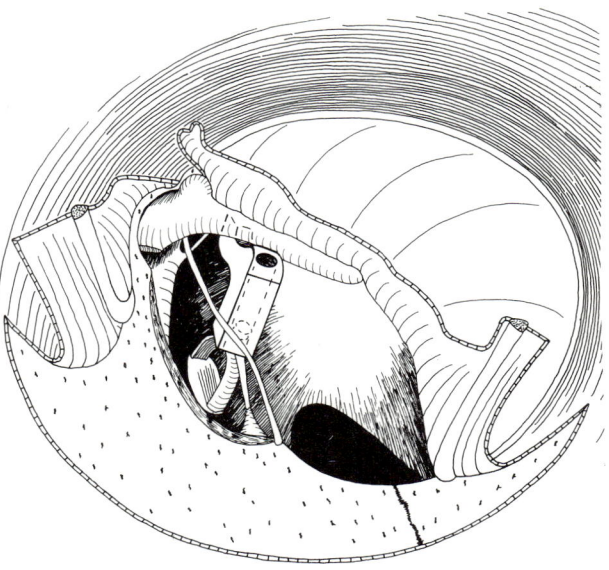

Fig. **835** The Wehr prosthesis with one notch in the proper position

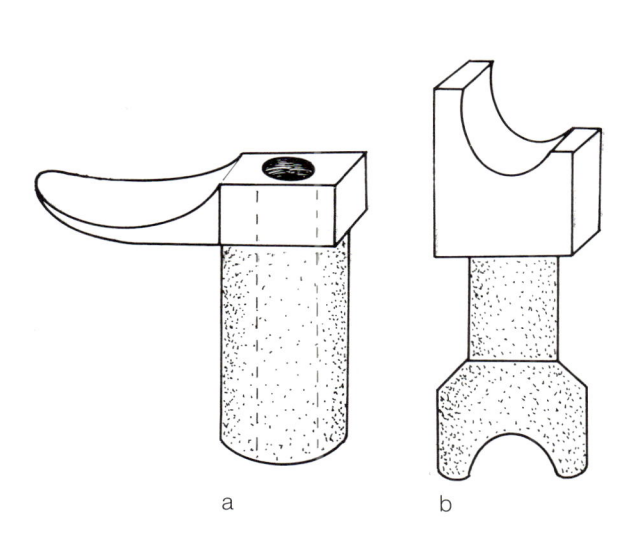

Fig. **836a** The small Goldenberg prosthesis with a hydroxyapatite head and a Plasti-Pore shaft. **b** The Blackspanner prosthesis

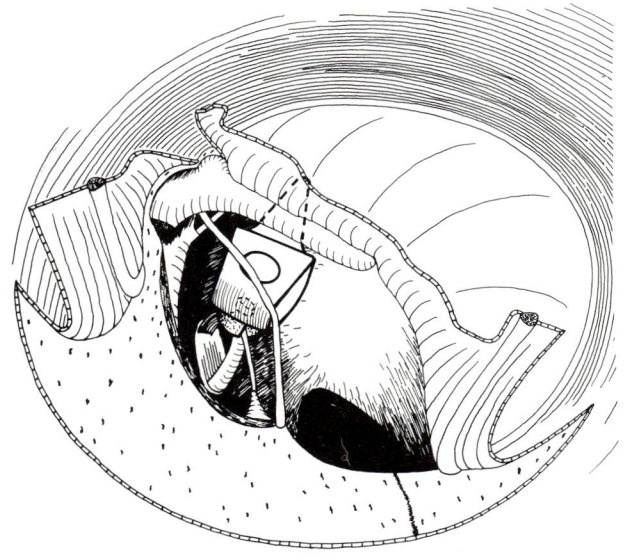

Fig. **837 The Goldenberg prosthesis.** The hydroxyapatite head is placed underneath the malleus handle. The Plasti-Pore shaft is trimmed to the head of the stapes and the stapedial tendon

trimming. The fluoroplastic shaft can be angled according to the angulation between the head of the stapes and the malleus handle.

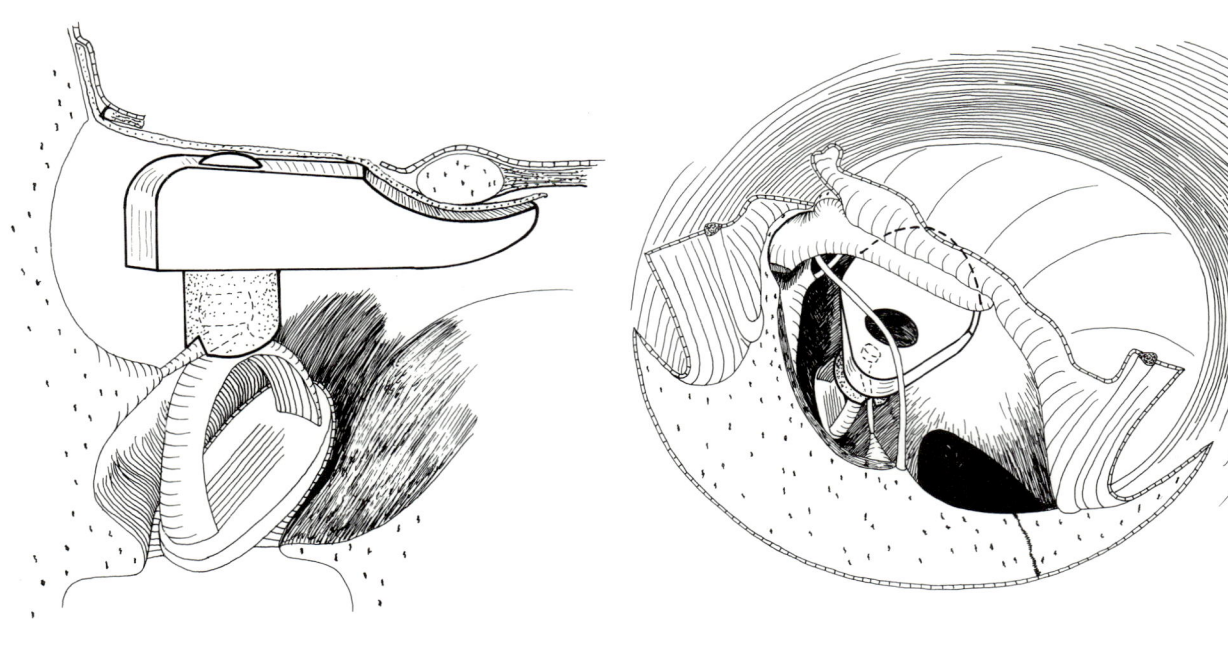

17 Type 2 Tympanoplasty with Biocompatible Materials

Fig. **838** Side view of the Goldenberg prosthesis underneath the malleus handle

Fig. **839** The Goldenberg prosthesis, with a large, wedge-shaped platform and a hole to see the head of the stapes

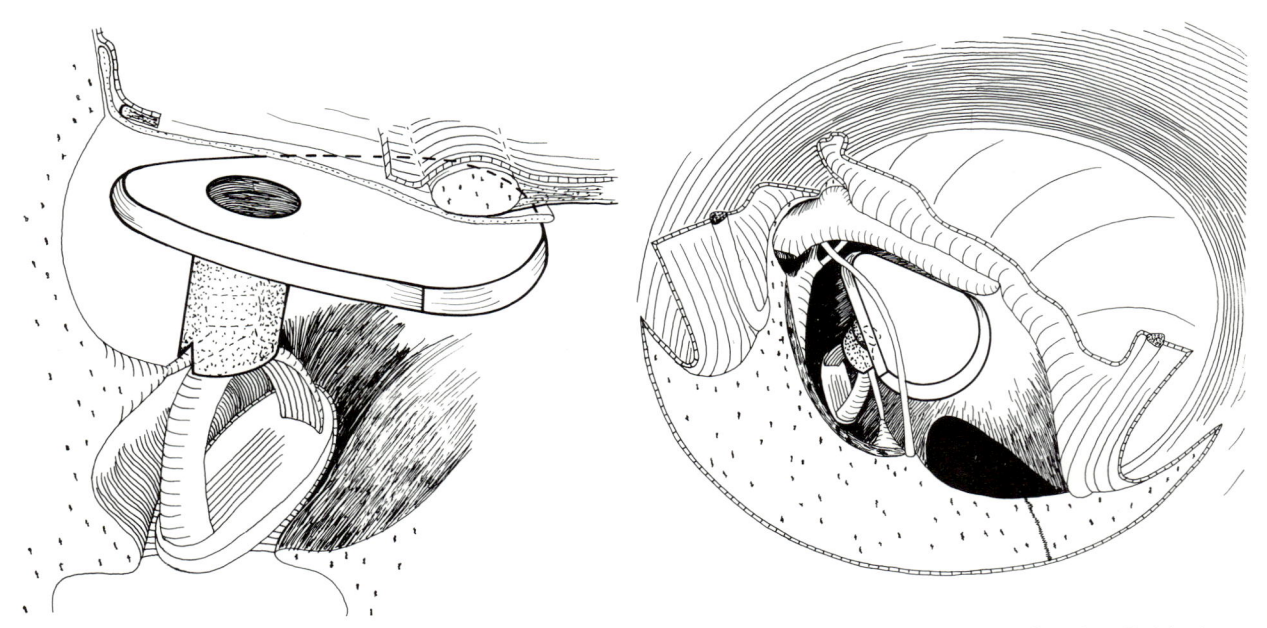

Fig. **840** Side view of the Goldenberg wedge-shaped prosthesis, in position under the malleus handle and under the drum

Fig. **841** An alternative position for the Goldenberg wedge-shaped prosthesis, parallel to the malleus handle

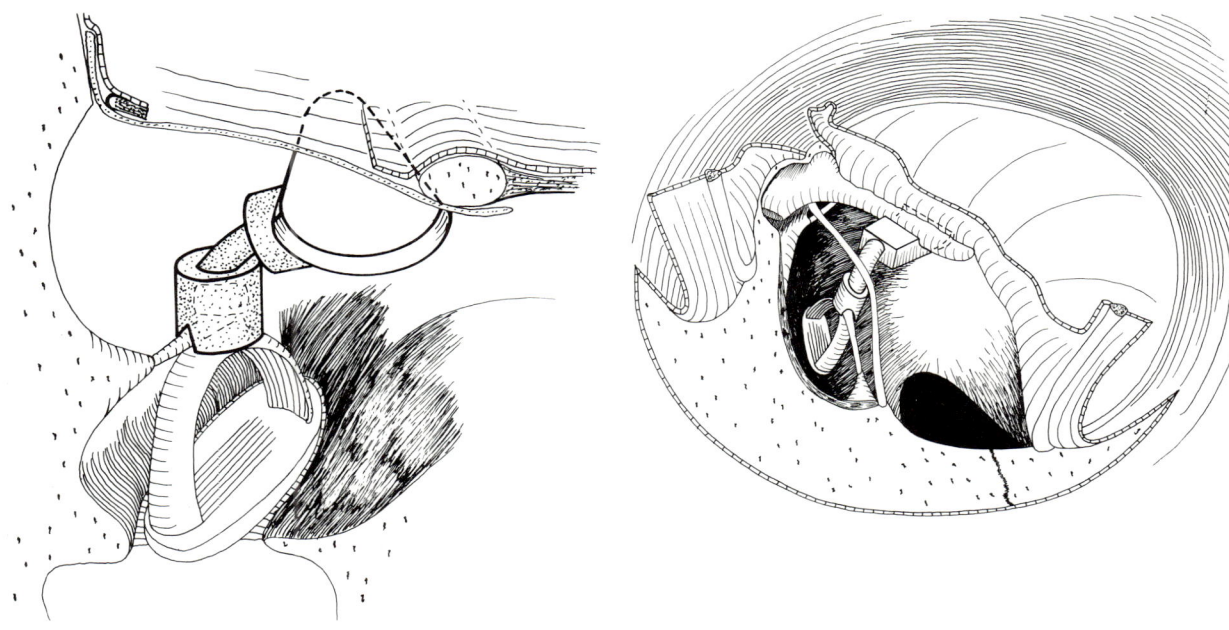

Fig. **842** Side view of the Goldenberg prosthesis, showing the angulation of the Plasti-Pore shaft

Fig. **843** The Black spanner prosthesis. The hydroxyapatite head is placed underneath the malleus handle. The fluoroplastic shaft is angled, and the crural notch is adapted to the head of the stapes

Glass Ionomer Cement

Glass ionomer cement is obtained by the reaction of a glass powder with a polyacrylic acid. The base component is a calcium aluminosilicate glass. In otology, glass ionomer cement (Ionos, Seefeld, Germany) is used to reconstruct the posterior bony wall and to obliterate the mastoid cavity (Geyer and Helms 1990, Babighian 1992). The inner coil of the cochlear implant and the electrode are fixed by cement.

To prepare the cement, the acid is forced into the glass powder–filled capsule by means of an activator, and mixed for 10–15 seconds. Using the applicator, the viscid paste obtained is pressed out of the capsule. The paste is workable for about five minutes. During this interval, the cement is transferred to the site of surgery, where it binds firmly to the bone. Using the paste, two ossicles can be connected, a defective long process of the incus can be restored by cement paste, or a defect of the posterior bony annulus or lateral attic wall can be repaired (Babighian 1992).

An Ionos ossicle has been manufactured, consisting of a 5-mm PORP prosthesis (Fig. **844**) and a 7-mm TORP prosthesis. The ossicle can be shaped

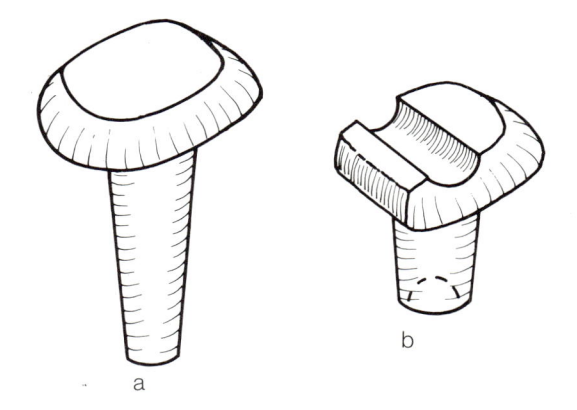

Fig. **844** **Glass ionomer cement prostheses. a** The head of the prosthesis is relatively large, and usually has to be shaped to a smaller size. **b** An example of a shaped prosthesis for interposition between the malleus handle and the head of the stapes

with a diamond drill. During drilling, it is best to hold it between two fingers. The prosthesis has good compatibility, is rapidly covered by middle-ear mucosa, has no biodegradability, and is not bioactive. Helms uses it routinely, but no clinical data on hearing results have yet been published. In the short term, there have been no extrusions in a group of 90 patients treated with the implant (Geyer and Helms 1990).

Metals

Metals as interposition grafts have seldom been used in type 2 tympanoplasty, but titanium prostheses have recently been introduced. During the 1960s, and at the beginning of the 1970s, Gerlach and Palva used steels wires (Gerlach 1971, Palva et al. 1971). Wire and gold prostheses are today used as interposition grafts (Pusalkar and Steinbach 1992). A recent investigation by Hüttenbrink (1992a) showed that wire has an excellent sound-transmission effect.

Titanium Prostheses

Magnan (1992) constructed TORP and PORP prostheses made entirely of titanium, including a special wire arrangement to allow the shaft of the prosthesis to be shortened or elongated before insertion (Audio-fit prosthesis, MXM Laboratories, Antibes, France). The head of the PORP prosthesis (Fig. **845**) measures 3×1×1 mm, and the outer shaft is 1 mm thick and ends with a bell-like acetabulum, to be placed on the head of the stapes. The shaft consists of two titanium tubes. The most distal tube is the inner one, going into the proximal, outer, tube. A titanium wire is fixed between the inner tube and the head of the prosthesis, allowing the two tubes to be held in the desired position and length. The spring effect provides easy insertion, without excessive pressure, maintaining the prosthesis on its leaning points during the postoperative healing process, whatever, the anatomic variations of the middle ear may be.

Babighian (1992), adapting the Magnan titanium spring-wire system, constructed a telescopic titanium–hydroxyapatite prosthesis (Audio-Micromed Company, Milano, Italy) (Fig. **846**). The head of the prosthesis and the main part of the shaft are made of hydroxyapatite. A titanium tube with a titanium spring-wire is placed in the head of the prosthesis. The advantage of this prosthesis is the possibility of shaping its head in relation to the conditions of the malleus handle and the drum.

The Gerlach Wire-Basket Prosthesis

Gerlach (1971) used a basket made of stainless-steel wire as an interposition graft between the head of the stapes and the drum. Gerlach demonstrated

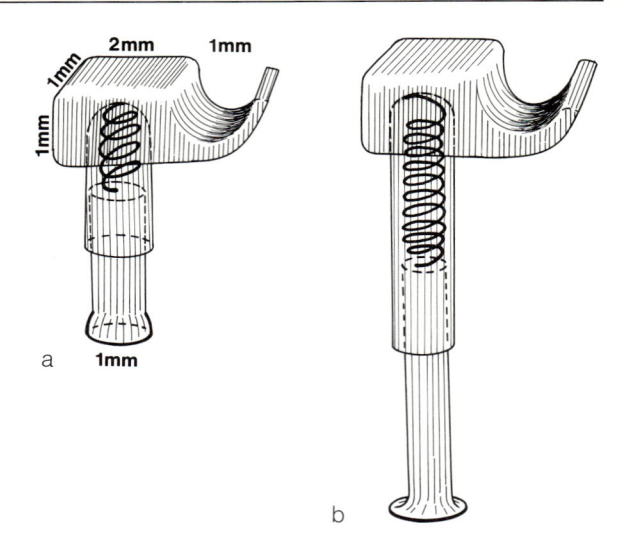

Fig. **845 Magnan titanium PORP and TORP prostheses,** with a special titanium wire that fixes the two shaft tubes into the desired position

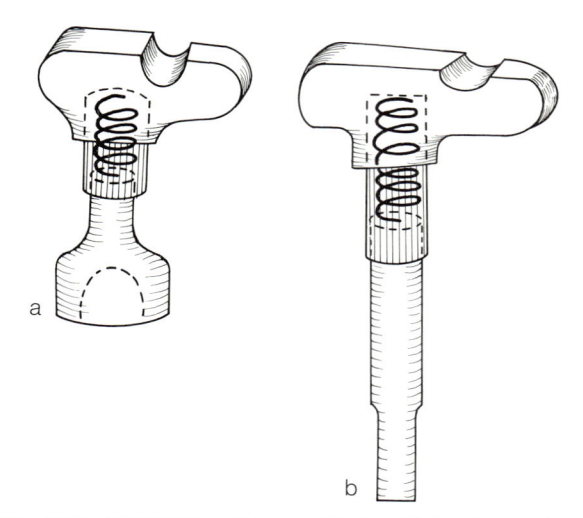

Fig. **846 Babighian telescopic prostheses,** made of hydroxyapatite and titanium. **a** The PORP has a hydroxyapatite notch for the head of the stapes. Both this and the TORP prosthesis **b**) can be elongated or shortened using the titanium wire system

good sound transmission with the wire. The energy can be transmitted to the stapes almost without loss. The basket form resembles the physiological condition, with a large surface laterally at the drum and a small one at the stapes. Different sizes of the basket prosthesis can be made.

Gerlach made his prosthesis as follows. Two ends of a wire sling are plaited together, and one end is cut off (Fig. **847a**). The wire of the sling is cut, and the same plait is performed with the two wire ends, but this second plait is made around the

2–4 mm–thick shaft of an instrument. The thickness depends on the diameter of the wire basket desired. One end of the wire is cut off. (Fig. **847b**). The two remaining wires are plaited together to form the bottom of the basket. One end is cut off, and the other is curved in such a way that the basket can be fixed to the neck of the stapes (Fig. **847c**). To help with the last plait, and to produce a well-shaped basket, performing the last plait around the end of a pin might be recommended.

The basket is fixed around the neck of the stapes (Fig. **848**). A double-cup forceps, or the forceps used in stapedectomy to fix the wire to the long process of the incus, can help to attach the wire to the stapes. Gerlach did not feel there was a problem with exteriorization of the prosthesis, as with other wire prostheses, in cases of retraction of the drum. He sometimes placed a thin Silastic sheet on the wire to prevent extrusion. Gerlach considered that cartilage or cortical bone plates were too heavy and too unstable. However, these prostheses have not been used, although placing cartilage slides, as used by Sheehy to cover a PORP-prosthesis (Figs. **811-813**), or using a perichondrium–cartilage plate to fix the tragal graft, as recommended by Glasscock (Fig. **617**), could offer a new variation on this interesting wire-basket prosthesis (Fig. **849**).

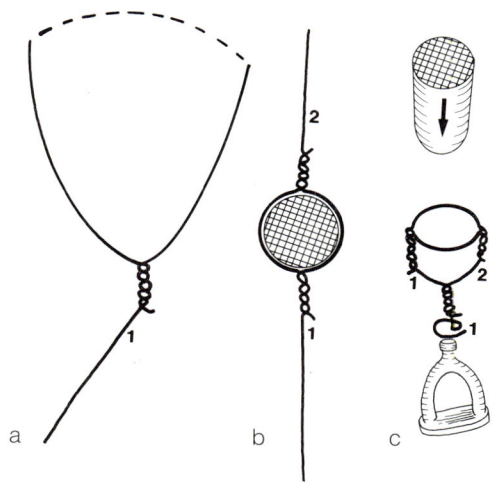

Fig. **847 Preparation of a Gerlach wire-basket prosthesis. a** Two ends of a wire sling (1) are plaited together, and one wire is cut. **b** The upper two wires (2) are plaited together around the 2–4 mm-thick shaft of an instrument. **c** Each of the two remaining wires is now plaited together, forming the bottom of the basket. The end of one wire (1) will fix the basket prosthesis around the neck of the stapes. The end of a pin (arrow) can be placed in the basket while working with the wires

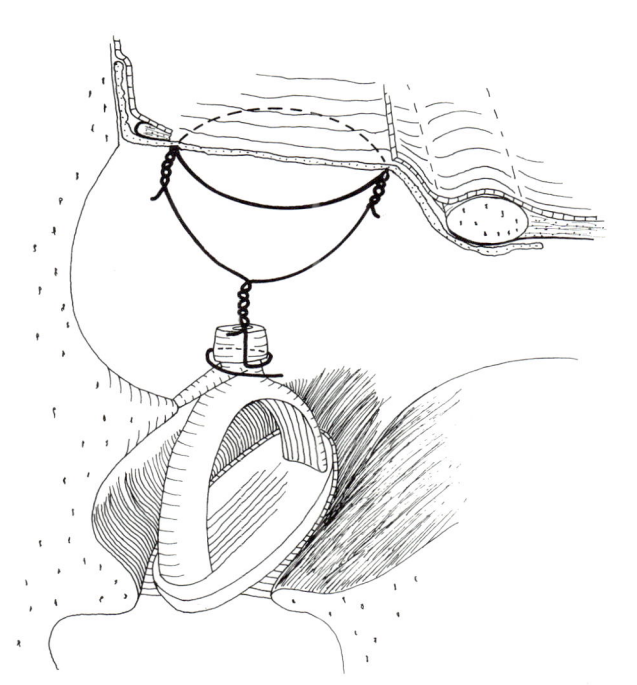

Fig. **848** The Gerlach wire basket is fixed onto the head of the stapes. The platform is underneath the drum or the fascia

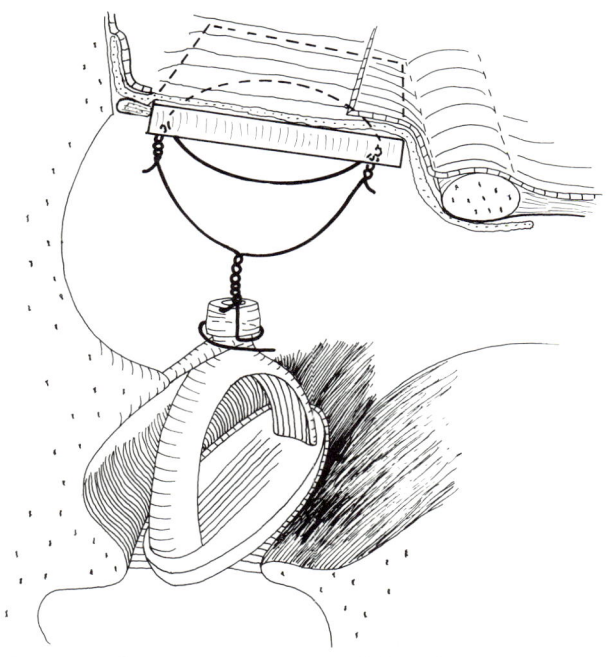

Fig. **849** Suggested covering of the wire-basket prosthesis with a slice of tragal cartilage placed between the malleus handle and the posterior bony annulus

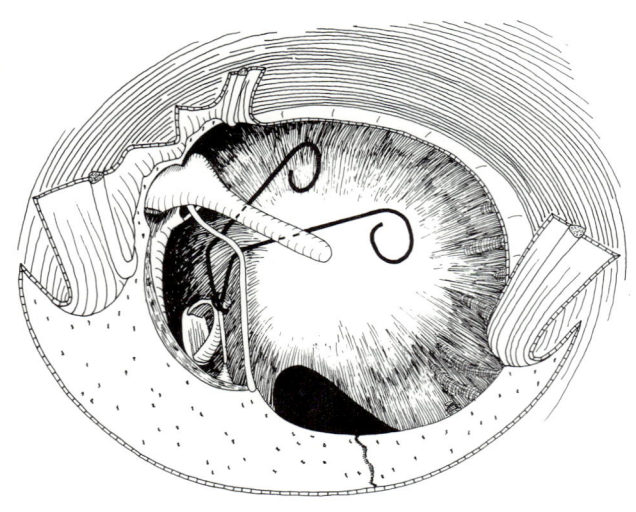

Fig. 850 **The Palva two-legged wire prosthesis** fixed onto the neck of the stapes and placed underneath the malleus handle. One leg points toward the Eustachian tube orifice, and the other toward the hypotympanum

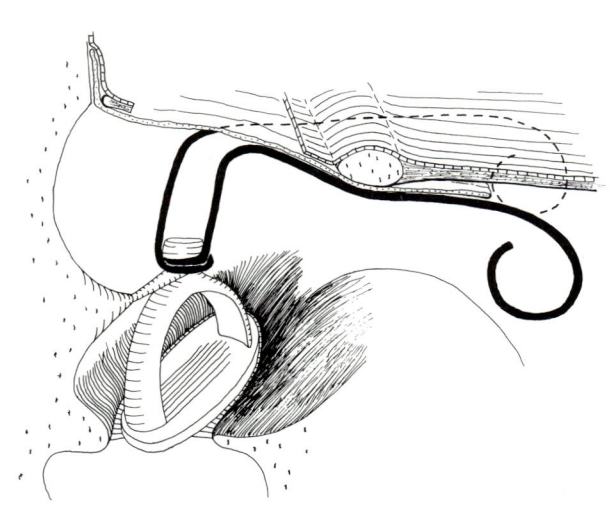

Fig. 851 Side view of the Palva two-legged prosthesis, showing its position under the drum

Palva Two-Legged and Three-Legged Wire Prostheses

From 1964 to 1969, Palva used two-legged or three-legged wire prostheses in a total of 169 ears. In the two-legged prosthesis consisting of stainless-steel wire, in cases with the stapes present, the wire is anchored to the neck of the stapes by a loop (Fig. **850**). The legs of the wire are placed under the malleus handle, one in the area of the Eustachian tube orifice, and the other in the hypotympanum (Figs. **850, 851**). Fascia, placed with the swing-door technique as an underlay graft, covers the wire. Often a large piece of Silastic is placed on the wire legs. (Palva et al. 1971). In the absence of the malleus handle, a bony plate is often placed on the wire.

In Palva's study, the ears were regularly checked, with a minimum observation period of one year. The wire prosthesis extruded in 8% of the ears. Keratin debris accumulated around the bar wire, and the prostheses had to be removed an average of two years after the operation. The hearing results were good, especially in ears covered with bony plate. Palva abandoned this prosthesis, but routine covering of all prostheses with cartilage plates was not attempted, and might be recommended. The usefulness of wire in ossiculoplasty should be reconsidered. The wire should be carefully and systematically covered with cartilage plates (Fig. **852**), cartilage slices, or composite cartilage–perichondrium grafts (Tolsdorff 1991) and one might try to use them in selected cases in connection with the Heermann palisade cartilage technique (Fig. **631**).

Gold Prostheses

Gold is biocompatible, stable, well tolerated, and easy to shape and adapt. Because of the softness of pure gold, the major problem with the metal has been now to manufacture a miniature prosthesis of the precise shape, size, purity, and with the amount of rigidity, required.

Two models of gold prosthesis have been produced and used by Pusalkar and Steinbach (1991). One is the antenna prosthesis, used as a TORP, (Fig. **853c, d**). The other is the bell prosthesis, used as a PORP (Fig. **853a, b**). Both are made of 0.4 mm pure gold wire. The platform is a rectangular wire. The rectangle can be pushed under the handle of the malleus, or can be interfaced with a cartilage plate or cartilage–perichondrium graft or fascia, or other combined grafts.

The bell prosthesis is an incus replacement prosthesis. The bell-shaped shaft is placed on the

Metals 301

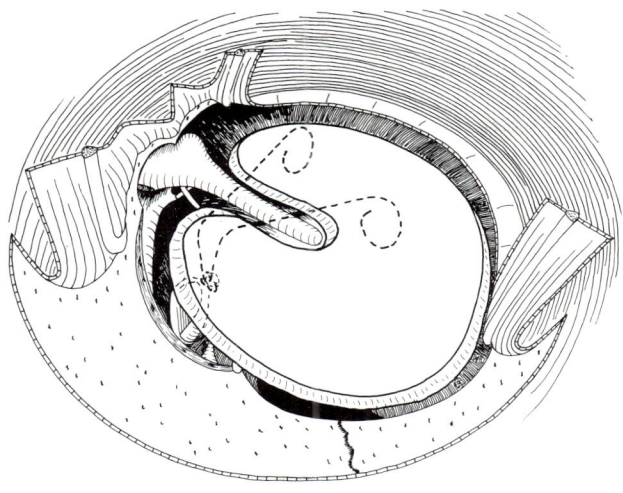

Fig. 852 Suggested covering of the Palva two-legged prosthesis with a large slice of autogenous tragal cartilage in a total perforation, with the malleus handle present

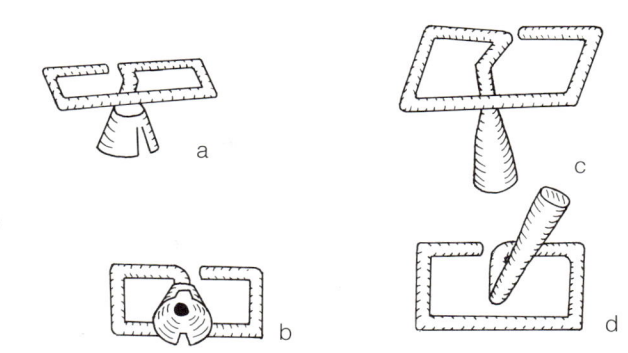

Fig. 853 **Gold prostheses** (Pusalkar and Steinbach). **a, b** Bell prostheses as PORPs. **c, d** Antenna prostheses as TORPs

head of the stapes, with the platform wire under the malleus handle (Fig. 854). It is usually covered by tragal cartilage plate (Fig. 855). The prosthesis is malleable, and the angle betweeen the shaft and the platform can change in all directions, as can the height. There are three sizes of bell prosthesis, ranging in height from 3.5 to 2.0 mm. The rectangular platform measures 4×2.5 mm.

The mean hearing gain in 40 cases of bell prostheses 9-30 months after surgery was 40 dB. Two prostheses were extruded.

The use of wire prostheses is once again becoming popular in the 1990s.

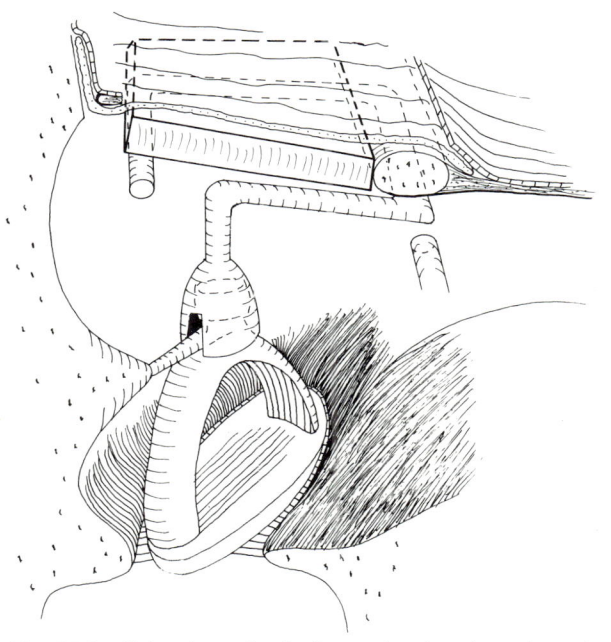

Fig. 854 Side view of a bell prosthesis, placed on the head of the stapes. The wire platform is underneath the malleus handle

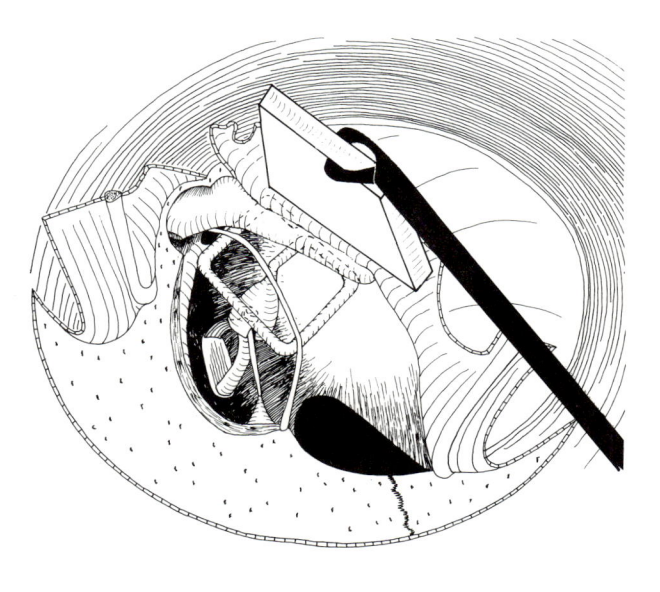

Fig. 855 The bell prosthesis covered by a piece of cartilage

18 Transposition and Pexis in Type 2 Tympanoplasty

Transposition

Transposition of the ossicles is an ossiculoplasty procedure in which the transposed ossicle, usually the malleus, remains in some communication with its surrounding tissue — either with the remnant of the tympanic membrane around the umbo, or the anterior malleolar ligament, or the tensor tympani tendon. These procedures roughly correspond to pedicled grafts.

Malleostapedial Transposition

This procedure was first published by Miodonski (1956), and was later practiced, with some modifications, by Hall and Rytzner (1959), Rubinstein et al. (1962), Portmann (1963), Sheehy (1965), and Szpunar (1967). Several methods of malleostapedial transposition have been used.

1. **Malleus neck to the stapes head.** This is the most often used transposition. It is used in combination with canal wall–down mastoidectomy in attic cholesteatoma. An anteroinferior drum remnant and an intact stapes should remain. After finishing the canal wall–down mastoidectomy and resection of the malleus head, which is usually invaded or resorbed by cholesteatoma, the anterior malleolar ligament and the tendon of the tensor tympani muscle are cut (Fig. **856**). The attachment of the drum to the anterior aspect of the malleus handle is loosened, and only the umbo is still attached to the drum. The entire malleus handle is rotated in a posterior direction, and placed on the head of the stapes. There is no need to create a hole on the undersurface of the neck of the malleus to fit the head of the stapes. The neck is positioned too low in relation to the facial prominence, where osseous fixation can take place. It is important to liberate the umbo almost totally from the drum, to avoid bending and traction of the malleus handle towards its original position (Fig. **857**).

This type of malleostapedial pexis can, in fact, be as good as interposition in selected cases with canal wall–down mastoidectomy, when the attachment of the malleus has to be cut so as to remove cholesteatoma located under the anterosuperior part of the drum. The malleus handle has to be almost totally loosened, and can easily be transferred onto

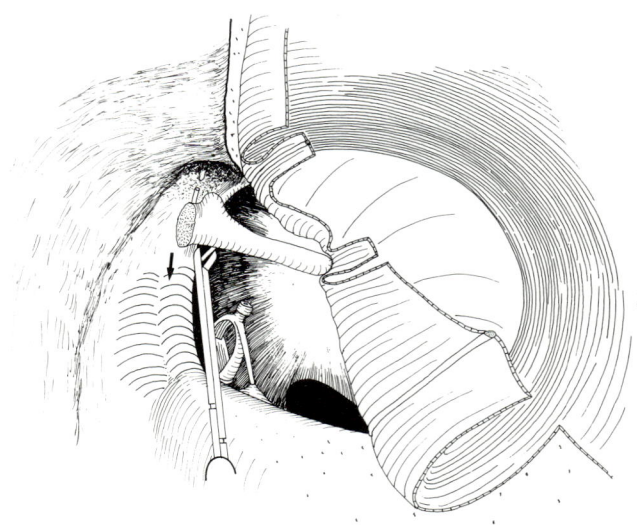

Fig. **856** Situation in a canal wall–down mastoidectomy with resection of the malleus head. The anterior malleolar ligament is cut, the tendon of the tensor tympani muscle is cut, and the tympanic membrane is separated from the anterior border of the malleus handle

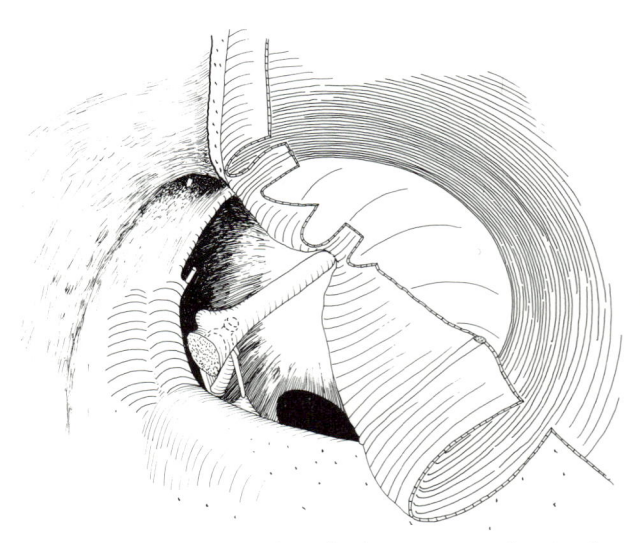

Fig. **857** The malleus handle is transposed onto the head of the stapes. The neck is touching the head of the stapes

Transposition

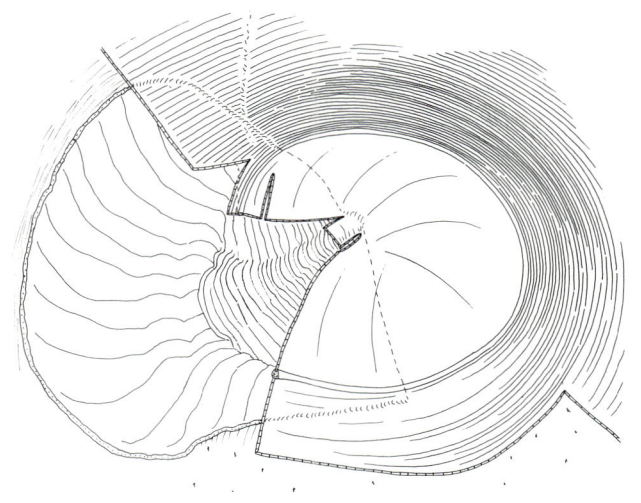

Fig. 858 The fascia is placed under the drum remnant and on the umbo, as well as on the malleus handle. It covers the lateral semicircular canal and the medial wall of the attic. The epithelial flaps are replaced

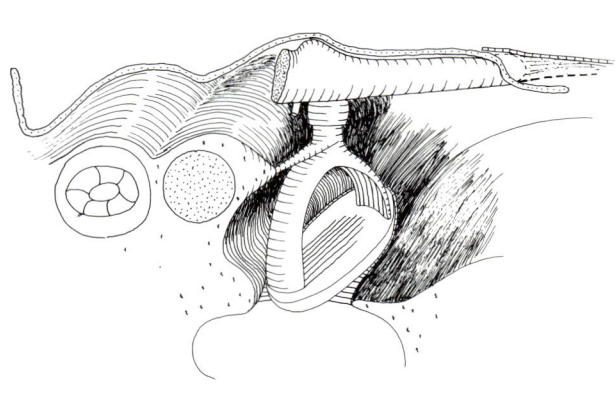

Fig. 859 Side view of the transposition of the neck of the malleus onto the stapes. The fascia is covering the malleus handle and the lateral semicircular canal, as well as the medial wall of the attic

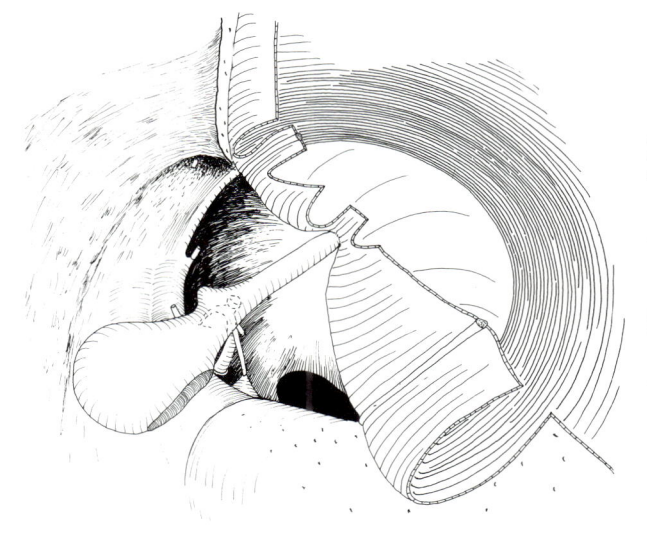

Fig. 860 Transposition of the entire malleus onto the stapes

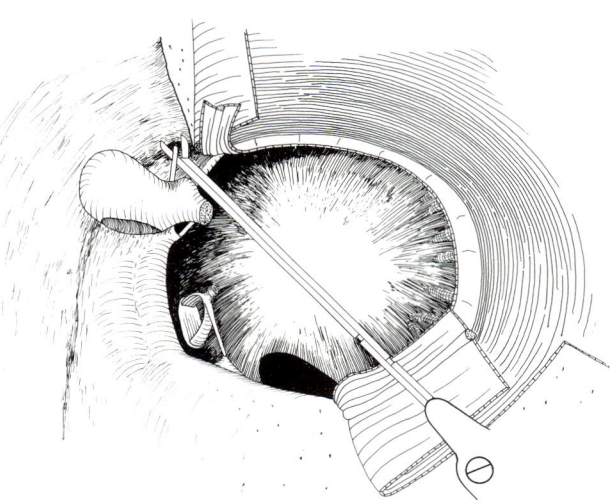

Fig. 861 Situation in a total perforation, canal wall–down mastoidectomy and missing malleus handle. The anterior mallear ligament is cut, and the malleus head is transposed onto the head of the stapes

the head of the stapes. The fascia is placed under the drum remnant, but lies on the malleus handle and the medial attic wall (Fig. 858). The fascia covers the facial nerve canal and the lateral semicircular canal. The tympanic cavity is low but safe, and any residual cholesteatoma in the anterior attic is easily identified (Fig. 859).

A method of interposing the entire malleus with its head on the stapes has been described (Szpunar 1967) (Fig. 860), but is not to be recommended, as it involves a considerable risk of bony fixation of the malleus head to the lateral semicircular canal. The method also seems to be unphysiological.

2. **Malleus head to the stapes head.** When the malleus handle is absent and there is total perforation, in tensa-retraction cholesteatoma, and in canal wall–down mastoidectomy, only the malleus head with its neck remains. It is still fixed to the tendon of the tensor tympani muscle (Fig. 861). Transposition of the head of the malleus onto the head of the stapes can be performed after cutting the ante-

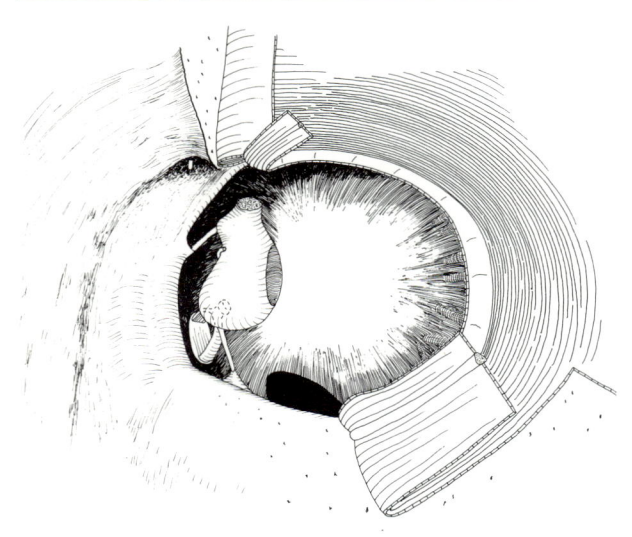

Fig. 862 The malleus head is transposed onto the head of the stapes. It is attached by the tendon of the tensor tympani muscle

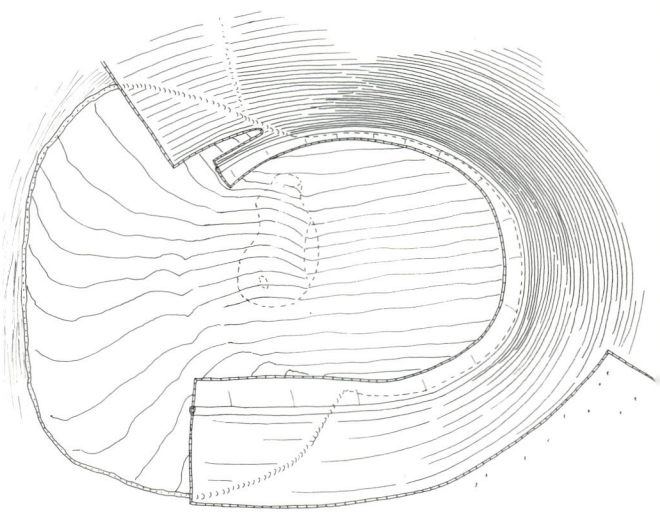

Fig. 863 The fascia covers the total perforation, the transposed malleus head, the medial wall of the attic, and the lateral semicircular canal. The skin flaps are replaced

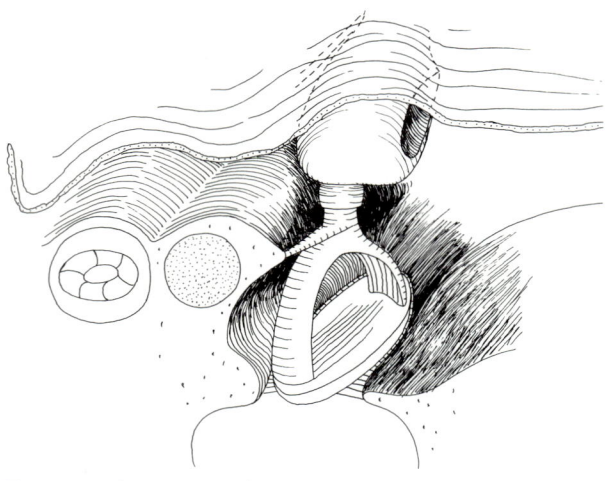

Fig. 864 Side view of the malleus-head transposition, allowing a high tympanic cavity. The fascia lies on the head of the malleus and on the prominence of the facial nerve

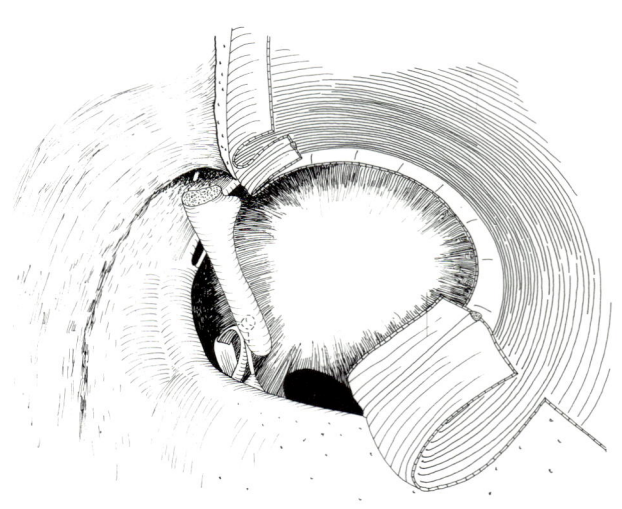

Fig. 865 The transposition of the umbo onto the stapes. The anterior mallear ligament is cut, and the malleus handle is turned towards the stapes

rior mallear ligament (Fig. **862**). This transposition in fact resembles an interposition, except that the malleus neck is fixed with the tendon. This may maintain the distance between the interposed malleus head and the facial prominence, avoiding bony fixation. The fascia covers the total perforation as a underlay graft (Fig. **863**), and also covers the malleus head and medial wall of the attic. The tympanic cavity is low (Fig. **864**).

3. **Umbo to the stapes head.** In total perforation, in tensa-retraction cholesteatoma, and after canal wall–down mastoidectomy, a resection of the malleus head often has to be performed, and only the malleus handle is still present. In a few selected cases, transposition of the umbo onto the head of the stapes can be performed after resection of the mallear ligament (Fig. **865**). The malleus is fixed by the tendon of the tensor tympani muscle, which holds it separate from the facial prominence, and allows some distance to remain between the malleus handle and the prominence of the horizontal part of the facial nerve (Fig. **866**). This method is

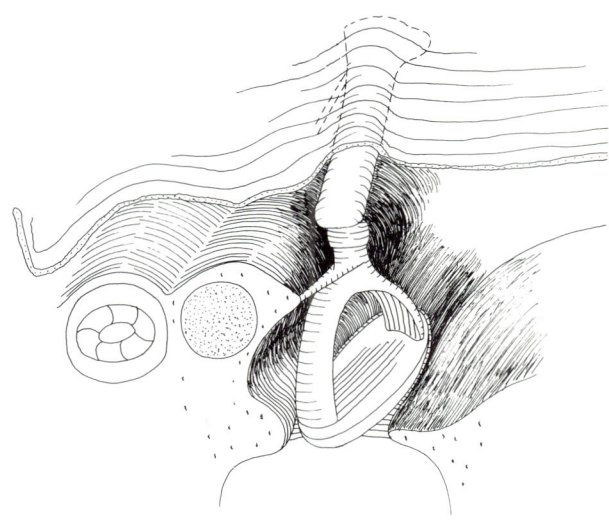

Fig. 866 Side view of the transposition of the umbo, showing the low tympanic cavity

not physiological, and any type of bone or cartilage interposition on the head of the stapes, with preservation of the malleus handle in its original position, is preferable.

Turner (1969) reported excellent results one year after canal wall–down mastoidectomy and transposition of the malleus (with the neck to head method). He achieved absolute hearing levels within 15 dB in 26 out of 40 cases and within 30 dB in 37 cases. These results are definitely better than those published in myringostapediopexy (Juers 1960, Pennington 1966). Turner termed this transposition method a malleostapediopexy.

Pexis

In pexis, the drum or malleus handle can be connected, without interposition, to the remaining part of the ossicular chain, particularly the head of the stapes. The various types of pexis can be classified as follows.

1) *Myringoincudopexy*. The drum is connected either a) to the remaining long process of the incus, or b) to the lenticular process still attached to the head of the stapes.
2) *Incudostapediopexy*, including methods of connecting or overbridging small defects in the long process of the incus to the head of the stapes. The aim of this method is to reestablish a complete ossicular chain.
3) *Malleostapediopexy* means creating a connection, usually with wire, between the malleus handle and the head of the stapes. There is a gradual transition to interpositions, in this method, especially in cases in which the connection created between the head of the stapes and the malleus handle consists of a very thin prosthesis of bone or biocompatible material, and the graft is in contact only with the stapes and the malleus handle and has no contact with the drum at all. This could be classified as a pexis, but the term interposition is better here, simply because something is interposed between the two ossicles.

Myringoincudopexy

A typical myringoincudopexy situation occurs in resection of an intact long process of the incus (Fig. 867) that has good contact with the stapes. The remnant of the long process of the incus is covered by fascia (Fig. 868), establishing a myrin-

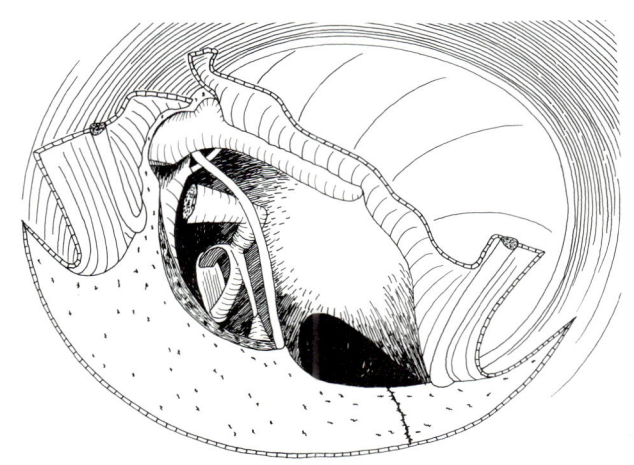

Fig. 867 **Myringoincudopexy** in a posterior perforation and intact posterior ear-canal wall. The long process of the incus is resected

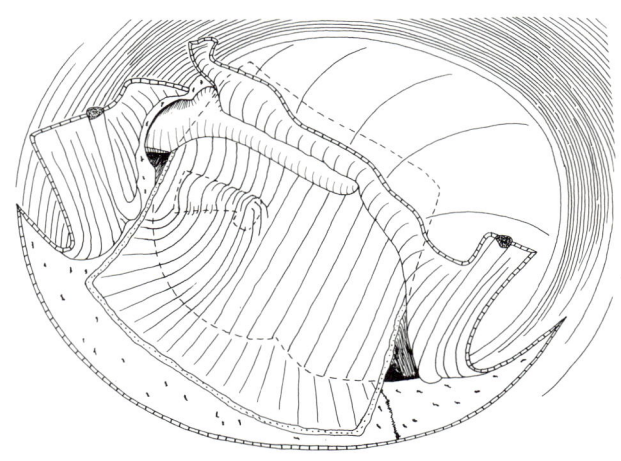

Fig. 868 The fascia is placed under the drum and on the remnant of the long process of the incus, and the flap is returned

Fig. **869** Side view of the myringoincudopexy, showing the low position of the drum posteriorly and good contact with the long process of the incus

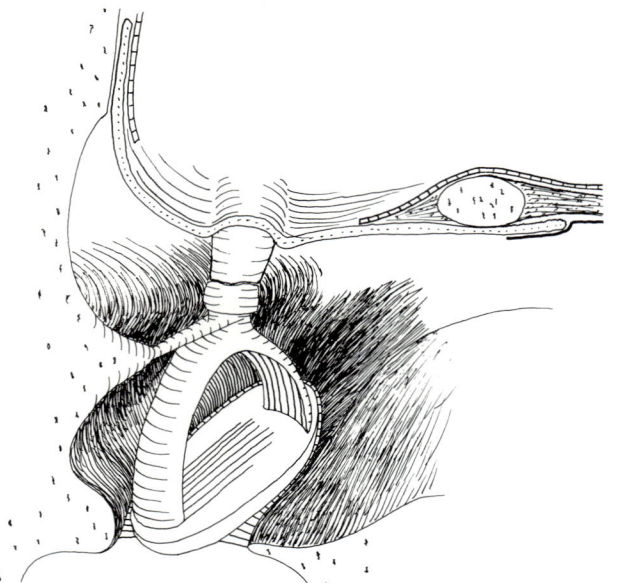

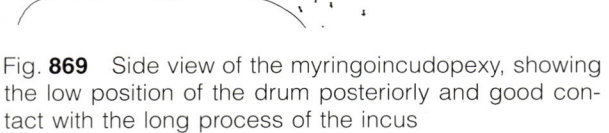

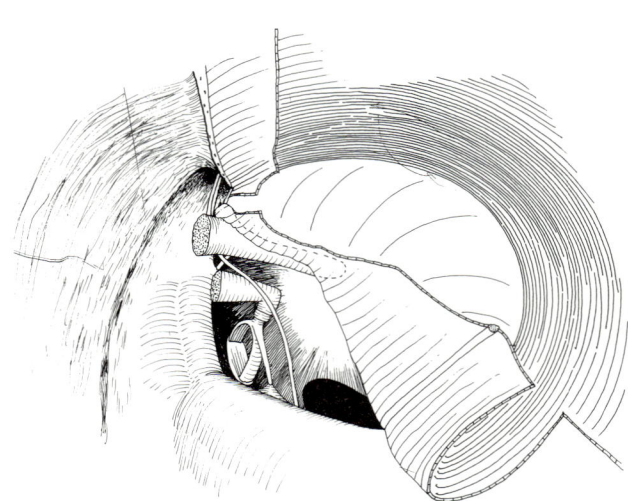

Fig. **870** Myringoincudopexy in a canal wall–down mastoidectomy. The posterior bony wall is removed, and the incus body and head of the malleus are resected. The attic and aditus are cleaned

goincudopexy. The connection takes place at a level lower than that of the normal drum (Fig. **869**), but the resultant hearing can be normal and stable.

The situation shown in Figure **867**, with an intact posterosuperior bony canal wall, is a rare one. Resection of the intact long process of the incus instead of disarticulation of the incus is sometimes used in bony or tympanosclerotic fixation of the incus body or malleus head, or both. More often, resection of the long process of the incus is used in attic cholesteatoma with severe erosion of the incus body. The long process of the incus is resected at an early stage of the operation, eliminating surgical trauma to the inner ear during the drilling and dissection in the attic. Though most surgeons disarticulate the lenticular process from the stapes, some prefer the type of resection shown in Figure **867**. In cases with bony fusion between the lenticular process and the head of the stapes, resection of the long process of the incus is necessary. It is performed by a small punch placed between the long process of the incus and the bony annulus, which has to be drilled away. The punch can also be introduced between the malleus handle and the long process of the incus (Fig. **712**).

Most often, resection of the long process of the incus takes place in connection with canal wall–down mastoidectomy and cleaning of the attic. In fact, this method was very often used before incus interposition was introduced, and it is still popular with many surgeons. During canal wall–down mastoidectomy and before cleaning the attic, the long process of the incus is resected by a punch, the incus body is removed, the bridge is safely drilled away, the head of the malleus is resected, and the attic is cleaned for cholesteatoma (Fig. **870**). After this fast procedure, an underlay fascia is placed on the remaining long process of the incus and under the drum remnants. The fascia covers the upper part of the malleus handle, the facial prominence, the lateral semicircular canal, and the medial attic wall (Fig. **871**). The tympanic cavity is lower than normal, but the malleus handle is also positioned somewhat medially, resulting in a small difference between the level of the long process of the incus and the malleus handle, and a quite even drum. Ears of this type can have excellent hearing and remain safe (Fig. **872**).

Myringoincudopexy may result from a situation in which the lenticular process is fused to the head of the stapes, and cannot be removed without risk to the inner ear from excessive movement of the mobile stapes (Fig. **873**). If the stapes is high and the malleus handle is positioned anteriorly, or retracted, or both, or if the malleus handle is less mobile than normal for any reason, it may be reasonable to carry out a myringostapediopexy, by placing fascia on the remnant of the lenticular process and establishing firm contact with it (Fig. **874**). The lenticular process in this situation is

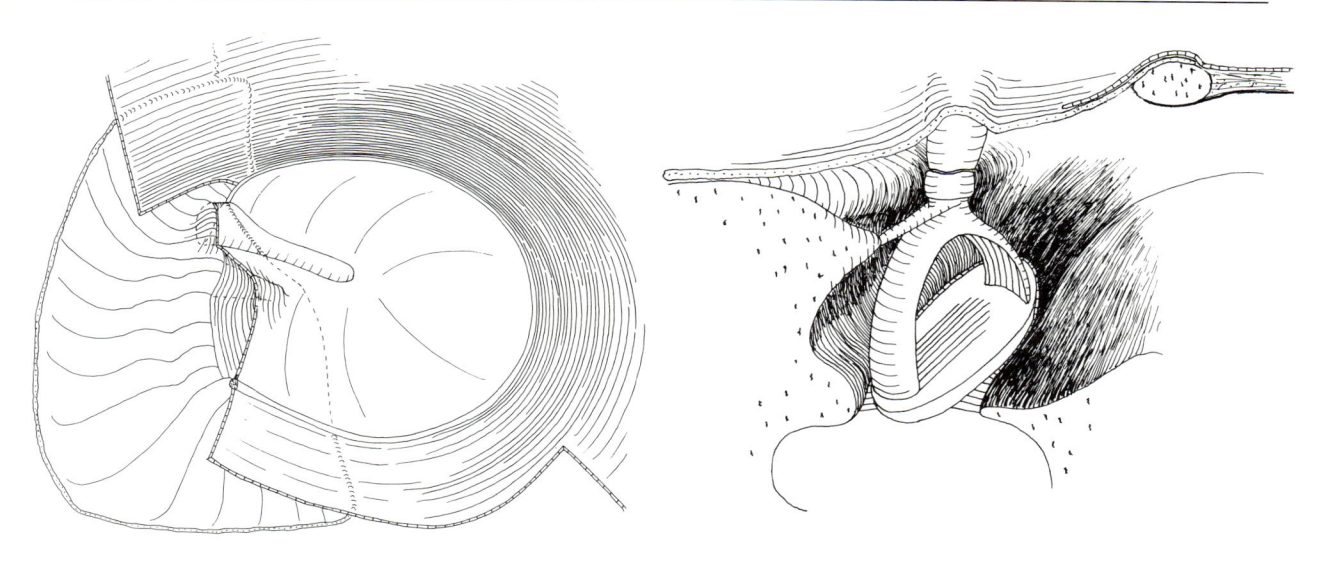

Fig. 871 The perforation is covered with fascia as an underlay graft. The skin flaps are returned, and the connection between the fascia and long process of the incus—the myringoincudopexy—is visible

Fig. 872 Side view of myringoincudopexy in canal wall–down mastoidectomy. The fascia has good contact with the remnant of the long process, and is placed on the prominence of the facial nerve. The tympanic cavity is lower then normal

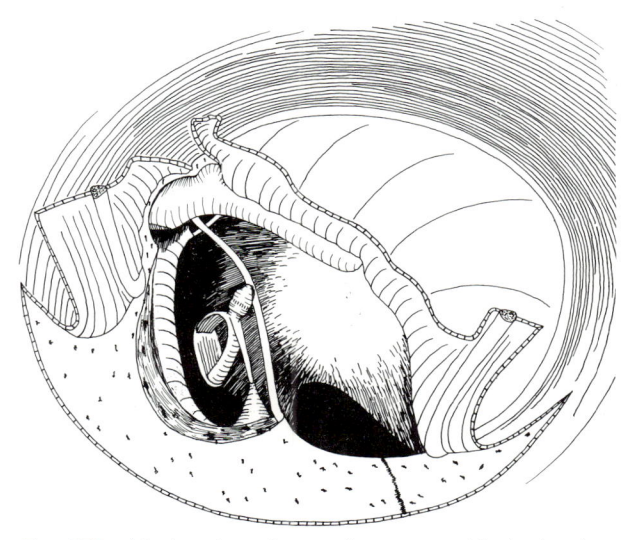

Fig. 873 Myringoincudopexy in a case with the lenticular process firmly fused with the head of the stapes. It cannot be removed, and will be covered by a fascia graft

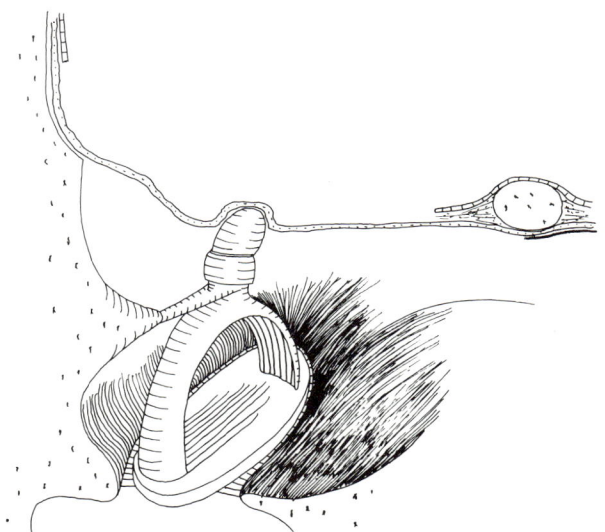

Fig. 874 Side view of the myringoincudopexy. The fascia is brought into contact with the lenticular process, and will be attached to it. The drum is in a lower position than normal

nearly at the same level as the malleus handle, partly because a larger part of the bony annulus is drilled off by more extensive otoslcerotic drilling, and partly because of the anterior positioning and retraction of the malleus. There is therefore no overhang, and a safe ear with no retraction can be achieved. The majority of surgeons interpose a small bony or cartilaginous autograft onto the lenticular process instead of performing myringoincudopexy.

Incudostapediopexy

Several methods are used to connect a defective long process of the incus with the stapes. The goal is to keep the ossicular chain intact and avoid extrusion of the incus. Some of these methods are interpositions rather than pexis procedures.

Incudostapediopexy with Bone and Cartilage

*1. Insertion of a piece of bone between the head of the stapes and a partly **dislocated** but anatomically intact long process* (Hough 1959). A roughly-shaped small piece of bone with a small groove for the stapes head (Fig. **875**), or a precisely-shaped bony cylinder with holes on both sides of the cylinder (Fig. **876**) can be placed between the head of the stapes and the subluxated incus with an intact lenticular process. In total luxation of the incus, the lenticular process can be pushed laterally under the drum with a relatively long piece of bone (Fig. **877**). Sound transmission now emanates directly from the drum—a myringoincudostapediopexy has been established.

Instead of cortical bone, a prosthesis made of homograft ossicles, cartilage, or a hollow shaft prosthesis of Plasti-Pore, ceramic, or hydroxyapatite, can be used. Cortical bone or shaped allogenous ossicle seems to be the best choice. Inserting a polyethylene tube (Fig. **807c**) produces a good primary result, but the hearing later deteriorates due to pressure necrosis or pressure resorption of the lenticular process and the head of the stapes (Kley 1964, 1966).

*2. Insertion of a piece of bone between **defective** long process of the incus and the head of the stapes.* Depending on the position of the remnant of the long process of the incus and the bone piece, there are three, in principle different, interpositions: a) bone can be placed *under* the remnant of the long process of the incus (Figs. **877-879**); b) bone can be placed *around* the incus, or the incus can be placed into a hole in the interposed bone; and c) bone can be placed *onto* the incus remnant.

a) *Under the incus remnant.* After elevation of the defective long process of the incus, a piece of bone with a small groove can be inserted between the head of the stapes and the incus remnant (Fig. **878**). This piece will remain sitting obliquely on the head of the stapes, due to the pressure of the elevated incus on the bone. The bone may become resorbed with time, resulting in loss of the initial hearing gain. On the other hand, if there is no firm contact, with some pressure between the interposed piece of the bone and the two ossicles, the bone piece will move without any corresponding movement in the

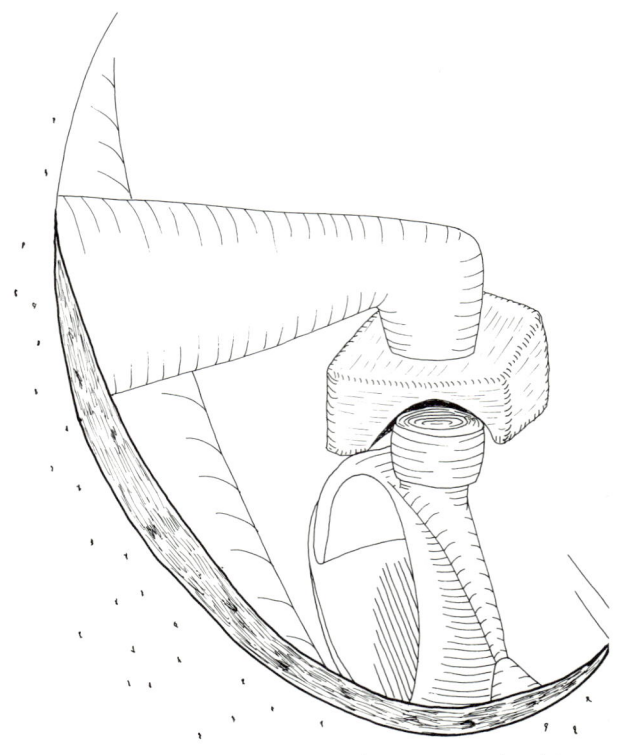

Fig. **875** **Incudostapediopexy** in a case of subluxation of the incus, with a normal lenticular process. A small piece of bone with a groove for the head of the stapes is interposed between the head of the stapes and the lenticular process

stapes. This technique is therefore unreliable in the long term.

A more sophisticated prosthesis (or method) has been developed in order to achieve better contact with the incus. A groove is drilled in a larger piece of bone to adapt it to the undersurface of the remnant of the long process of the incus (Fig. **880**). However, the problem of separate movement of the prosthesis and poor contact with the stapes is not solved with this prosthesis either. To strengthen the pexis, a piece of fascia can be placed onto or around the long process of the incus (Fig. **881**). The pexis can also be strengthened with ionomer cement (Fig. **882**) placed onto the long process of the incus, at the edge of the piece of the cortical bone. The amount of ionomer cement used should be very small.

Recently, a prosthesis made of hydroxyapatite (Smith and Nephew, Richards Company), as suggested by Applebaum (1990), has been introduced for reconnecting the incus and the stapes in patients with defects of the incudostapedial joint. A groove

Pexis 309

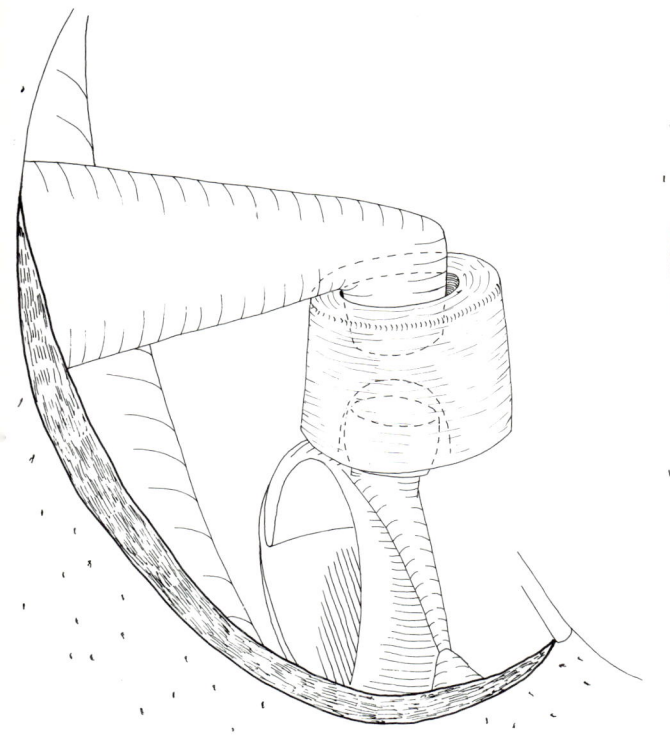

Fig. 876 Incudostapediopexy using a shaped bony cylinder with a hole for the lenticular process and for the head of the stapes

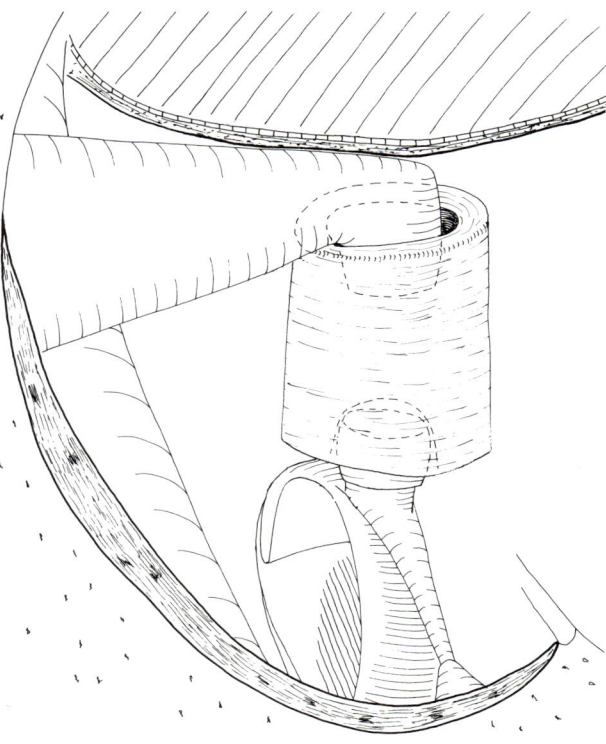

Fig. 877 Complete luxation of the incus, with a normal lenticular process. A cylinder of bone with holes for the lenticular process and the head of the stapes is placed between the long process of the incus and the head of the stapes. The incus is elevated to touch the drum, allowing sound transmission via the drum, the long process of the incus, the bony cylinder and the stapes

for the incus and a hole for the head of the stapes are created, but the groove should be shaped and widened at one end so as to be able to bring the prosthesis under the long process. The problem of placing the hydroxyapatite prosthesis is the same as described above for bone prostheses (Fig. **883**). It is possible to observe the position of the head in relation to the prosthesis through the hole made for the head of the stapes.

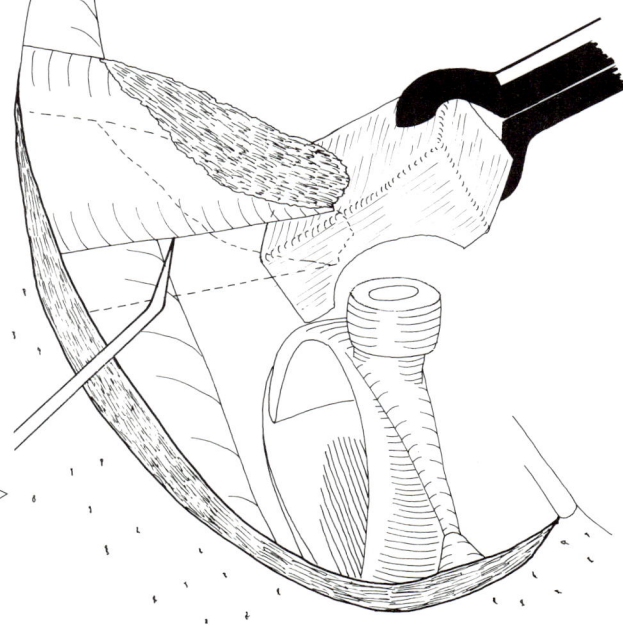

Fig. 878 Incudostapediopexy in a case with a defective long process of the incus. A small piece of bone with a groove for the head of the stapes is carefully placed on the head of the stapes after elevation of the incus remnant with a hook

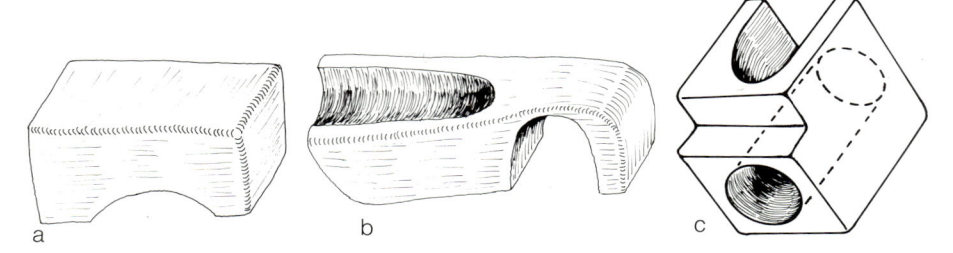

Fig. 879 Prosthesis for an incudostapediopexy for reconstruction of the incudostapedial joint. **a** A small bony prosthesis, with a groove for the head of the stapes. **b** A larger prosthesis, with a groove for the head of the stapes and a larger groove for the remnant of the long process of the incus, to be placed under the long process. **c** The Applebaum incudostapedial joint prosthesis, with a hole for the head of the stapes and a groove for the long process of the incus

Spencer (1976) used a prosthesis made of tragal cartilage. A piece of 2.5×3.0 mm tragal cartilage with attached perichondrium on both sides is used and shaped. On one side, the perichondrium is partly elevated (Fig. 884), and a groove is cut with a beaver knife. This provides a trough for the long process of the incus. The remnant of the lenticular process is elevated from the head of the stapes and turned inferiorly, but not removed, providing a larger and flatter surface on which to place the tragal cartilage prothesis (Fig. 885). After placement of the cartilage prosthesis under the remnant of the incus and on the head of the stapes, the perichondrium flap is folded back, closing the pocket and providing a good chance for fixation of the graft to the incus.

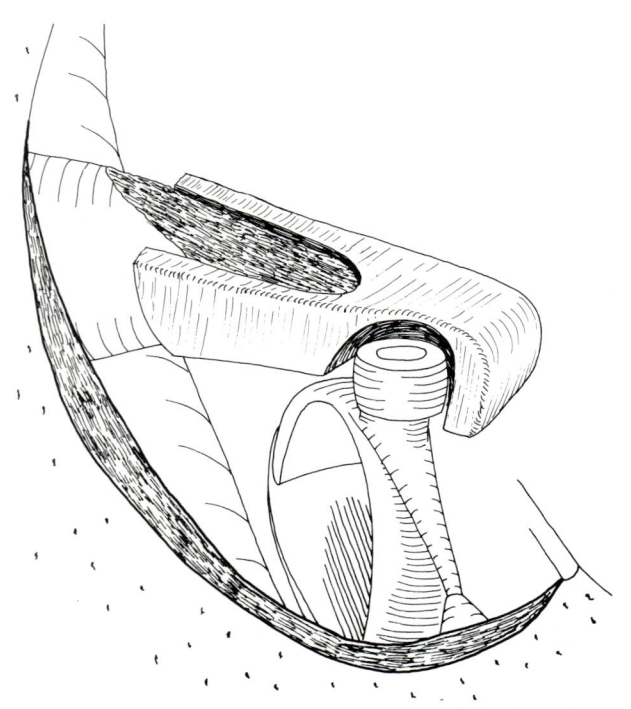

Fig. 880 Incudostapediopexy in a defective long process of the incus, using a specially-shaped bony prosthesis with a groove for the head of the stapes and a larger groove for the incus, to be placed under the incus remnant and on the head of the stapes

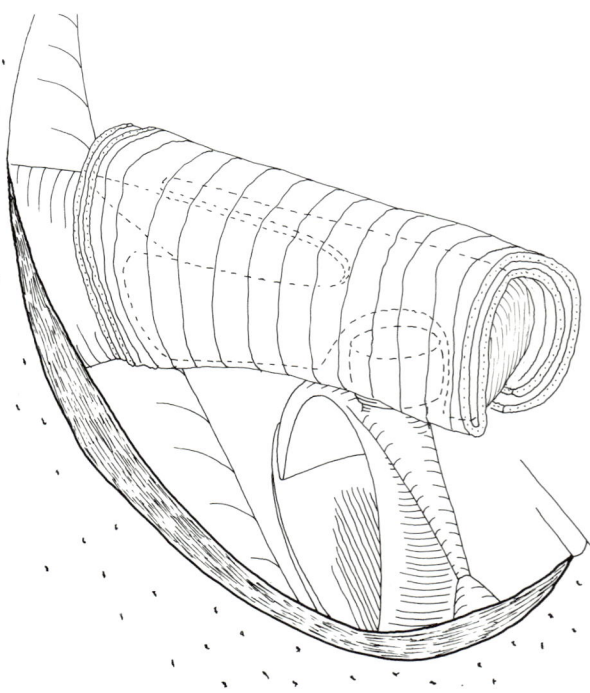

Fig. 881 The incudostapediopexy is covered with fascia

Pexis 311

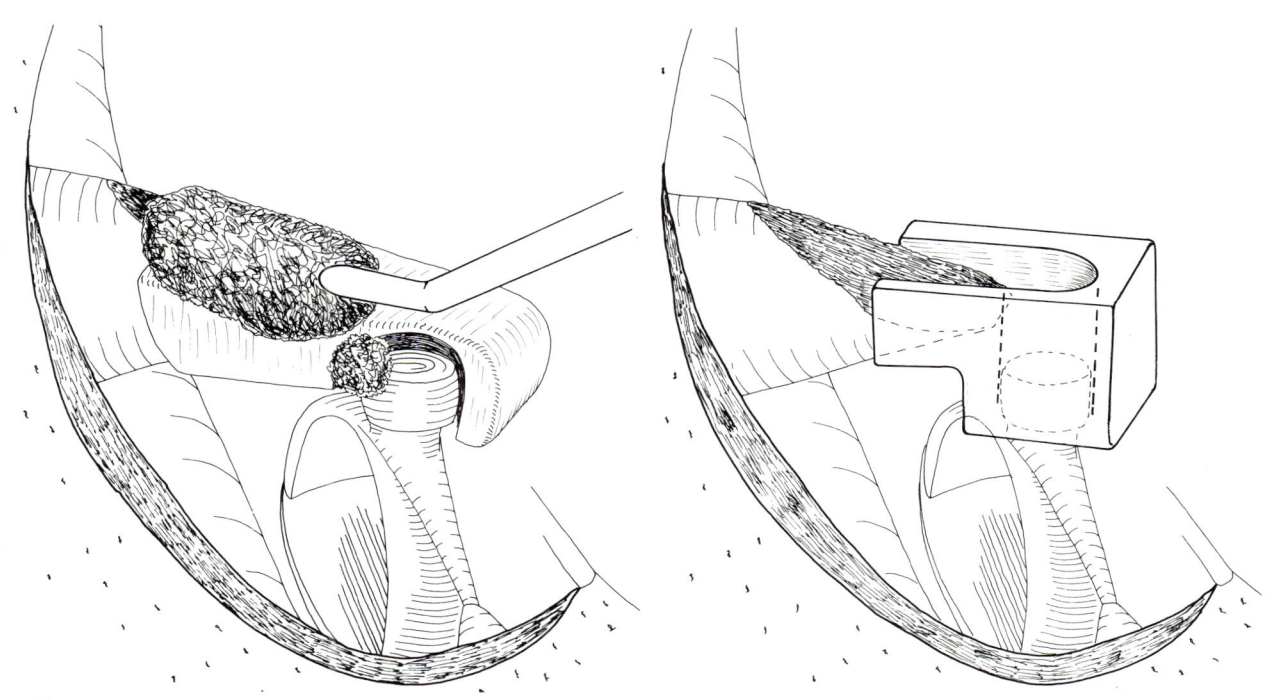

Fig. 882 Fixation of the pexis with ionomer cement placed on the remnant of the bony process of the incus and the cortical bone

Fig. 883 **The Applebaum hydroxyapatite incudostapedial joint prosthesis.** The prosthesis is placed on the head of the stapes, with its groove under the remnant of the incus

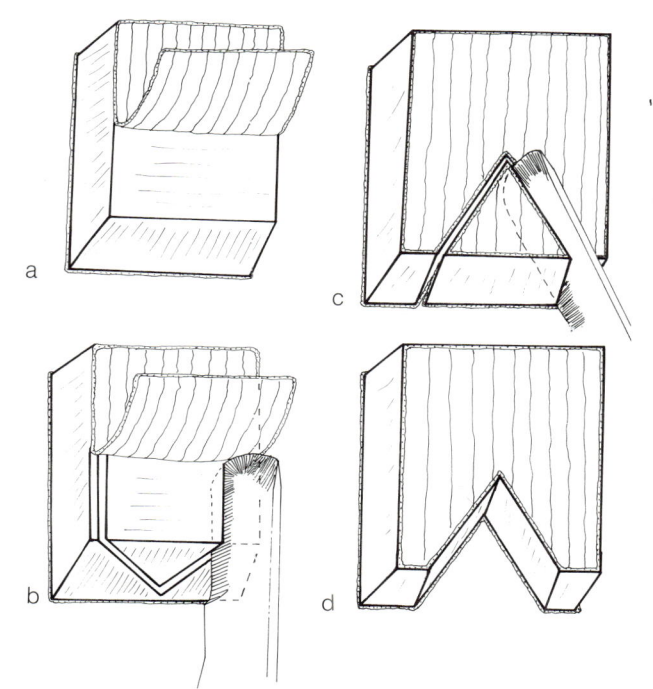

Fig. 884 Tragal cartilage prosthesis for reconstruction of the incudostapedial joint, an incudostapediopexy. **a** Perichondrium is elevated from a piece of tragal cartilage. **b** A groove is cut with a beaver knife in one half of the tragal cartilage. **c, d** Preparation of another cartilage prosthesis for incudostapediopexy, with a wedge cut off the tragal cartilage

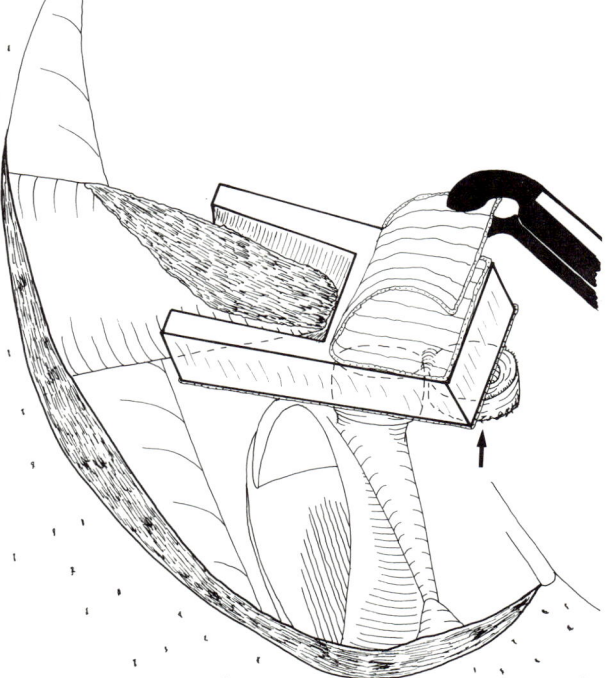

Fig. 885 **The Spencer tragal cartilage prosthesis** for incudostapediopexy. The prosthesis is placed on top of the head of the stapes and underneath the remnant of the long process of the incus. The tragal perichondrium is replaced, creating a pocket around the remnant of the long process of the incus

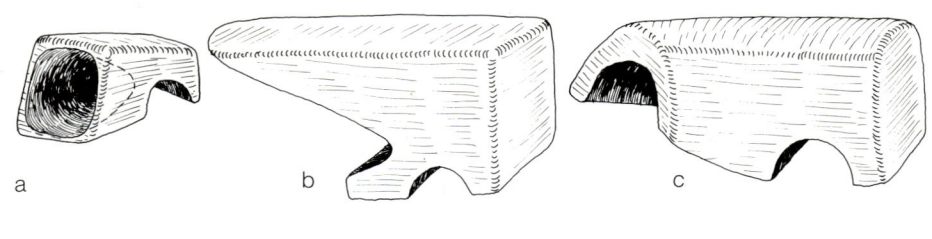

18 Transposition and Pexis in Type 2 Tympanoplasty

Fig. 886 Prostheses shaped from cortical bone or ossicles for incudostapediopexy in reconstruction of the incudostapedial joint. **a** A large hole for the remnant of the long process of the incus, and a groove for the head of the stapes. **b** A groove for the head of the stapes and a wedge-like excavation for the remnant of the long process of the incus. The prosthesis is placed on the incus. **c** A small groove for the head of the stapes and a large groove to be placed on the remnant of the long process of the incus

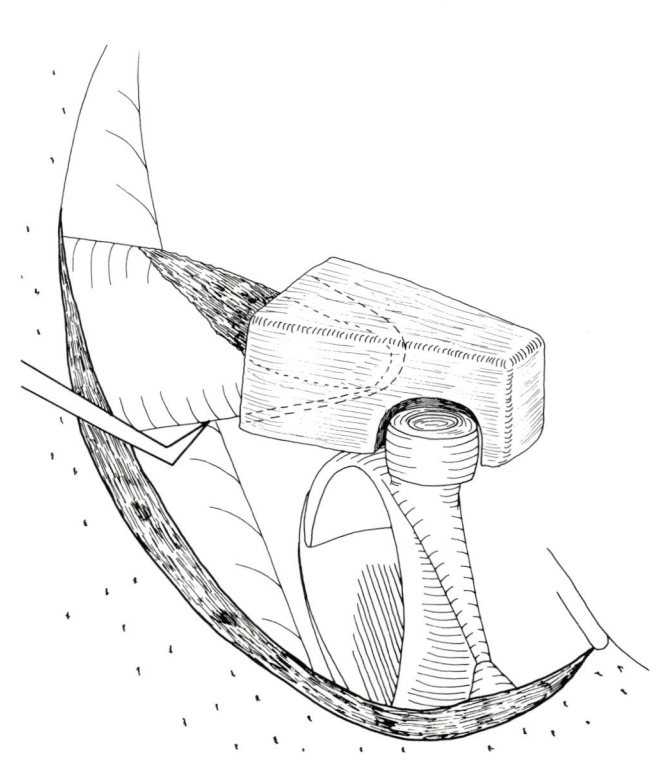

Fig. 887 An incudostapediopexy with a prosthesis placed on the head of the stapes and attached with a hole to the remnant of the long process of the incus

b) *Around the incus remnant.* A large hole is drilled in a piece of cortical bone or allogenous incus so that it can be attached to the remnant of the long process (Fig. **886**). The prosthesis is shaped in such a way that it is in contact with the head of the stapes via a groove and with the long process of the incus via a hole (Fig. **887**). The long process of the incus is gently elevated with a hook, and the prosthesis is pushed onto its end. The hole in the bone prosthesis should be sufficiently large from the very beginning, avoiding unnecessary elevation of the incus. The groove, or the hole for the head of the stapes, should be low so that the prosthesis can easily slip into it. This method is technically the most difficult to perform, but is the most physiological and reliable in the long term. Polyethylene prostheses based on the same principles have been used (Fig. **807a, d**), but they did not work over the long term due to the rigidity of the polyethylene and bone resorption occurring in the incus remnant and stapes around the edges of the prosthesis.

In a larger defect of the long process of the incus, Spencer (1976) used a piece of tragal cartilage fitted carefully to the remnant of the incus. A wedge is cut out of a piece of cartilage covered with perichondrium on both sides (Fig. **884**). The prosthesis is placed on the head of the stapes, with the wedge adapted to the remnant of the incus (Fig. **888**). This method is in some respects a cartilage interposition, as described above (Fig. **792**), especially with Spencer's recommendation to use a larger piece of cartilage so as to be able to bring it into contact with the malleus handle as well (Fig. **888**).

Pexis 313

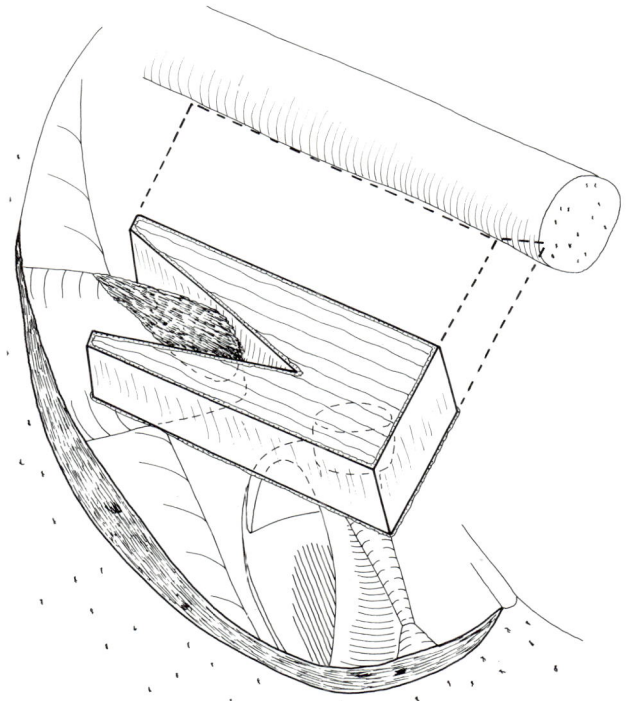

Fig. **888** The Spencer tragal cartilage prosthesis on the head of the stapes. The wedge of the prosthesis is brought into firm contact with the remnant of the long process of the incus. The dotted line indicates a larger tragal prosthesis in contact with the malleus handle

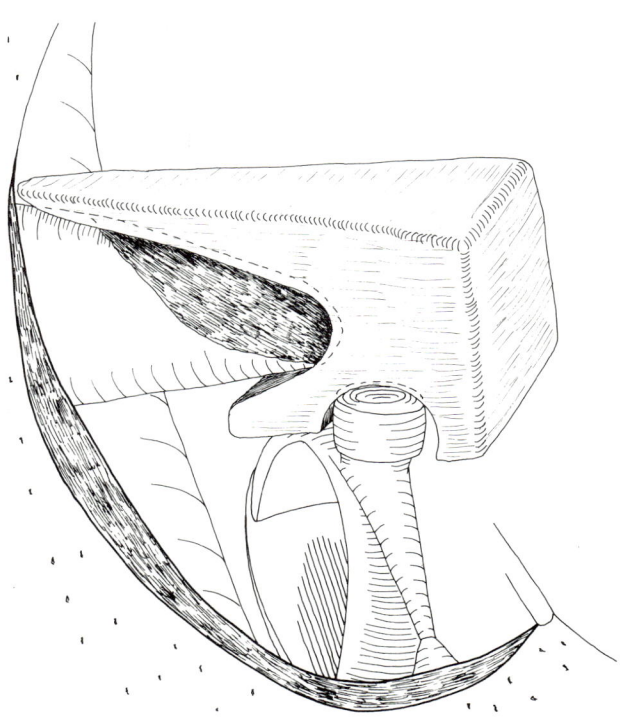

Fig. **889** An incudostapedial prosthesis of cortical bone or ossicle placed on the head of the stapes and on the remnant of the long process of the incus

c) *Onto the incus remnant.* A piece of bone is placed on the remnant of the long process of the incus and the head of the stapes. Autogenous bone, or allogenous ossicles of various sizes, can be used, and the pieces can be shaped in various ways. These methods resemble the interposition methods, and even though the aim of the methods is to reconstruct the incudostapedial joint, the hope is that sound transmission can also occur via the drum and a relatively high prosthesis. In a fairly large piece of bone (1×2 mm) or an allogenous ossicle, a groove is drilled for the head of the stapes and another, larger groove for contact with the defective incus (Fig. **886**). The second groove is made in such a way that a bony edge can sit underneath the remnant of the long process of the incus, improving the connection with the incus (Fig. **889**).

Another, more sophisticated, way of shaping the ossicle has been performed, using a large groove in a relatively large piece of bone or an allograft ossicle (Fig. **886**). The graft rides on the incus remnant and the head of the stapes (Fig. **890**).

As seen in Figure **881**, fascia can be placed onto or around a pexis with bone, facilitating the formation of fibrous tissue and stabilization of the pexis.

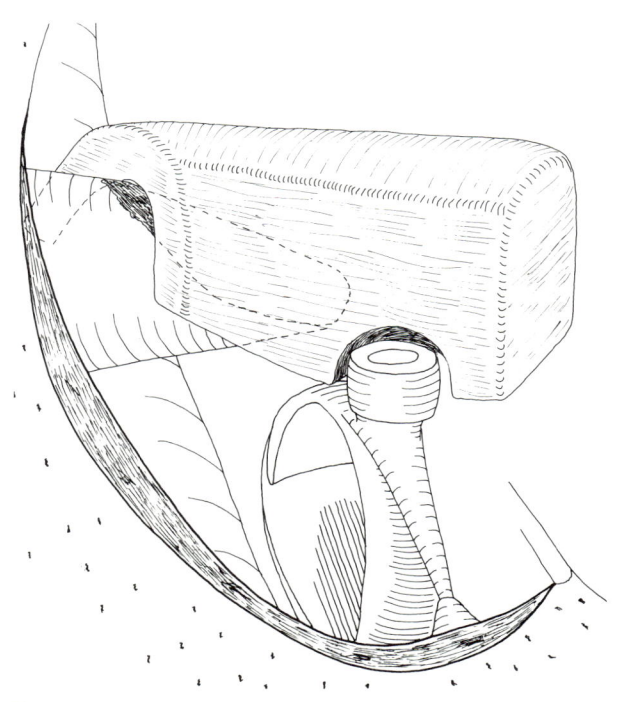

Fig. **890** An Incudostapediopexy, with a prosthesis placed on the head of the stapes and, with a large groove, on the remnant of the long process of the incus

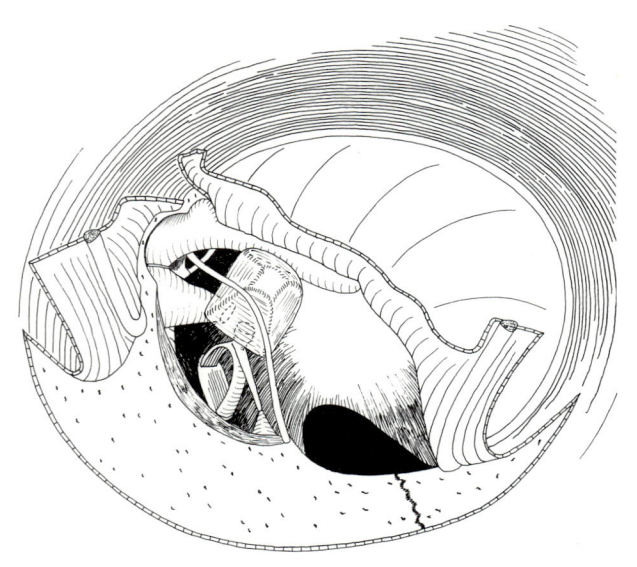

Fig. 891 **Sadé's small tripod prosthesis,** consisting of a pyramid of cortical bone or allogenous ossicle. The pyramid is placed on the remnant of the long process and the head of the stapes and has contact with the malleus handle

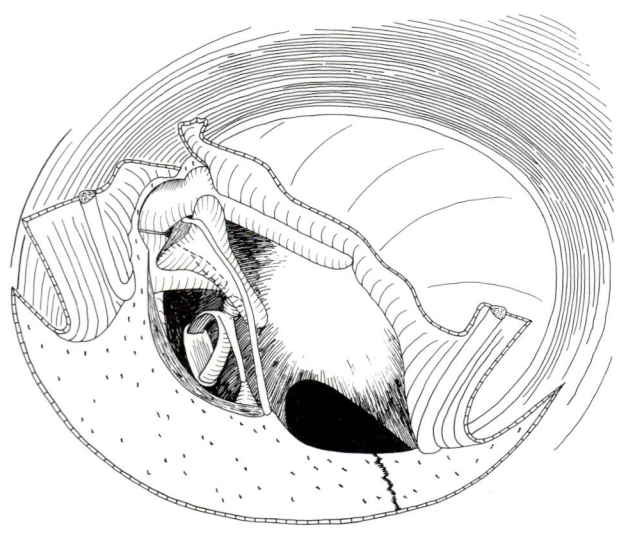

Fig. 892 **Sadé's long tripod prosthesis,** placed on the long process of the incus, has contact with the head of the stapes and the malleus handle

All of the pexis procedures using pieces of cortical bone or ossicles illustrated in Figures **879, 880, 887, 889,** and **890,** or using hydroxyapatite prostheses (Fig. **883**), can be stabilized with small amounts of ionomer cement placed on the edges of the long process of the incus and the piece of cortical bone (Fig. **882**).

Sadé (1987) uses a small tripod prosthesis, a pyramid made from cortical bone or allogenous ossicles. The pyramid is supported simultaneously at three points: the stapes, the incus remnant, and the side of the malleus handle (Fig. **891**).

A long tripod prosthesis or a prolongation made of cortical bone or allogenous malleus is placed obliquely on the long process of the incus, bridging the defective incus with the stapes (Figs. **892, 893**). The prosthesis also has contact to the malleus handle. Sadé (1987) achieved the best one-year results using the small tripod method.

To bridge incudostapedial defects, cartilage can be used in a way similar to that devised by Spencer. The cartilage prosthesis, with a groove placed underneath the incus remnant (Fig. **885**), can be turned 180° and placed on the incus remnant. The prosthesis rides on the incudostapedial defect.

Incudostapediopexy with ionomer cement. Babighian (1992) uses ionomer cement to repair the ossicular chain in the following pathologies and in the following ways:

1) Reshaping the eroded long process of the incus following chronic otitis, or in post-stapedectomy cases. A drop of ionomer cement is brought onto the defective long process of the incus. With a small elevator (Fig. **894**) the drop is pulled inferiorly towards the head of the stapes, remodeling the lenticular process. A new layer of ionomer cement is placed on the previous one if the connection to the stapes seems to be inadequate (Fig. **895**).

2) Fixation of a malleoincudal disjunction after traumatic ossicular dislocation. After posterior and superior tympanotomy, either with a retroauricular or an endaural approach, an atticotomy is performed (Figs. **216-222, 896**). The superior aspect of the malleus head is located, and the incus body is repositioned and fixed to the malleus head by a small amount of ionomer cement. The cement is carefully laid down on the articular side of the ossicle using a small elevator (Fig. **896**). The defect in the attic wall can be closed with the ionomer cement, by spreading it over a relatively large area of the defect and drilling the superfluous cement away with a diamond drill under constant irrigation. The ossicle should be protected by Silastic during application of the cement to the atticotomy.

Pexis 315

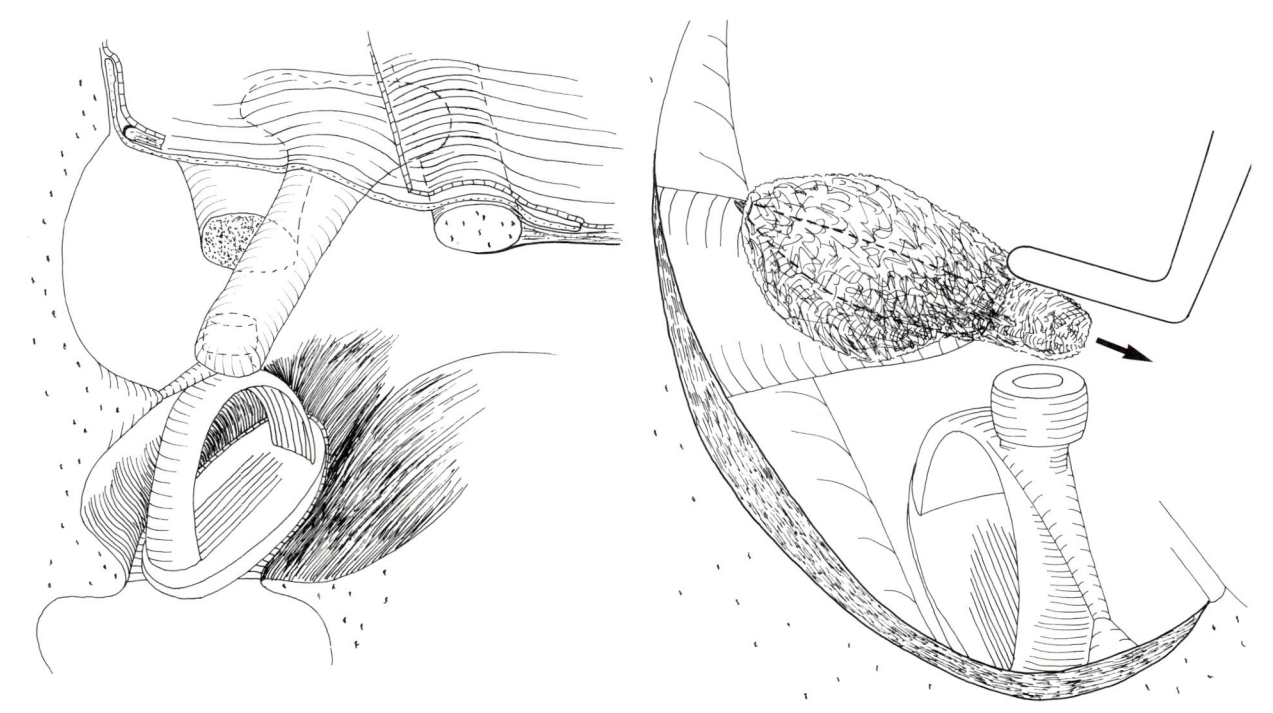

Fig. 893 Side view of the large tripod prosthesis, showing its contact with the head of the stapes, the defective long process of the incus, and the malleus handle

Fig. 894 **Babighian's technique for reshaping the defective long process of the incus with ionomer cement.** A drop of cement is placed on the remnant of the incus and pulled by rougine towards the head of the stapes

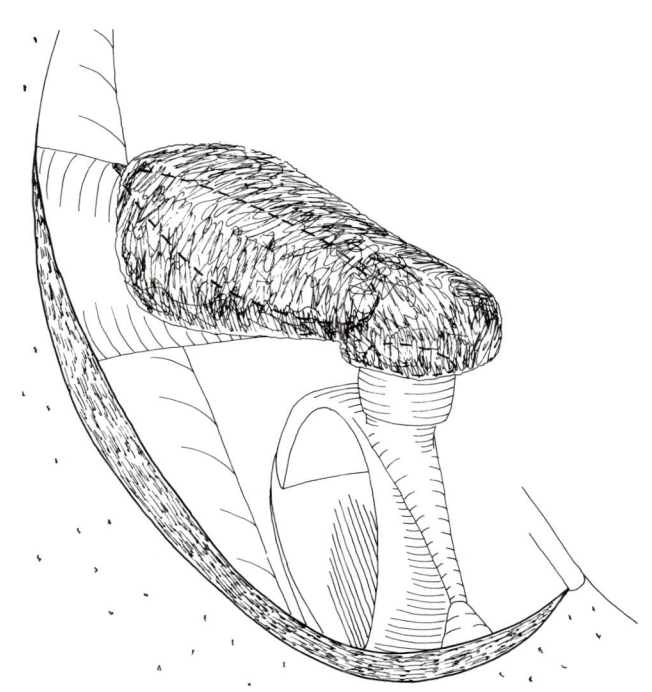

Fig. 895 The lenticular process is reshaped and connected with the head of the stapes using ionomer cement

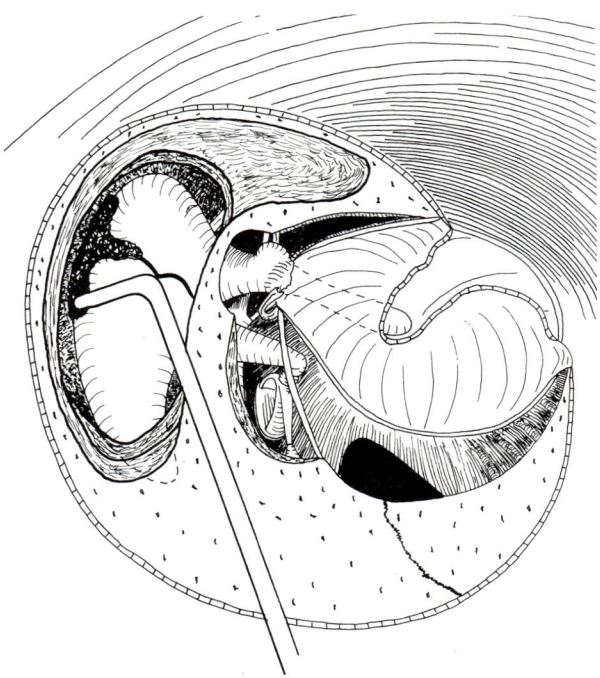

Fig. 896 Fixation of the posttraumatic malleoincudal disjunction. After atticotomy, the head of the malleus is glued to the incus body by placing a thin layer of ionomer cement on their superior aspects and at the incudomalleolar junction

Babighian (1992) also repairs bony wall defects of the posterior and lateral attic walls and anterior ear-canal walls. The cement should be covered with fascia or cartilage, and only small bony defects should be covered by ionomer cement, so as to avoid granulation. In large reconstructions of the bony ear-canal wall, granulation tissue formation and epithelialization problems occur with the areas of the ear canal covered.

The author has used ionomer cement to repair posterior bony annulus defects, but there seems to be no need to cover an atticotomy with cement or bone pieces in posttraumatic cases with normal tubal function. If the bridge is preserved (Fig. **904**), there will be no retraction, because of the atticotomy.

3) Babighian (1992) also attempted to glue an intact allogenous incus to the malleus, and eventually to the head of the stapes, with ionomer cement. This fascinating transplantation of an entire ossicle to produce a completely intact ossicular chain is a new and interesting event in tympanoplasty, although Gundersen, in the early 1960s, inserted an accurate polyethylene model of a normal incus (Gundersen 1964). This polyethylene incus is held in place with a small steel clip, which grips the neck of the malleus. Articulation with the head of the stapes is ensured through a small polyethylene tube.

Fixation of the small bony pieces used in incudostapediopexies with ionomer cement can be very useful, and may improve the pexis methods (Fig. **882**). Ionomer cement will surely have a place in ossicular reconstruction in the future.

Incudostapediopexy with wires. Steel wires have been used to connect the incudostapedial joint defect (Fig. **897**). An eye is fitted to the long process of the incus, and the wire is connected to the stapes head (Oppenheimer and Harrison 1963); good results have been seen with this method. But if the wire is too tight around the stapes head or the long process of the incus, there may be resorption of the bone, and the wire may slip out of position. The wire can be tightened on the lateral or medial aspects of the incus remnant (Fig. **897**), providing various distances to the head of the stapes and probably producing various effects on the hearing.

A stainless-steel wire is fixed with a loop to the remnant of the long process, and the other end is inserted into the excavated head of the stapes like the arm of a record player (Fig. **898**). Oppenheimer and Harrison (1963) achieved good results with this method, but very little has been published on wire prostheses in general, and there are no long-term results are available for these techniques at all. It is not known whether it is better to place the wire above or under the incus remnant (Fig. **898**).

Gold and platinum wires have been used in a similar way (Mehmke 1966). Mehmke used 0.2–0.3 mm–thick gold wire anchored to the incus in a spiral shape (Fig. **899**). Gold clips which can be pressed over the long process and the head of the stapes, have also been used by Mehmke in patients with a defective lenticular process.

Combinations of stainless-steel wire and polyethylene have also been used to repair incudostapedial defects.

Generally, it can be concluded that not enough is known about the long-term functioning of these prostheses connecting the incudostapedial joint. The steel-wire prosthesis is very interesting, and should be used and investigated more than it has been so far.

Holes and grooves in the incus remnant. Recently, Hüttenbrink (1992 b) developed a drill that enabled him to drill small holes through the neck of the malleus. This type of drilling improves the fixation technique for wire, and may lead to a renaissance of the wire pexis methods.

After performing experiments on cadavers with small drills with diameters of 0.5 and 0.35 mm with the new Shea Micro Drill (Treace Company, Memphis), the present author has found that small holes can be created in the long process of the incus. The following methods can be used in incudostapediopexies. Small holes of various diameters can be drilled through the remnant of the long process of the incus. Stainless-steel wire, gold wire, or any other type of wire, can be tightened medial to the long process of the incus and brought medially towards the stapes head and down to the footplate (Fig. **900**). The wire can also be tightened lateral to the remnant of long process of the incus and brought laterally towards the stapes head. Though medial tightening seems to be technically more difficult, it allows better movement of the stapes than the method of tightening the wire laterally on the long process of the incus, which is easier to perform. The size of the hole (Fig. **900**) depends on the minimum size of the drill, and also determines the thickness of the wire used. It will be possible to use holes of 0.2 mm and a wire thickness of 0.135 mm, like the wires in stapes surgery.

In addition to holes, small grooves can be drilled along the incus remnant, especially on its posterosuperior aspect, enabling the wire to lie in the groove and allowing better and more stable stapes movement (Fig. **901**). A groove can also be created medially at the distal end of the remnant of

Pexis 317

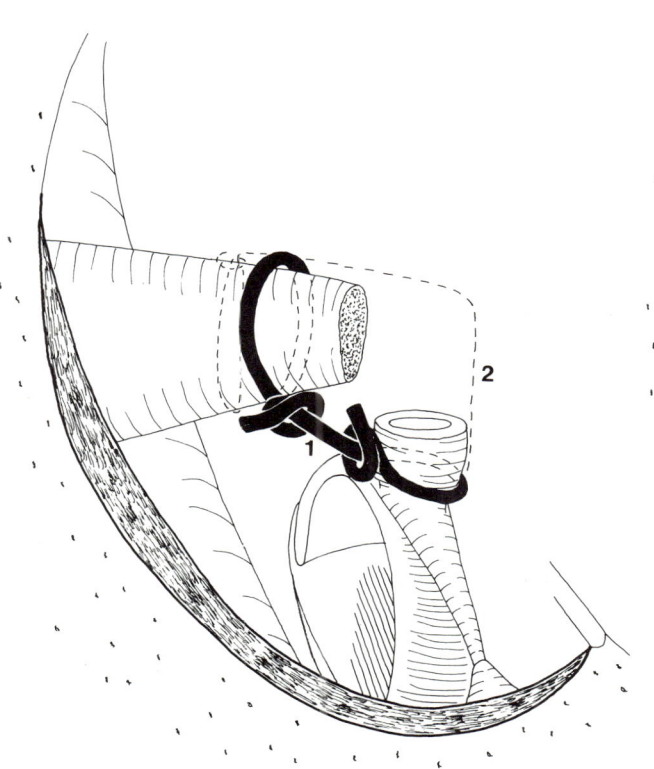

Fig. 897 **An incudostapediopexy with a wire** between the remnant of the long process of the incus and the neck of the stapes. The prosthesis is tied medially (1) or laterally (2) onto the long process of the incus

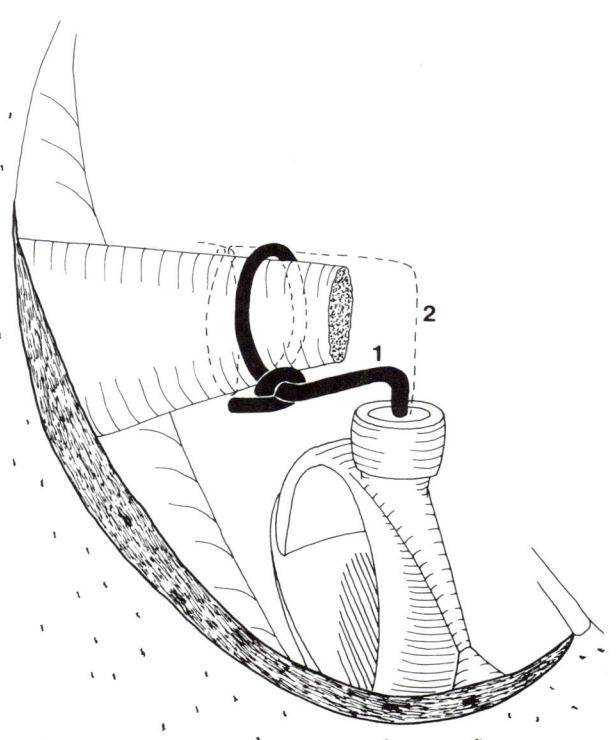

Fig. 898 The record-player arm type of incudostapediopexy with a wire. The wire is attached to the long process of the incus and tied either medially (1) or laterally (2). The connection with the head of the stapes takes the shape of a record-player arm

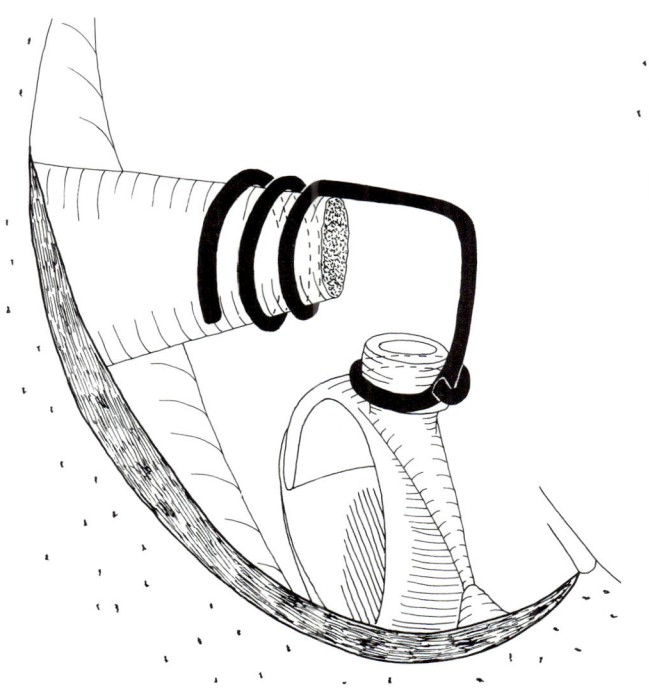

Fig. 899 Mehmke's wire incudostapediopexy, where the wire is fixed to the remnant of the long process in a spiral

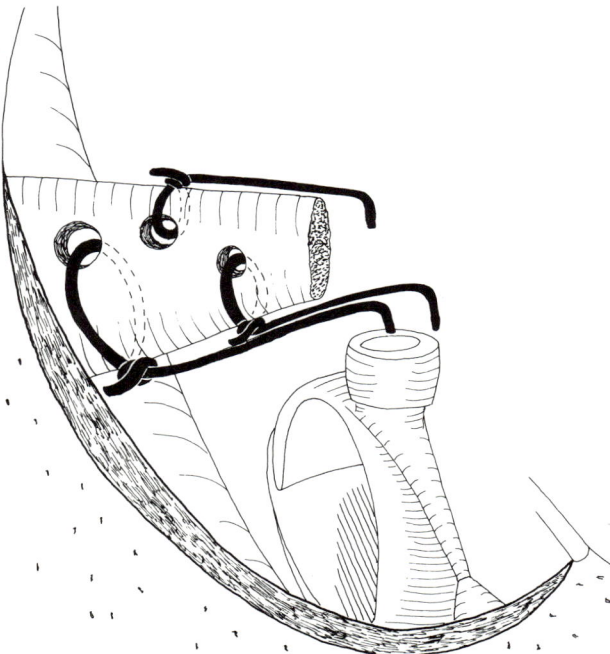

Fig. 900 Proposal for incudostapediopexy using wires and holes in the remnant of the long process. The wires are tied medially or laterally to the incus

the long process of the incus to support the wire movement (Fig. **902**).

Holes and grooves also provide better tightening of the prostheses to the incus remnant. Instead of tying a knot, another hole can be drilled into or through the thicker distal end of the long process (Fig. **903**), or even into the incus body itself. The same tightening principles as those used in stapedectomy can be applied when fixing wire prostheses in incudostapediopexy. Finally, the holes in the bones could be produced by a laser beam.

Fixation of pexis wires with ionomer cement. On temporal bones, the author has carried out wire fixation using small amounts of ionomer cement in incudostapediopexies (Figs. **904, 905**). The wire fixation can be performed either a) within the drilling hole in the incus remnant; b) along the long process of the incus; c) onto the head or neck of the stapes; or d) onto the anterior crus of the stapes. Fixation can also be carried out in the situations described above, without holes (Figs. **897-899**). If used carefully in small quantities and with careful measurement and shaping of the wire before starting the cement fixation, ionomer cement will surely improve the wire pexis techniques and make them easier to perform. Wire fixation with cement allows the holes to be larger, means they can be placed more proximally towards the incus body. Ionomer cement can also attach the wire to the incus remnant without a hole, as in fixation of a cochlear electrode.

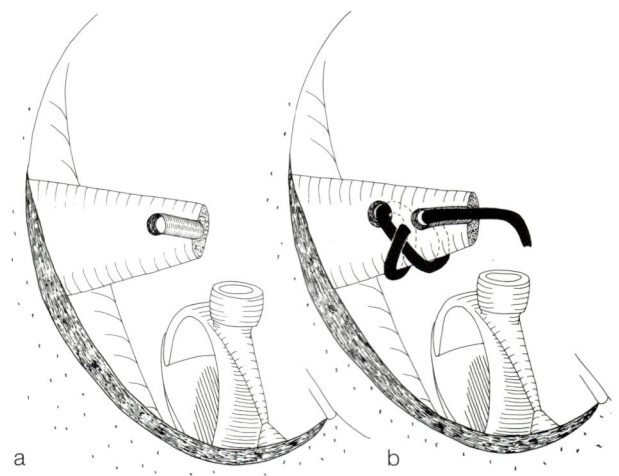

Fig. **901** Proposal for incudostapediopexy using a hole through the incus remnant and a groove for stabilization of the wire. **a** A hole and a groove are created. **b** A second hole is made for fixation of the wire, which goes through the first hole and then through the groove to the stapes

Pexis 319

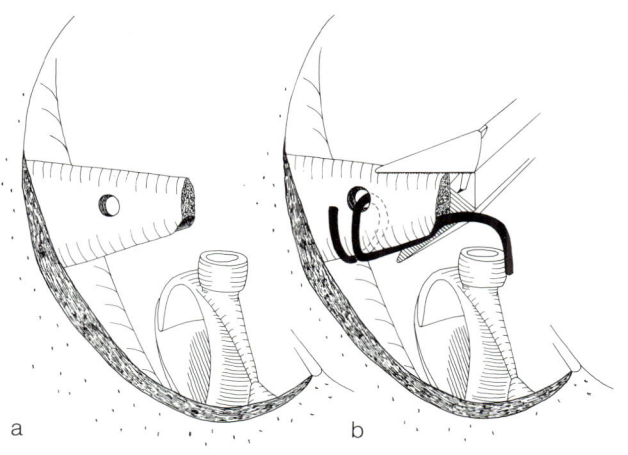

Fig. **902a** An Incudostapediopexy with a hole through the incus remnant and a groove medially in the distal part of the incus remnant. **b** The wire goes through the hole along the medial aspect of the long process of the incus, and along the groove towards the head of the stapes

Fig. **903** Proposal for a wire incudostapediopexy, with the wire being fixed using an extra hole. **a** A hole and a groove are made distally in the long process of the incus, and another hole is made proximally. **b** The wire is placed through the distal hole and along the groove, and is fixed in the proximal hole using a forceps

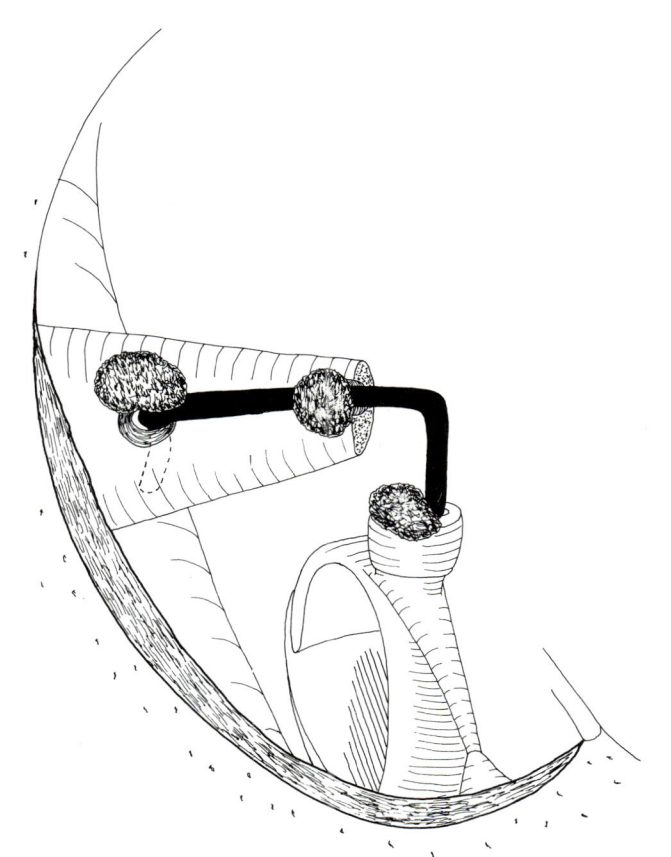

Fig. **904** Proposals for wire fixation in a hole at the end of the incus remnant and to the head of the stapes using ionomer cement

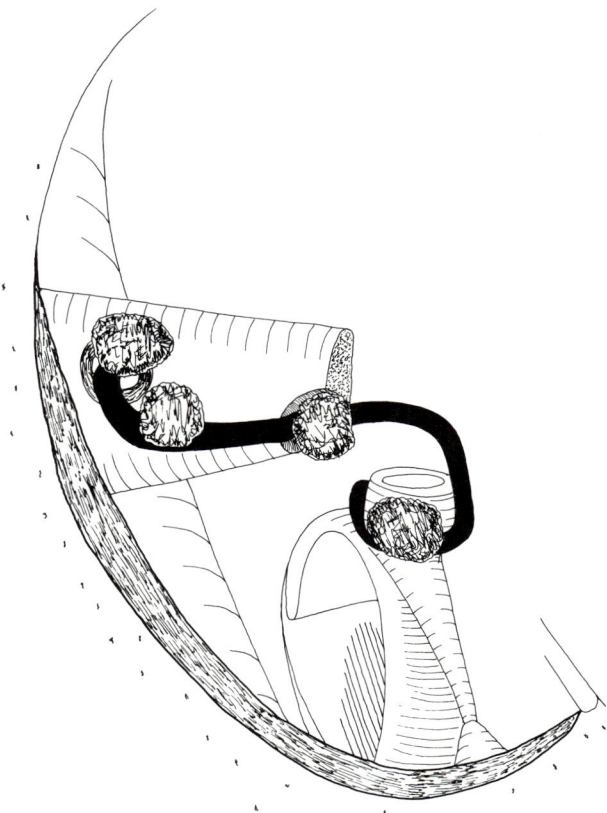

Fig. **905** Proposals for wire fixation to the incus remnant (within a hole, along and at the end of the remnant) and to the neck of the stapes, using ionomer cement

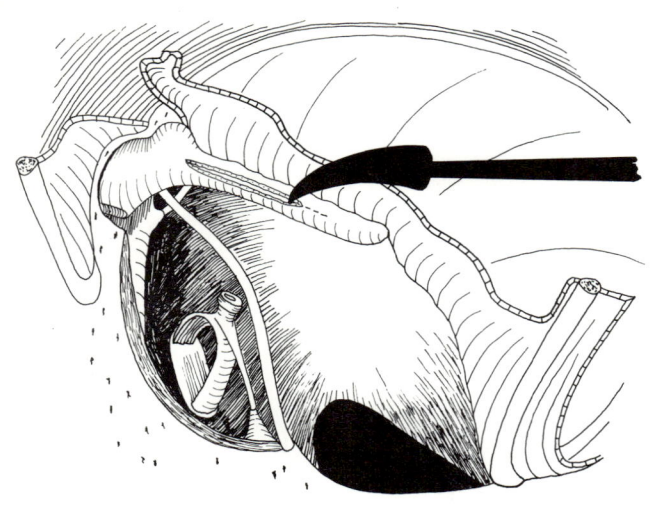

Fig. 906 Malleostapediopexy with a wire. An incision is made through the periosteum on the posterior aspect of the malleus handle

Malleostapediopexy

Generally, "malleostapediopexy" is the term for a wire connection between the malleus handle and the stapes. As mentioned above, some surgeons use "malleostapediopexy" to refer to transposition of the malleus handle onto the stapes. Wire malleostapediopexy was used by Oppenheimer and Harrison (1963), Mehmke (1966) and also Bellucci (1966). The metal wire may be made of tantalum, stainless steel, platinum, or gold. The malleus handle is connected with the stapes head.

An incision is made in the periosteum of the posterior aspect of the malleus handle using a small sickle knife (Fig. 906). The periosteum is elevated together with the lamina propria, liberating the upper half of the malleus handle (Fig. 907). A stainless-steel wire, 0.3 mm thick, is cut to an appropriate length. A loop is made at the malleus end, with another loop at the stapes end. The wire is inserted onto the malleus handle with a forceps (Fig. 908). It is pressed tightly to the malleus handle with the forceps, and its end is at the same time pushed up under the malleus handle with a curved rugine (Fig. 909). The stapes loop is brought carefully around the neck of the stapes and clamped together with alligator forceps — a technique similar to that used for wire fixation in stapes surgery (Fig. 910). A piece of cartilage or perichondrium, or an additional piece of fascia, covers the steel wire (Fig. 911). If used, the fascia is placed on the malleus handle.

Bellucci (1966) prefers an angled wire prosthesis, mainly for protection against strong stapes movements (Fig. 912).

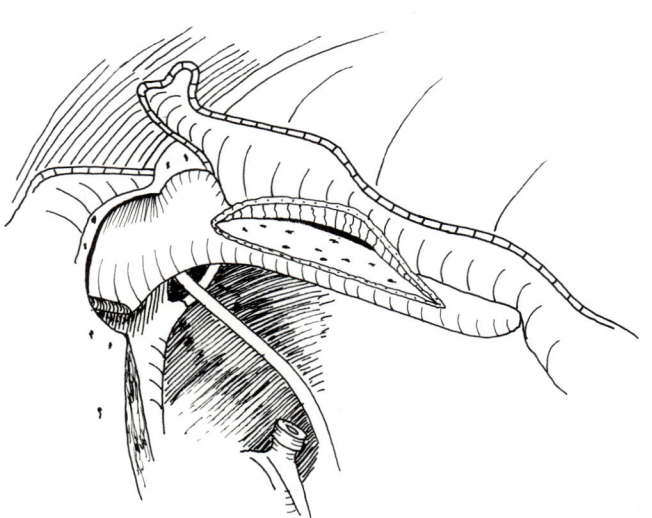

Fig. 907 The periosteum and lamina propria of the malleus handle are elevated, and a pocket is formed

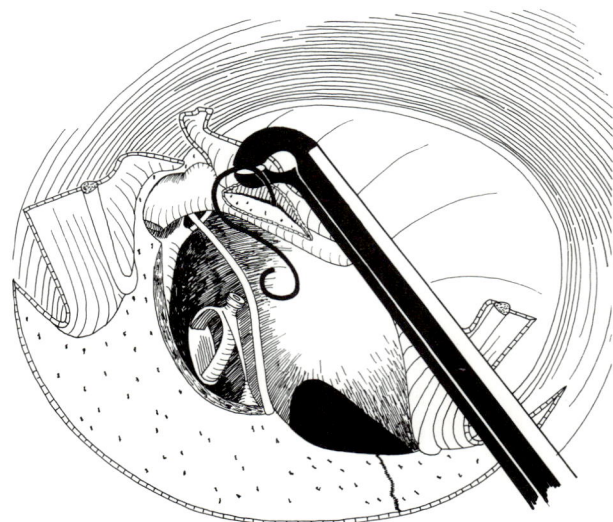

Fig. 908 A stainless-steel wire is placed on the malleus handle

Pexis

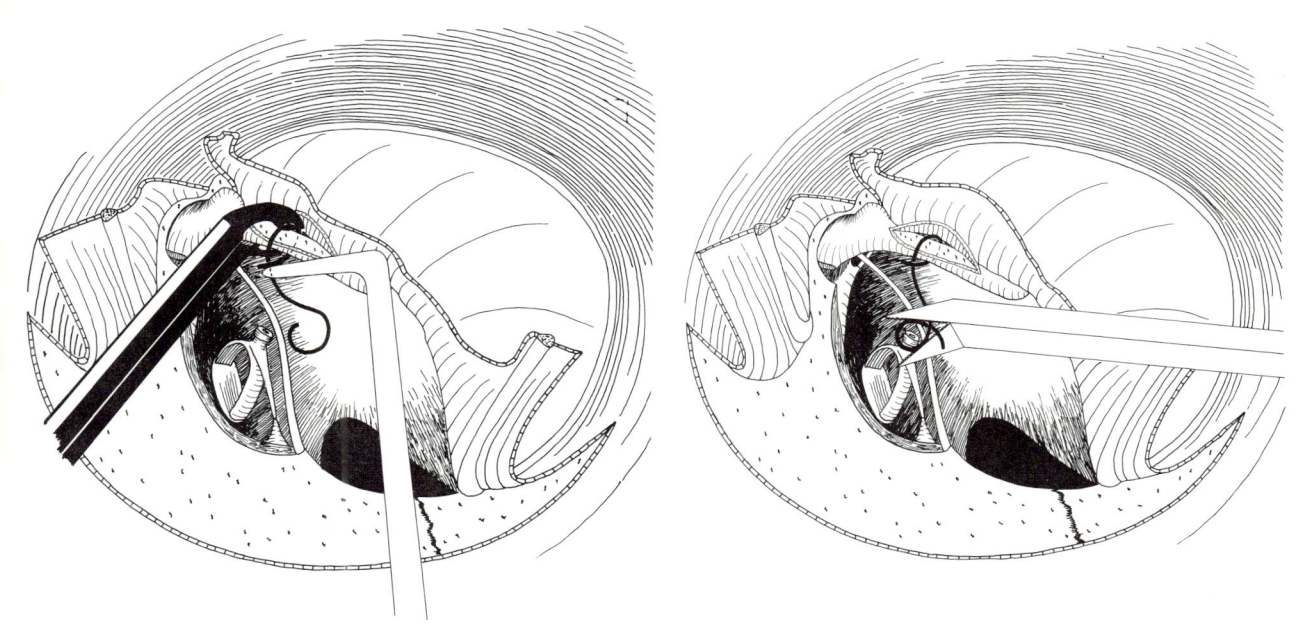

Fig. 909 The wire is fixed around the malleus handle

Fig. 910 The wire is fixed around the head of the stapes

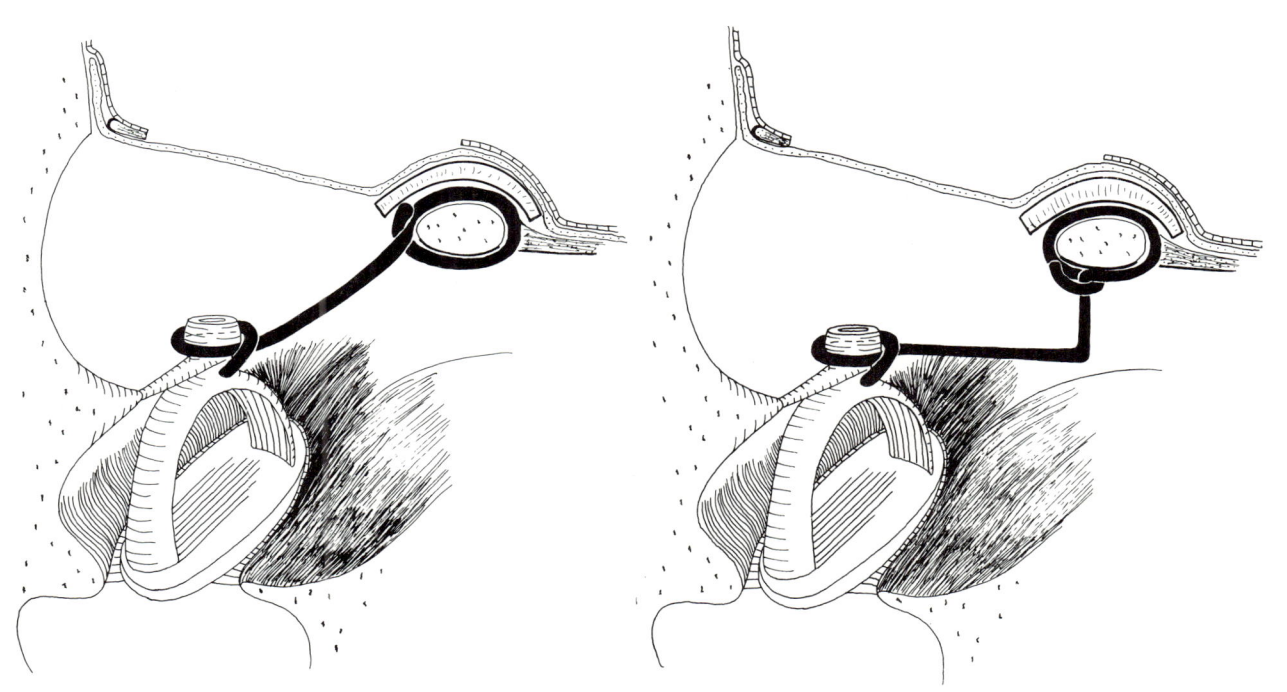

Fig. 911 Side view of the malleostapediopexy, showing the covering of the wire at the malleus handle with a small piece of cartilage

Fig. 912 **The Bellucci malleostapediopexy,** with the wire running rectangularly from the malleus to the stapes

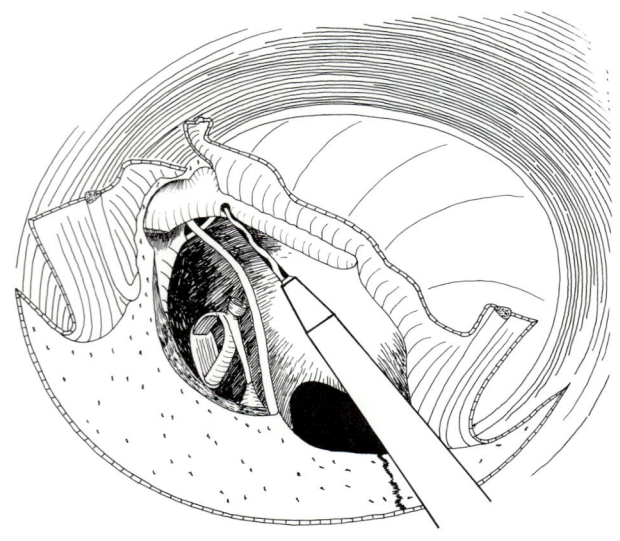

Fig. 913 **The Hüttenbrink malleostapediopexy.** A hole is drilled through the malleus handle with a small spiral drill

The Hüttenbrink malleostapediopexy. As mentioned above, Hüttenbrink (1992b) has developed a special thin drill with a diameter of 0.2 mm (Fischer Company, Freiburg, Germany) to drill a hole into the malleus handle just inferior to the attachment of the tendon of the tensor tympani muscle (Fig. 913). A relatively soft gold wire is passed through the hole and fixed to the malleus handle with a small loop. The stapes end of the wire is fixed to the neck of the stapes with a forceps (Fig. 914). This technique marks a considerable step forward in ossiculoplasty, as it improves wire fixation to the malleus, eliminates the possibility of adhesions around the interposition grafts, and provides firm attachment of the wire prosthesis to the malleus handle. Hüttenbrink (1992a) showed that due to the piston-like vibration of the ossicular chain, the position of the wire loop around the malleus handle has no influence on sound amplification. However, it is essential that the prosthesis is attached firmly to the malleus, as in this method.

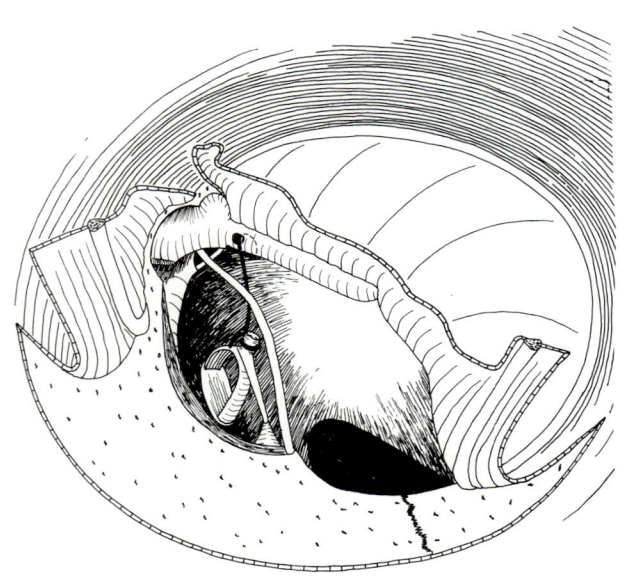

Fig. 914 A gold wire is fixed at the malleus handle and the stapes

Myringostapediopexy

The tympanomeatal flap or fascia graft is applied directly onto the head of the stapes. This technique was used as early as 1901 by Matte. Zöllner and Wullstein used myringostapediopexy very often during the 1950s. Juers (1954) gave the method its name, and Hamberger and Liden (1958) achieved good hearing results with transcanal myringostapediopexy.

It is well know that spontaneous myringostapediopexy, with atrophy and retraction of the eardrum resulting in resorption of the long process of the incus, is a common sequela after secretory otitis and long-lasting tubal dysfunction. In our studies of treated secretory otitis media during the late 1960s, myringostapediopexy was found in 10% of the ears (Table 1, p. 132). Hearing was still very good in the vast majority of these cases, but the retractions may later progress down to the head of the stapes, and the migration of keratin from the retraction pockets may deteriorate.

When a myringostapediopexy is carried out without canal wall–down mastoidectomy via a transcanal tympanoplastic procedure in patients with posterior perforation and with the stapes and malleus handle present, the fascia has to be placed deeply onto the head of the stapes and fixed to the stapes with small Gelfoam balls. This type of tympanoplasty causes a posterior retraction pocket (Fig. 915), and excessive drilling of the posterior bony annulus should therefore be performed to widen the access to the retraction pocket (Fig. 916). This exposes the horizontal portion of the facial nerve, and part of the lateral semicircular canal can even be seen. Posteroinferiorly, the chorda tympani has to be liberated. The drilling opens the aditus ad antrum, again producing possible retractions. After the perforation has been covered with an underlay fascia graft, it should be carefully fixed to the head of the stapes (Fig. 917). After the epithelium flaps have been replaced, the low position of the posterior part of the eardrum is evident (Fig. 918). Myringostapediopexy is therefore a very rare procedure in ears with an intact canal wall. In such cases, interposition is preferable to myringostapediopexy.

With canal wall–down mastoidectomy, myringostapediopexy can be performed in selected cases with high stapes (Fig. 919), and an anteriorly positioned or absent malleus handle. In such cases, it can be a safe and stable operation. Among 282 patients with cholesteatoma and with intact stapes who were treated using a one-stage operation between 1965 and 1980, myringostapediopexy was performed in 17 cases (Tos 1982). The mean abso-

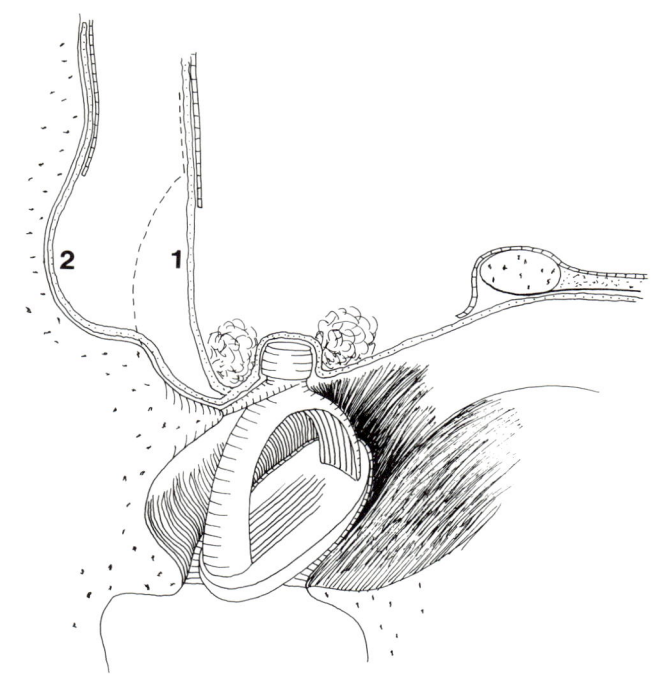

Fig. 915 Myringoincudostapediopexy, showing the necessity of drilling the posterior bony ear canal. 1) The situation without drilling. 2) The myringostapediopexy after drilling. The fascia is in contact with the head of the stapes

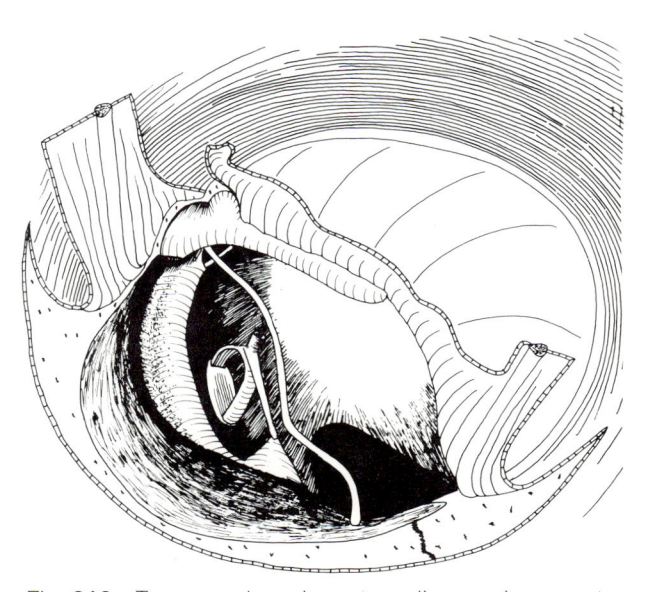

Fig. 916 Transcanal myringostapediopexy in a posterior perforation. Extensive removal of the posterosuperior bony annulus is carried out, exposing the prominence of the facial nerve and part of the lateral semicircular canal. The chorda is mobilized

lute hearing 11-15 years after the operation was 37.3 dB, compared to 34.8 dB in a group with interposition with autogenous incus and 45.0 dB in a group with interposition of other grafts. Our method of choice was interposition of autogenous incus, and these 17 patients were selected cases with high stapes and an established and well-functioning myringostapediopexy.

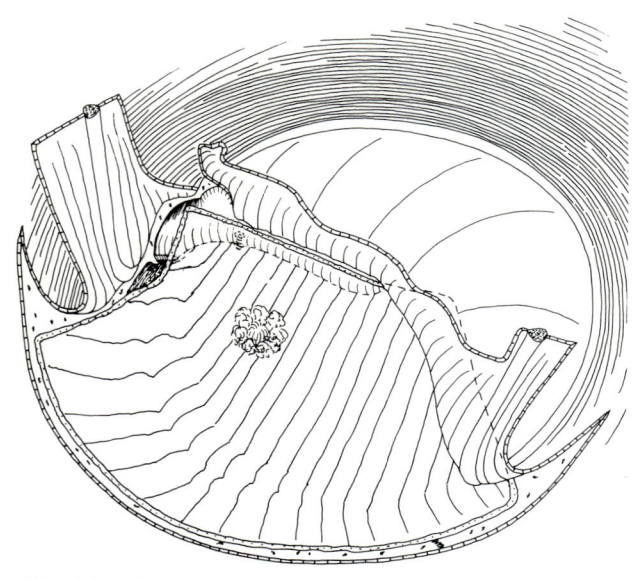

Fig. **917** Myringostapediopexy with fascia. Fascia is placed under the malleus handle and on the head of the stapes, and fixed around it

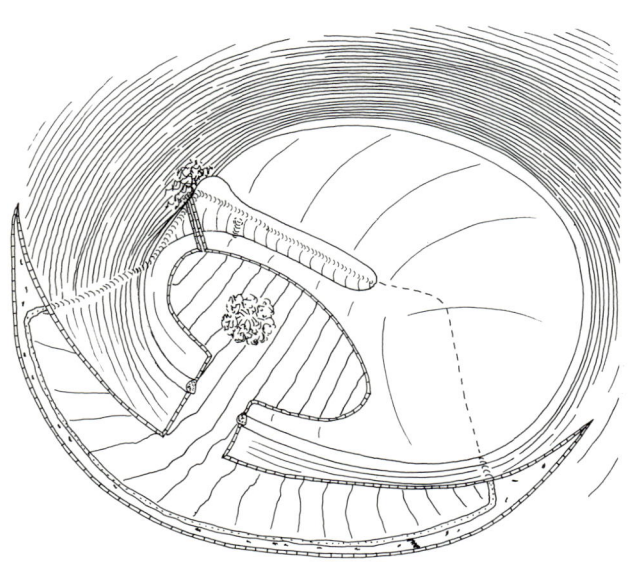

Fig. **918** The skin flaps are replaced

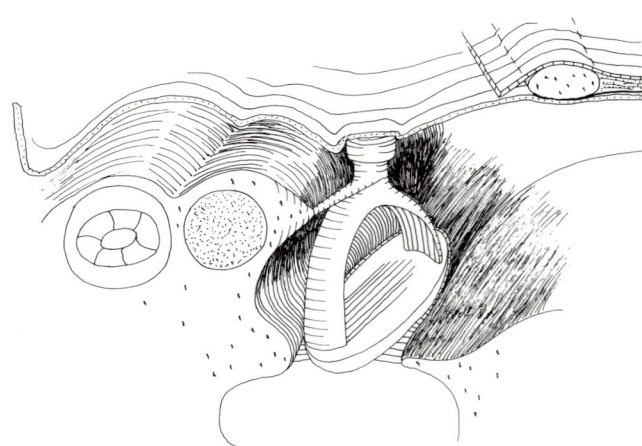

Fig. **919** Side view of the myringostapediopexy in canal wall–down mastoidectomy. In a high stapes, the fascia is placed onto the head of the stapes and lies on the prominence of the facial nerve and lateral semicircular canal. The tympanic cavity is small

19 Tympanoplasty in Partial Defects of the Stapedial Arch

In chronic middle-ear disease and its sequelae, the stapedial arch can be completely normal, or partly or totally resorbed. In the first group, a type 2 tympanoplasty is performed, and in the latter group a type 3 tympanoplasty with a columella is performed. In the middle group, with partial defects of the stapes, the graft should be shaped so as to fit exactly onto the remaining part of the crura, and the tympanoplasty used is sometimes type 2, and sometimes type 3.

In our studies of chronic middle-ear disease and its sequelae (Tos 1979), partial defects of the stapes were found in 5% of the ears, ranging from 3% in the group with sequelae of otitis to 10% in the tensa-retraction cholesteatoma group (Table **2** p. 243).

Various defects of the stapedial arch were found (Tos 1975) (Fig. **920**), and the shaping of the ossicles or cortical bone grafts should be related to the defects of the stapedial arch (Fig. **921**).

The most common defect is absence of the stapedial head. The remainder of the neck is usually tapered, and after cleaning and scarification, the height of the neck becomes further deminished, so that it is with the stapedial tendon. The remnant of the long process of the incus should be shaped and placed asymmetrically on the top of the stapedial neck (Fig. **921 a**). A better alternative is to drill a relatively deep but small groove for the stapedial arch. The graft rides on the arch. This minimizes the risk of osseous fixation of the graft to the pyramid eminence and facial prominence.

Absence of the head and neck of the stapes, or the lateral part of the stapedial arch (Fig. **920 a–b**) is also a relatively common pathological situation. The arch may be defective, while there is still bony

Fig. **920** Missing parts of the stapedial arch. **a, b** Head and neck. **c, d** Lateral part of the arch. **e–g** Anterior limb

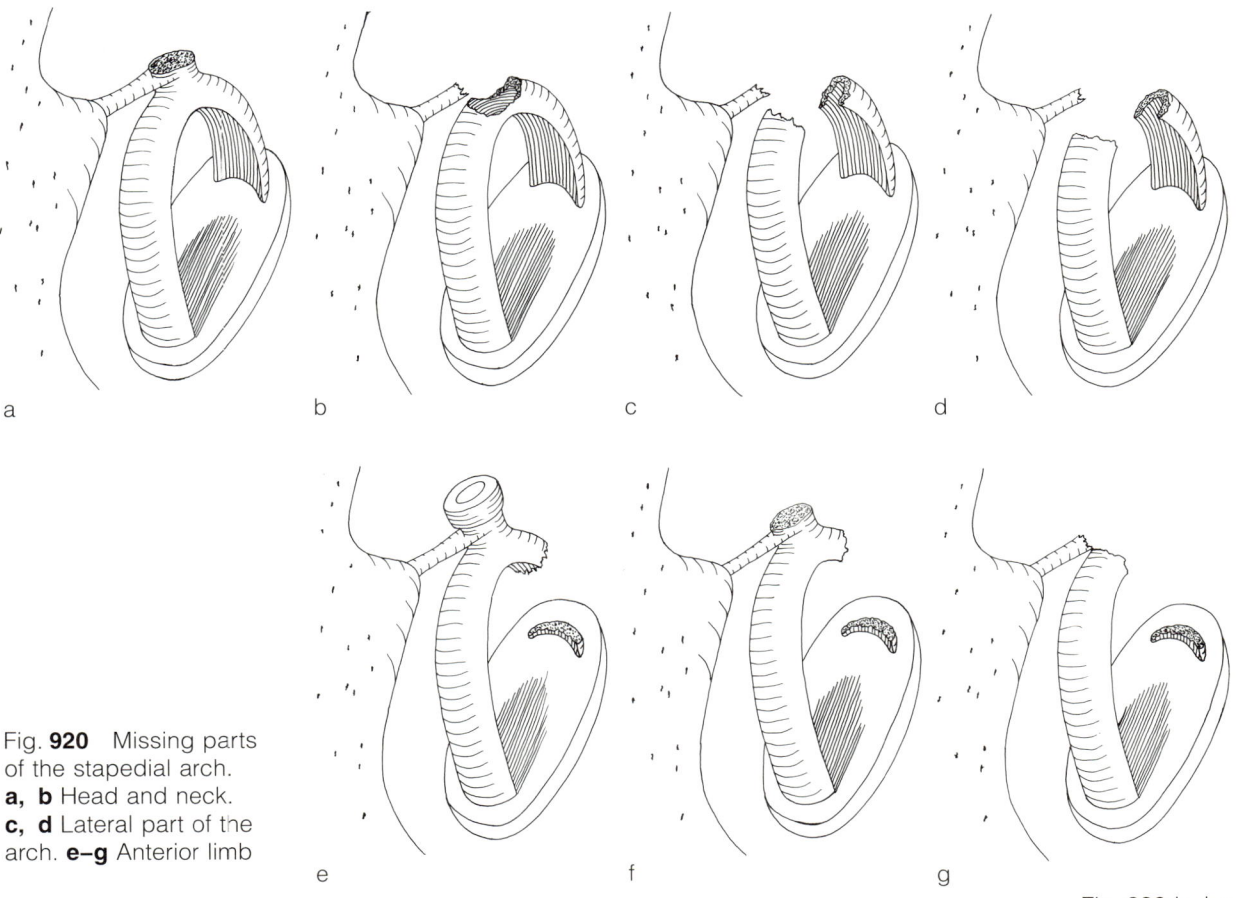

Fig. **920 h–j** ▷

Fig. **920 h–j** Posterior limb

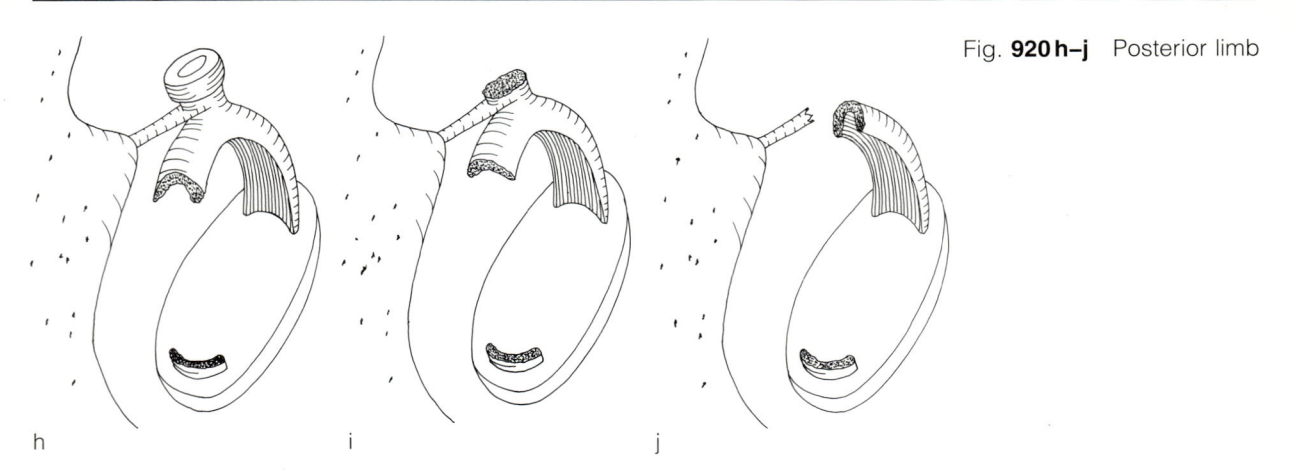

h   i   j

contact between the limbs (Fig. **920 b**), but often the limbs are destroyed laterally and there is no contact between them (Fig. **920 c, d**). In any case, the level of the remaining stapedial arch is below the level of the pyramid eminence. A riding incus, with a deep groove in the remnant of the long process, is the best prosthesis for such defects (Fig. **921 c, d**).

An absent anterior or posterior limb of the stapes is also seen (Fig. **920 e–j**). The head and neck of the stapes may be intact (Fig. **920 e, h**), and in such situations, interposition of a small shaped, incus prosthesis should be an appropriate solution (Figs. **922, 923**). With careful shaping, it should be possible to avoid fixation of the graft, especially as the head of the stapes is higher than the pyramid eminence. The weight of the graft in relation to the missing limb of the stapes, and late resorption of the remaining limb, may be problematic, but when the anterior limb is missing, the weight problem is less acute; the stapedial tendon supports the posterior limb against tilting, and the direction of forces from the graft towards the posterior limb resembles a columella effect (Fig. **923**). When the posterior limb is absent, there are no weight or resorption effects, and the direction of the forces involved is not a straight columella effect (Fig. **923**).

When both the head and a limb of the stapes are missing (Fig. **920 f, i**), and when only one limb is present (Fig. **920 g, j**), it is better to use a columella from the malleus handle to the footplate (Fig. **921 e–h**). The incus, or a piece of cortical bone, can be shaped in such a way that contact can be established between the footplate and the remnant of the anterior or posterior limb of the stapes (Fig. **921 e–h**). This is done by drilling a groove on the side of the incus columella.

Analysis of older statistics relating to patients who underwent surgical treatment from 1963 to 1971 (Tos 1975) shows that bony fixation to the facial prominence occurs particularly in ears with partial defects on the stapes. Since 1972, the author has systematically shaped the incus or cortical bone in patients with partial defects of the stapedial arch in the manner described above, and the results have considerably improved.

Using cartilage prostheses in ears with partial defects of the stapes may lead to difficulties in fixation of the cartilage to the neck of the stapes; on the other hand, however, the problems of bony fixation do not arise when using cartilage.

The riding cartilage prostheses of the Utech type (Fig. **790**) or Glasscock type (Fig. **791**) can be applied when the stapedial head and neck are missing. The author has used a tragal cartilage prosthesis (Fig. **924**) produced as follows. Two legs are cut out of a piece of tragal cartilage. The prosthesis is placed on the defective stapedial arch. It rides on the arch, and the legs stand on the footplate. This prosthesis is a combination of the type 2 and type 2 interposition grafts, like the incus prostheses (Fig. **921 e–h**).

In artificial prostheses produced from biocompatible materials, especially hydroxyapatite, deep keyhole notches can be cut out on each side of a Plasti-Pore shaft, allowing the shaft to ride on the remaining stapedial arch (Figs. **814, 824–842**). The hydroxyapatible platform can face either the drum or the malleus handle.

The Kraus modified Schuring ossicular implant (Smith and Nephew, Richards Company), with a fluoroplastic shaft and a specially-designed dual strut riding on the stapes, is suitable for partial

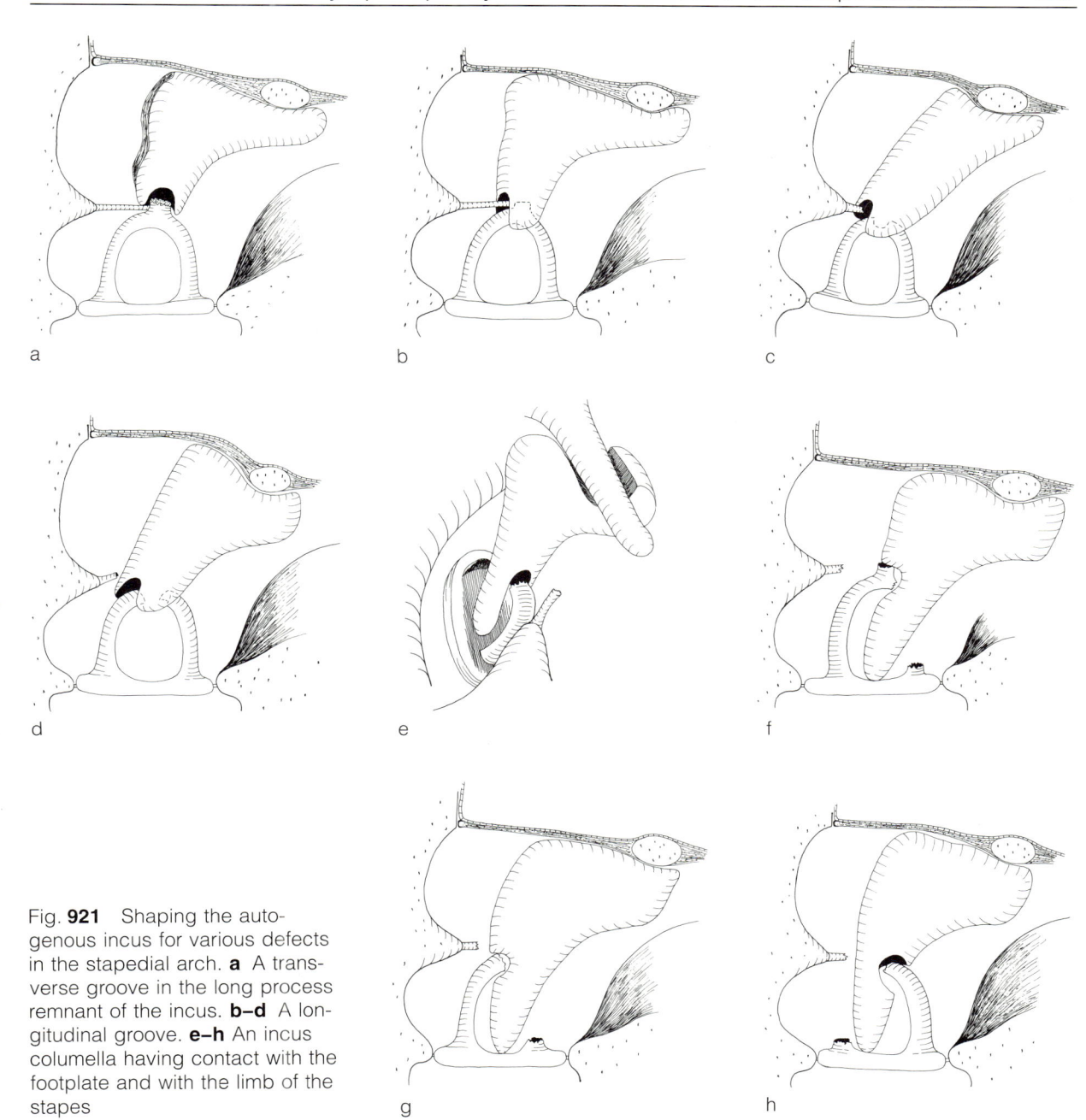

Fig. 921 Shaping the autogenous incus for various defects in the stapedial arch. **a** A transverse groove in the long process remnant of the incus. **b–d** A longitudinal groove. **e–h** An incus columella having contact with the footplate and with the limb of the stapes

defects of the stapedial arch (Fig. 925). The dual strut rides on the stapedial arch, the shaft can be shortened or elongated on the eardrum end, and a hydroxyapatite cap can be mounted on the shaft to face the undersurface of the drum after trimming on the shaft. Instead of hydroxyapatite, a piece of bone or incus remnant, or a tragal cartilage plate, can be used. In fact, this prosthesis is a modification of one of the few type 2 tympanoplasty prostheses that combine two prostheses. Originally, Schuring combined a Teflon Robinson piston, used in otosclerosis surgery, with an incus body. A hole is drilled in the incus body, and the shaft of the Teflon piston prosthesis is placed in the hole (Schuring et al. 1978). The cap is placed on the head of the stapes, and the incus is placed underneath the drum (Fig. 926).

The Goldenberg hydroxyapatite-Plasti-Pore prostheses are also based on the principle of combined prostheses. In type 3 ossiculoplasty, many combined prostheses have been described and are in use.

19 Tympanoplasty in Partial Defects of the Stapedial Arch

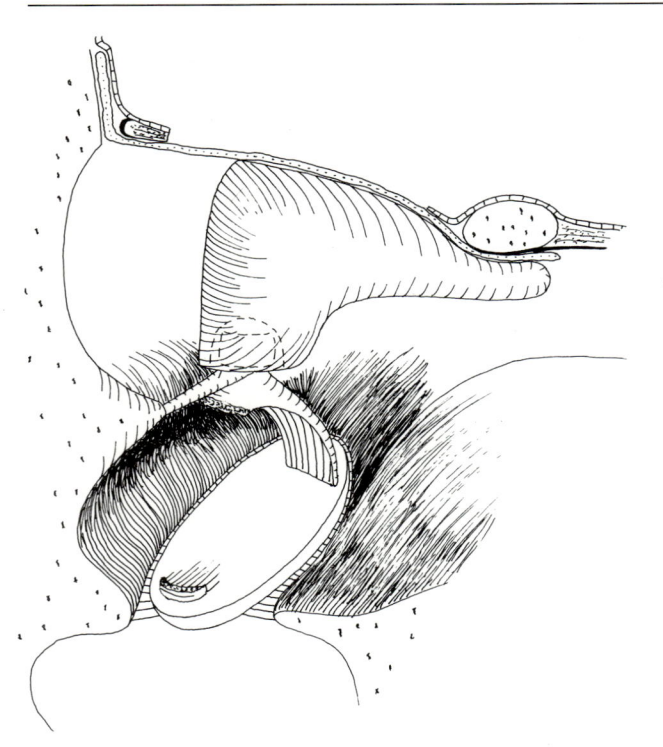

Fig. **922** Defect in the posterior limb of the stapes. A small incus prosthesis is shaped with a hole for the head of the stapes

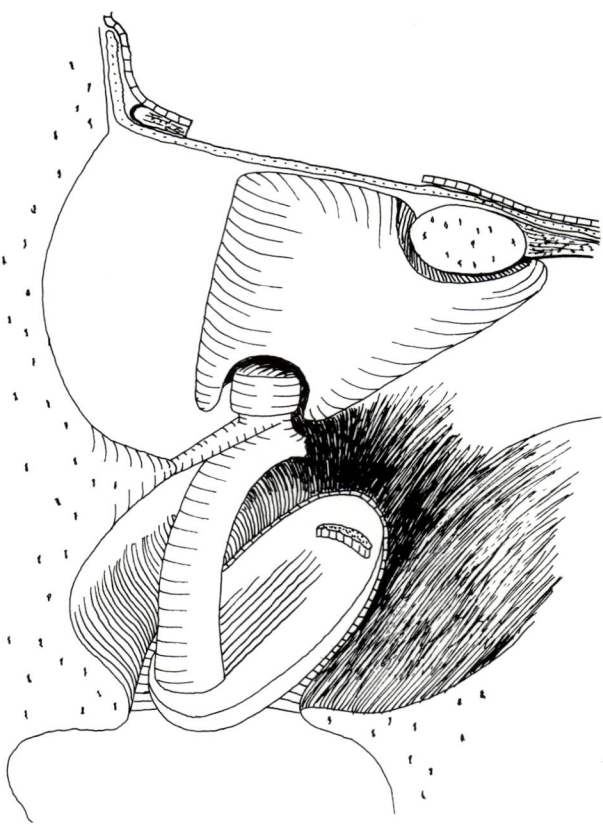

Fig. **923** Defect in the anterior limb of the stapes. A small incus prosthesis is shaped with a hole for the head of the stapes and a groove for the malleus handle

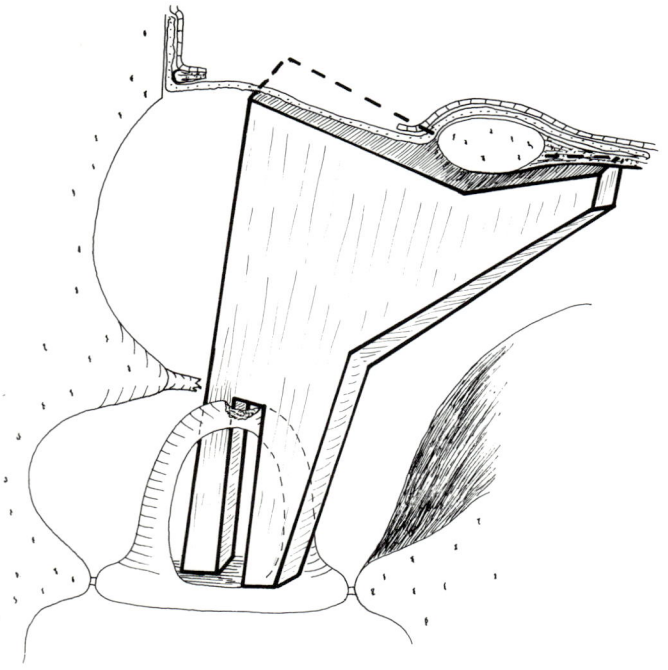

Fig. **924** Defect in the head and neck of the stapes. A tragal cartilage prosthesis is riding on the arch, in contact with the arch and the footplate

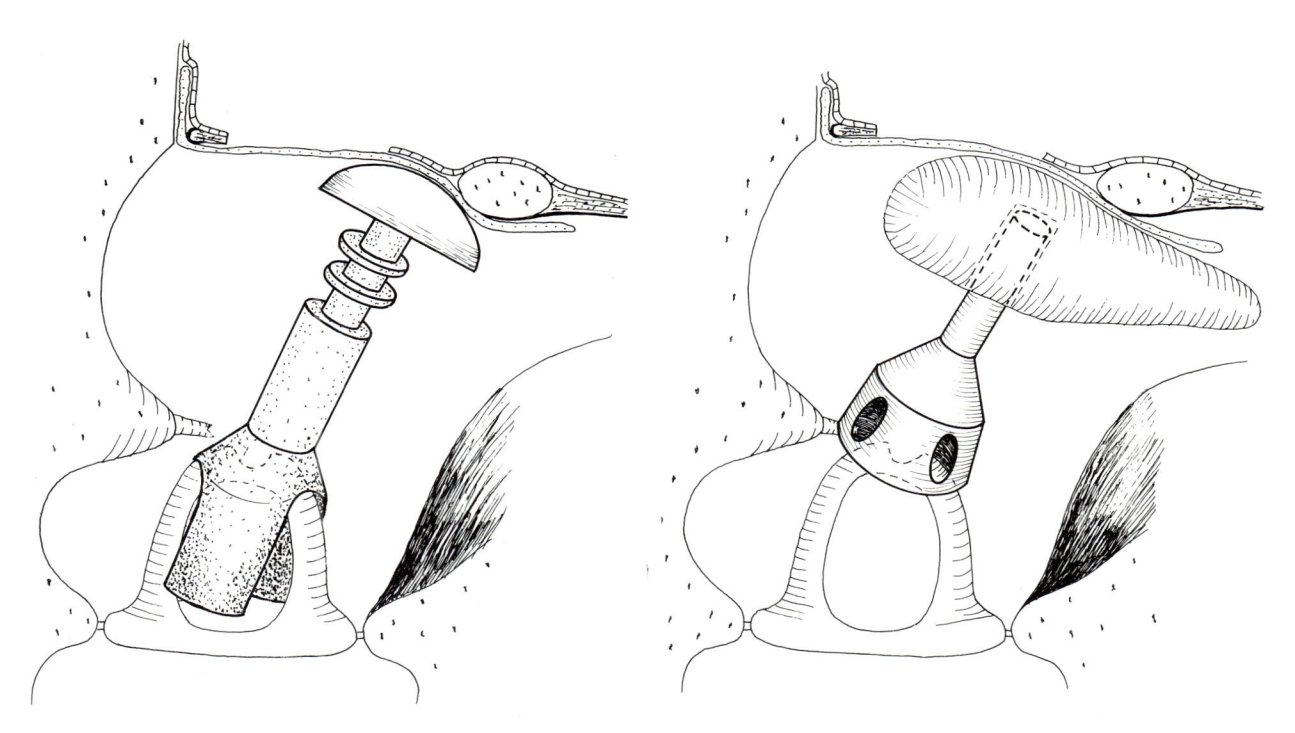

Fig. 925 **A Kraus modified Schuring ossicular implant** for a partial defect of the stapes. The dual struts ride on the defective stapedial arch. The fluoroplastic shaft is connected to a hydroxyapatite cap that is in contact with the drum and the malleus handle

Fig. 926 **Schuring's combined prosthesis,** made of a Teflon Robinson piston and an autogenous incus. The cup of the Teflon piston is placed on the defective stapedial arch, and the incus is connected to the drum and malleus handle

20 Tympanoplasty with the Malleus Handle Missing

The malleus handle is of great importance for the functioning of the tympanic membrane and for the success of myringoplasty. Several myringoplasty procedures have been developed with the aim of securing a solid attachment of the graft to the umbo in ears with total eardrum perforation. These procedures are designed to give the new eardrum a conical shape and to prevent it from becoming lateralized. In ears with a missing malleus handle, however, such procedures cannot be employed, and the postoperative function is therefore generally poorer than with ears that have an intact malleus handle.

The overall incidence of ears with missing malleus handle is 7% (Table **2**, p. 243, ranging from 15% in tensa-retraction cholesteatoma to 1% in sinus cholesteatoma and 0% in attic cholesteatoma. In noncholesteatomatous ears the incidence is about 10%. In nearly all cases, the missing malleus handle is associated with total or subtotal perforation of the ear drum (Tables **3, 4,** p. 244).

A correlation between ears with a missing malleus handle and the condition of the remaining ossicular chain (Table **5**) shows that malleus handle defect as the only ossicular pathology occurs in 11% of tensa-retraction cholesteatomas, 4% of granulating otitis media, and in 3% of sequelae to otitis media.

A missing malleus handle combined with a defect of the long process of the incus, but with the stapes present, was found in 8% of tensa-retraction cholesteatoma patients and in 4–6% of the sequelae to otitis group.

The third combination, a missing malleus handle with a defect of the long process and a defect on the stapedial arch, was a less common pathology.

There are several possible forms of tympanoplasty in ears with a missing malleus handle, depending partly on the rest of the pathology in the ossicular chain. The various types of tympanoplasty are:

1. Myringoplasty of the total perforation.
2. Disruption of the chain and incus interposition.
3. Interposing cartilage plates onto the intact incudostapedial joint.
4. Using cartilage plates in a disrupted chain.
5. Interposition of other prostheses.
6. Allogenous drum–malleus graft.
7. Reconstruction of the defective malleus handle–malleoplasty.

Table **5** Frequency of different types of ossicular defect in 1100 consecutive cases with chronic middle-ear diseases

Defects of the ossicular chain	Cholesteatomas			Granulating otitis	Sequelae of otitis	Adhesive otitis
	Attic n = 152 (%)	Sinus n = 166 (%)	Tensa n = 108 (%)	n = 165 (%)	n = 429 (%)	n = 80 (%)
Malleus handle only	–	–	11	4	3	–
Malleus handle + incus–stapes present	–	1	8	4	5	6
Malleus handle + incus–stapes absent	–	3	6	2	1	3
Incus–stapes present	59	50	44	41	29	47
Incus–stapes absent	16	37	20	13	4	21
None (intact)	26	10	12	38	57	23

8. Construction of a new malleus–myringoplasty (Schiller 1979)

Procedures 1–4 are mainly malleus bypass procedures, and rely on sound transmission from the drum to the incudostapedial joint or to the stapes, and only partly on possible connection with, or movement of, the remnant of the malleus. Procedure 5 is entirely a malleus bypass procedure—a prosthesis goes from the drum directly to the head of the stapes.

Myringoplasty in Total Perforation

In patients with an intact incudostapedial joint and a missing malleus handle (Fig. **927**) a myringoplasty can be performed, establishing a contact between the fascia and the incudostapedial joint—a kind of myringoincudopexy. The myringoplasty technique, either as onlay or underlay grafting, is modified to take account of the missing malleus handle.

In the onlay technique, the skin incision is made about 2 mm laterally to the annulus (Fig. **927**). The epithelium from the annulus is removed all the way round, and the three superior epithelial flaps are elevated: the posterosuperior flap, the malleus flap, and the anterosuperior flap (Fig. **928**). Since the malleus handle is missing, the elevation of the superior epithelial flaps, especially the malleus flap, should be extended far more superiorly than with a normal malleus handle (Fig. **491**).

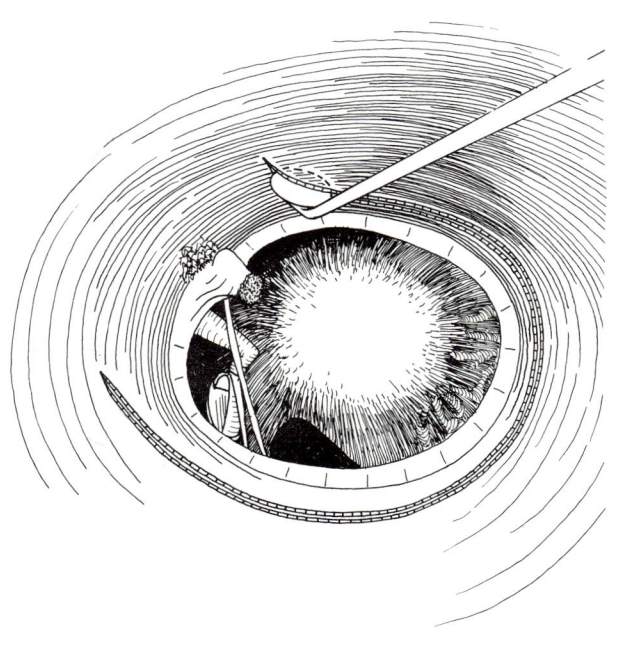

Fig. **927** Missing malleus handle, intact incudostapedial joint and total perforation. A circumferential incision is made from the 11-o'clock to the 1-o'clock position, about 1 mm lateral to the annulus

The entire Shrapnell's membrane region and the neck of the malleus should be exposed. Fascia is placed on the long process of the incus, the incudostapedial joint, and the malleus remnant (Fig. **929**). The epithelial flaps are replaced

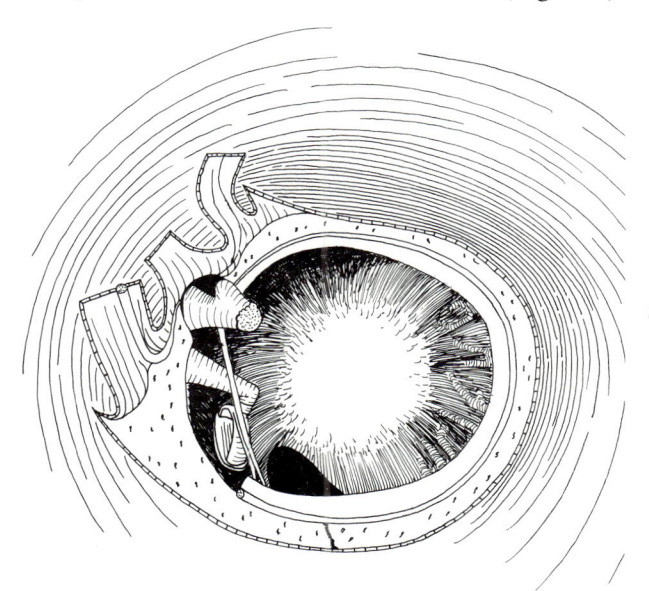

Fig. **928** Three superior epithelial flaps are elevated; a posterosuperior flap, a malleus flap with Shrapnell's membrane, and an anterosuperior flap. The epithelium from the drum remnant and annulus is removed

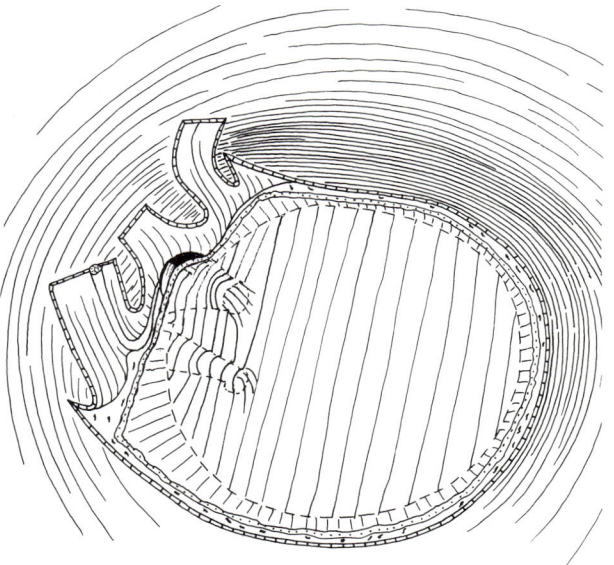

Fig. **929** Fascia covers the remnant of the malleus and the long process of the incus as an onlay graft

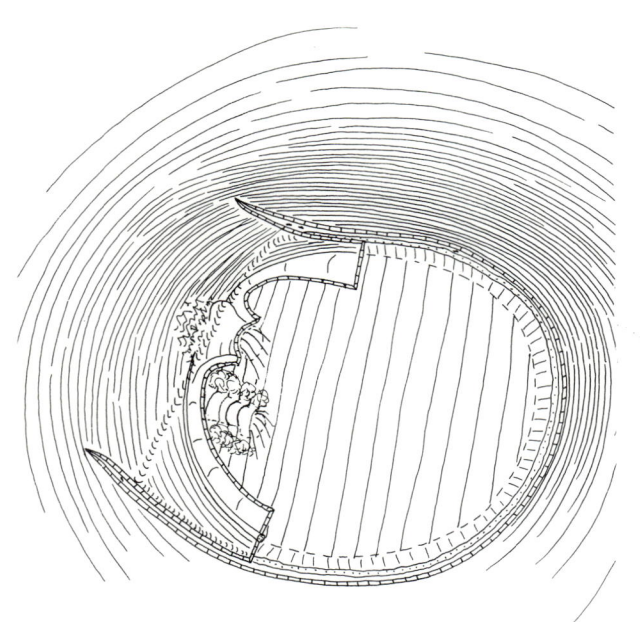

20 Tympanoplasty with the Malleus Handle Missing

Fig. 930 The epithelial flaps are replaced, and the connection with the long process of the incus—the myringoincudopexy—is secured by placing small Gelfoam balls around the incudostapedial joint

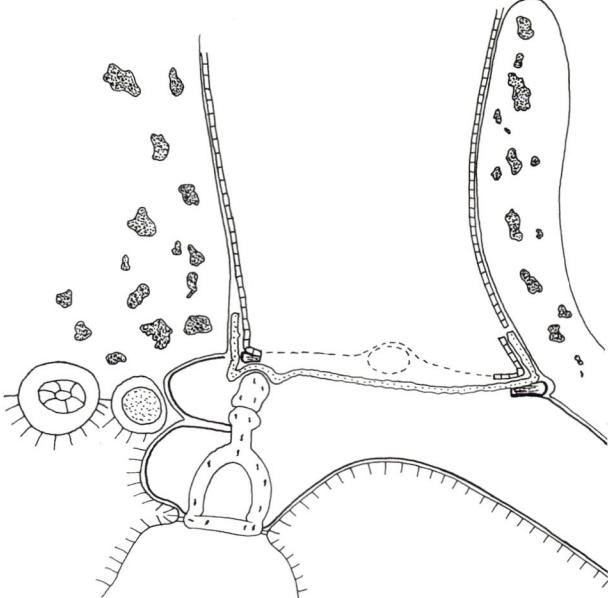

Fig. 931 Side view of onlay grafting in total perforation with a missing malleus handle. The fascia is placed on the long process of the incus and the incudostapedial joint

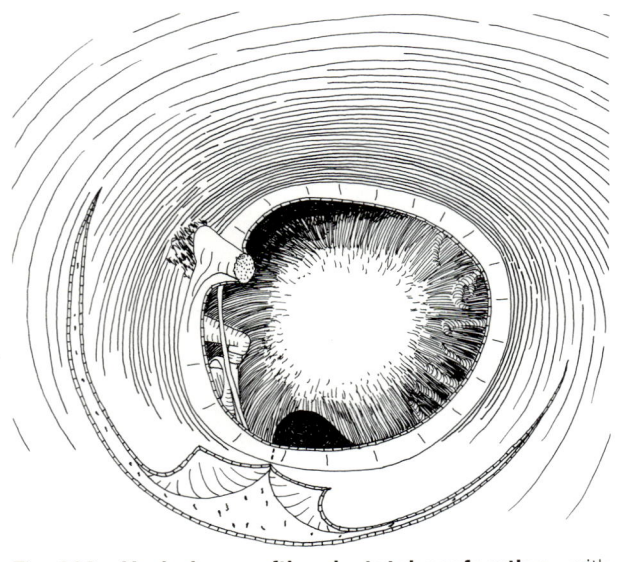

Fig. 932 **Underlay grafting in total perforation,** with a missing malleus handle but an intact incudostapedial joint. A lateral circumferential incision is made from the 12-o'clock to the 6-o'clock position

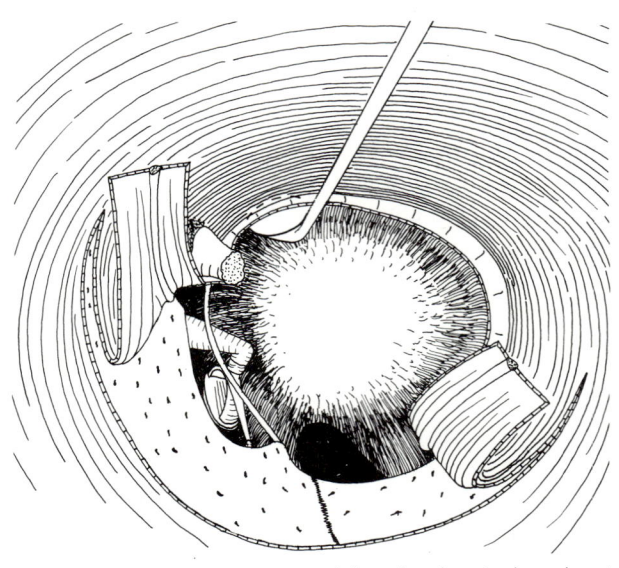

Fig. 933 The tympanomeatal flap is elevated and cut at the 9-o'clock position, as in the swing-door technique. The mucosa under the anterior annulus is removed

(Fig. 930). Sound transmission runs mainly via the incudostapedial joint, and the position of the drum is somewhat lower than normal (Fig. 931). The drum does not have a conical shape, and there is a risk of insufficient energy transmission to the stapes, despite excessive movement of the new tympanic membrane.

In the underlay grafting technique, after a circumferential incision, the tympanomeatal flap is elevated (Fig. 932). The flap and the annulus are cut at the 9-o'clock position, and the annulus is further elevated as in the swing-door technique (Fig. 933). Otosclerosis drilling is performed, especially in cases with posteriorly positioned stapes, to enlarge

Myringoplasty in Total Perforation

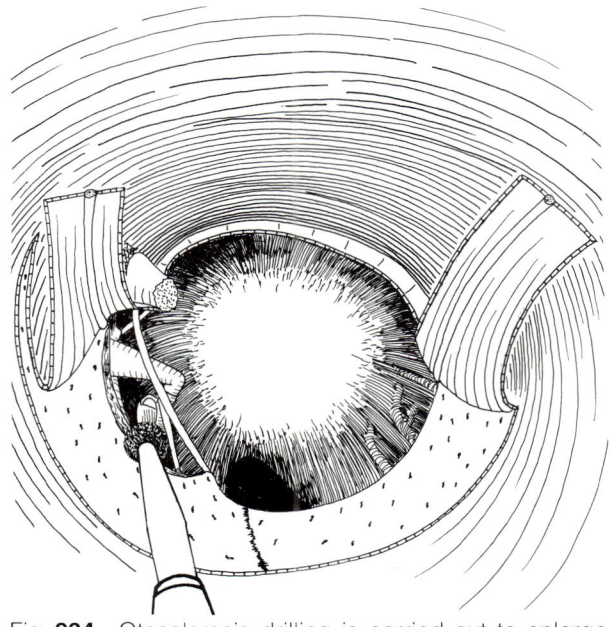

Fig. **934** Otosclerosis drilling is carried out to enlarge the posterosuperior area of the drum and improve contact with the incudostapedial joint

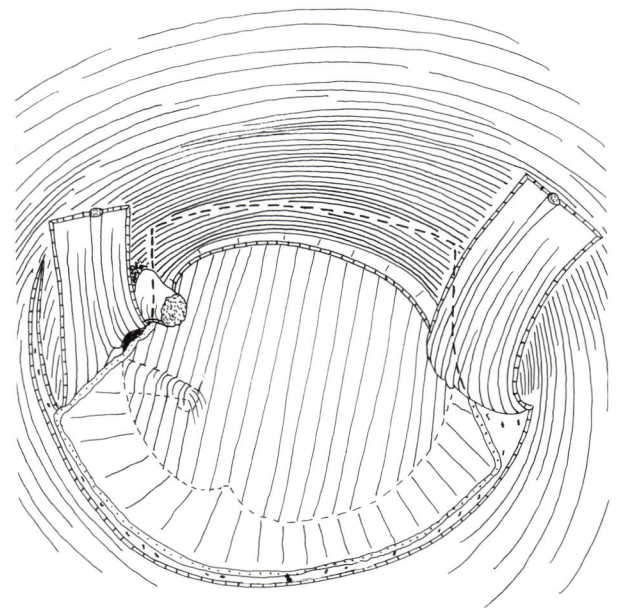

Fig. **935** The fascia is placed as an underlay graft far anteriorly under the annulus, and under the remnant of the malleus

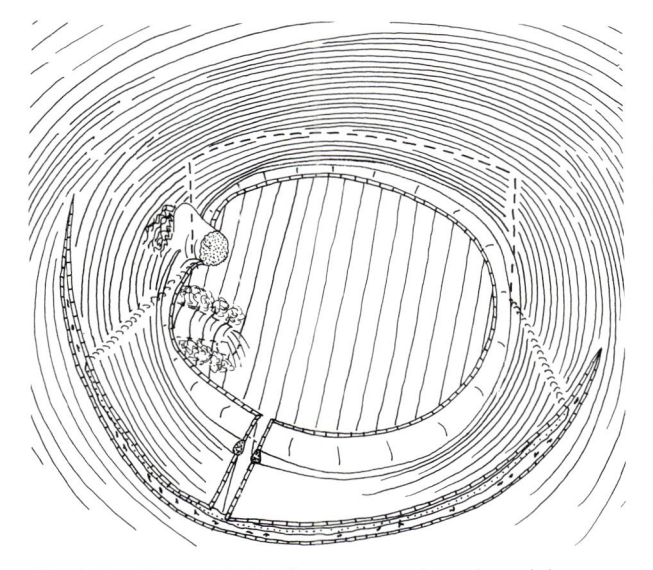

Fig. **936** The epithelial flaps are replaced, and the connection of the fascia to the incudostapedial joint is secured by placing small Gelfoam balls around the joint

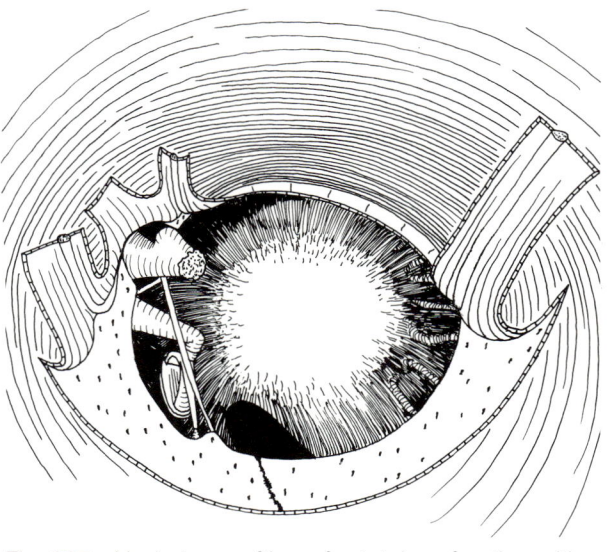

Fig. **937** Underlay grafting of a total perforation with a missing malleus handle. The fascia is placed on the remnant of the malleus. The malleus flap, including the Shrapnell's membrane, has to be elevated more extensively

the posterosuperior drum area (Fig. **934**). Fascia is placed under the annulus anteriorly and under the malleus remnant (Fig. **935**), and the epithelial flaps are returned. Care is taken to fix the fascia firmly to the incudostapedial joint using small Gelfoam balls (Fig. **936**). In placing the fascia under the malleus remnant no further elevation of the epithelium is needed (Fig. **934**).

When the fascia is placed on the malleus remnant, the epithelium from the Shrapnell's membrane region has to be elevated (Fig. **937**). The fascia covers th Shrapnell's membrane region and the incudostapedial joint (Fig. **938**), and the epithelial flaps are replaced. The fascia lies on the malleus remnant (Fig. **939**).

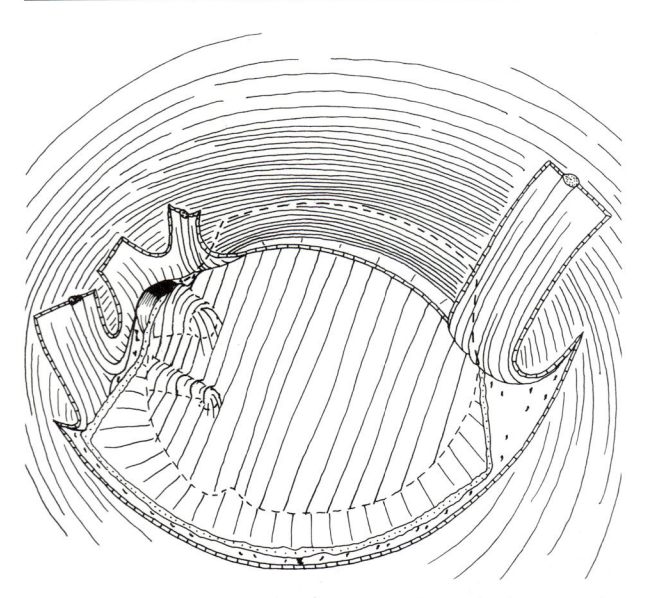

Fig. **938** The fascia is placed underneath the anterior annulus and on top of the malleus remnant and incudostapedial joint

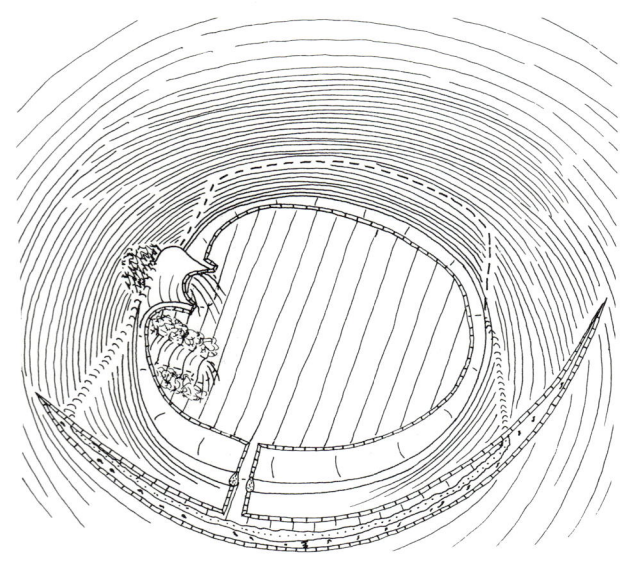

Fig. **939** The epithelial flaps are replaced, and the connection to the incudostapedial joint is secured with small Gelfoam balls placed around the joint

Disruption of the Ossicular Chain and Interposition of the Incus

Some surgeons prefer to disrupt the incudostapedial joint, extrude the incus, and interpose it, as in type 2 tympanoplasty. This type of situation also occurs in cases with a defective long process of the incus in combination with a missing malleus handle (Fig. **940**), which is, in fact, more common than a missing malleus handle without a defect in the long process of the incus (Table **5,** p. 330).

After a circumferential skin incision in the ear canal, elevation of the tympanomeatal flap and the annulus as in the swing-door technique is performed (Fig. **941**). After otosclerosis drilling of the posterosuperior bony annulus, the incus is extruded and interposed in such a way that the short process of the incus has some contact with the remnant of the malleus (Fig. **941**). This is usually achieved if the incus is placed far anteriorly. The remenant of the long process points anteriorly. Prior to the interposition, the malleus remnant is scarified so as to facilitate the formation of a fibrous connection between the incus and the malleus. This somewhat unstable assembly can be glued together with fibrin glue. The perforation is closed using fascia as an underlay graft (Fig. **942**). The epithelial flaps are returned, and care is taken that the interposed incus remains in position (Fig. **943**). It is fixed with Gelfoam balls.

A missing malleus handle with a disrupted incudostapedial joint is the most common ossicular pathology involving a missing malleus handle. Analysis of our results in surgery for a missing malleus handle (Tos and Arndal 1992) showed considerably better and more stable long-term hearing in cases where the incudostapedial joint remained intact (Fig. **929**) than in cases where it was disrupted and a type 2 tympanoplasty with interposition of incus (Fig. **943**) was performed. Preserving the ossicular chain intact is therefore recommended.

Disruption of the Ossicular Chain 335

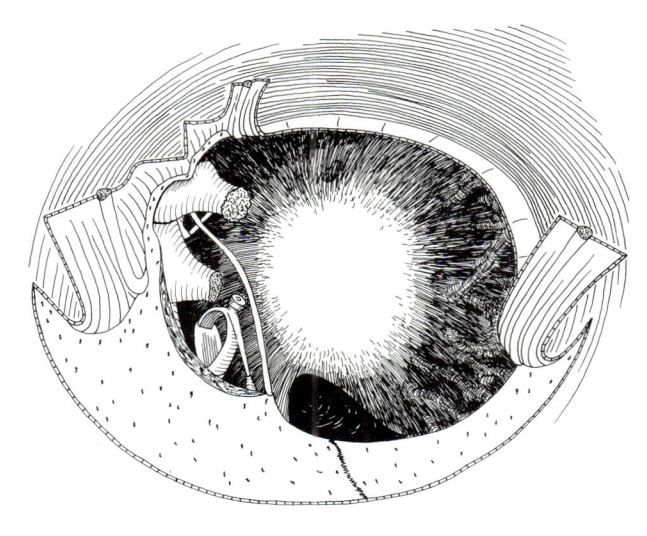

Fig. **940** A total perforation with a missing malleus handle and missing long process of the incus. The tympanomeatal flaps are elevated posteriorly and superiorly, and the perforation is closed using the underlay grafting technique

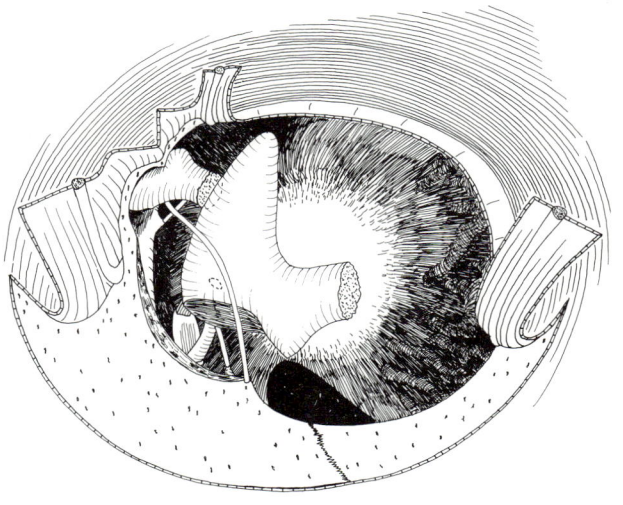

Fig. **941** The incus is interposed with a small hole on the superior aspect of the body. The short process points anteriorly and has contact with the remnant of the malleus handle. The remnant of the long process points inferiorly

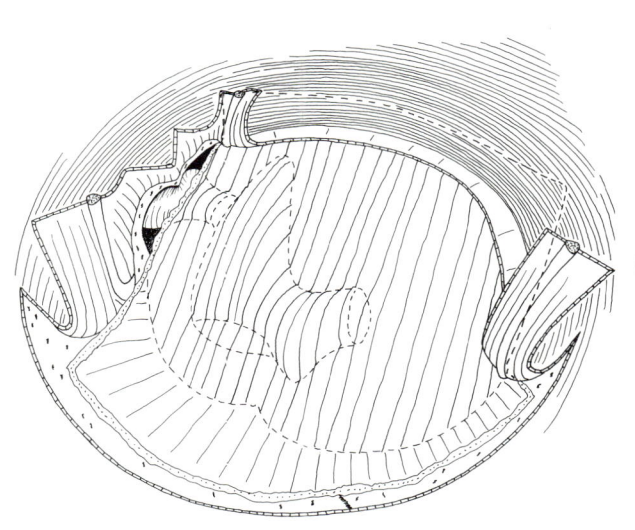

Fig. **942** Fascia is placed as an underlay graft far anteriorly under the annulus, covering the incus and the remnant of the malleus handle

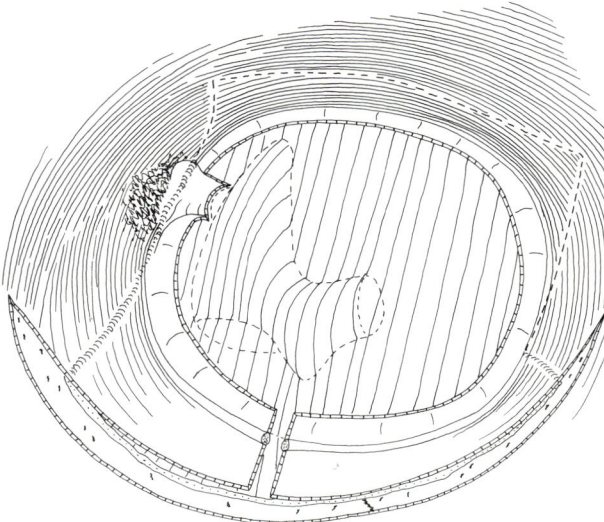

Fig. **943** The epithelial flaps are replaced

Interposition of Cartilage Plates

With the recognition that maintaining an intact ossicular chain produces better long-term results than disrupting it in cases with a missing malleus handle, and that better results can be achieved with a normal malleus handle than with a missing malleus handle, several techniques have been developed in an effort to compensate for the missing malleus handle. One of these is to enlarge the contact area and improve the connection between the drum and the intact incudostapedial joint.

Sheehy (1972) recommends interposition of a tragal cartilage plate onto the intact ossicular chain (Fig. **944**). A relatively long plate of tragal cartilage is placed under the posterosuperior bony annulus and onto the incudostapedial joint. The plate is directed anteroinferiorly, towards the 5-o'clock position. Fascia covers the total perforation and the cartilage as an onlay graft (Fig. **945**). The flaps are returned (Fig. **946**). The cartilage plate is carefully fixed with Gelfoam balls. This technique is simple, and seems to be the most physiological one (Fig. **947**). In the author's experience this technique has produced better long-term results than the previously used techniques.

There are some other techniques using cartilage plates with an intact incudostapedial joint and a missing malleus handle. A composite tragal cartilage–perichondrium graft is one of the suggested

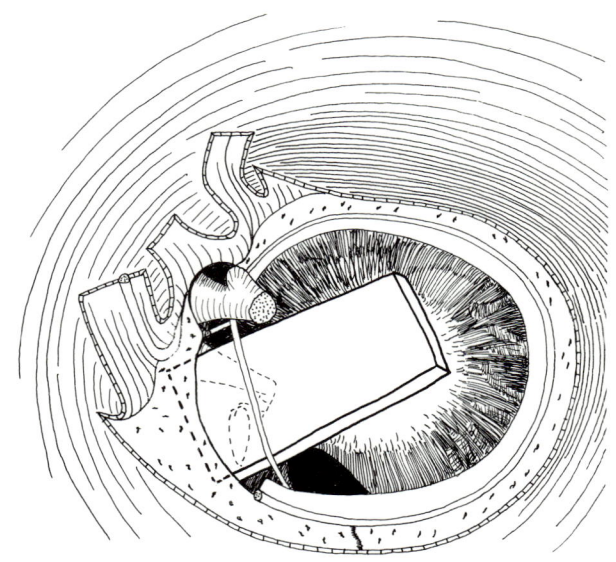

Fig. **944** A total perforation with a missing malleus handle and an intact incudostapedial joint. The ear is prepared for onlay fascia grafting. A plate of tragal cartilage is placed on the incudostapedial joint. It points in an anteroinferior direction, and posterosuperiorly it lies under the bony annulus (Sheehy)

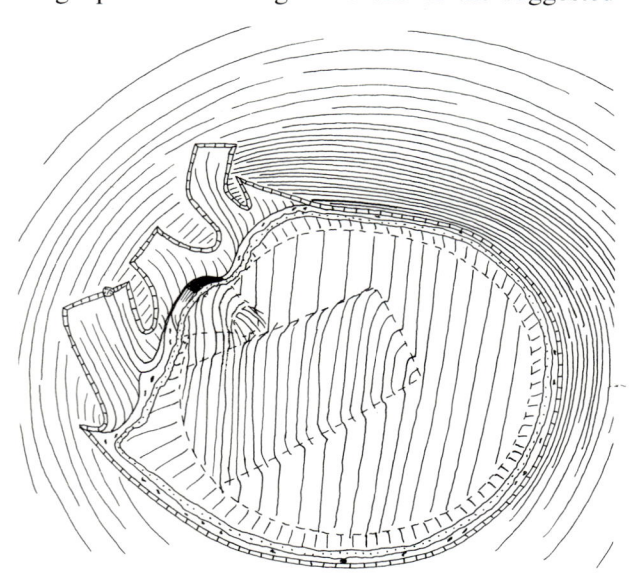

Fig. **945** The fascia covers the annulus and the tragal plate, as well as the remnant of the malleus, as an onlay graft

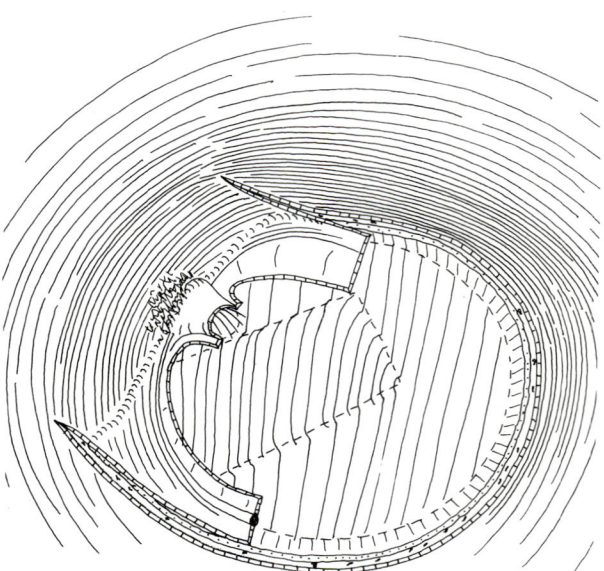

Fig. **946** The epithelial flaps are replaced

Interposition of Cartilage Plates

solutions (Tolsdorff 1991). A large piece of tragal cartilage with perichondrium is removed. The perichondrium on one side, and the peripheral part of the cartilage are removed, but a large island of cartilage is left attached to the perichondrium from the opposite side (Fig. **948**). After the epithelium has been elevated around the annulus and superior epithelial flaps have been created, the composite cartilage–perichondrium graft is placed as an onlay graft onto the annulus (Fig. **949**). The cartilage side of the composite graft faces the tympanic cavity in such a way that there is a good contact between the cartilage and the intact incudostapedial joint. The perichondrium is placed on the annulus and the denuded bone (Fig. **950**), and finally the epithelium flaps are replaced.

Similar techniques were described by Goodhill (1967) (Figs. **614, 615**) and Glasscock (1973) (Figs. **618, 619**). Cartilage palisade techniques (Heermann 1970) are also suitable for tympanoplasty in ears with a missing malleus handle.

Another simple technique is placement of a tragal cartilage plate with perichondrium onto the intact incudostapedial joint and the bony annulus at the 6-o'clock position (Fig. **950**). This technique can be used either with an underlay or onlay fascia grafting. The technique is similar to the Sheehy cartilage plate technique and the Heermann annulus–stapes cartilage plate.

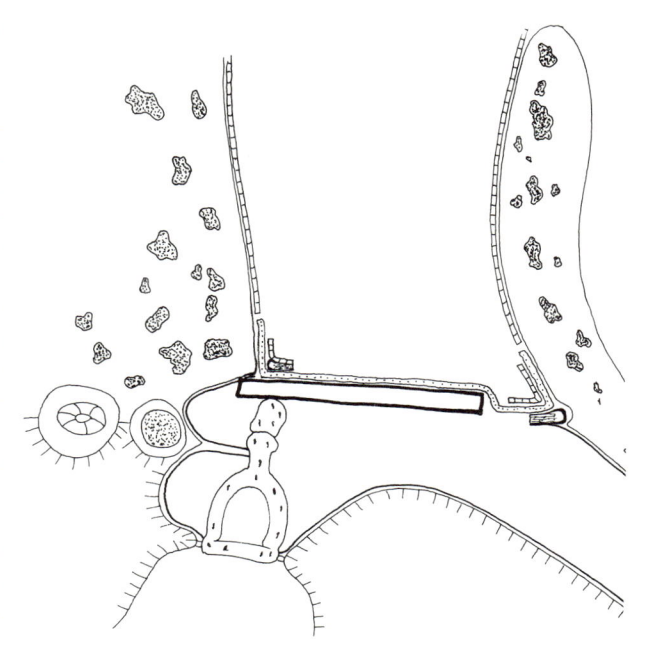

Fig. **947** Side view of myringoplasty and tragal cartilage plate interposition, illustrating the placement of the plate underneath the bony annulus and on the of the long process of the incus

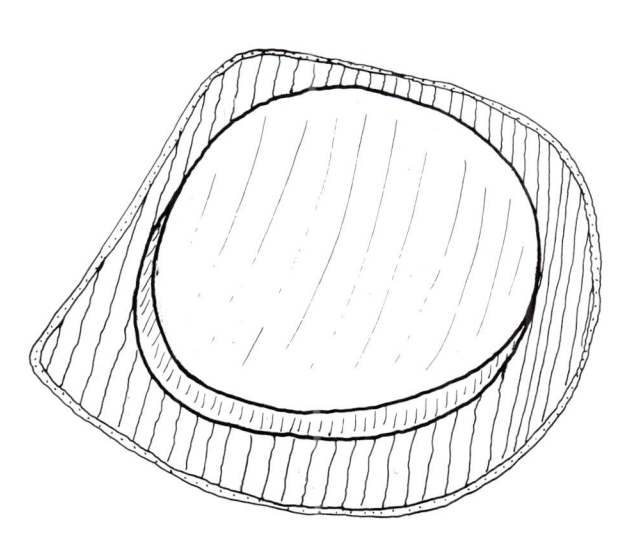

Fig. **948** A tragal cartilage–perichondrium composite graft to cover a total perforation

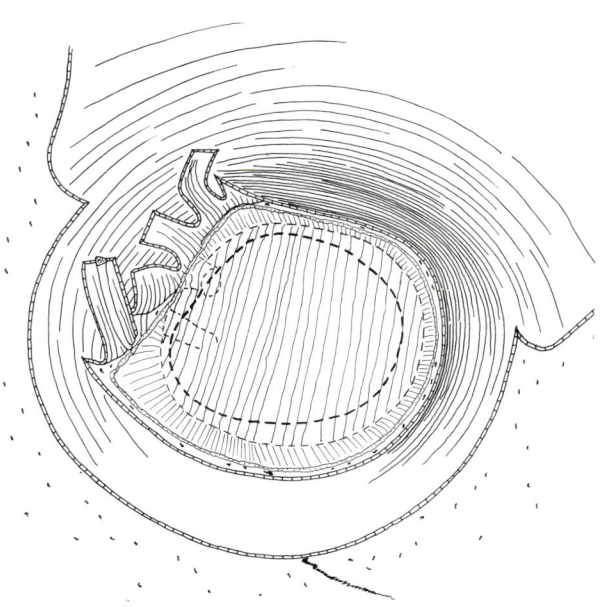

Fig. **949** The composite cartilage–perichondrium graft is in place in a case with total perforation and a missing malleus handle. The plate has some contact with the remnant of the malleus and the incudostapedial joint. Perichondrium covers the denuded bone and the annulus

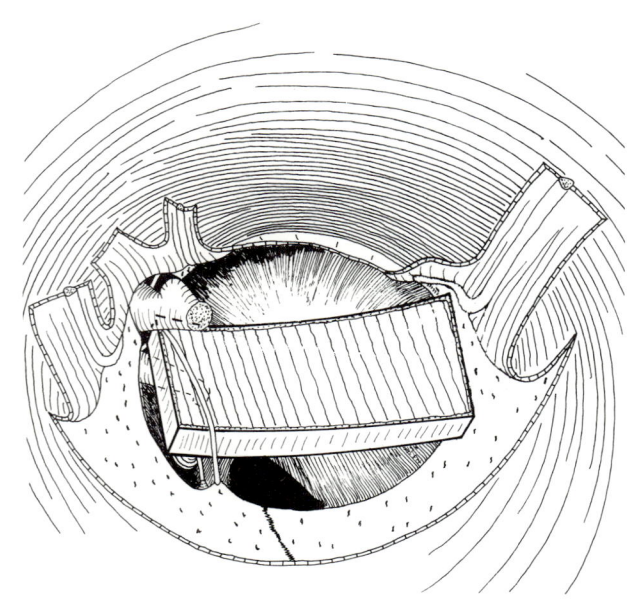

Fig. 950 A tragal cartilage plate with perichondrium placed on the intact incudostapedial joint and on the bony annulus in a case with a missing malleus handle

Cartilage Plates in a Disrupted Ossicular Chain

When the malleus handle and long process of the incus are missing, the thumb touch technique can be used as described above (Fig. 621). A piece of cortical bone or allogenous incus is specially shaped (Fig. 951) to be placed as a graft between the head of the stapes and the composite cartilage–perichondrium graft. A small protrusion is drilled out on the head of the bony prosthesis to be placed into the hole on the cartilage plate. After measuring the size of the cartilage plate needed, the plate is cut, leaving the perichondrium attached to one side of the tragal cartilage. The hole in the cartilage plate can be created with a drill (Fig. 952). The composite graft is placed with the cartilage facing the tympanic cavity (Fig. 953). The thumb-touch graft is carefully placed onto the head of the stapes and into the hole made in the cartilage plate (Fig. 953), and the perichondrium is placed on the denuded bone as an onlay graft and adapted to the epithelium edges. The epithelial flaps are replaced (Figs. 954, 955).

A relatively large cartilage plate (4 mm) can be placed on the head of the stapes and on the anteroinferior bony annulus (Heermann et al. 1970). The plate lies between the long process of the incus and the malleus handle (Fig. 956). The plate can be placed on the bony annulus, with the perforation being covered as an underlay graft, or it can be placed on top of the fibrous annulus, with the perforation being covered as an onlay graft.

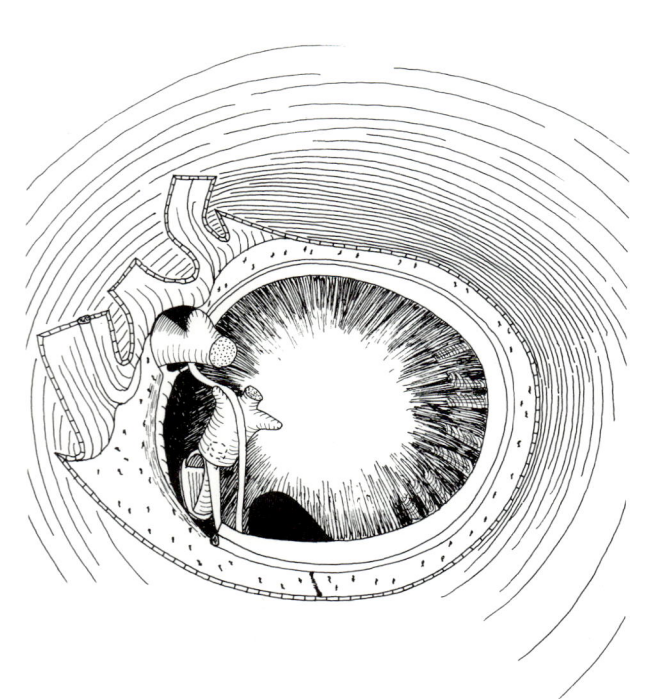

Fig. 951 **The thumb touch technique in total perforation,** with a missing malleus handle and long process of the incus. The epithelium flaps are elevated, and a specially-shaped incus or cortical prosthesis is placed on the head of the stapes

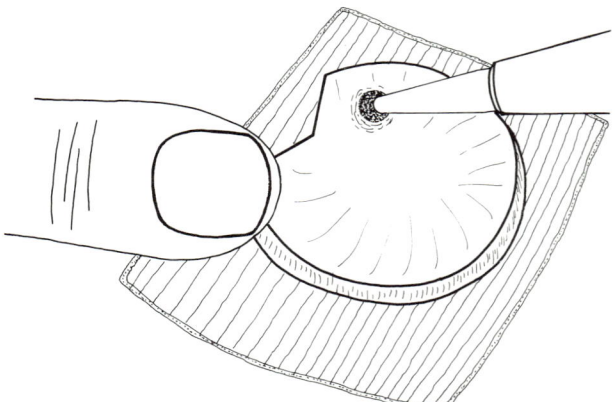

Fig. 952 A tragal cartilage–perichondrium composite graft. A superior wedge of the cartilage is cut. Posterosuperiorly, a hole for the bony prosthesis is drilled

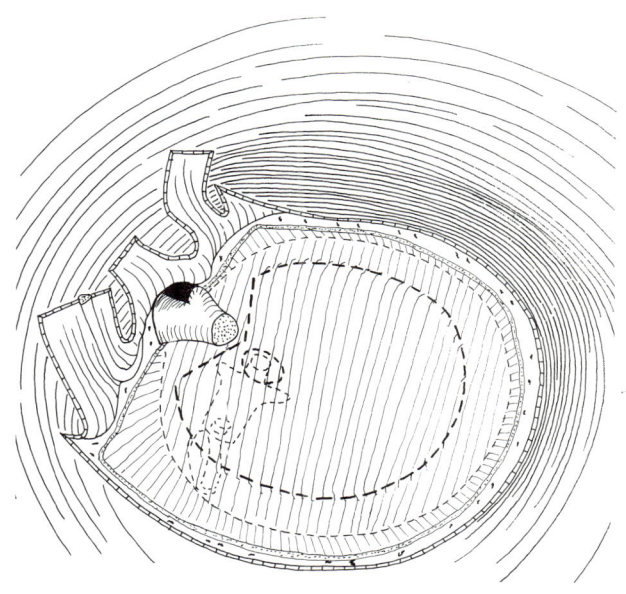

Cartilage Plates in a Disrupted Ossicular Chain

Fig. **953** The composite graft is placed on the denuded bone and annulus. The thumb touch prosthesis is placed on the head of the stapes and into the hole in the cartilage plate. The perichondrium covers the annulus and the denuded bone

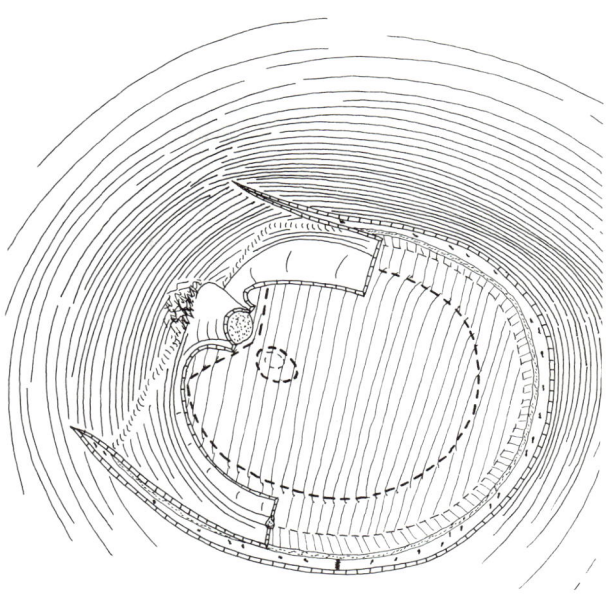

Fig. **954** Epithelial flaps are replaced

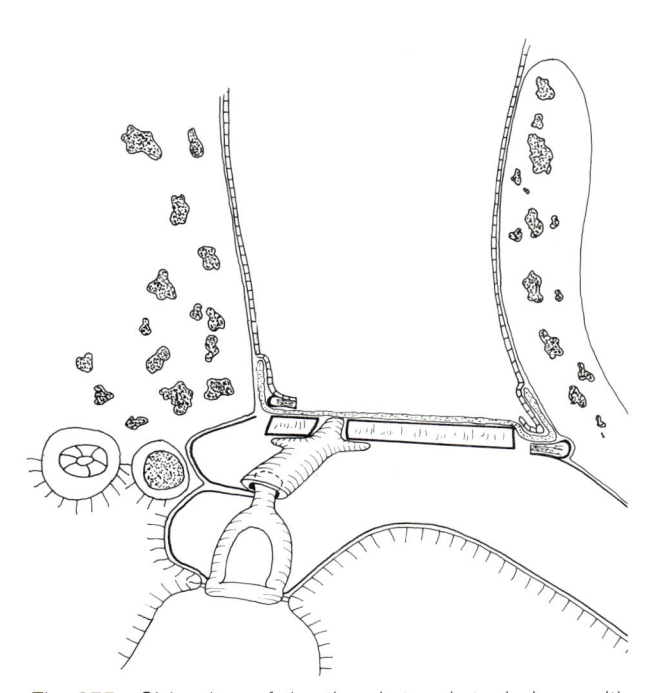

Fig. **955** Side view of the thumb touch technique with the cartilage–perichondrium composite graft. The bony prosthesis lies with its hole on the head of the stapes and with its protrusion in the hole of the cartilage

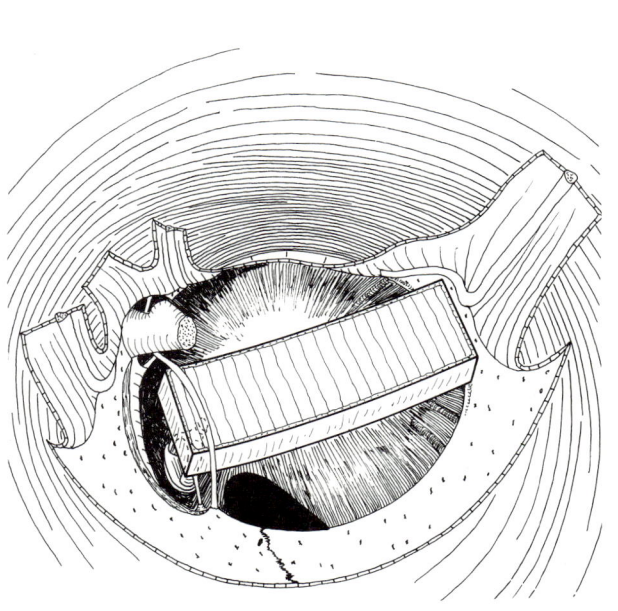

Fig. **956** An annulus stapes cartilage plate (Heermann), with the attached perichondrium, is placed on the head of the stapes and on the bony annulus at the 5-o'clock position in a case with a total perforation and missing malleus handle and long process of the incus

Interposition of Other Prostheses

Several combined prostheses have been described to bridge the defect produced by the missing malleus handle and missing long process of the incus. By shaping the incus, cutting the short process of the incus and using the slender long process, good contact with the tympanic membrane can be achieved (Fig. **957**). Palva used a two-legged steel wire covered with a bony plate (Fig. **958**). Instead of bony plate, a piece of cartilage can be used and the total perforation can be closed with an underlay or onlay graft.

Various prostheses with a large platform are used in ears with a missing malleus handle. Platforms made of hydroxyapatite face the undersurface of the drum or fascia, such as the Goldenberg prosthesis (Fig. **841**). Other platforms, especially those made of Plasti-Pore, are covered with cartilage slides in a manner similar to that used by Sheehy (Fig. **812**). PORPs with a fixed cartilage platform, as described by Jackson et al. (1983), are suitable in cases with a missing malleus handle. The cartilage platform should be made larger than the platform of the prosthesis (Figs. **815, 816**) so as to have good contact with the undersurface of the drum.

Fig. **957** A shaped allogenous incus, with a hole in the remnant of the short process, is placed on the head of the stapes. The entire long process, with the lenticular process, points anteriorly and has good contact with the drum

Allogenous Drum–Malleus Graft

In patients with a missing malleus and an intact ossicular chain (Fig. **927**), disarticulation of the chain and extrusion of the incus and malleus head so as to implant the drum and malleus is sometimes performed, but it is doubtful whether the results with this method can be better than with much more simple methods that leave the chain intact and place a cartilage plate onto the intact chain (Figs. **944, 949**). When the malleus handle and long process of the incus are missing in combination with a total perforation, an allograft drum–malleus transplantation is reasonable. This can be performed using an endaural or retroauricular approach. Harvesting the drum–malleus graft is described above (pp. 229–231). A drum–malleus graft with an attached tympanomeatal flap (Fig. **670**) or without one (Fig. **668**) can be used.

In the endaural approach, in cases without cholesteatoma, placing the new drum onto the patient's annulus is preferable. By combining the technique using three superior epithelial flaps and the technique of outward elevation of annulus epithelium, good epithelial covering of the allogenous annulus can be achieved. These methods are illustrated above (Figs. **510–512** and **678–679**).

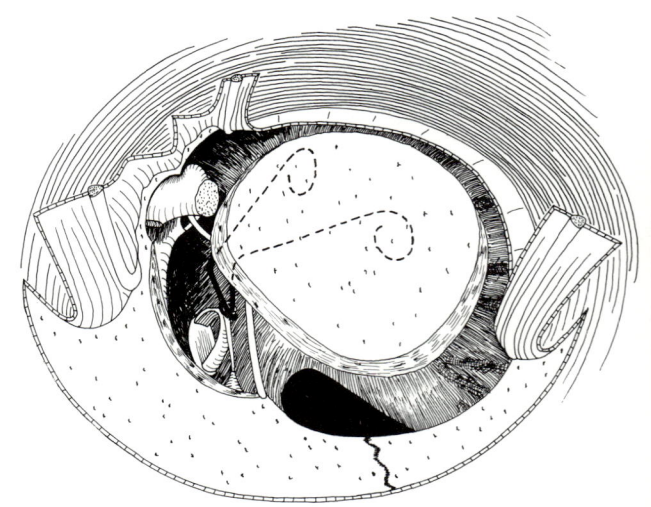

Fig. **958 The Palva two-legged wire technique** in a total perforation with a missing malleus handle and long process of the incus. The two-legged wire is fixed to the head of the stapes, with one leg pointing to the Eustachian tube and the other towards the hypotympanum. The wire is covered with a bony plate

After the bed for the allograft drum has been prepared, the incus is extruded, the tendon of the tensor tympani muscle and the anterior malleolar ligament are cut, and the malleus head can be pulled out of the attic and removed (Fig. **959**). The tympanic cavity is filled with Gelfoam moistened with antibiotics, and the incus is shaped, with a hole in the body being made to fit the head of the stapes. The shortened short process points anteriorly, and the long process remnant points inferiorly. The drum–malleus allograft is then brought into the tympanic cavity, and the malleus head is gently pushed up into the attic. After adjustment of the allogenous drum onto the host annulus, the position of the ossicles is checked (Fig. **960**) and the epithelial flaps are replaced (Figs. **961, 962**).

Other allograft drum-malleus techniques can be applied, such as those of Brandow (1969, 1976) (Figs. **671–674**), Perkins (1979) (Figs. **676–681**) or Marquet (1971) with an attached tympanomeatal flap (Figs. **683–685**).

No late results have been published documenting whether transplantation of an allograft drum is better than other techniques, but it seems more physiological, particularly with the conical shape of the allogenous drum. If allogenous drum transplantation is justified, patients with a missing malleus handle must be much more suitable for allogenous transplantation than those with an intact malleus handle.

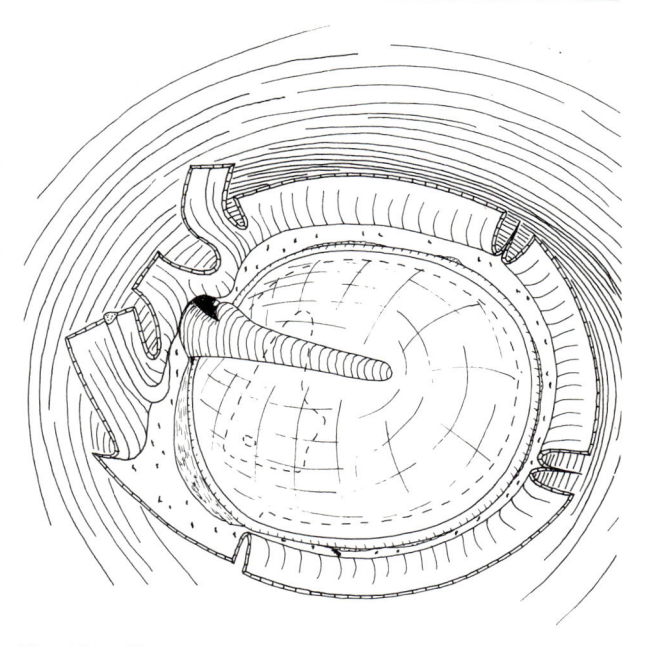

Fig. **960** The drum–malleus allograft, without periosteum from the surrounding tympanomeatal flap, is placed on the host annulus. The allogenous malleus is in place in the attic, and the autogenous incus is interposed

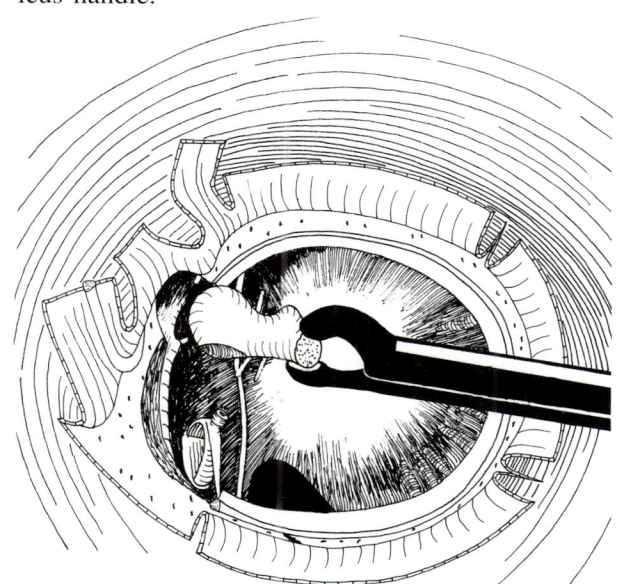

Fig. **959** Removal of the malleus remnant in a case with a missing malleus handle and total perforation. The three superior epithelial flaps are elevated, and the epithelium is elevated outward from the drum remnant and the annulus in order to cover the transplanted drum–malleus allograft

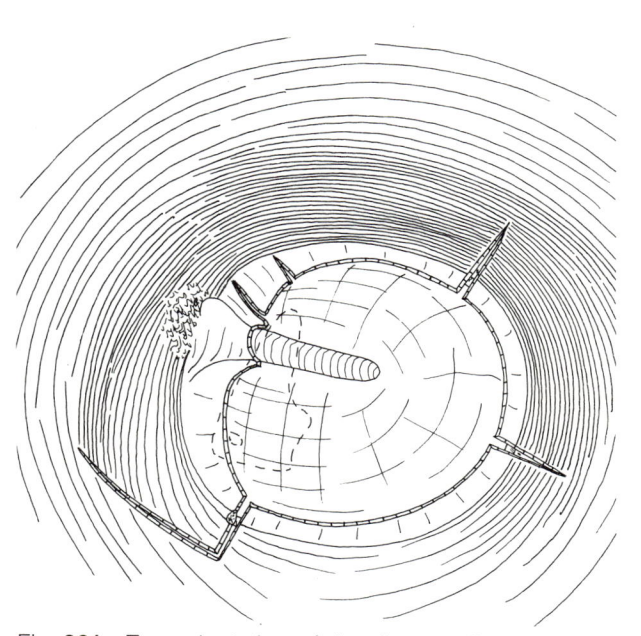

Fig. **961** Transplantation of the drum-malleus allograft is completed, and the epithelial flaps are replaced

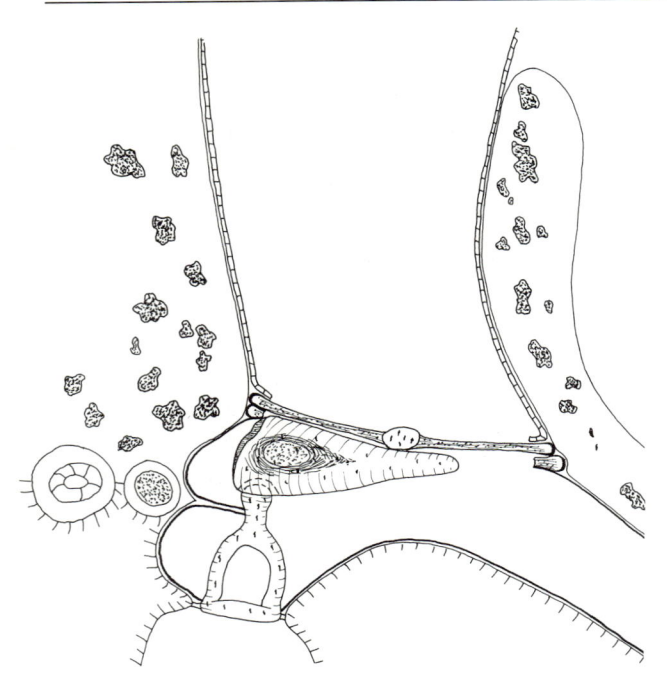

Fig. 962 Side view of the allogenous drum–malleus transplantation on the host annulus. The autogenous incus is interposed between the stapes and the allogenous drum and malleus handle

Malleoplasty of the Defective Malleus Handle

Reconstructing a defective malleus handle is possible, and in fact the technique is not difficult. The author has performed it several times using an endaural approach with the ear speculum, as follows. It is relatively easy to shape an appropriate allogenous malleus handle out of an allogenous malleus (Fig. 963). It should fit exactly onto the host malleus remnant. The hole for the malleus neck should be deep enough, and a groove should be made for the tendon of the tensor tympani muscle (Fig. 964) and possibly for the anterior malleolar ligament, so as to be able to push the allogenous handle sufficiently far onto the host malleus remnant.

After preparing the bed for the fascia, the allogenous malleus handle is pushed onto the malleus remnant, which is stabilized by counterpressure from a hook (Fig. 965). The junction is fixed with fibrin glue, and can be embedded with a thin fascia or perichondrium, or periosteum. The fascia can be placed as an onlay graft over the annulus, but beneath the malleus handle. The superior part of the fascia has two small tongue-like prolongations, which are pulled, on each side of the malleus, into the ear canal. The tongues cover the malleus handle (Fig. 966). The anterior tongue is folded posteroinferiorly, and the posterior tongue anteroinferiorly on the malleus handle, thus completely covering the allogenous malleus handle and securely embedding the malleoplasty in the fascia (Fig. 967). After replacing the epithelial flaps, careful packing should be carried out to avoid dislocation of the malleus handle. Another way of cover-

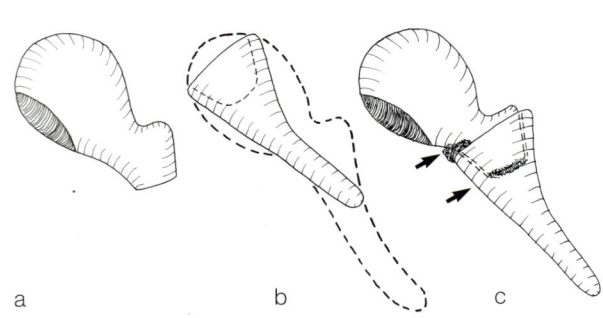

Fig. 963 Shaping a malleus handle from an allogenous malleus. **a** The remnant of the host malleus, with the missing malleus handle. **b** A hole is drilled in the head of the allogenous malleus, and the neck is reduced to the size of the malleus handle. **c** The allogenous malleus is placed on the host malleus remnant. A suggested placement of a small amount of ionomer cement into the acetabulum of the allogenous malleus handle, or medially at the border between the malleus remnant and the allogenous malleus handle, or both, is shown (arrows)

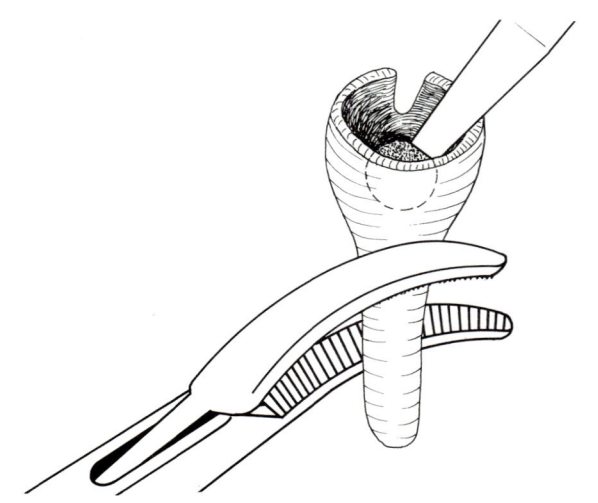

Fig. 964 Preparation of the allogenous malleus graft by drilling a large hole into the head of the malleus, with a groove for the tendon of the tensor tympani muscle

Malleoplasty of the Defective Malleus Handle 343

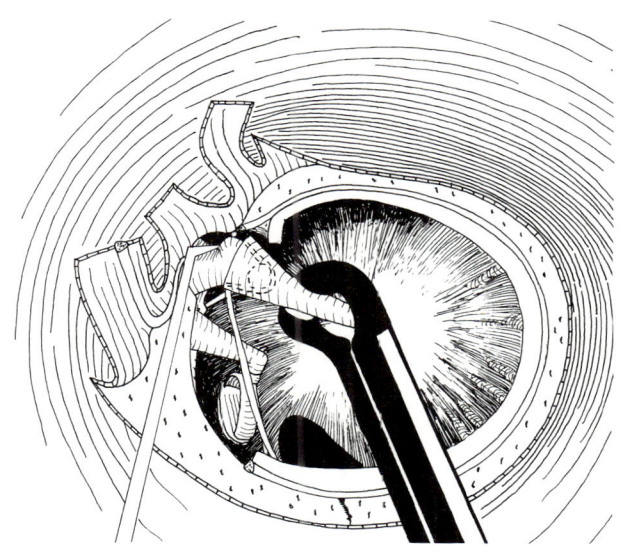

Fig. **965** The malleus handle allograft is pushed onto the remnant of the host malleus

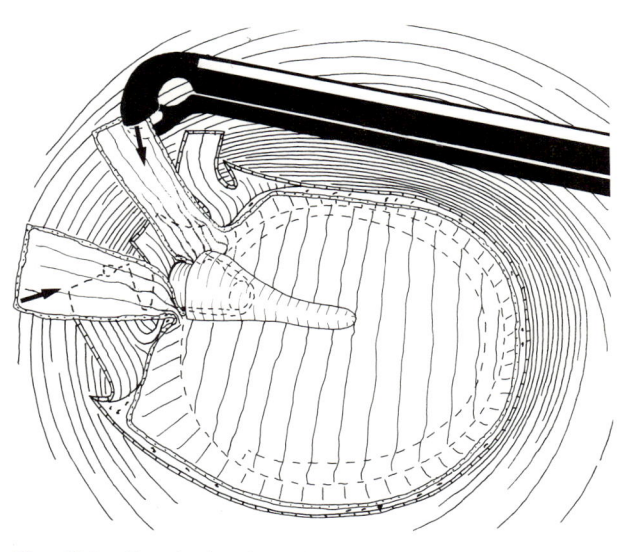

Fig. **966** Fascia is placed on top of the annulus, but underneath the reconstructed malleus handle. The two tongues of fascia cover the allogenous malleus handle and the connection between the host malleus and the allogenous malleus

ing the malleus handle is to use a double perichondrium graft (Fig. **610**).

A firm bony connection of the malleoplasty can be achieved with this method, which is an optimal result, but even fibrous healing stabilizes the drum level. In addition to malleoplasty, a myringoincudopexy, as shown previously (Fig. **929**), can be performed.

In ears with a missing malleus handle and missing long process of the incus, a malleoplasty, in combination with incus interposition, can be performed. The advantage of this is that the malleus neck can be drilled thin for easier insertion into the hole of the allogenous malleus handle. After the malleoplasty, interposition of the incus connected to the new allogenous malleus handle can be performed.

During the 1970s, the author used Hystoacryl in two cases to glue the allogenous malleus onto the host malleus remnant. In both cases, granulations occured due to the Hystoacryl, and both ears suffered eardrum perforations. This was not the case with using fibrin glue.

Using ionomer cement is easier. A very small amount of ionomer cement can be placed on the bottom of the acetabulum of the new malleus handle just before it is attached to the remnant of the host malleus. It fixes the allograft to the malleus (Fig. **963c**). Immediately after this, a small amount of ionomer cement can be placed onto the medial aspect of the autogenous–allogenous border. Ionomer cement should make malleoplasty easier

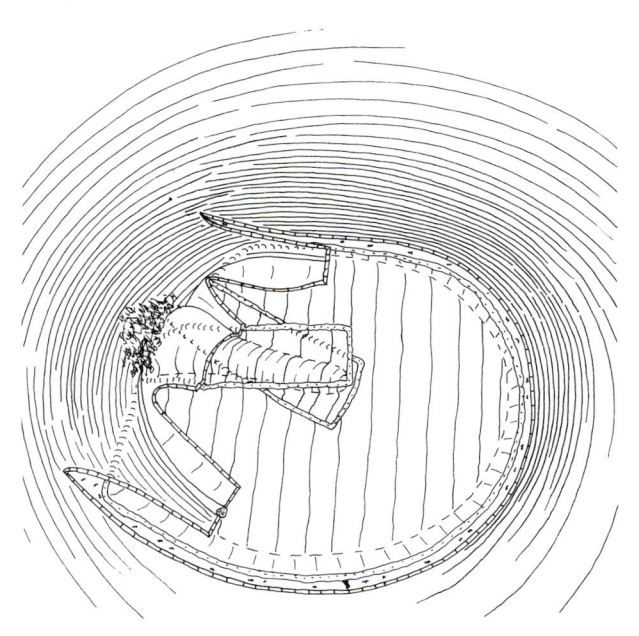

Fig. **967** The two fascia tongues are in position. The anterior tongue is pulled posteroinferiorly, and the posterior tongue anteroinferiorly. The skin flaps are replaced

and more popular than it is now, and tympanoplasty should become more conservative, with more frequent preservation and repair of existing structures than is the case today.

Malleomyringoplasty

Schiller (1979) introduced the construction of a new malleus. The malleus replacement prosthesis is placed between the two fascia layers when the fascia is still attached to the temporalis muscle. This complicated method has several stages:

1) Harvesting the bone in a retroauricular incision. In a retroauricular incision, a piece of 2×2×4 mm cortical bone is removed, either by chiseling or drilling, depending on whether mastoidectomy is used or not. The bone should be solid, with no fractures. The harvesting of bone using a chisel is illustrated above (Figs. **771, 772**). The use of a drill for compound grafts is illustrated below (Figs. **1076** and **1077**).

2) Shaping the malleus replacement prosthesis (Fig. **968**). The prosthesis should be 5 mm long, 1 mm wide and 2–3 mm high. First, the platform of the prosthesis is shaped with a small diamond drill (Fig. **968**). The shaft is then shaped, and a small hole is drilled through it (Fig. **969**).

3) From the retroauricular incision, the temporalis fascia is exposed (Fig. **248**), but the fascia can also be exposed using a separate incision superior to the auricle (Fig. **230**). The prothesis is mounted within the two layers of fascia. A 4-mm incision is made in the superficial layer, which consists of loose areolar tissue. This tissue is elevated from the deep fascia layer with a pair of scissors, and a pocket is created. A small hole is cut in the middle of the pocket (Fig. **970**). The prosthesis is placed between the superficial and the deep layer of the fascia, and the shaft of the prosthesis points out of the hole (Fig. **971**). A stainless steel wire is mounted in the hole. The fascia is elevated from the temporalis muscle, and the total composite graft is removed with scissors.

4) The bed for the onlay graft myringoplasty is created by making the three superior epithelial flaps and removing the epithelium lateral to the annulus (Fig. **972**). After it is trimmed to the proper size, the fascia is brought into the tympanic cavity, and the wire prosthesis is connected to the limb of the stapes (Fig. **973**). The fascia is carefully fixed with Gelfoam balls all the way round the annulus, and the epithelial flaps are returned. The myringoplasty can be performed as an onlay graft or an underlay graft. Schiller recommends carrying out this technique in one stage.

The method is complex, but is the method of choice when there is an old radical cavity without any ossicles, combined with otosclerosis or other fixations of the footplate. The reconstruction of the drum and the malleus should be performed in the first stage, as shown by Schiller, and in the second stage the platinectomy or platinotomy can be performed and the prosthesis fixed to the new malleus handle.

For two-stage procedures combined with stapedotomy or stapedectomy, various other malleus replacement grafts can be used, e.g., an incus-like graft placed between the two layers of fascia (Schiller 1979). The lenticular process protrudes out of the composite graft, and lies under the drum, to be connected with a wire prosthesis.

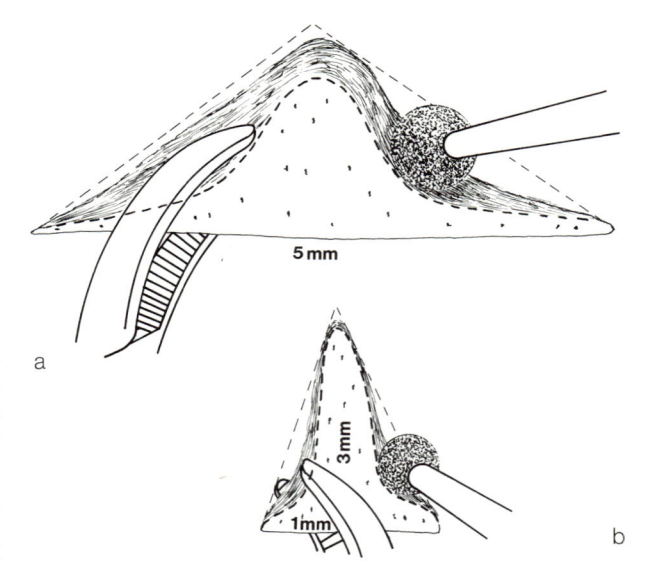

Fig. **968** **Schiller's technique for drilling a malleus replacement prosthesis** from a large piece of cortical bone (**a**). The prosthesis should be 5 mm long, 3 mm high, and 1 mm broad. **b** Superfluous bone is drilled off

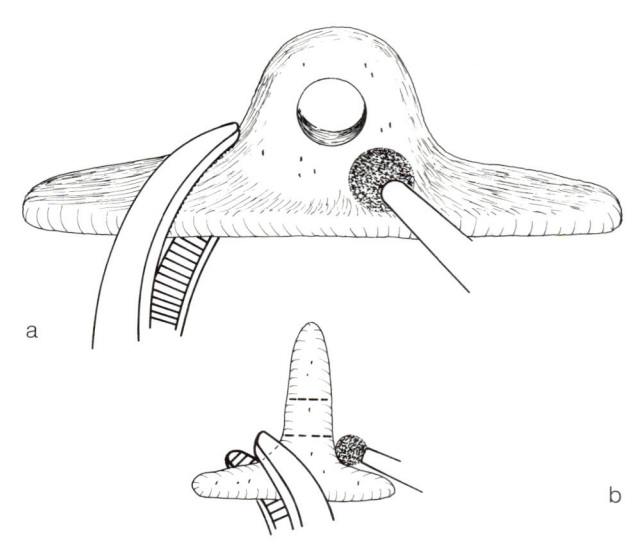

Fig. **969** The final shaping of the malleus replacement prosthesis. **a** A hole is made on the shaft for the wire. **b** The platform is drilled thin so as to be placed between the two fascia layers

Malleomyringoplasty

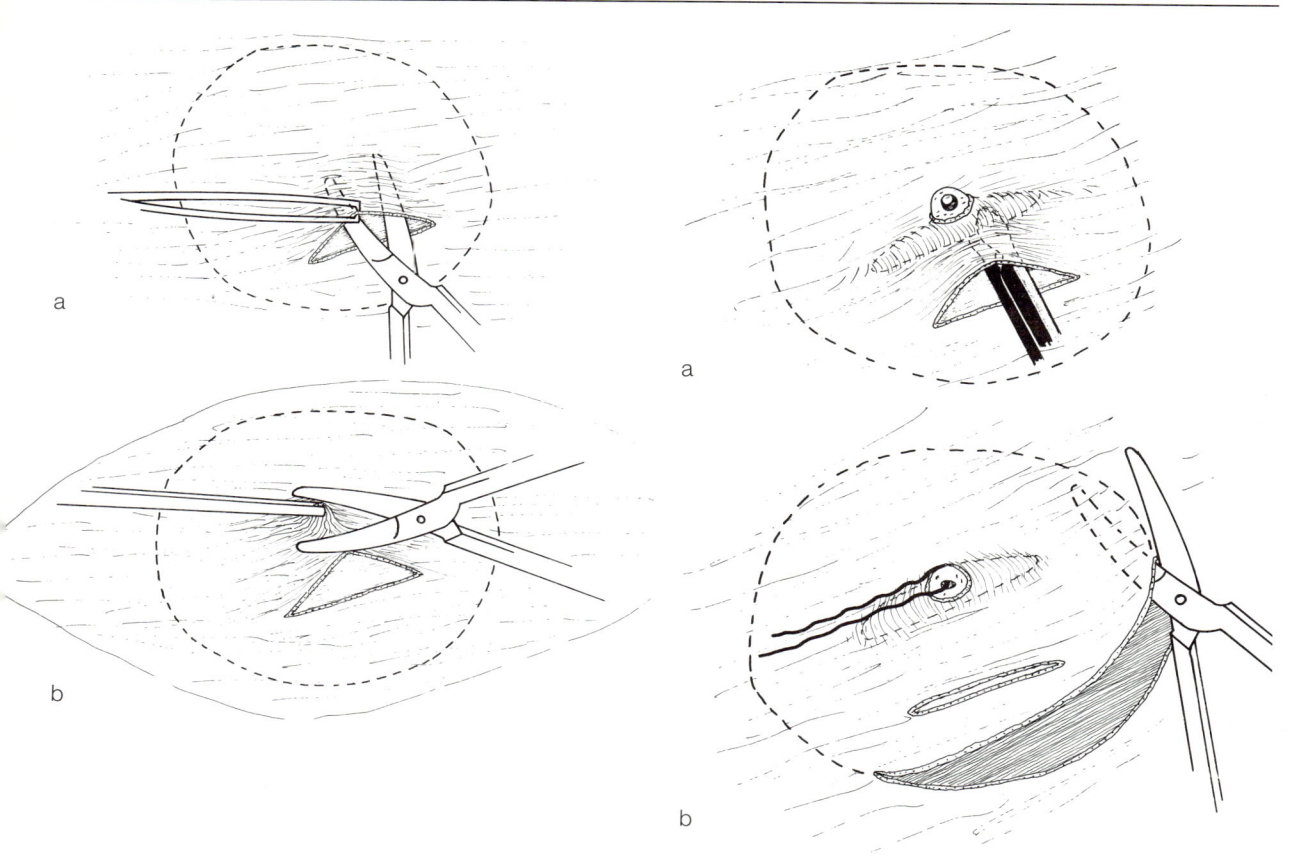

Fig. 970 Preparation of the composite fascia–bone graft. **a** A 4-mm incision is made on the superficial layer of the fascia. A pocket is created between the superficial and deeper layers of the fascia with a pair of scissors. **b** The superficial layer is elevated with a forceps, and a small hole is cut for the shaft of the prosthesis

Fig. 971a The malleus replacement prosthesis is placed in the pocket between the two fascia layers. The shaft points out through the hole. **b** A wire is brought through the hole of the prosthesis, and the fascia is excised and will be trimmed to the appropriate size

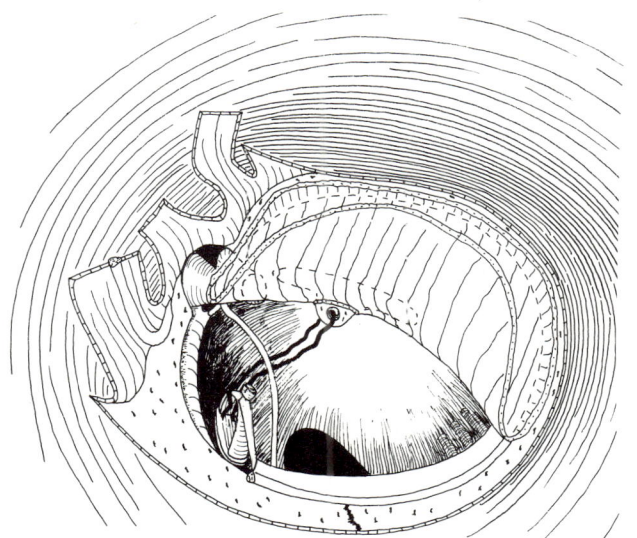

Fig. 972 The malleus replacement prosthesis and the fascia graft are placed on the annulus and drum remnant. The wire is fixed to the anterior limb of the stapes

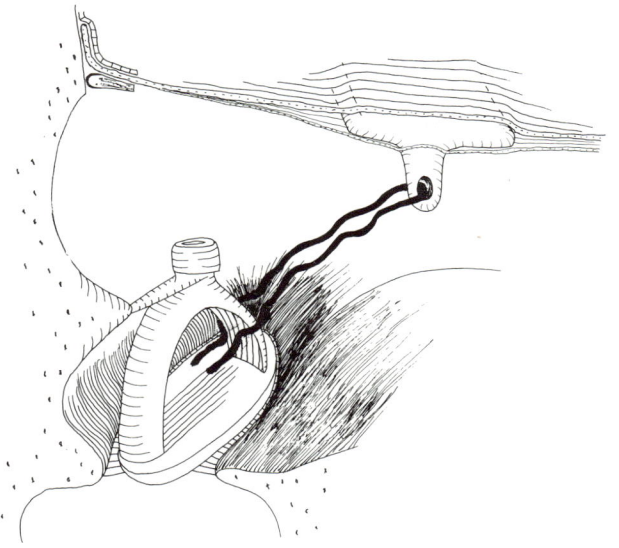

Fig. 973 The malleus replacement prosthesis lies between the two fascia layers. Through the hole of the prothesis shaft, a wire connects the posterior limb of the stapes with a new malleus

Preservation of the Malleus Handle

As seen in Tables **2–5**, a missing malleus handle is not often the result of disease; unfortunately, it is quite often removed by surgeons. Formerly, when radical mastoidectomy was carried out, the malleus handle was always removed. Before the days of tympanoplasty this was understandable, because it served no purpose. Today, however, one should always consider preserving the handle of the malleus, together with the anterior remnant of the tympanic membrane in all cases where it is thought possible to reconstruct the sound conduction mechanism—and this is in fact nearly always possible. The author hardly ever removes a malleus handle, and it is hard to understand why so many surgeons do this.

In noncholesteatomatous disease, it is always possible to remove any retracted epithelium membrane and leave the malleus handle in situ. The malleus handle is never resorbed in attic cholesteatoma. There can be ingrowth of the attic cholesteatoma around the neck of the malleus and under the drum remnant, but the malleus handle can be mobilized by cutting the tendon of the tensor tympani muscle and elevating it. This makes entire malleus handle and the undersurface of the drum remnant completely visible, and any keratinized squamous epithelium can be cleaned. There is definitely no need to remove the malleus handle in attic cholesteatomas (Fig. **974**). If any doubt still remains about a complete removal of the cholesteatoma membrane under the anterior part of the eardrum, the drum can be detached from the malleus handle as shown in Figure **951**. The malleus handle is in contact with the drum only at the umbo, and it can be transpositioned onto the stapes. After cleaning of the region, it can also returned to its original place.

In sinus cholesteatoma, the matrix is originally located in the tympanic sinus and posterior tympanum. It can continue under the malleus handle and the anterior part of the drum. In these cases, too, the malleus handle can be cleaned from both sides by elevating the drum anteriorly to the malleus (Fig. **975**). This allows the undersurface of the malleus handle and the anterosuperior part of the drum to be visualized, and keratinized squamous epithelium can be removed. In this situation, the malleus is only attached at the umbo, but this connection can also be disrupted and the drum undersurface further inspected. There is no need to remove the malleus handle when treating sinus cholesteatoma.

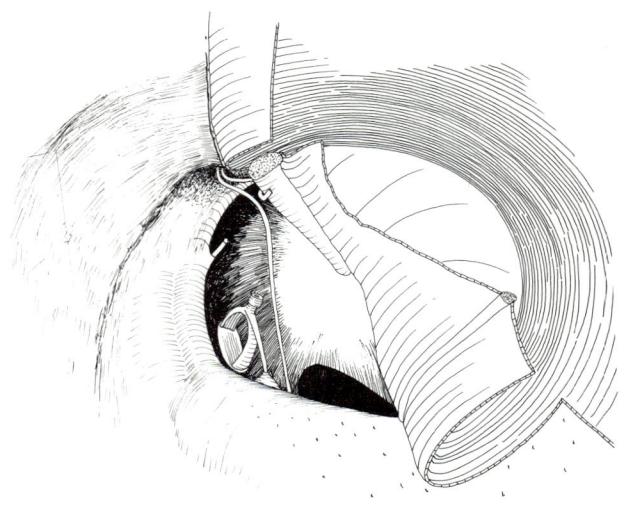

Fig. **974** Cleaning the malleus handle and the undersurface of the drum in an attic cholesteatoma. The head of the malleus is resected, the tendon of the tensor tympani muscle is cut, and the malleus handle and the neck are elevated

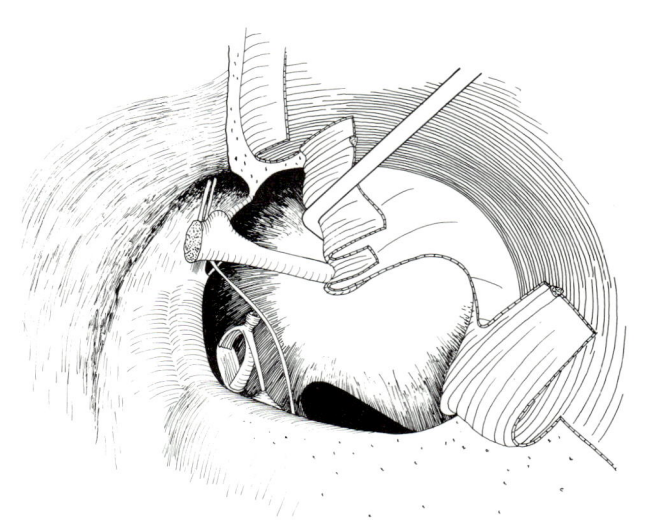

Fig. **975** Cleaning the malleus handle in sinus cholesteatoma. After canal wall–down mastoidectomy, the drum is elevated from the anterior aspect of the malleus, allowing inspection of the anterior tympanum. The malleus can be cleaned. It has little contact with the drum at the umbo region

Preservation of the Malleus Handle

In tensa-retraction cholesteatoma there is, by definition, a total perforation or total retraction of the drum, which is to be removed, so that the malleus handle—if not resorbed—will protrude into the tympanic cavity, without any drum connection. This type of malleus can easily be cleaned (Fig. 976). The umbo can be elevated and the undersurface can be seen. There is definitely no need to remove the malleus handle.

In ears without a malleus handle, there are many more problems in myringoplasty and reconstruction of the ossicular chain, and the results are poorer, in comparison with ears with otherwise the same pathology, but with the malleus handle intact. It is therefore worthwhile to preserve the malleus handle.

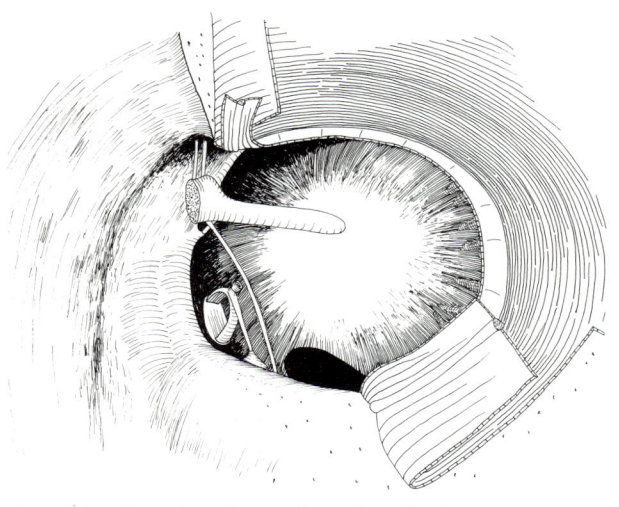

Fig. 976 Cleaning the malleus handle in tensa-retraction cholesteatoma with total perforation. The malleus handle is connected to the bone with the tendon of the tensor tympani muscle and anterior malleolar ligament. It can be cleaned of keratinized squamous epithelium from all sides, and there is no need to remove it

21 Type 3 Tympanoplasty with the Stapes Absent

In ears with a missing or severely defective stapedial arch, a columella between the footplate and the malleus or tympanic membrane is used. Columellae made of the following materials can be applied: autogenous and allogenous incus, autogenous cortical bone, allogenous stapes, autogenous and allogenous cartilage malleus handle, teeth, synthetic biocompatible materials such as polyethylene, Teflon, Plasti-Pore, porous plastic, fluoroplastic, bioinert ceramics, bioactive ceramics, glass, cement, and metals. All these materials are described above (pp. 285–301). Only the specific technical problems related to the various columellae and materials, and to the particular pathology caused by an absent stapes, are described here.

Prognosis with Columellae

Compared with type 2 tympanoplasty with interposition in ears with the stapes present, the outcome and long-term prognosis is much poorer in type 3 tympanoplasty with columella and the stapes absent. All statistics comparing the results of type 3 and type 2 clearly demonstrate better postoperative hearing and fewer reoperations with type 2 than with type 3 tympanoplasty. There are epidemiological, pathogenetic, pathological and functional explanations for these differences.

Analysis of our consecutive surgical series shows a high incidence of ears with missing stapedial arches in cholesteatoma cases (16% in attic, 40% in sinus, and 35% in tensa-retraction cholesteatomas; see Table 2, p. 243). In the group with sequelae of otitis, the stapedial arch was missing in only 5% of the ears. Type 3 columellae are therefore more often associated with more extensive surgery, especially mastoidectomy, than type 2 tympanoplasty procedures with interposition. Type 2 tympanoplasty without mastoidectomy is the most common procedure.

Pathogenetically, the disease is more pronounced and has a longer history at presentation in ears with a missing stapedial arch than in those with the stapes present. It is well established that bone resorption occurs in contact with keratinized squamous epithelium, either in active cholesteatoma or in a retraction pocket with debris accumulation. In sinus cholesteatoma originating from a posterosuperior retraction, the stapedial arch is most commonly resorbed. During the development of sinus cholesteatoma, the following stages can be recognized: atrophy and retraction in the posterosuperior part of the drum, myringoincudipexy, resorption of the long process of the incus, myringostapediopexy, and resorption of the head, neck, and arch of the stapes. Resorption of the stapedial arch can therefore, in most cases, be considered as a more progressive stage of the same process.

Pathological changes in the tympanic cavity are usually more severe in ears with a missing stapedial arch than in those with the stapes present. There are greater alterations in the middle-ear mucosa, and there is always pathology in the posterior part of the tympanic cavity. The risk of fixation of the columella by adhesions is greater than in ears with the stapes present. Keeping the posterior part of the tympanic cavity ventilated is more difficult when the stapedial arch is missing than when it is present.

It is of course well known that, physiologically, a columella can never replace the function of a mobile stapes.

Variations in Columella Placement

Many factors influence the choice, size, shaping, and placement of the columella.

1) Mastoidectomy or no mastoidectomy? In ears with tympanoplasty, only the position of the malleus handle determines the shape and size of the columella (Fig. 977).
2) Canal wall–up or canal wall–down mastoidectomy? In canal wall–down mastoidectomy, there is usually no air space, or a vibrating membrane, superior to the columella (Figs. 978, 979), and the columella should therefore be directed more anteroinferiorly so as to provide better contact to the vibrating part of the drum, which is smaller (Fig. 980) than in ears with canal wall–up mastoidectomy or without mastoidectomy. In canal wall–down mastoidectomies, the bridge, which usually determines the

Variations in Columella Placement

Fig. **977** Various positions of the malleus handle and various angles between the posterior bony annulus, footplate, and malleus handle. The handle requires various sizes and shapes of columellae

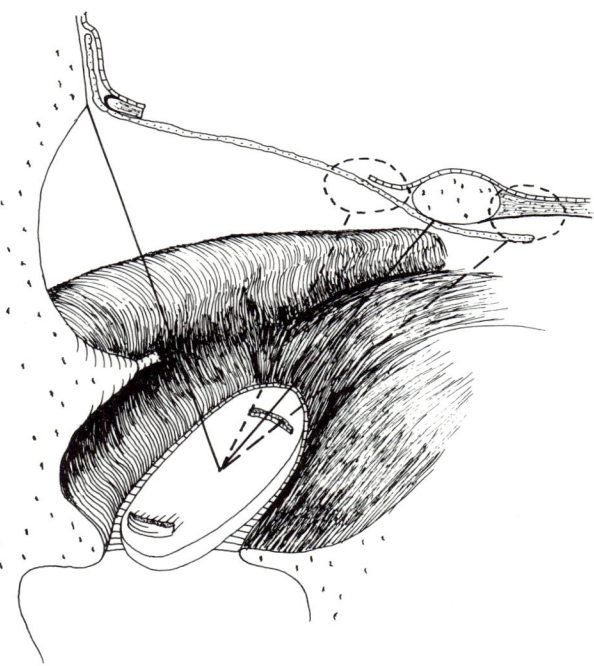

Fig. **978** A thin incus columella in a canal wall–down mastoidectomy situation, placed under the malleus handle and directed anteriorly

Fig. **979** Side view of the thin incus columella in canal wall–down mastoidectomy

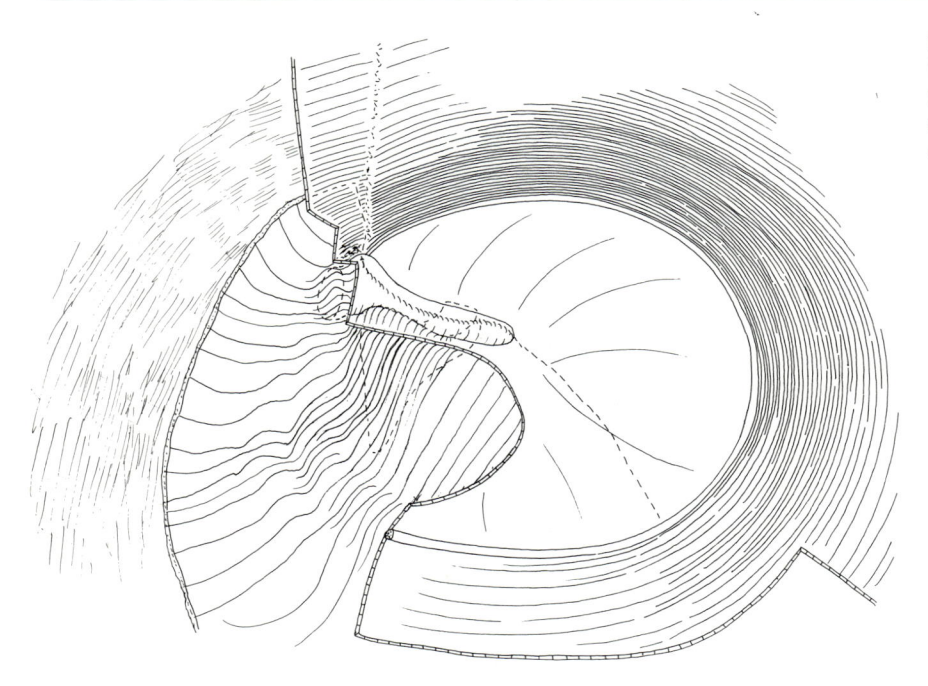

Fig. **980** The fascia covers the columella, the facial prominence, the attic, and the lateral semicircular canal. The epithelial flaps are replaced

height of the superior part of the tympanic cavity, is missing. The columella therefore has to be shorter with canal wall–down than with canal wall–up mastoidectomy or no mastoidectomy.
3) Intact or missing malleus handle? Generally, the head of the columella should be larger in patients with no malleus handle than in those with a normal malleus, in order to increase the contact area with the drum.
4) The distance from the footplate to the malleus handle often varies, as does the angle between the posterior bony annulus and malleus handle and the center of the footplate (Fig. **977**). In an anteriorly-positioned malleus handle, the distance to the footplate is longer, and the angle larger, than in a posteriorly-positioned malleus. The columella should be shaped in relation to these distances.
5) The size of the oval window niche. When there is a narrow niche caused either by thick mucosa or prominent bone on the promontorial side, the columella should be thin, so as to avoid fixations.
6) A prominent horizontal part of the facial nerve, causing a narrow and oblique oval-window niche. The columella should be thin and directed inferiorly. Sometimes it is almost impossible to place a columella on the center of the footplate.

Autogenous Incus Columella

If the stapedial arch is missing, the long process of the incus is also resorbed. A columella of autogenous incus therefore consists mainly of the short process of the incus, which is placed on the middle of the footplate and the incus body, with its articular surface in contact either with the undersurface of the malleus handle, or with the undersurface of the drum, or in contact with both structures. The latter situation is the most common one. The remnant of the long process wither points anteriorly (Fig. **981**) or inferiorly (Fig. **982**); most of the columella is placed parallel to the malleus handle, and only the most distal part of the long process remnant is shaped and positioned just under the lower part of the malleus handle. The incus body and the long process remnant can be placed parallel to the malleus handle (Fig. **983**).

When the autogenous incus columella is placed under the malleus handle, with the long process remnant directioned anteriorly, the incus has to be shaped so as to fit the malleus handle (Fig. **984**). When there is a short distance to the malleus handle, part of the incus body and the entire long process should be drilled away. When there is a long distance, half of the incus with the long process remnant is drilled away. A hemi-incus prosthesis is formed (Goodhill 1967) and placed obliquely between the footplate and the malleus handle (Fig. **985**).

Variations in Columella Placement

Fig. **981** The incus columella, with the short process placed on the footplate. The long process remnant is directed anteriorly and placed under the malleus handle

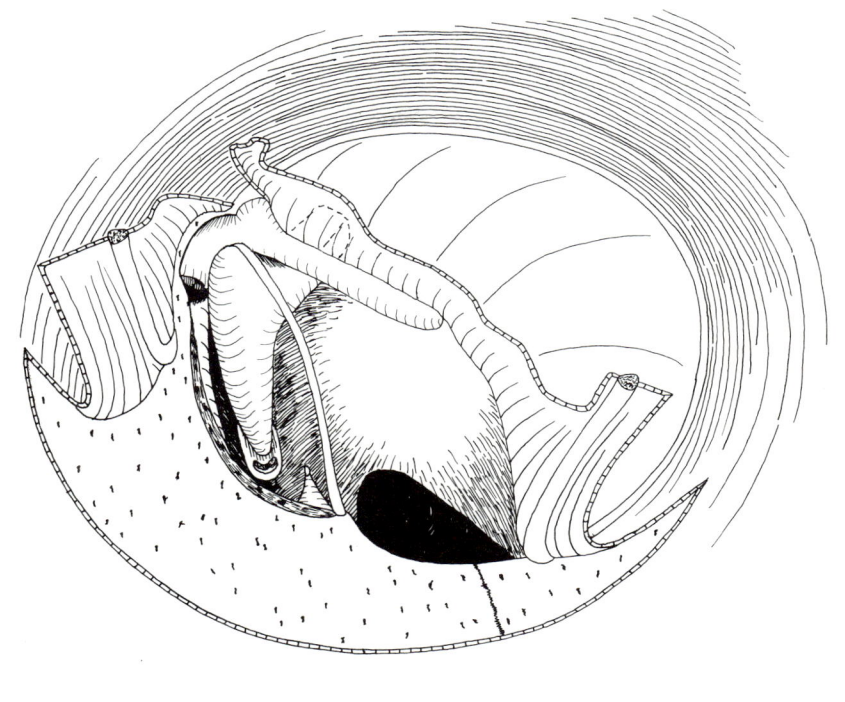

Fig. **982** The incus columella, with the short process placed on the footplate. The long process remnant is directed inferiorly, parallel to the malleus handle, and the most distal part is shaped and placed under the malleus handle

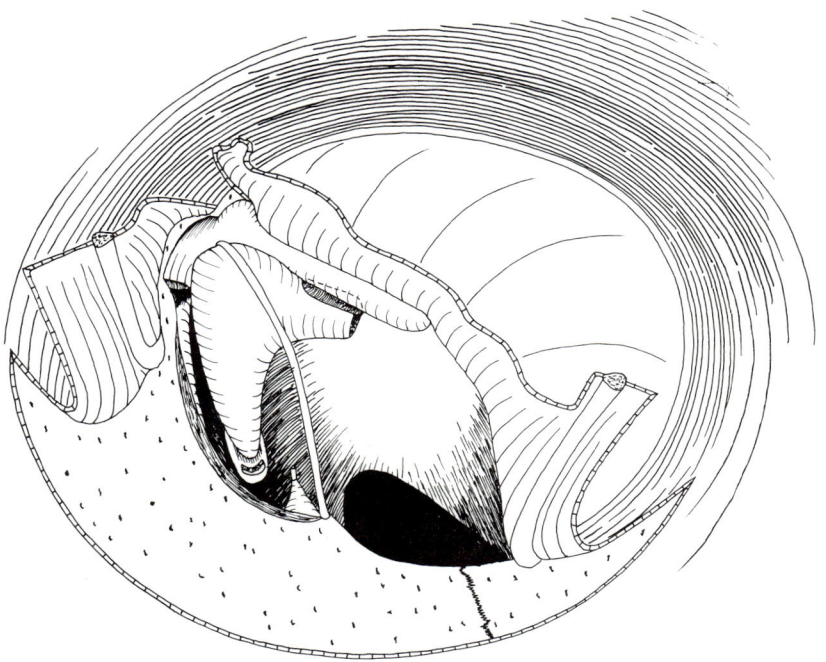

When the malleus handle is in a normal position, some of the incus body has to be drilled away (Fig. **984b**), but this type of columella is still in broad contact with the drum and malleus handle (Fig. **986**).

In addition to providing sound transmission to the footplate, an incus columella can prevent retraction of the posterosuperior part of the drum. This is the case in ears with a posterior and normally positioned malleus handle (Figs. **985, 986**). The incus body is broadly in contact with the drum, and the distance between the posterior bony annulus and the columella is short. A retraction posterosuperior to the prosthesis is thus prevented, in contrast to the hemi-incus prosthesis (Fig. **985**), which only provides a small area of contact with the relatively large and unsupported posterosuperior part of the drum. This posterosuperior drum area may retract

21 Type 3 Tympanoplasty with the Stapes Absent

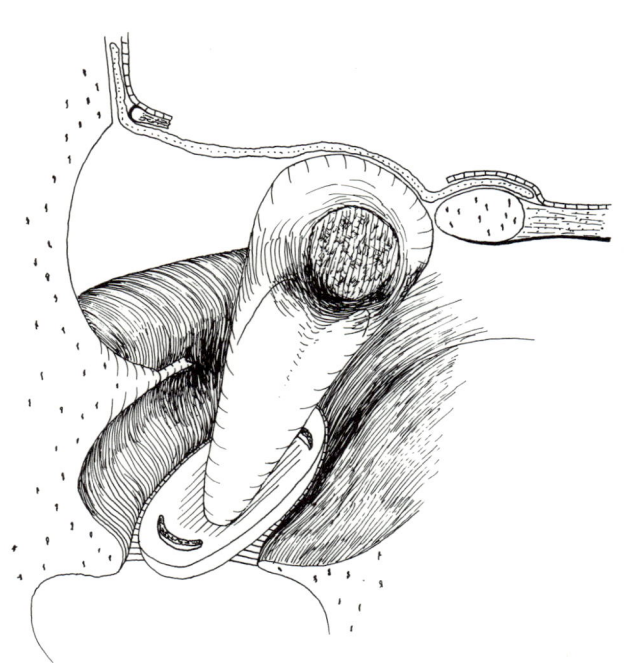

Fig. 983 The incus columella, with the short process placed on the footplate. The whole long process remnant is placed parallel to the malleus handle

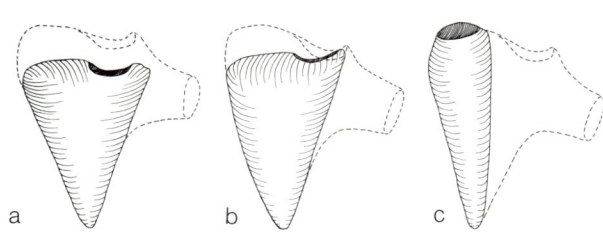

Fig. 984 Various ways of shaping the autogenous incus with a defective long process. The short process is placed on the footplate, and the incus body and the long process are drilled off to various degress. **a** Extensive drilling in a situation with a short distance between the footplate and the malleus handle. **b** Minor drilling of the incus in a situation with a normal distance to the malleus handle. **c** Half of the incus body, with the long process remnant, is drilled away in cases with a long distance between the footplate and the malleus handle (hemi-incus prosthesis)

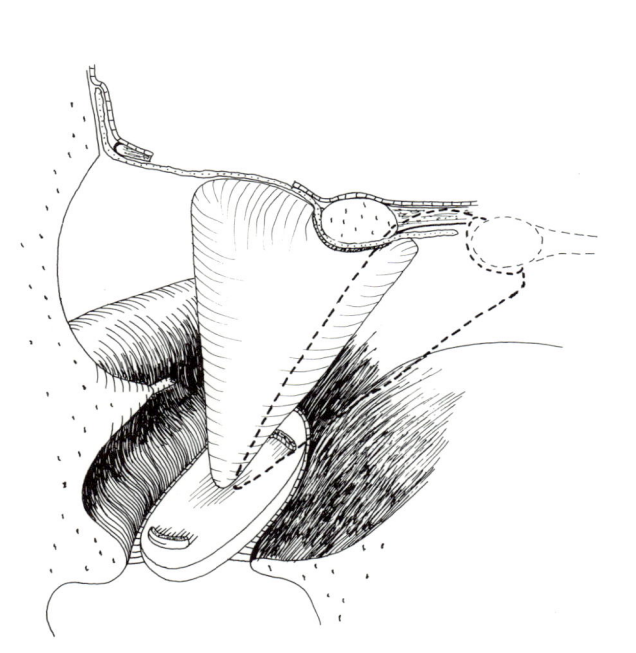

Fig. 985 A small incus columella with the short process, placed on the footplate. The incus body is in firm contact with the drum and the malleus handle. The dotted line illustrates the hemi-incus prosthesis in a case with a long distance between the footplate and the malleus handle

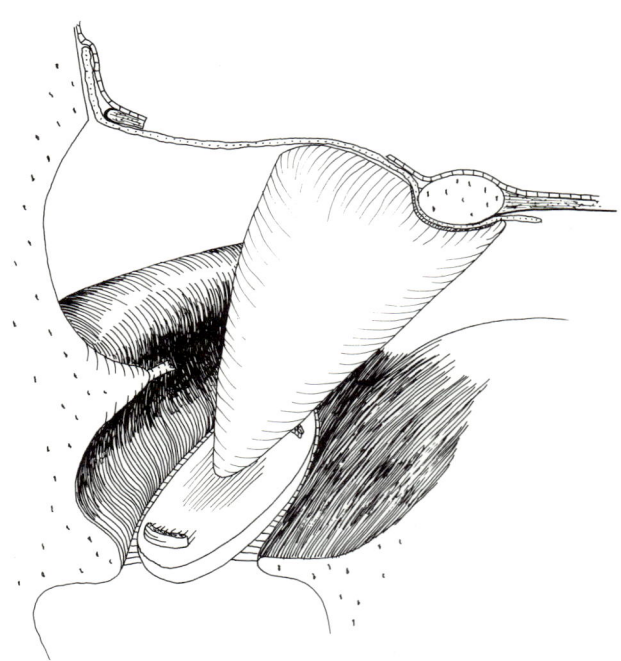

Fig. 986 A normal position of the malleus handle and an incus columella with broad contact to the drum and the malleus handle

behind and onto the posterior surface of the columella, reducing the vibrating area of the drum and fixing the prosthesis (Fig. **987**).

When shaping and placing the platform, the incus, or any other bony prosthesis, a compromise between preventing retraction and providing good function needs to be achieved.

Another compromise relates to the thickness of the incus columella in the oval-window niche. Placing an "untouched" short process of autogenous incus with its mucosa, without any drilling of the short process (as shown in Figures **981–983, 986, 988**) is a common procedure when the oval-window niche is of normal width. If there is sufficient distance to the walls of the niche, an unshapen and compact columella can hardly be resorbed or osseously fixed. There will be no new formation of bone with secondary bony fixation, and usually this type of "untouched" columella becomes covered with mucosa. If there is any narrowing of the niche, the columella should be drilled thin (Figs. **977, 989**).

Columellae in the shape of a "7", with a thin shaft at a 60° angle, or L-shaped columellae with the shaft at an 80–90° angle, to the head of the prosthesis, which is also relatively thin, are often used (Fig. **989**). The head is placed either under, or parallel to, the malleus handle. T-shaped prosthesis, with a thin shaft perpendicular to the platform, are also commonly used (Fig. **990**). The platform is usually directed in an anteroposterior direction. Grooves can be made on the platform of the 7-shaped and T-shaped prostheses while they are being trimmed.

Some surgeons use polyethylene or Teflon sleeve, or a Silastic tube placed on the thin shaft, to prevent bony fixation of the prosthesis in the oval-window niche (Fig. **991**). Fixation can be prevented in this way, but ischemic bony necrosis may occur at the footplate end of the columella. Often, the tube itself increases the thickness of the shaft. The author has seldom practiced covering the shaft of the incus columella, but regularly uses 4×2 or 3×2–mm thin Silastic pieces placed on the facial nerve side and the promontory side of the oval-window niche (Fig. **992**). When well-ventilated ears underwent repeat surgery, the Silastic was still in place, with no adhesions. In poorly-ventilated ears, the Silastic was embedded in fibrous tissue or a mucosa-like membrane, with partial or total obliteration of the oval-window niche. There is no scientific proof that Silastic sheeting of the niche has any significant effect in preventing obliteration of the niche.

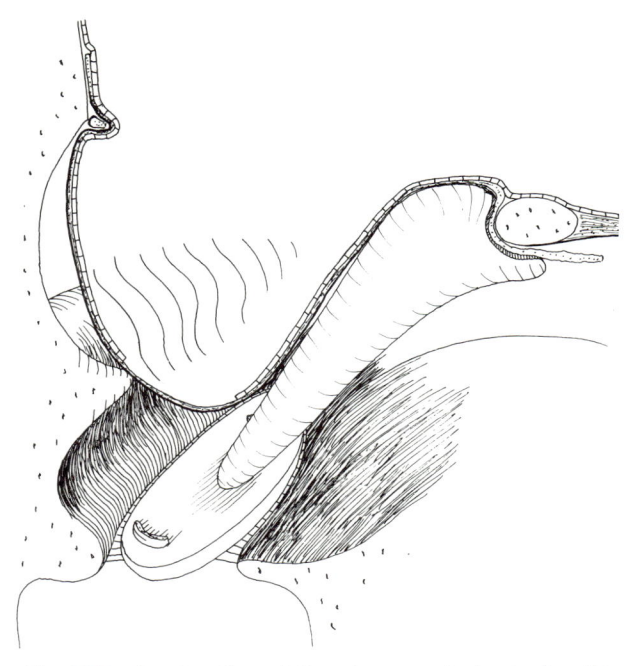

Fig. **987** A retraction of the drum posterior to the thin columella

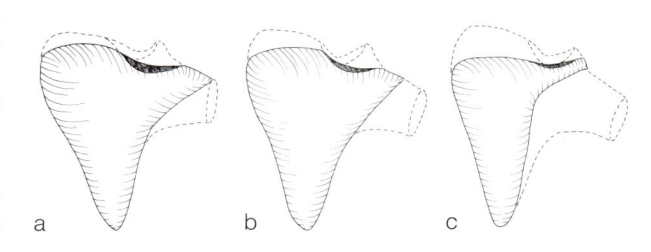

Fig. **988** Shaping of the incus columella, especially its long-process remnant. **a** The long process is included in the columella. **b** The long process is drilled off. **c** Part of the incus body and the long process are drilled off

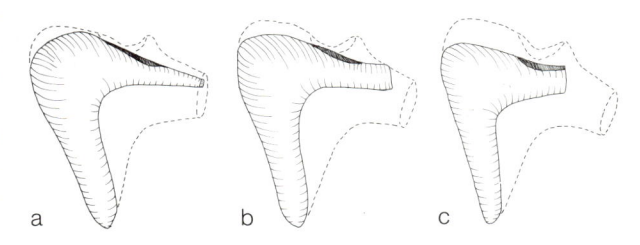

Fig. **989** 7-shaped and L-shaped incus prostheses, with considerable drilling of the short process of the incus in cases with a narrow oval-window niche. **a, b** The angle between the horizontal and vertical parts is about 60°. **c** The angle is about 80–90°

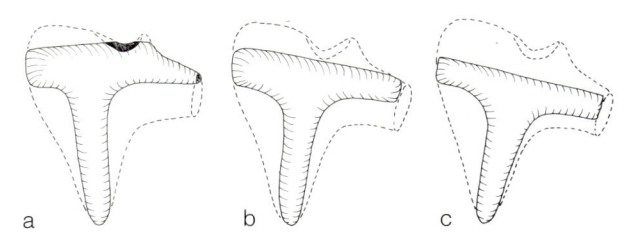

Fig. 990 An incus T-prosthesis. The short process of the incus is made thinner, and the horizontal part is flat, **a** with or **b, c** without grooves for the malleus handle

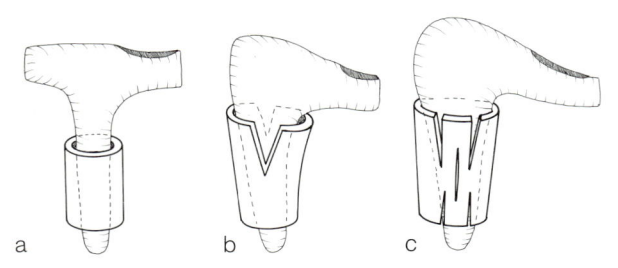

Fig. 991a Polyethylene, **b** Teflon, and **c** Silastic tubes placed on a thin short process of the incus to prevent fixation of the columella in the oval-window niche. Small incisions are made in the sleeves to release the pressure on the bone (**b, c**)

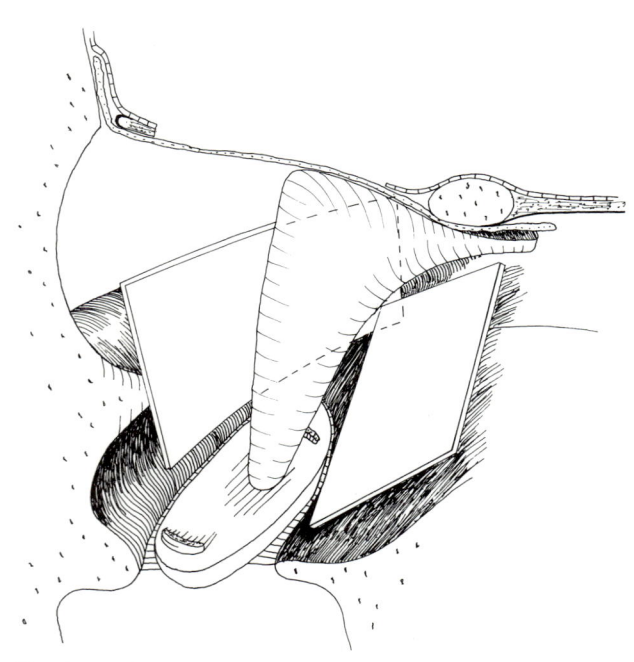

Fig. 992 Placement of small pieces of thin Silastic sheeting on the promontorial side and the facial nerve side of the oval-window niche, preventing bony fixation of the columella

Allogenous Incus

All shaping based on using the short process of the incus as the columella can also be performed in allogenous incus, in the same way as that shown in Figures **977–991**. In addition to the short process columella, allogenous incus can also be used to create a long process columella. The long process is thinner as well as longer than the short one, and it is therefore usually not necessary to drill it thinner (Fig. **993**). It can be placed in the niche as it is.

The lenticular process can be drilled off, or it can be left untouched and placed on the footplate. An allogenous incus prosthesis with the lenticular process placed on the footplate is usually used in ears with high tympanic cavities (Figs. **994, 995**). If the lenticular process is directed posteriorly, the incus body and the short process should be drilled off (Fig. **993**).

In ears with a laterally-positioned drum and a missing malleus handle, with or without blunting, the entire allogenous incus has to be used. It is placed with its lenticular process on the footplate (Fig. **996**). The top of the incus body reaches the lateralized drum, and the short process is directed anterosuperiorly.

Sometimes even the entire incus is not long enough to establish stable contact with a severely lateralized drum. In these rare cases, the author has used a 4×5–mm piece of tragal cartilage–perichondrium composite graft, with perichondrium attached to the drum side and a large perichondrium attached to the incus side. After the cartilage plate has been placed between the incus and the drum, the 2-mm long stripes of perichondrium cover the medial and lateral sides of the incus body, and stabilize the prosthesis (Fig. **997**).

Often, the lenticular process is drilled off the long process of the incus, which is placed on the middle of the footplate. The body and the short

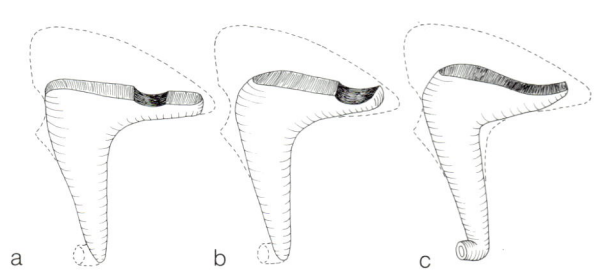

Fig. 993 Shaping an allogenous incus columella with its long process placed on the footplate. **a, b** The lenticular process is removed, or **c** is left intact. The head of the incus and short process are drilled off to various degrees

Variations in Columella Placement 355

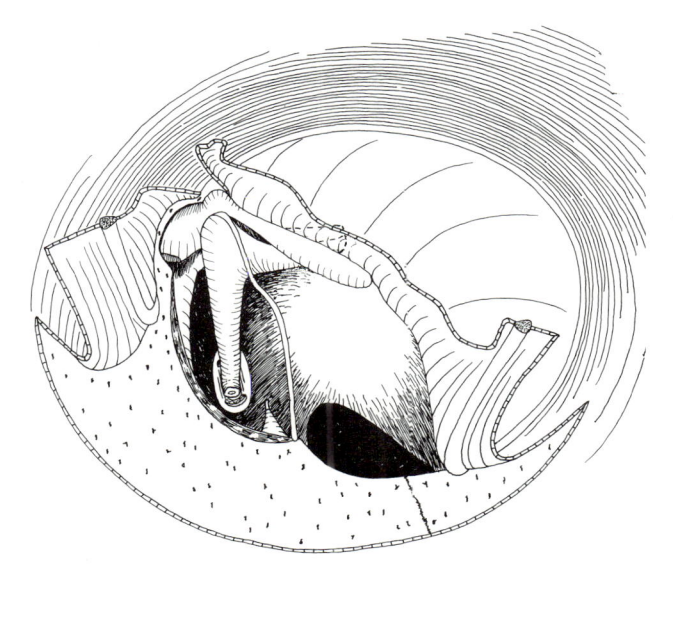

Fig. **994** A shaped allogenous incus columella, with the lenticular process placed on the footplate and the short process under the malleus handle

Fig. **995** Side view of the allogenous incus columella. The lenticular process is placed on the footplate. The short process is drilled thin so as to be placed under the malleus handle. The prosthesis has broad contact with the drum

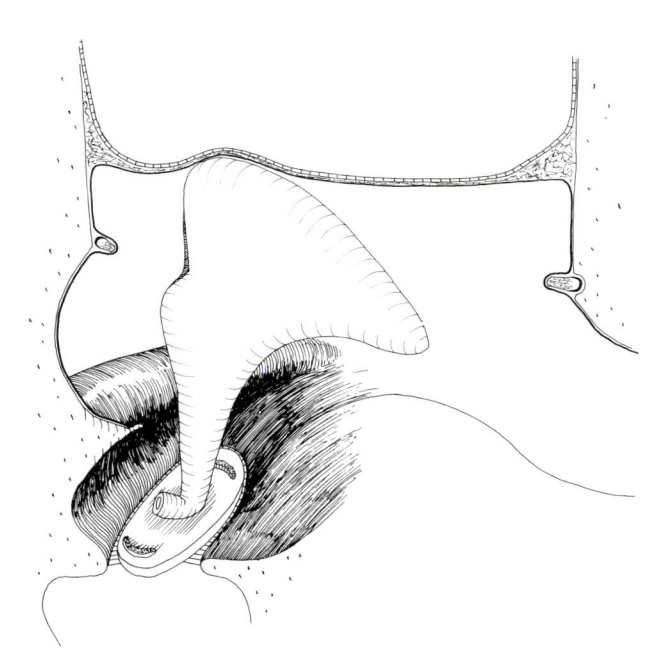

Fig. **996** The entire allogenous columella in a case with a laterally-positioned drum and a missing malleus handle. The lenticular process is placed on the footplate. The incus body touches the drum

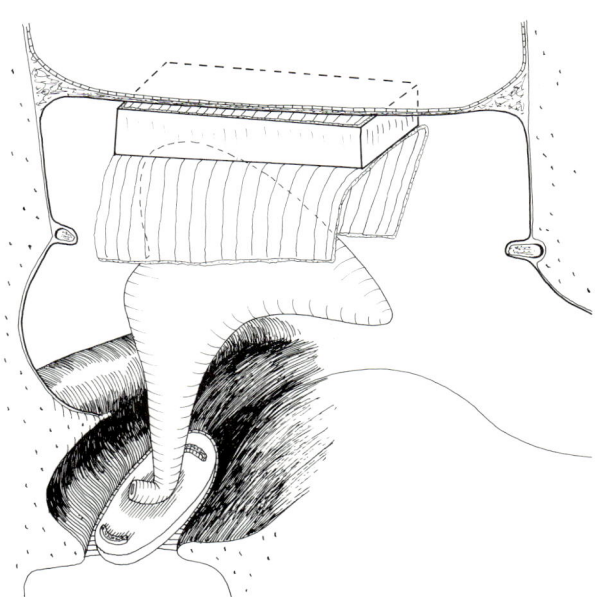

Fig. **997** Additional interposition of a cartilage plate with perichondrium between the drum and the allogenous incus in cases with extensive lateralization of the drum. The perichondrium surrounds the incus body, stabilizing the prosthesis

process are shaped to the appropriate shape and length. The short process can be placed under the malleus handle (Fig. **998**), or parallel to it. In the latter case, the long process of the incus is shortened so as to achieve the exact length for the prosthesis (Fig. **999**).

Cortical Bone

Cortical bone is often used in type 3 tympanoplasty, as it is easy to harvest and shape. Since resorption of the stapedial arch is often associated with cholesteatoma, a mastoidectomy is performed and a large piece of bone is usually taken to produce a columella. Harvesting cortical bone and shaping an interposition graft are shown in Figures **771–773** above. When the thin columella is being shaped, care should be taken not to crush or fracture it with the surgical clamps, or other prosthesis-holding forceps. The drilling should be carried out gently with a diamond burr (Fig. **1000**). Cortical-bone prostheses are L-shaped, 7-shaped, or T-shaped, like the shaped incus prostheses shown in Figures **989–991**. Sometimes—especially when an appropriate piece of cortical bone is unavailable—a stick-like columella can be placed between the footplate and the malleus handle (Fig. **1001**). Sound transmission with this type of columella is good, but there is a risk of a posterior drum retraction (Fig. **1002**). In

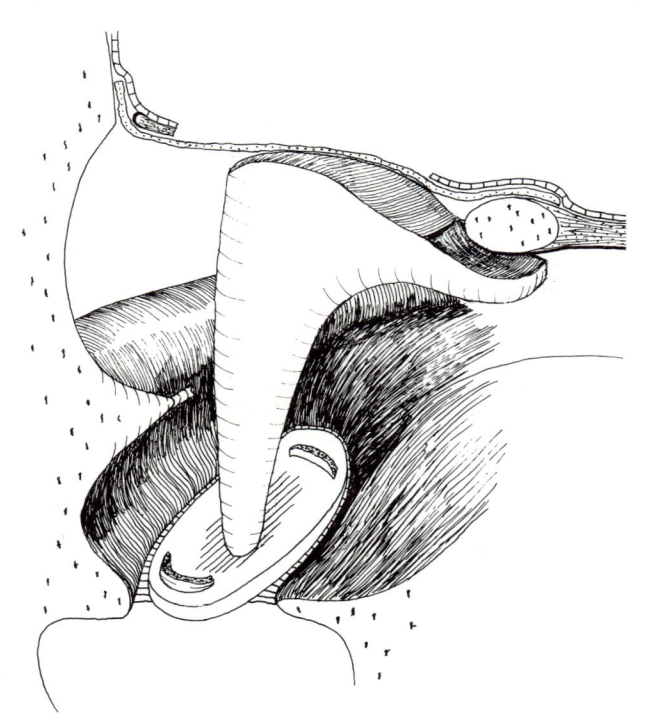

Fig. **998** An allogenous incus columella, with the long process placed on the footplate. The lenticular process is drilled off. The short process is shaped and placed under the malleus handle

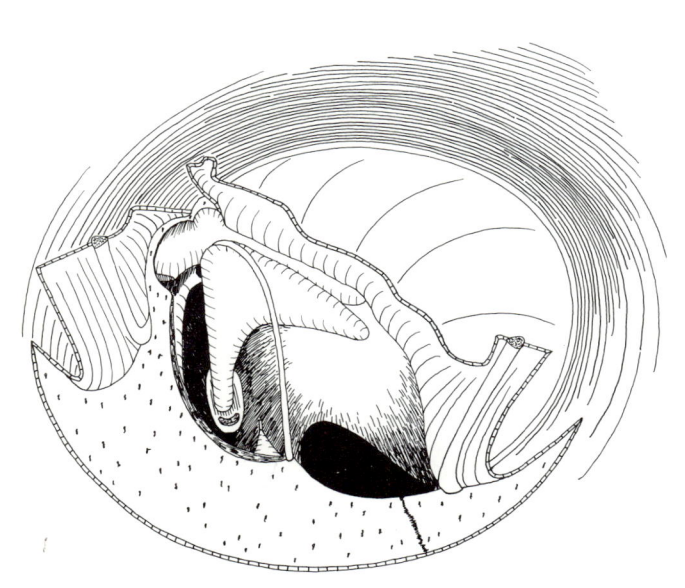

Fig. **999** An allogenous incus columella, with the long process placed on the footplate and the body and short process parallel to the malleus handle

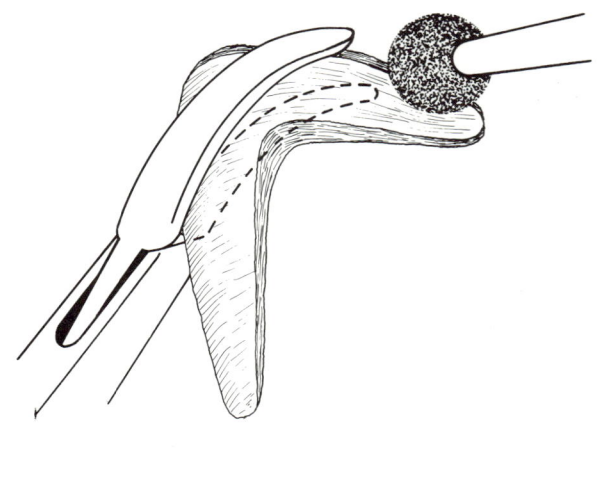

Fig. **1000** Shaping a thin cortical-bone L-prosthesis. The cortical bone is gently fixed with a surgical clamp at the junction between the horizontal and vertical parts of the prosthesis

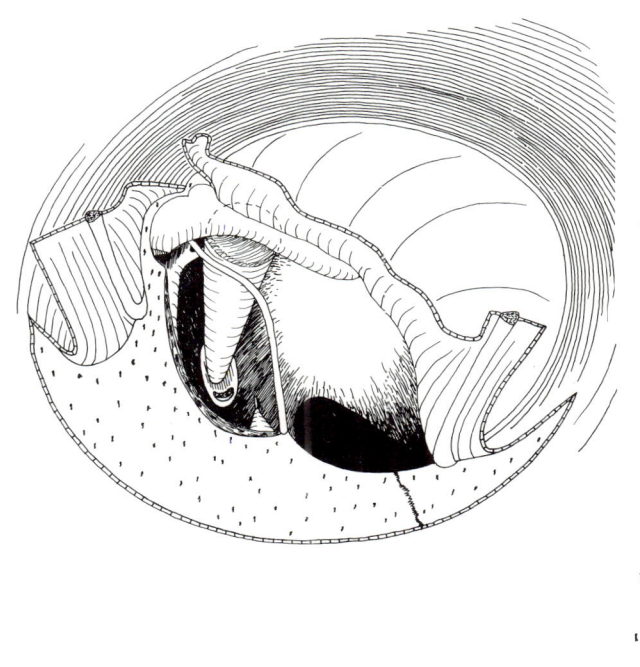

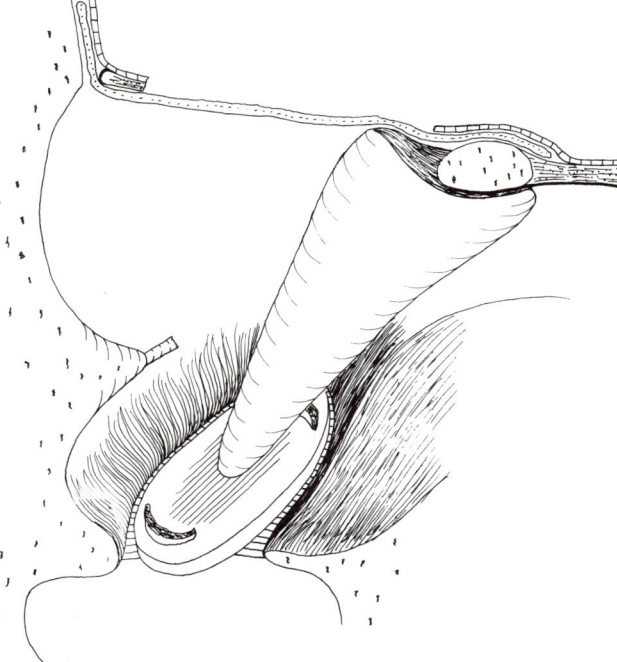

Fig. **1001** A stick-like columella of cortical bone placed between the malleus handle and the footplate

Fig. **1002** Side view of the stick-like columella, with a groove for the malleus handle

general, the shaping and placing of a cortical-bone columella are similar to those described and illustrated for autogenous or allogenous incus columella.

Autogenous and Allogenous Malleus Columella

The malleus head, with its neck, can easily be shaped into a mushroom-like columella (Fig. **1003**), and this type of columella is particularly suitable in canal wall–down mastoidectomy when the malleus head and neck have been removed. A columella made of the malleus handle has also been used. In a canal wall–down mastoidectomy situation in which only the malleus handle is present and the tendon of the tensor tympani muscle has been transected, using an allogenous malleus handle as the columella elevates the autogenous malleus handle (Fig. **1004**).

With a severely lateralized drum, the entire allogenous malleus is placed between the footplate and the drum (Fig. **1005**). This is in fact the largest distance that can be bridged by a single ossicle.

A columella between the eardrum and the footplate can be established by transposing the auto-

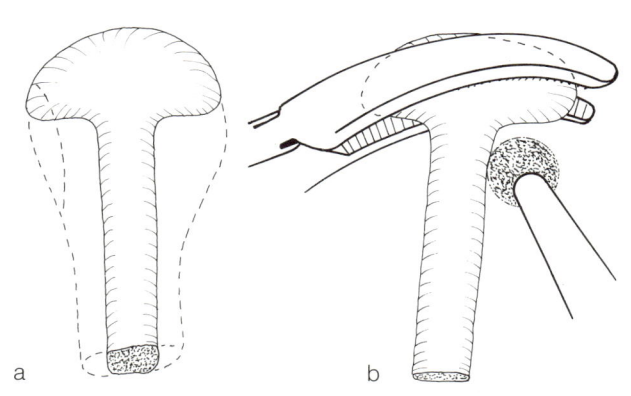

Fig. **1003** Shaping a mushroom-like columella from the head and the neck of the malleus

genous malleus handle (Fig. **1006**). The malleus handle is loosened from the drum, except at the umbo region, and its neck is placed on the footplate. The malleus handle has a tendency to be pulled back to its origin position, and may be displaced from the footplate. This method should therefore be restricted to a very few selected cases.

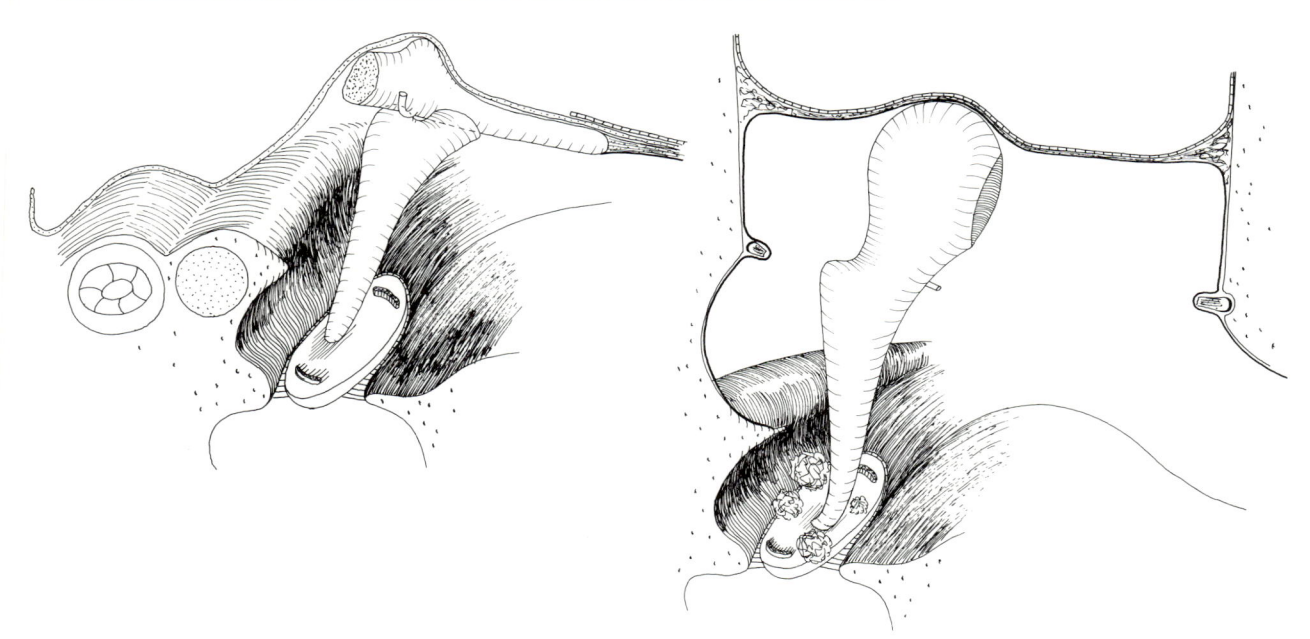

Fig. **1004** A Malleus-to-malleus columella in a situation with a canal wall–down mastoidectomy and a mobile autogenous malleus handle, which can be elevated with a columella of allogenous malleus handle

Fig. **1005** The entire allogenous malleus is placed between the footplate and a severely lateralized ear drum

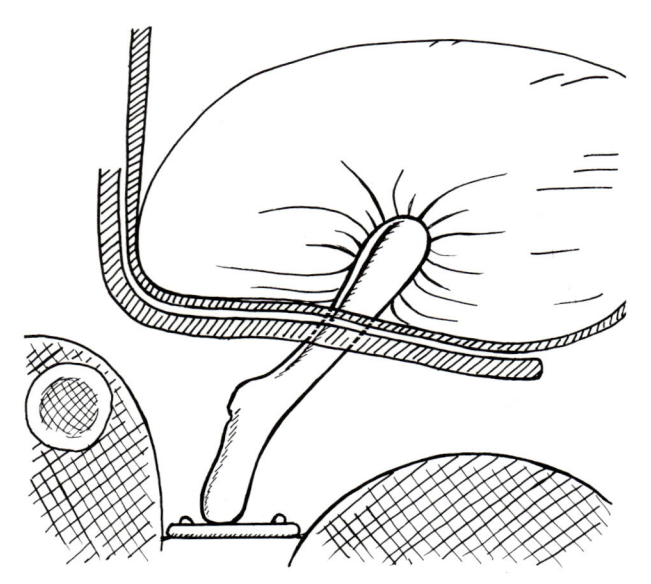

Fig. **1006** Transposition of the autogenous malleus handle onto the footplate. The malleus handle is freed from the drum as far as the umbo region

Allogenous Stapes Columella

An allogenous stapes columella was first used in stapes surgery as early as 1960 (Glaninger and Neuhold 1968). Glaninger used an allograft replacement after stapedectomy for otosclerosis. Two patients had previously undergone radical surgery, and also fixation of the footplate. Tobeck (1962) used frozen allograft stapes in otosclerosis. Hyldyard et al. (1968) used autoclaved stapes.

In surgery for chronic otitis, Marquet (1971) applied an allograft stapes with the capitulum placed on the patient's footplate as a simple columella (Fig. **1007**). Fascia can be placed on the allograft footplate, but Marquet placed an allograft drum on it.

From 1975, to 1977, the present author systematically used a stapes–incus assembly (Tos 1978 a) as follows. The allograft stapes is placed with its capitulum on the patient's footplate, and surrounded by Gelfoam balls. On top of the allograft stapes footplate, an allograft incus is placed, with its long process pointing forward and downward, and with fascia placed on top. The short process of the allograft incus points downward and backward. This method is used in association with reconstruction of the ear canal and obliteration during total reconstruction of old radical cavities (Fig. **1008**), or in canal wall–down mastoidectomy with fascia placed on the facial nerve prominence and the

Variations in Columella Placement 359

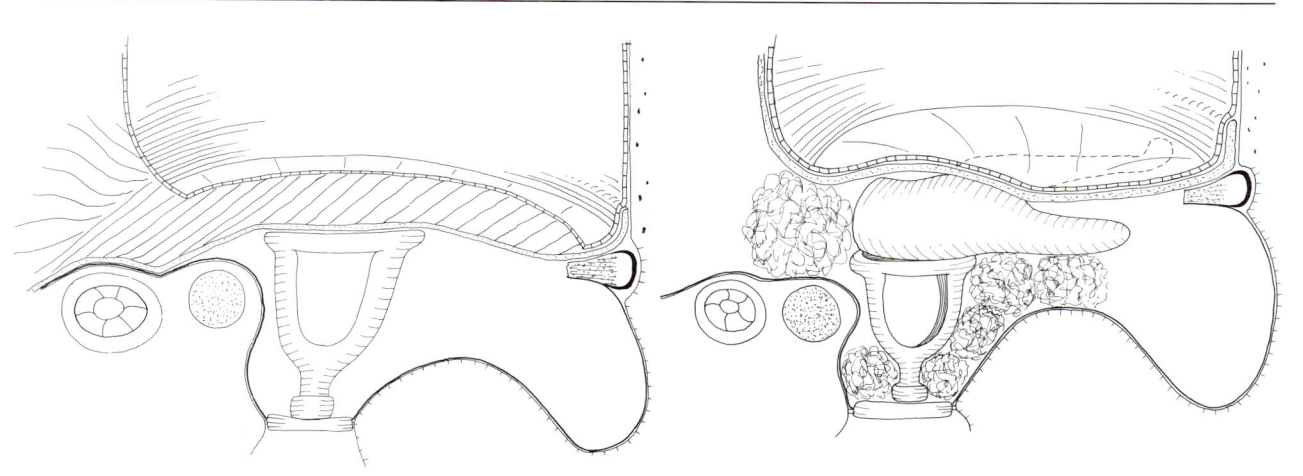

Fig. **1007** An allogenous stapes placed with its capitulum on the footplate in a canal wall–down mastoidectomy. The fascia covers the facial nerve prominence

Fig. **1008** An allogenous stapes–incus assembly. The incus is placed on the allogenous stapes footplate, and the ear canal is reconstructed with a large underlay fascia graft

lateral semicircular canal (Fig. **1009**). Compared with the incus columella, the allograft stapes provided somewhat better results.

In ears with an intact bony canal wall and malleus handle, an autogenous incus is placed between the allogenous footplate and the malleus handle (Fig. **1010**). Instead of the incus, a 5×4 mm piece of tragal cartilage with attached perichondrium is placed between the allogenous footplate and the malleus handle (Fig. **1011**). Placing an autogenous tragal cartilage is an improvement on the stapes columella techniques, especially in the canal wall–

down situation (Fig. **1012**). A larger piece of tragal cartilage (6×6 mm) with perichondrium is placed on the allogenous footplate, providing a large area of contact with the drum and preventing retraction of the drum. The allogenous footplate is hidden beneath, and supported by, the tragal cartilage, which may be in contact with the facial nerve prominence without affecting the hearing.

The author occasionally uses allograft stapes in a special technique, as follows (Tos 1978b). The footplate of the allogenous stapes is reduced in size and placed on the host footplate. This footplate-

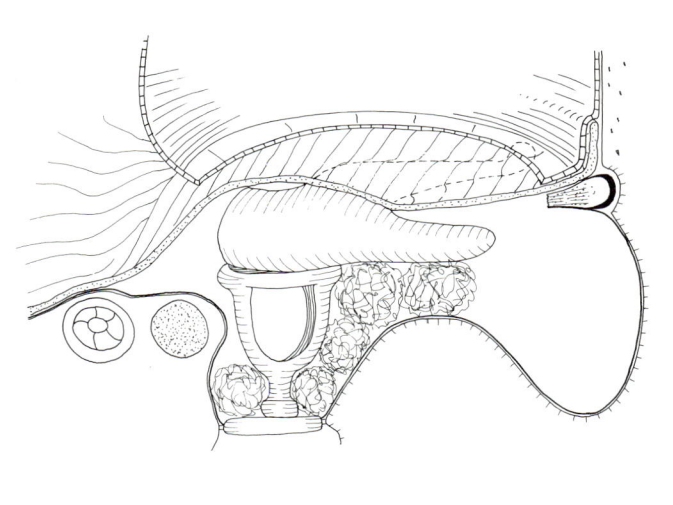

Fig. **1009** A stapes–incus assembly in a canal wall–down mastoidectomy. The fascia covers the total perforation, the incus, and the attic region. The allogenous stapes is stabilized with Gelfoam balls

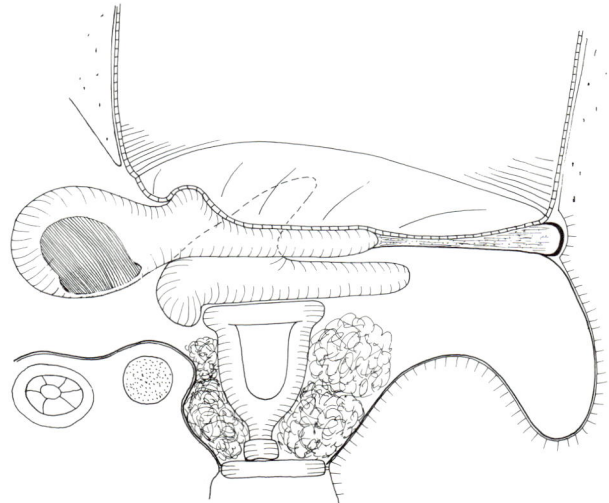

Fig. **1010** An allogenous stapes–incus assembly when the malleus is present. A shaped incus is placed between the allogenous stapes footplate and the malleus handle

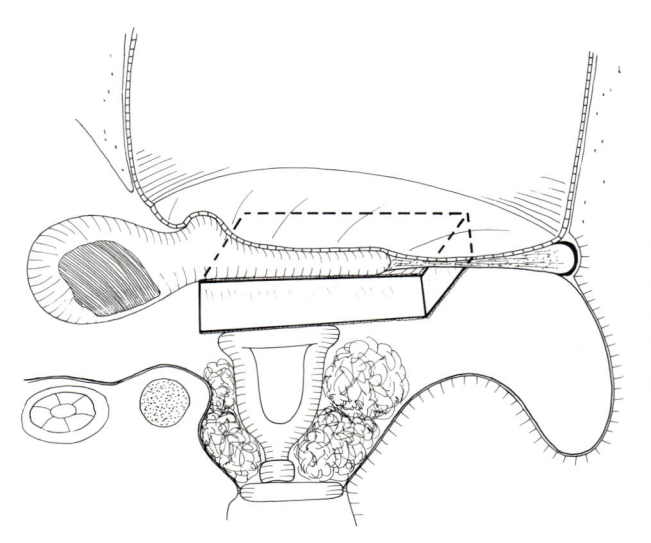

Fig. **1011** An allogenous stapes–cartilage assembly. A piece of cartilage with perichondrium is placed between the allogenous stapes footplate and the malleus handle

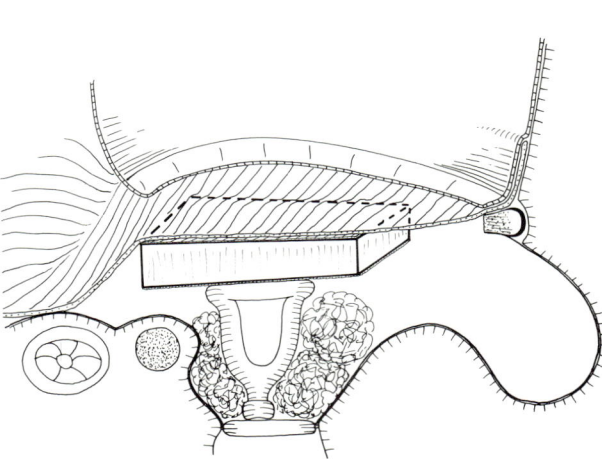

Fig. **1012** An allogenous stapes–cartilage assembly in a situation with a missing malleus handle and canal wall–down mastoidectomy. A cartilage plate is placed on the allogenous stapes footplate, and the total perforation and attic region are covered with a fascia graft

to-footplate method is intriguing, and converts a type 3 tympanoplasty into a type 2 tympanoplasty. The allogenous stapes footplate has to be reduced in size, and this is carried out by holding the stapes with two fingers, without gloves, and drilling the edges of it with a small diamond drill. The drilling should be very careful, so as not to fracture the crura or the footplate (Figs. **1013, 1014**). A right allograft stapes is used for the right ear, ad a left one for the left ear, and a bank of reduced right and left stapes bones can be established for the purpose. A diminished allogenous stapes is placed with its footplate on the host footplate and fixed by Gelfoam balls, or with a fibrin glue. After the stapes has been placed solidly on the footplate, a reduced and shaped incus can be placed between the stapes and the malleus handle (Fig. **1015**).

In ears without ossicles, e.g., during reconstruction of old radical cavities, an allogenous incus with a hole for the head of the stapes can be placed on the allogenous stapes (Fig. **1016**).

Placing tragal cartilage on the transplanted stapes has been shown to have several advantages in footplate-to-footplate techniques: the cartilage is not heavy, it does not tilt the stapes, and it can be placed on the facial nerve prominence without becoming fixed. The tragal cartilage can be placed between the malleus handle and the head of the allogenous stapes. A hole is drilled in the tragal cartilage with a small diamond drill, to serve as the acetabulum for the head of the stapes (Fig. **1017**).

In canal wall–down mastoidectomy and footplate-to-footplate stapes transplantation, e.g., in partial reconstructions of old radical cavities, using tragal cartilage has been shown to be a good method. A larger piece of cartilage is used, a small hole is drilled in the middle of the cartilage, and the cartilage is placed on the homogenous stapes. It can be fixed to the facial prominence by Gelfoam. A piece of fascia is used to cover the cartilage, tympanic cavity, and the attic (Fig. **1018**).

Allogenous stapes can be used together with another small columella made of ossicles or cortical bone (Fig. **1019**). A hole is drilled through the allogenous footplate, and a thin piece of bone is inserted through the hole. This composite columella is connected with the malleus handle. Moon (1976) used this type of columella after stapedectomy for tympanosclerosis.

Variations in Columella Placement

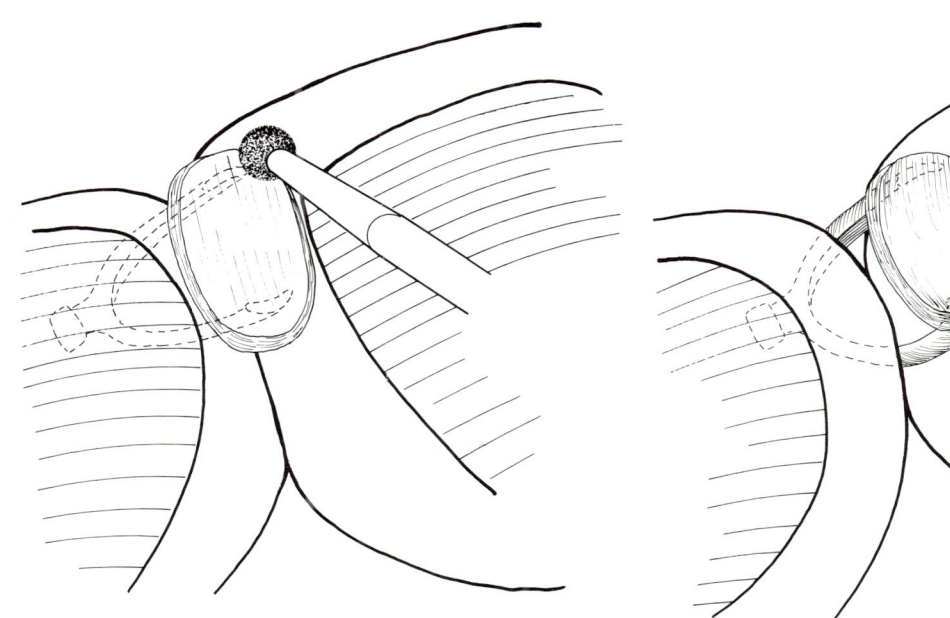

Fig. **1013** Reducing the size of an allogenous stapes footplate for footplate-to-footplate implantation. The crura of the stapes are held with two fingers, without gloves

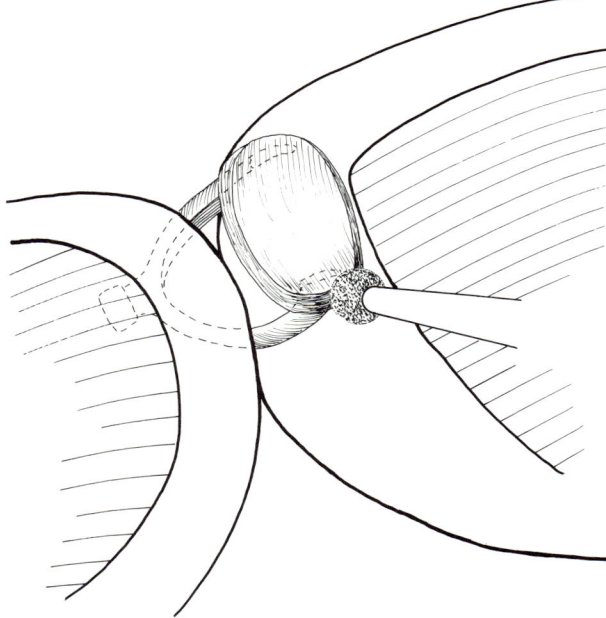

Fig. **1014** The edges of the allogenous footplate are drilled off, to be placed on the patient's footplate

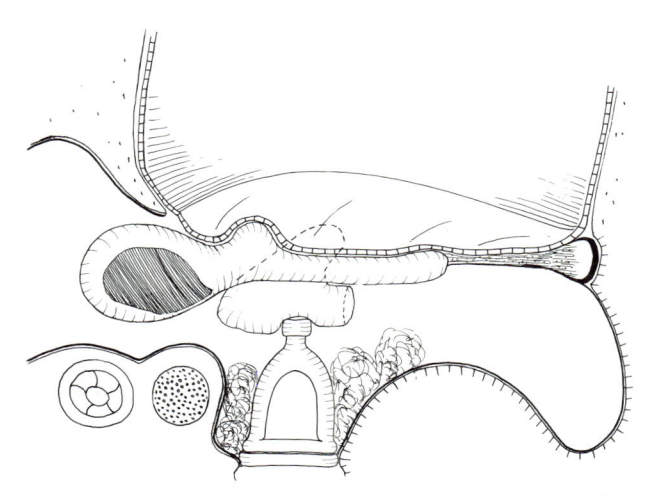

Fig. **1015** Footplate-to-footplate placement of an allogenous stapes. A shaped incus is interposed between the head of the allogenous stapes and the malleus handle. The stapes is fixed by Gelfoam balls

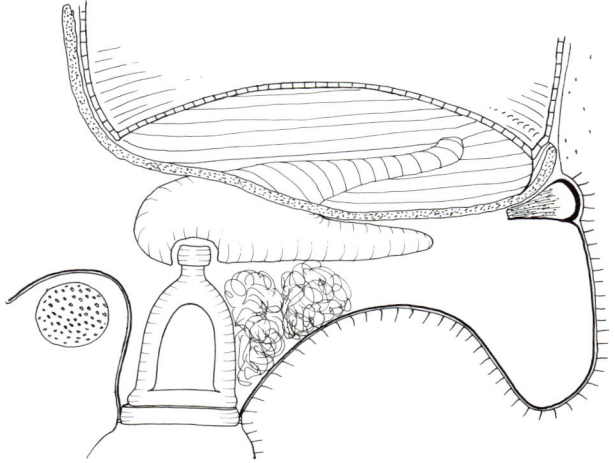

Fig. **1016** Footplate-to-footplate implantation of an allogenous stapes. An allogenous incus is placed on the head of the stapes. The total perforation is covered with a large fascia graft, also reconstructing the ear canal

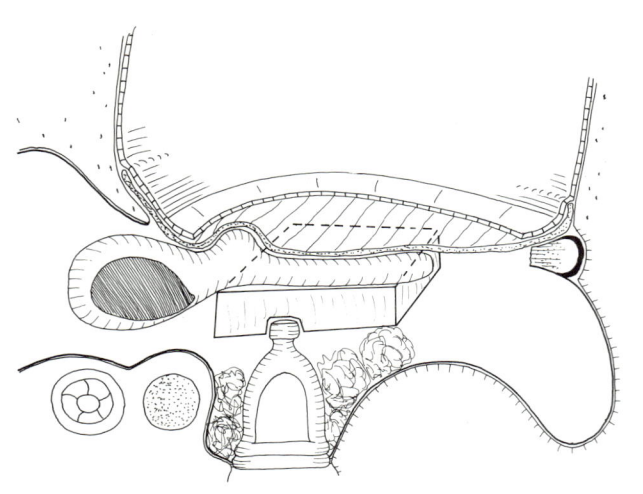

Fig. **1017** Footplate-to-footplate implantation of an allogenous stapes. A piece of tragal cartilage is interposed between the head of the allogenous stapes and the malleus handle

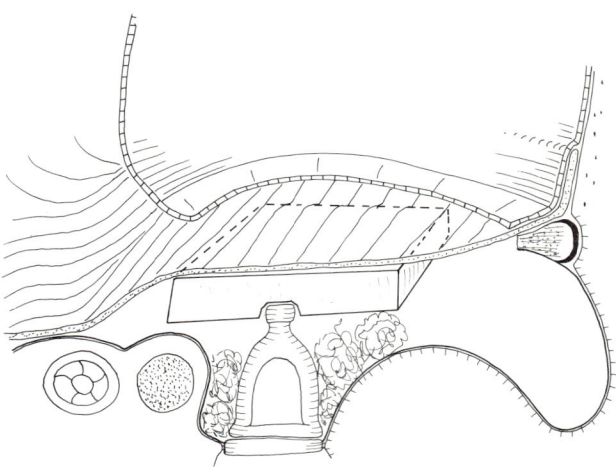

Fig. **1018** Footplate-to-footplate implantation of an allogenous stapes in a situation without a malleus and with canal wall–down mastoidectomy. A relatively large piece of tragal cartilage with a hole is placed on the head of the allogenous stapes. The perforation, tragal cartilage, and attic region are covered with fascia

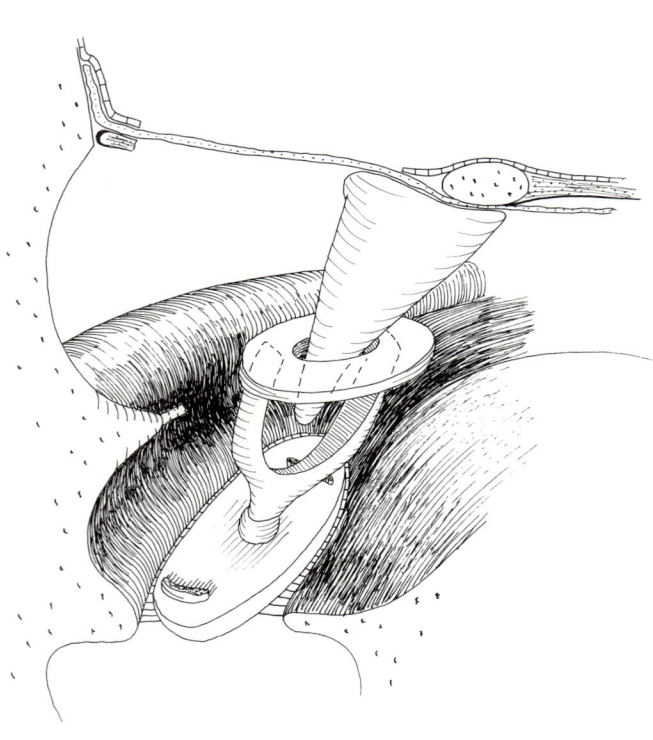

Fig. **1019** An allogenous stapes is placed with its head on the footplate. A small columella connecting the malleus handle is placed into the hole on the allogenous stapes footplate

Cartilage Columella

Cartilage columellae have been used since the beginning of the tympanoplasty area. Jansen (1963) was the first to use a cartilage columella made of allogenous septal cartilage. He used a T-shaped columella placed on the footplate, with the horizontal part in contact with the bony annulus posteriorly, and with the malleus handle anteriorly (Fig. **1020**). Jansen sometimes placed stainless-steel wires through the shaft and horizontal part of columella, but most often the septal columella was used without wires.

For ossiculoplasty, autogenous tragal and conchal cartilage, autogenous and allogenous septal cartilage, autogenous and allogenous costal cartilage, as well as cartilage from the meniscus, has been used in a way similar to that described above with type 2 tympanoplasty (pp. 277–284).

Tragal and Conchal Cartilage Columella

Pfaltz used tragal and conchal cartilage in 1962, mainly as a columella after stapedectomy for otosclerosis, but also occasionally in surgery for chronic otitis media (Pfaltz and Piffko 1968). Goodhill (1967) used conventional columellae prepared from autogenous tragal cartilage, shaped with a knife to match the footplate region and placed in contact with the fascia, tragal perichondrium, or malleus handle. These cartilage struts were unstable and soft (Fig. **1021**). Goodhill more often used a car-

Variations in Columella Placement

Fig. 1020 **Jansen's T-shaped allogenous cartilage prosthesis.** The horizontal part is placed under the bony annulus and under the malleus handle

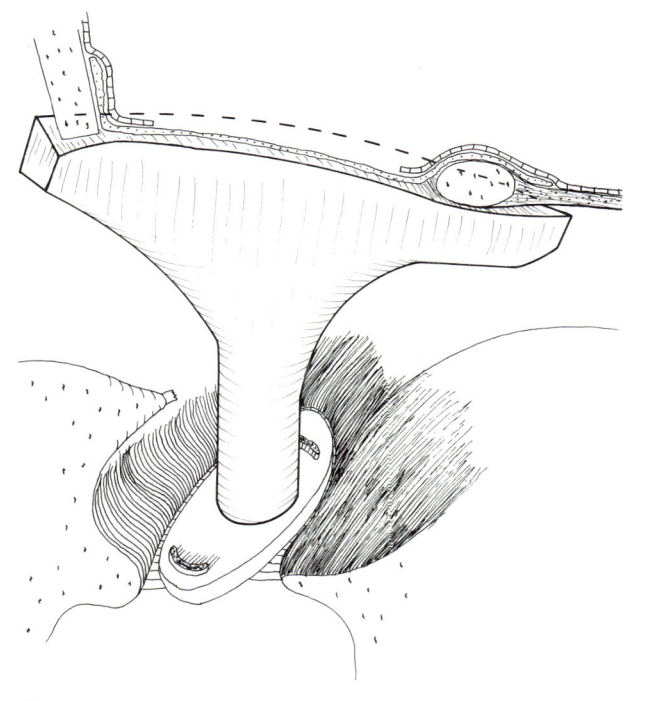

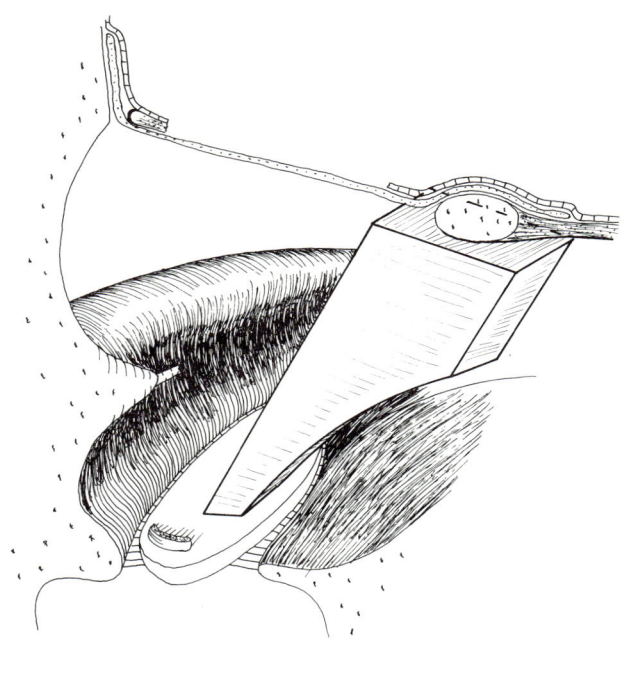

Fig. 1021 **Goodhill's tragal cartilage strut** placed as a columella between the footplate and the malleus handle

tilage–perichondrium composite T-columella (Fig. **1022**), prepared as follows. A large piece of tragal cartilage with attached perichondrium on both sides is harvested as described above (Fig. **265**). The perichondrium is partly elevated from the anterior and posterior side of the cartilage, except at its lateral edge (Fig. **1023**). Using a scalpel, a T-shaped cartilage prosthesis is cut out. The perichondrium is still firmly attached to the horizontal part of the columella (Fig. **1023**). The Goodhill cartilage–perichondrium T-columella is then trimmed and placed on the footplate. The direction of the horizontal part of the platform depends on the situation. If there is an anteriorly-positioned malleus handle with a long distance to the footplate, the columella can be placed under the malleus handle, the horizontal part being directed anteroposteriorly, and the perichondrium covers the superior and inferior areas of the tympanic cavity (Fig. **1024**). If the columella is turned 90°, the horizontal part is then directed superoinferiorly, and the perichondrium is in contact with the posterior and anterior annulus, respectively. The horizontal part is positioned parallel to the malleus handle in this situation (Fig. **1025**). A fascia graft covers the perichondrium so as to close the perforation.

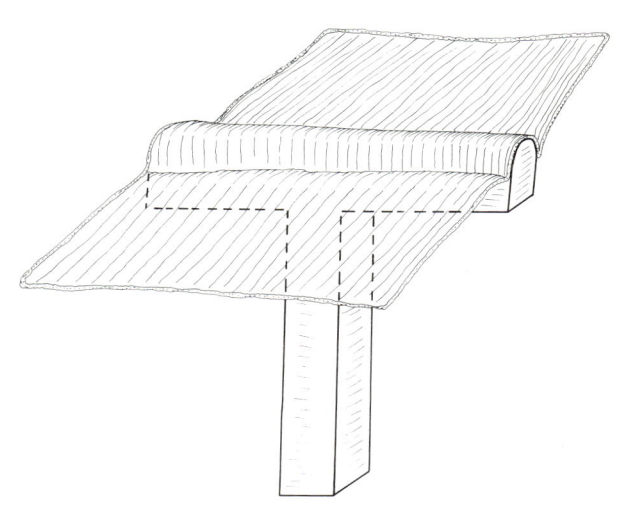

Fig. **1022 Goodhill's tragal cartilage–perichondrium compound T-columella,** with the perichondrium attached to the horizontal part of the columella

21 Type 3 Tympanoplasty with the Stapes Absent

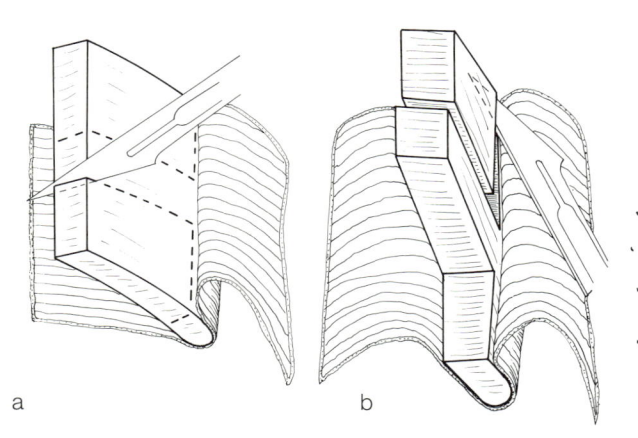

Fig. 1023 Preparing a tragal cartilage–perichondrium T-columella. **a** The perichondrium is partly elevated. **d** The cartilage is cut off with a scalpel

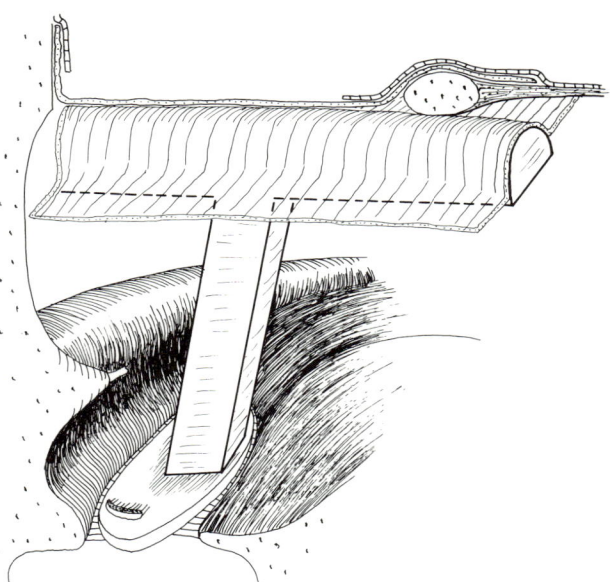

Fig. 1024 The Goodhill cartilage–perichondrium T-columella is placed on the footplate, with its horizontal part directed postero-anteriorly. The perichondrium is placed under the drum remnant, and the perforation is covered by a fascia graft

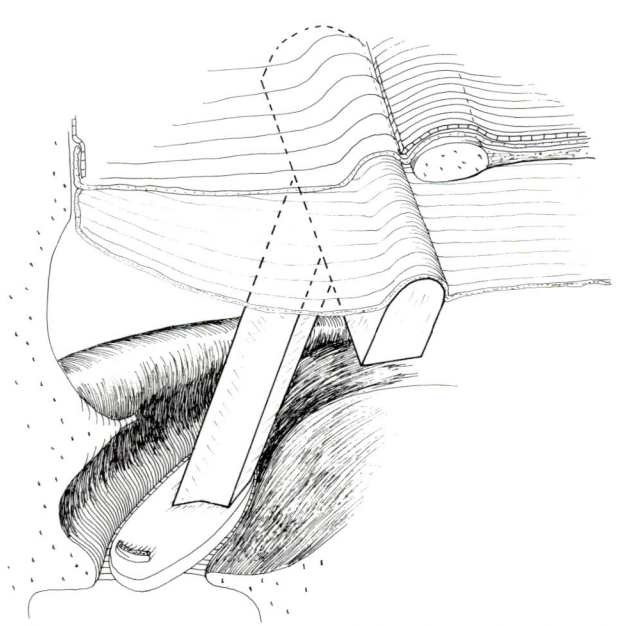

Fig. 1025 The cartilage–perichondrium T-columella placed on the footplate, with the horizontal part placed parallel to the malleus handle. The perichondrium is attached to the posterior bony annulus

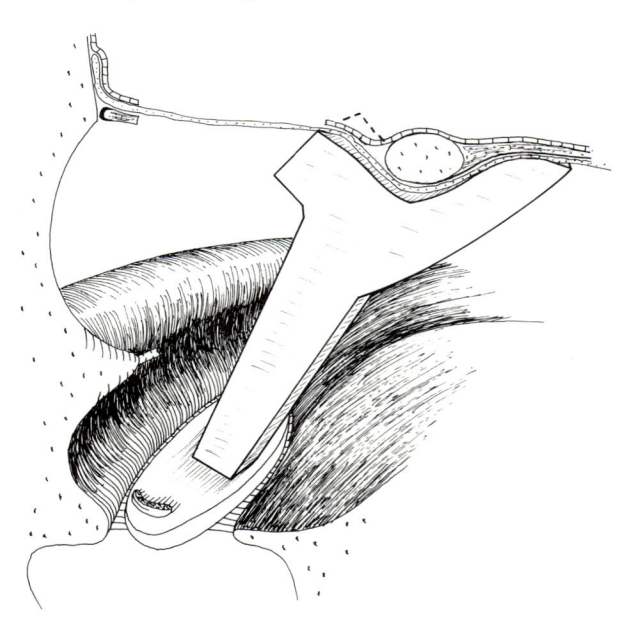

Fig. 1026 **Glasscock's tragal cartilage strut columella.** A groove is made for the malleus handle

Shea and Glasscock (1967), using tragal cartilage struts as columellae, placed them either under the malleus handle (Fig. **1026**) or under the drum. The struts had small platforms. Recognizing the problem of strut displacement occuring before the strut is securely attached, Shea and Glassock recommend complete filling of the middle ear with absorbable gelatine sponge after the strut is positioned. To avoid fixation of the perichondrium to the facial nerve prominence, the perichondrium should be removed from the columella before use.

Smyth's Septal Cartilage Columellae

Smyth constructed the boomerang strut, made of homogenous septal cartilage acquired through nasal septum surgery (Fig. **1027**) (Smyth et al. 1971). The cartilage was stored in 70% alcohol at 5° Celsius and washed in normal saline for one hour before use. Recognizing that even a septal cartilage strut is sometimes too soft, Smyth systematically inserted a stainless-steel wire into the cartilage columella in a way suggested by Jansen. Two pieces of stainless-steel stapedectomy wire are inserted, at an 80° angle to each other, into a 6×6–mm piece of septal cartilage (Fig. **1027**). The strut is then cut with a No. 11 scalpel in such a way that the stainless-steel wires are covered with thin layer of cartilage. To avoid later extrusion of the shaft wire, it should be inserted from the footplate end, stopping 1 mm short of the horizontal part of the prosthesis (Fig. **1027**). In this way, contact between the wire and the drum is avoided. Jansen's T-struts and Smyth's L-struts are strengthened with wires in the same way (Fig. **1028**).

A boomerang strut, similar to that used by Jansen (1963) was often placed by Smyth and Kerr (1967) on top of the malleus handle (Fig. **1029**). The horizontal part of the T-prosthesis points in an antero-inferior direction, while posteriorly, the horizontal part touches the bony annulus (Fig. **1030**).

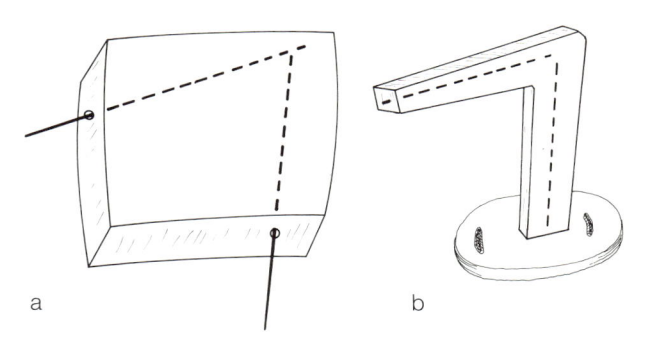

Fig. **1027** **Smyth's boomerang septal cartilage strut,** strengthened with steel wires placed at 80° to each other

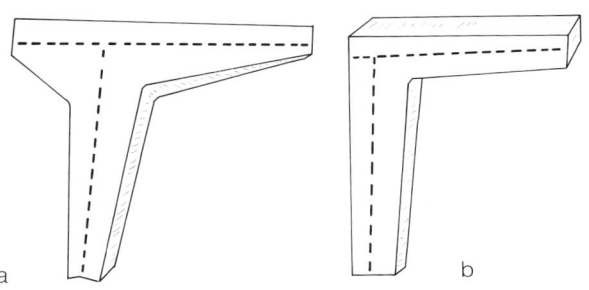

Fig. **1028a** **The Jansen T-cartilage columella,** and **b** the **Smyth L-columella,** both strengthened with wires

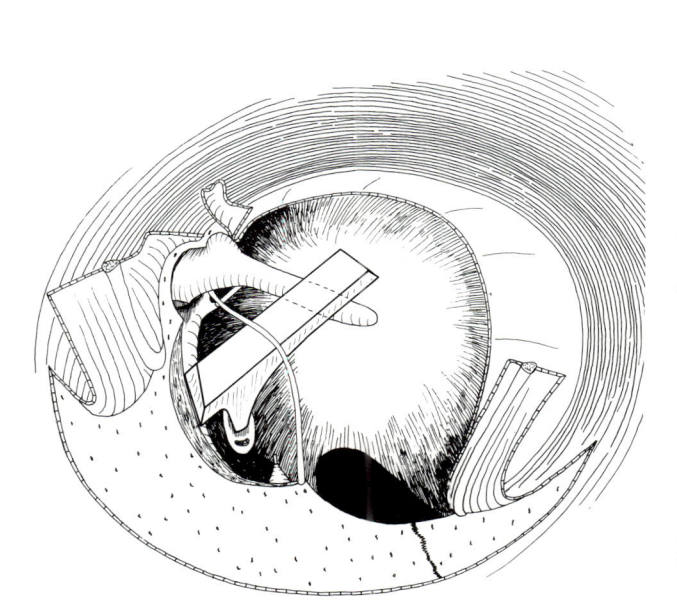

Fig. **1029** The T-shaped cartilage columella placed on the malleus handle in a case of total perforation

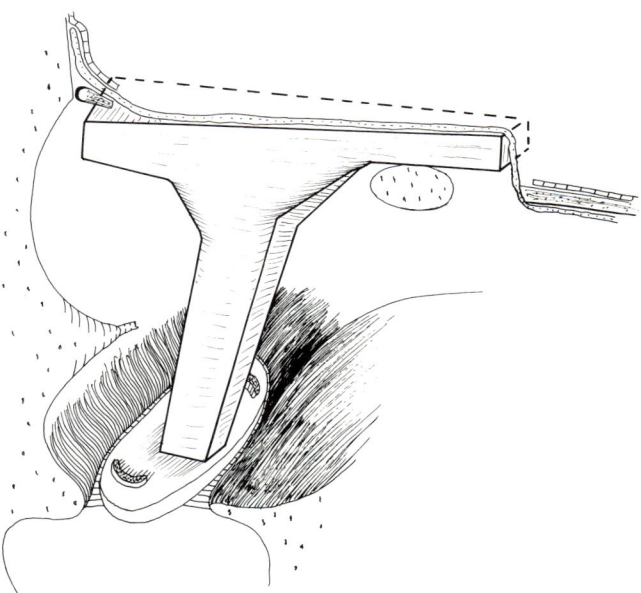

Fig. **1030** Side view of the T-columella placed on the malleus handle

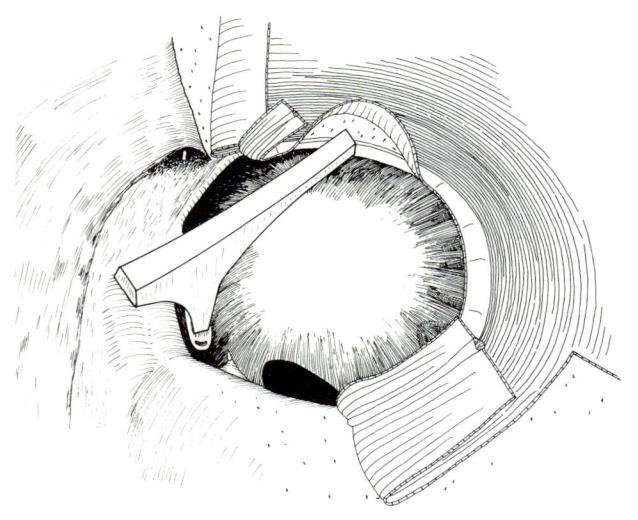

Fig. 1031 A long T-prosthesis columella, with its horizontal part placed on the anterior annulus in a situation with a canal wall–down mastoidectomy and a missing malleus

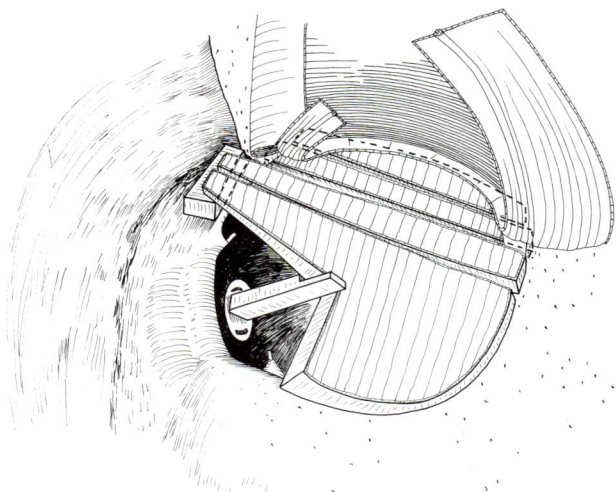

Fig. 1032 **The Heermann L-shaped cartilage annulus–tensor tympani plate,** in a case with canal wall–down mastoidectomy and a missing malleus. The two anterior cartilage palisades are placed underneath the inferior bony annulus and on top of a piece of cartilage placed on the tensor tympani muscle prominence. The large L-shaped columella is placed on the inferior bony annulus. The columella is connected with the footplate by a cartilage strut

In patients with a missing malleus handle, usually in situations after canal wall–down mastoidectomy, the horizontal part of the T-shaped prosthesis lies anteriorly on the bony or fibrous annulus (Fig. 1031).

In palisade myringoplasty with tragal and conchal cartilage, Heermann (1991) applies a large L-shaped plate of cartilage placed inferiorly onto the inferior part of the bony annulus in ears with missing stapedial arch and malleus, in canal wall–down mastoidectomy situations. Superiorly, the plate is placed on a small piece of cartilage—an architrave—positioned on the tensor tympani muscle. This L-shaped annulus–tensor tympani plate is connected with the footplate using an L-shaped cartilage strut (Fig. 1032). The columella lies securely between the footplate and the cartilage plate.

Don and Linthicum (1975) proved histologically that implanted autogenous tragal and allogenous septal cartilage remains viable and is covered by mucosa. In addition, the integrity of the prosthesis is assured in the short term (6–18 months). Over the long term (1–19 years), the histological fate of cartilage prostheses is unpredictable, however. Steinbach and Pusalkar (1981) and Stein-

bach et al. (1992) found that L-shaped cartilage columellae broke at the angle between the vertical and horizontal limbs. They found fibrous degeneration and disappearance of the cartilage in many prostheses removed after surgery. They recommend that the perichondrium should be intact and included in the columella for purposes of nutrition on at least one side. Compared to implanted ossicles, the vascularity of the cartilage is much poorer, and the sound conduction decreases gradually with time.

Allogenous Costal Cartilage

Allogenous costal cartilage has better sound transmission properties than columellas produced from tragal or septal cartilage (Cole 1992, Zini 1992). The original thickness of the shaft in Cole's allogenous cartilage columella (Figs. 798–803) is 2 mm, and the footplate end of the shaft is therefore trimmed to match the size of the footplate (Fig. 1033). The head of the prosthesis has a diameter of 4 mm, and it can be placed under the drum if the malleus handle is missing, or under the malleus handle.

The Zini allogenous costal columella resembles the Jansen T-columella. The horizontal

Variations in Columella Placement

Fig. **1033 The Cole allogenous costal cartilage columella,** placed between the footplate and the drum

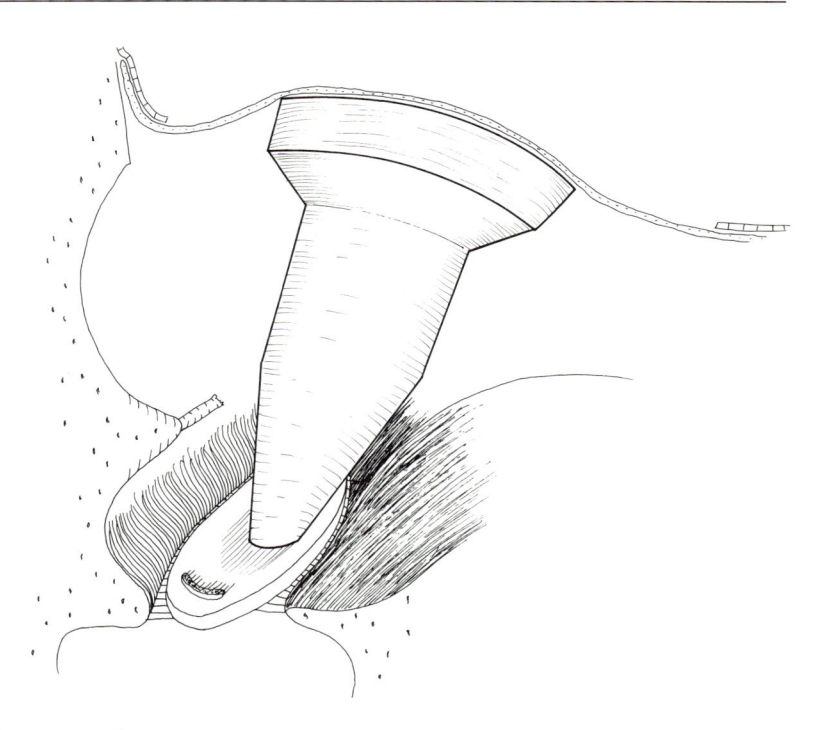

part is placed posteriorly under the bony annulus, and under the malleus handle anteriorly (Fig. **1034**). The sound transmission is excellent in this type of columella (Zini 1992), but long-term results are so far lacking.

Allogenous Dentin Columellae

Columellae have been created from teeth (Zini 1970, Gibb and Steward 1972), but have never become widely used, perhaps because they tend to decay. Various columella shapes can easily be produced, such as T-shaped, L-shaped, and 7-shaped columellae (Fig. **1035**).

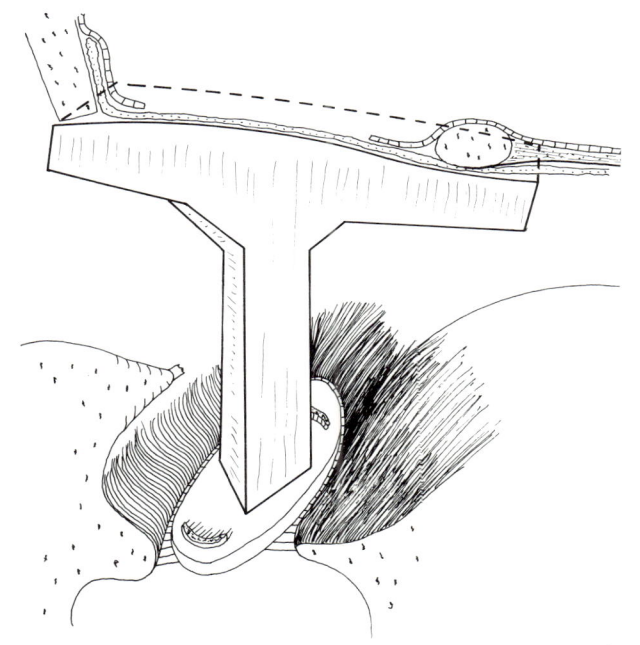

Fig. **1034 The Zini costal cartilage columella** is placed on the footplate, and its horizontal part is connected to the posterior bony annulus and the malleus handle

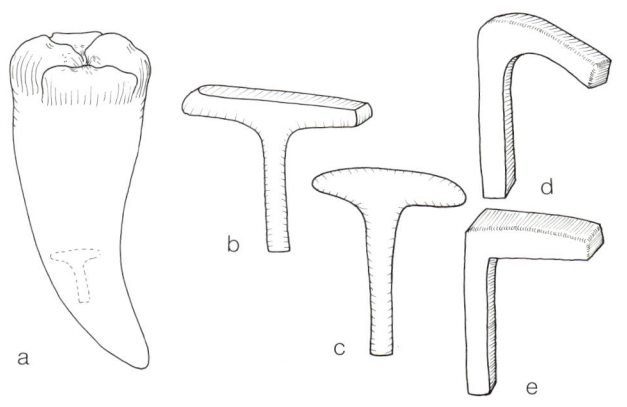

Fig. **1035** Various small columellae, shaped from a tooth (**a**). **b** The T-columella, **c** the mushroom-like columella, **d** the 7-shaped columella, and **e** the L-shaped columella

Columellae with Biocompatible Materials

Columellae made of synthetic biomaterials have been, and still are, widely used in middle-ear surgery. The characteristics of the materials and the fates of the prostheses are described above (pp. 285–298).

Polyethylene or compact *Teflon* columellae were tubes with a relatively small platform of shapes similar to those described above in type 2 tympanoplasty prostheses. The tubes had a sunflower-shaped or mushroom-shaped platform, and a groove for the malleus handle (Figs. **805**, **806**). Some columellae with a solid, thin Teflon shaft have also been used (Fig. **1036**). A Teflon footplate–malleus columella, to be fixed to the undersurface of the neck of the malleus (Tabor 1971), or a long Shea polyethylene stapes strut adapted with a large groove for the malleus handle, have been used as columellae (Fig. **1036**). Like the polyethylene and Teflon prostheses in type 2 tympanoplasty, columellae made of these materials have also been abandoned, due to the very high extrusion rates. Shafts of the polyethylene and Teflon columellae have been used for many years, and are still used, as composite graft prostheses together with the incus, cortical bone, or cartilage. Polyethylene or Teflon prostheses do not face the drum.

Porous plastic columellae. This group mainly consists of Proplast, Plasti-Pore, and Fluoroplastic. The first Shea Proplast columella consists of a 0.5 mm Teflon shaft, with a small disk of Proplast on the footplate and a larger Proplast disk facing the undersurface of the drum (Fig. **1037**). A Shea columella entirely made of Plasti-Pore (Smith and Nephew, Richards Company) has a thin platform. Shea (1976) never covers the platform with cartilage but many other surgeons do. The Tilt-Top TORP prosthesis (Smith and Nephew, Richards Company) allows the head of the prosthesis to be tilted. The head and distal part of the shaft are made of Plasti-Pore, and the proximal part of the shaft is made of polyethylene (Fig. **1037 c**).

To cover the Shea Plasti-Pore TORP prosthesis, Saraceno et al. (1978) created a tragal cartilage–perichondrium graft, fixed to the head of the prosthesis as follows. A 7×7–mm piece of tragal cartilage, with the perichondrium attached to the posterior and anterior sides, is excised (Fig. **1038**). The posterior perichondrium layer is slipped from the cartilage. A small incision is made in the center of the anterior perichondrium layer. After partial elevation of the anterior perichondrium layer, the shaft of the prosthesis is pushed through the hole in the perichondrium, allowing the head of the prosthesis to be placed between the cartilage and the perichondrium. The composite graft is placed on the footplate, with the cartilage underneath the drum and the posterior perichondrium layer on top of the posterior bony annulus, fixing and stabilizing the prosthesis (Fig. **1039**).

Jackson and Glasscock (1983) suture the cartilage plate onto the TORP and PORP (Figs. **815, 816**). Sheehy (1990) covers the head of the Plasti-Pore prosthesis with a cartilage slice (Figs. **811–813**).

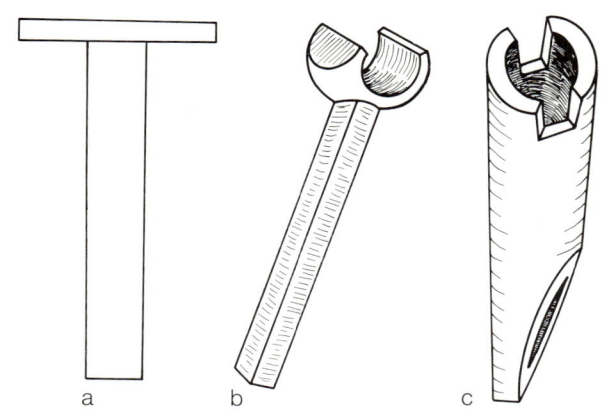

Fig. **1036** Teflon columellae. **a** the Guilford Teflon columella, with a solid shaft. **b** The Tabor Teflon footplate–malleus columella. **c** The Shea polyethylene stapes strut

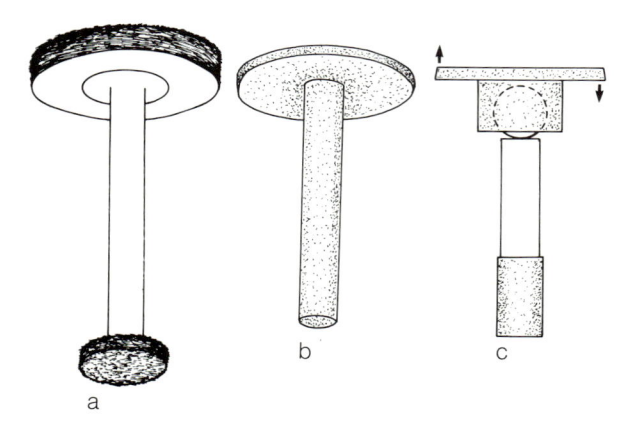

Fig. **1037a** The first Shea Proplast columella. **b** The Shea Plasti-Pore columella. **c** The tilt-top TORP prosthesis, made of Plasti-Pore and polyethylene

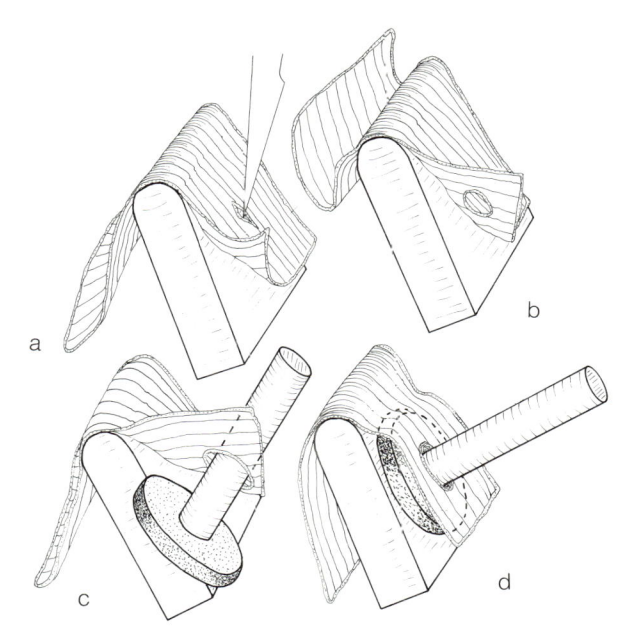

Fig. 1038 **Saraceno's technique** for fixing the tragal cartilage to the Plasti-Pore TORP columella. **a** The posterior perichondrium layer is elevated from the cartilage, and a small incision is made in the anterior layer. **b** The anterior perichondrium layer is partly elevated. **c** The shaft of the columella is pushed through the hole. **d** The platform of the prosthesis is in place between the tragal cartilage and the perichondrium

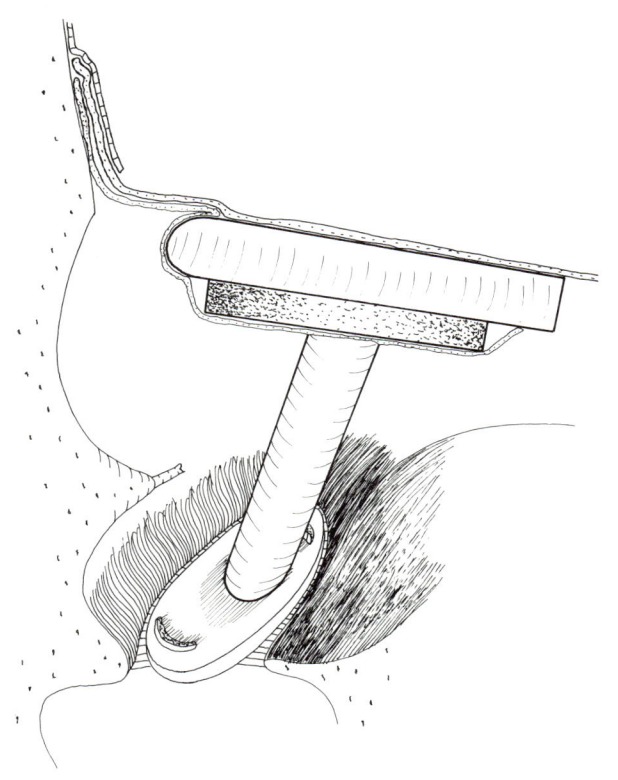

Fig. 1039 The Plasti-Pore columella, with the tragal cartilage–perichondrium covering, is placed between the footplate and the drum. The posterior perichondrium layer is placed on the posterior bony annulus, stabilizing the columella

In addition to the Sheehy TORP prosthesis, several other Plasti-Pore prostheses are used, such as the Austin off-centered TORP, the Fisch TORP, which also is off-centered, and the Causse TORP, with a large platform (Fig. **1040**).

Malleable Polycel columellae. Very interesting are malleable TORPs made of Polycel, containing a stainless-steel wire. The shaft is thin, and can easily be bent in various planes and at various levels (Fig. **1041**). The Hubbard footplate–malleus Polycel strut (Treace company, Memphis, USA) has a groove for the malleus handle. The shaft can be bent in all directions, and the TORP prosthesis can be trimmed to any length (Fig. **1042**). The head of the TORP can be tilted, so that the groove can fit the malleus handle exactly. Bending of Polycel shafts is done using two alligator forceps that hold the shaft in different positions (Fig. **1043**).

Several other polycel TORPs are used, e.g., the Brackmann modified TORP (Fig. **1041 d**). Brackmann recommends covering the platform of the prothese with cartilage.

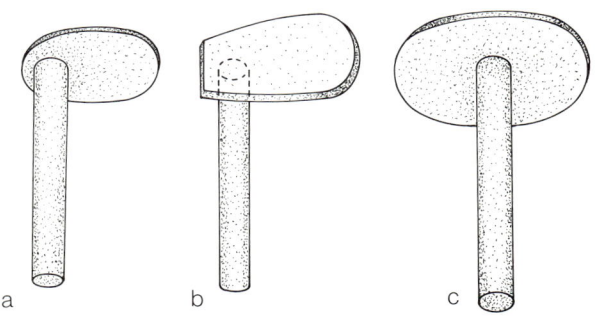

Fig. 1040 Plasti-Pore columellae. **a** The Austin off-centered TORP. **b** The Fisch off-centered TORP. **c** The causse TORP

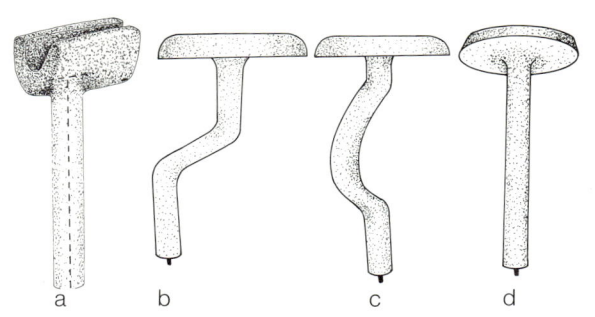

Fig. **1041** Malleable Polycel columellae fortified with stainless-steel wires. **a** The Hubbard footplate–malleus Polycel strut. **b, c** Various angulations of the columella shaft. **d** The Brackmann modified TORP

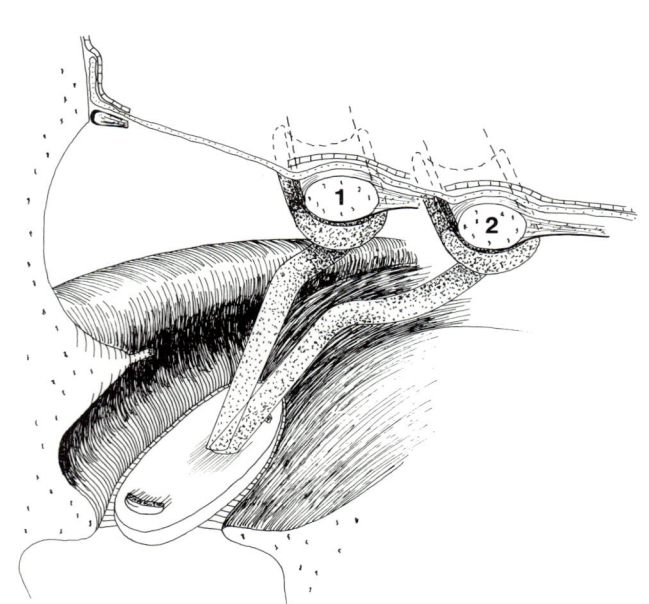

Fig. **1042 Hubbard footplate–malleus struts,** with the malleus handle positioned posteriorly (1) and anteriorly (2)

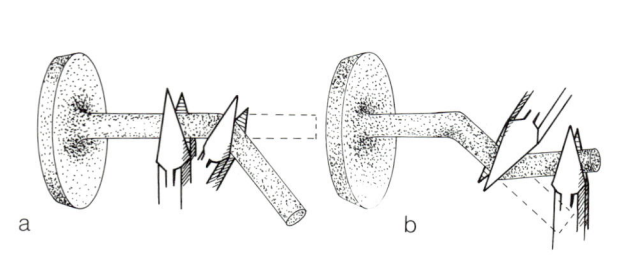

Fig. **1043** Bending a Polycel shaft with two alligator forceps. One holds holding the shaft while, the other bends it. **a** The first bend, **b** the second

To fix a cartilage plate onto the head of the prosthesis, the Moretz Peg-top TORP (Treace Medical Company) includes a peg on top of the platform of the prosthesis (Fig. **1044**). The cartilage plate is mounted on the prosthesis as follows. A 6×6-mm piece of tragal cartilage is harvested. With a needle punch, a hole is punched into the center of the cartilage plate. The peg-top TORP is placed in the cartilage hole. The cartilage plate is trimmed to the appropriate size with a knife, and the excess peg is sliced off with a knife. The shaft is bent, trimmed, and cut to the appropriate shape and length. The peg can be placed on the platform asymmetrically (Fig. **1045**), and tragal cartilage placed on top of the platform can be even larger. Both prostheses are used in situations in which the malleus handle is missing (Fig. **1046**).

Similar to the Moretz prosthesis, but with a new design, is the Passali–Livi TORP, consisting of a circular plate of allogenous cartilage and a Teflon piston, connected with a steel link (Fig. **1045 d**).

The polycel peg-stem total ossicular prosthesis (Shea and Moretz 1984; Treace Medical Company), with a peg on the distal end of the shaft, is interesting (Fig. **1047**). The head of the prosthesis is 4 mm in diameter, and the shaft 1 mm. The peg is 0.75 mm long and 0.3 mm thick. A microhole is drilled on the footplate and the peg is placed in the hole. The prosthesis actually includes a stapedotomy, and should only be used in very selected noninfective cases when there is an intact drum and good tubal function. No late results have yet been published for this method.

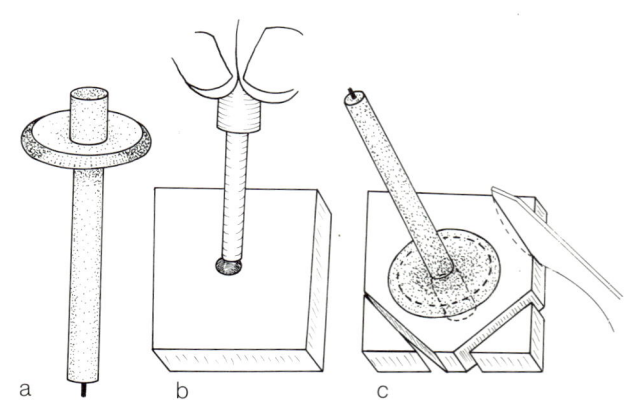

Fig. **1044a** The Moretz peg-top TORP. **b** A hole is punched into the center of a piece of tragal cartilage. **c** The peg-top TORP is inserted into the cartilage hole, and the cartilage is trimmed with a scalpel

Columellae with Biocompatible Materials

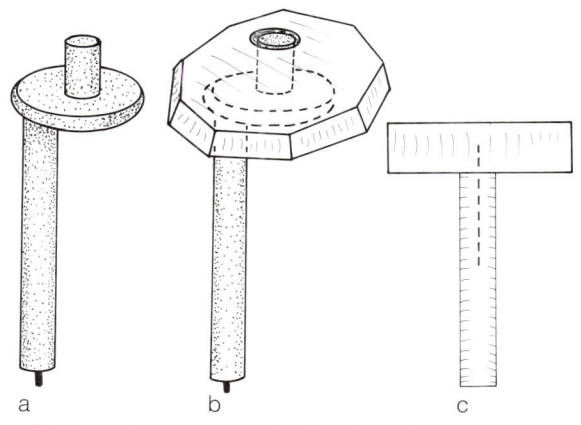

Fig. **1045a** An asymmetrically-placed peg on the Moretz peg-top TORP. **b** A large cartilage plate covers the platform, and the excess peg is sliced off. **c** A Passali–Livi TORP with a 1-mm thick allogenous cartilage plate measuring 4 mm in diameter, and a 0.6-mm thick teflon piston connected with a steel wire

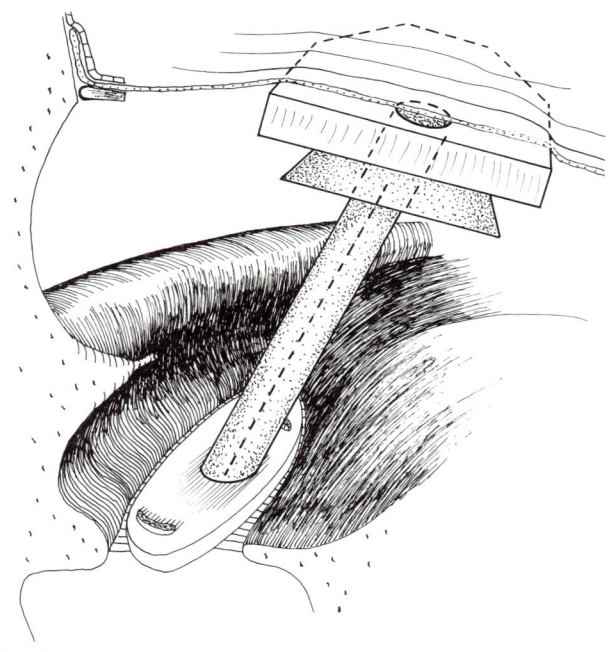

Fig. **1046** The Moretz peg-top TORP positioned between the footplate and the drum

Several types of PORP are shown above (Figs. **808–811**, pp. 286–287). All of these PORPs also have corresponding TORPs, which have the same head but a thin, long shaft without a hole.

Ceramic columellae. Columellae made of the bioinert aluminum-oxide ceramic material, Frialit (Fig. **1048**), are used by Jahnke (1988) and other surgeons. The columellae are L-shaped, or angled with 1–3 grooves in the platform. The grooves are shaped for the malleus handle, and can be widened to fit the malleus handle exactly (Fig. **1050**). The columella platform is often been covered with cartilage. The second generation of ceramics (Jahnke 1992) includes small holes at the distal end of the shaft to facilitate ingrowth of fibrous tissue into the shaft, stabilizing the prosthesis (Fig. **1049**). Jahnke (1992) recommends placing fibrous tissue on the footplate (Fig. **1049**) to achieve better anchorage of the ceramic columella to the footplate.

The Bioceram CORP-T columella (Yamamoto 1981) has a convex, smooth, and elliptical head (Fig. **1049c**). The shaft is 0.8 mm thick, with a 1-mm thick base to stabilize the prosthesis on the footplate. There are three lengths of CORP-T columellae available (5, 6, and 7 mm). Yamamoto uses CORP-T columella in connection with microslices of allogenous septal cartilage in canal wall–down mastoidectomy situations (Figs. **623–626**).

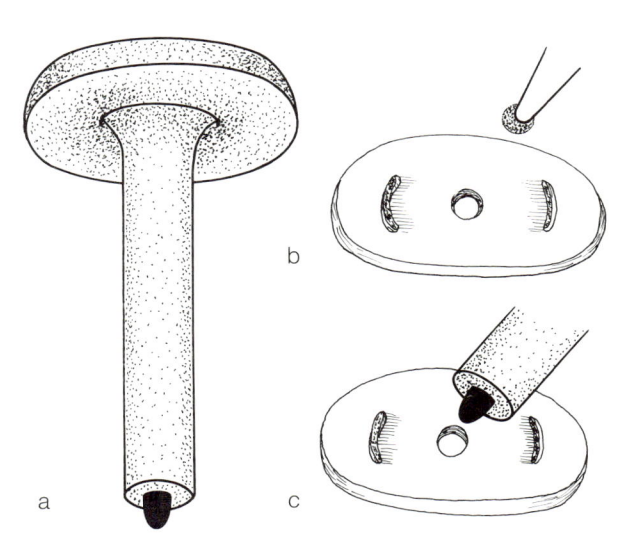

Fig. **1047a** The Polycel peg-stem total ossicular prosthesis. **b** A hole is drilled into the footplate using a diamond drill. **c** The peg of the prosthesis is inserted into the hole of the footplate

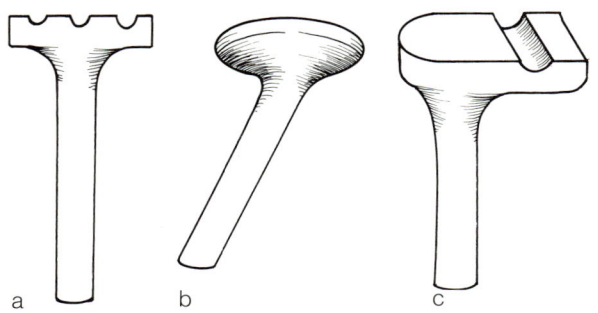

Fig. **1048a** The Frialit ceramic columella, with three grooves in the platform. **b** An angled-shaft columella. **c** An L-shaped columella, with one groove

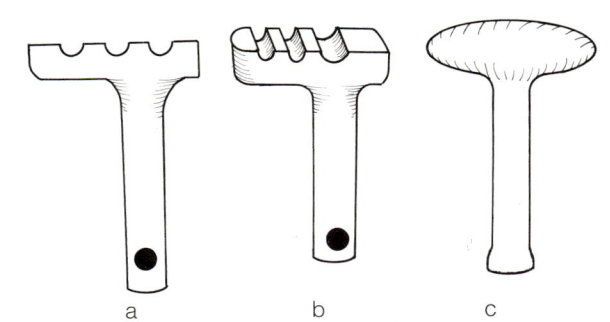

Fig. **1049a, b** Second-generation Frialit ceramic columellae, with holes in the distal ends of the shafts. **c** The Bioceram CORP-T columella, with a convex, smooth, elliptical head

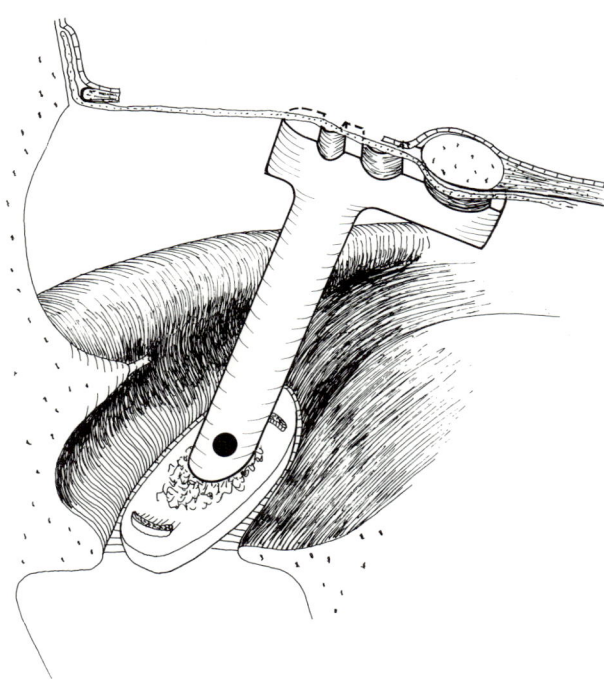

Fig. **1050** A Frialit ceramic columella placed between the footplate and the malleus handle. Between the columella and the footplate, fibrous tissue is placed to provide better anchorage of the columella to the footplate. A groove on the platform is widened to fit the malleus handle better

The CORP-T is inserted through the slit in the cartilage slice, as with the CORP-P(Figs. **825–827**). The head of the prosthesis protrudes through the cartilage slit, and it is covered with fascia (Fig. **1051**).

Columellae made of the bioactive glass ceramic material, Ceravital (Xomed Company, Jacksonville, USA), are widely used. The head of the prosthesis is not covered with cartilage, but with bone dust (Reck 1984, Gersdorff et al. 1986).

Dense hydroxyapatite columellae. Hydroxyapatite has become a very popular material, and many types of columellae have been designed and used. The advantage of columellae with a Plasti-Pore shaft and hydroxyapatite head is the malleability of the shaft, which can easily be trimmed and bent, while the hydroxyapatite head has good biocompatibility, and can also be shaped by drilling.

The Goldenberg (1990) incus–stapes prosthesis, with wire reinforcement of the Plasti-Pore shaft (Fig. **1052**), can easily be bent into the appropriate shape and position (Figs. **1053, 1054**).

The Black oval T-prosthesis (Smith and Nephew, Richards Company) with a rounded oval, 3×4-mm hydroxyapatite head and either a Plasti-Pore or fluoroplastic shaft reinforced with stainless-steel wire (Fig. **1052**), reduces extrusion of the prosthesis and allows retraction of the drum. The shaft has good malleability.

Several columellae are made entirely of hydroxyapatite: The Wehrs incus–stapes prosthesis (Wehrs 1987) has a single notch for short distances and a double notch for long distances between the malleus handle and the footplate (Fig. **1055**). The Wehrs columella is placed on the footplate, the malleus handle is elevated with a hook, and the head is gently pushed under the malleus handle (Fig. **1056**).

The Grote hydroxyapatite L-shaped incus–stapes prosthesis, with a 0.6-mm hydroxyapatite

Columellae with Biocompatible Materials 373

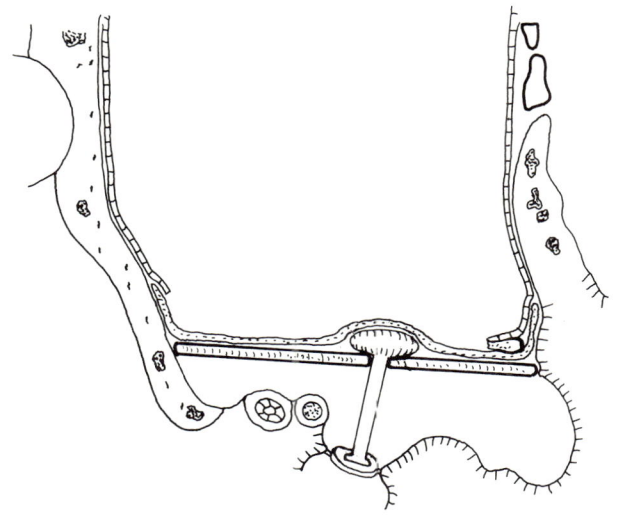

Fig. 1051 Placement of the CORP-T columella in a situation with no ossicles and canal wall–down mastoidectomy. A septal cartilage slice covers the tympanic cavity. The head of the prosthesis protrudes through the slit of the cartilage, and is covered with fascia

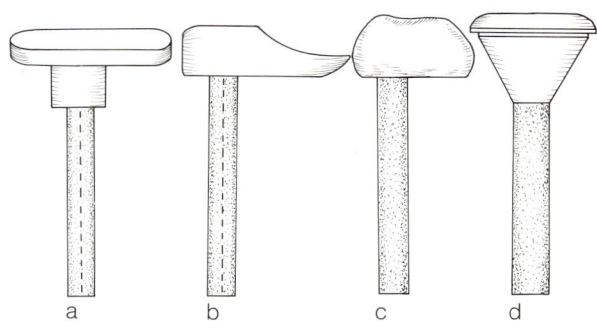

Fig. 1052 Hybrid hydroxyapatite Plasti-Pore or fluoroplast columellae. **a** The Goldenberg incus–stapes prosthesis, with a large hydroxyapatite platform and a Plasti-Pore shaft reinforced with a stainless-steel wire. **b** A similar Goldenberg prosthesis, with a small cup for the malleus handle. **c** The Black oval-top TORP prosthesis, made of hydroxyapatite and Plasti-Pore. **d** The Shea hydroxyapatite–fluoroplastic TORP

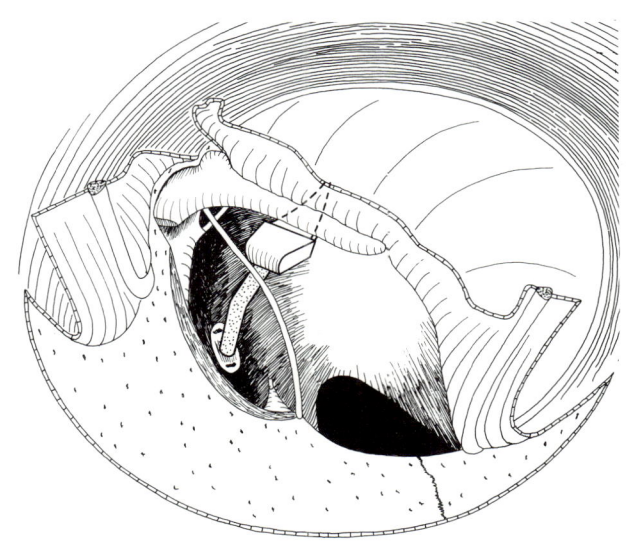

Fig. 1053 **The Goldenberg incus–stapes prosthesis,** placed between the footplate and the malleus handle. The small hydroxyapatite head is placed under the malleus handle like a hook, and the shaft is bent and angulated

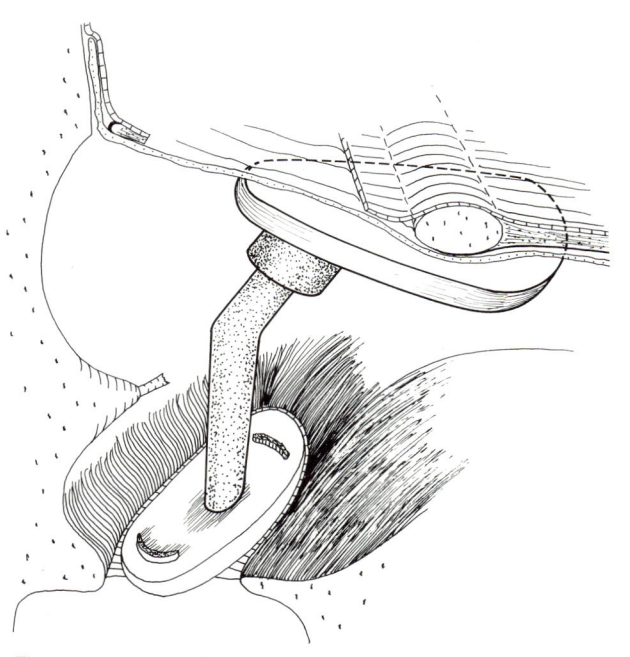

Fig. 1054 **The Goldenberg hydroxyapatite TORP,** with a relatively large platform placed under the malleus handle and an angulated Plasti-Pore shaft placed on the footplate

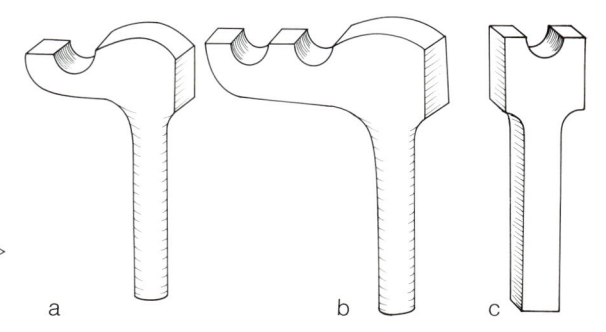

Fig. 1055 **The hydroxyapatite Wehrs prostheses,** ▷ **a** with one notch, and **b** with two notches. **c** The Kartush columella, made entirely of hydroxyapatite

shaft and a relatively large platform (Fig. **1057**), allows the length of the shaft to be tailored with a small chisel. The shaft is centered on the footplate, with an oval piece of Gelfoam wrapped around the shaft of the prosthesis (Fig. **1058**). The head of the columella is placed on the malleus handle (Grote 1989).

The Apoceram T-columella (Yanagihara et al. 1988) has a smoothly curved platform with cross-grooves on it (Fig. **1057**).

The Kartush incus–stapes strut prosthesis is made entirely of hydroxyapatite (Fig. **1055**). The head is designed to match the shape of the malleus handle (Fig. **1059**).

The Black spanner strut consists of a fluoroplastic shaft and a hydroxyapatite head (Smith and Nephew, Richards Company), which can be tailored to the malleus handle. The prosthesis is particularly suitable when the malleus handle is in an anterior position (Fig. **1060**). The shaft can easily be bent.

The *glass-ionomer cement* TORP (Ionos, Seefeld, Germany) (Fig. **844**) has a large head and a relatively thick shaft that can be drilled to the appropriate size using a diamond burr.

Metallic columellae. The titanium TORP (Fig. **845**) (Magnan 1992; MXM Laboratories, France) includes a special wire arrangement to allow the shaft of the prosthesis to be shortened or elongated before insertion (Fig. **1061**). The groove on the head of the prosthesis seems to be large in relation to the size of the malleus handle. It should

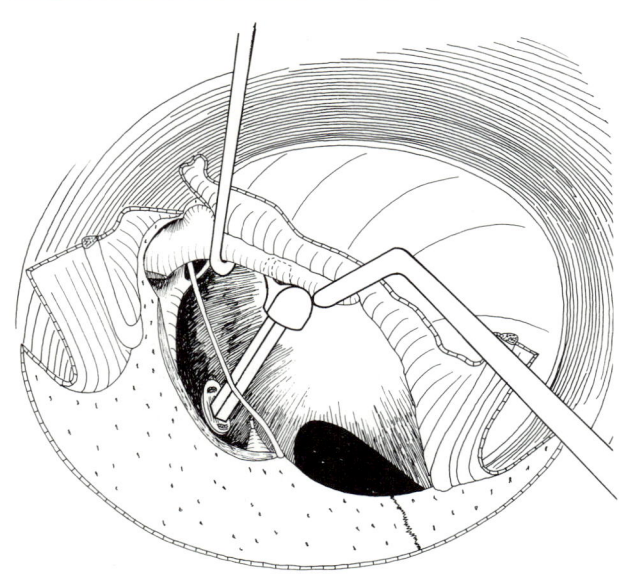

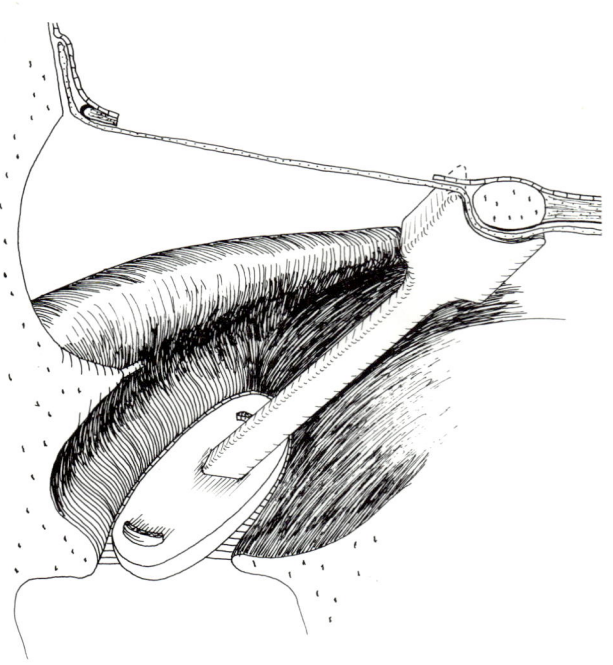

Fig. **1056** Placement of the Wehrs columella between the footplate and the malleus handle. The malleus handle is elevated with a hook, and the head of the prosthesis is gently pushed under it with a small rugine

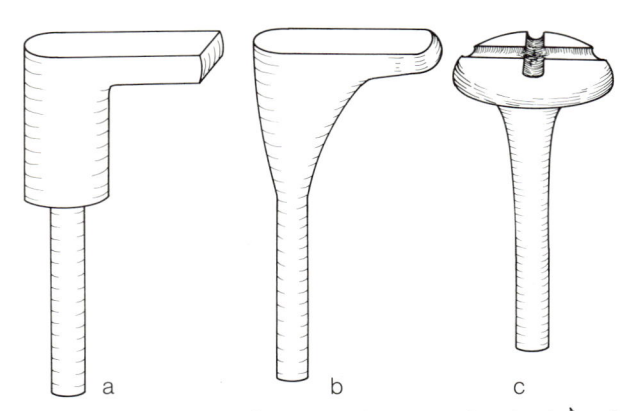

Fig. **1057a, b The Grote hydroxyapatite L-shaped incus–stapes prostheses. c** The Apoceram T-type prosthesis, with a cross-groove on the platform

Fig. **1058** The Grote L-shaped prosthesis is placed ▷ with its shaft on the center of the footplate, and with the head on the malleus handle. An oval piece of Gelfoam is placed in the oval window niche to stabilize the prosthesis

Fig. 1059 **The Kartush hydroxyapatite incus-stapes strut prosthesis,** in a situation with an anteriorly-positioned malleus handle

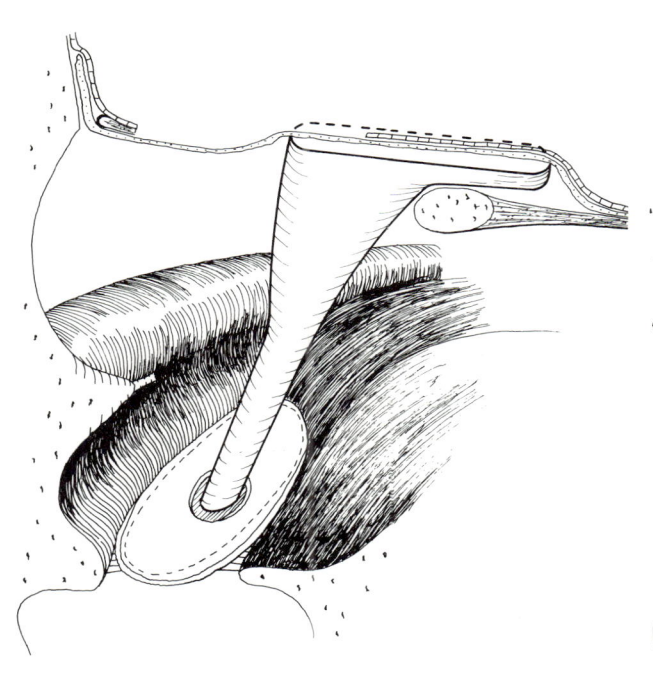

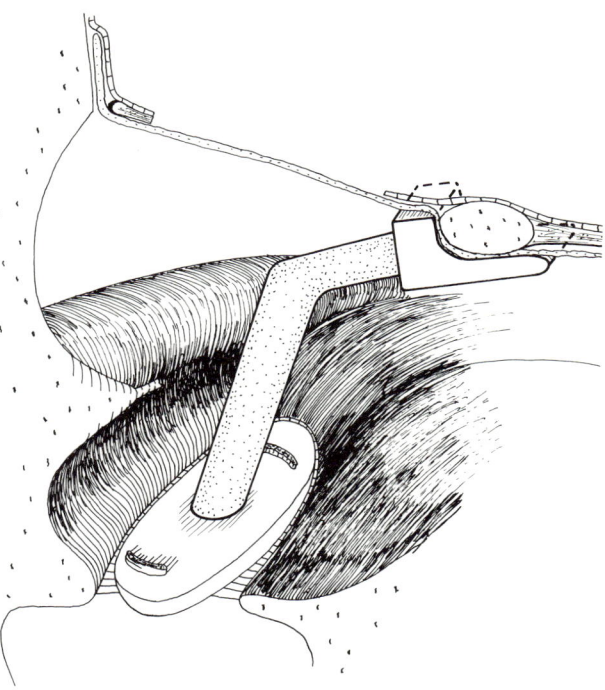

Fig. 1060 **The Black spanner strut,** with a hydroxyapatite head and a fluoroplastic shaft, in a situation with an anteriorly-positioned malleus handle. The fluoroplastic shaft is angled, and the hydroxyapatite head is trimmed to the malleus handle

be placed in the superior part of the malleus handle. No late results with this prosthesis have yet been published.

The Babighian telescopic TORP, including the Magnan wire system, has a hydroxyapatite shaft and head (Audio Micromed Company) (Fig. **846**). The hydroxyapatite can be trimmed and shaped (Babighian 1992).

Metallic wire columellae. The Palva three-legged columella, made of stainless-steel wire, is placed with one leg on the footplate. The other two legs are placed towards the hypotympanum and tubal orifice, respectively (Fig. **1062**). Palva abandoned the use of wires (Palva et al. 1971), but if they are covered with large cartilage plates as shown in Figure **852**, they may be used in selected cases.

The incus replacement prosthesis (IRP), with stainless-steel wire (Sheehy 1965) was first used in stapedectomy after horizontal canal fenestration, but has also been recommended as a columella when there is a mobile footplate. A periosteum incision is made on the posterior side of the malleus handle, and a pocket is created between the malleus handle and the drum remnant (Fig. **1063**). The IRP-prosthesis is placed on the malleus handle

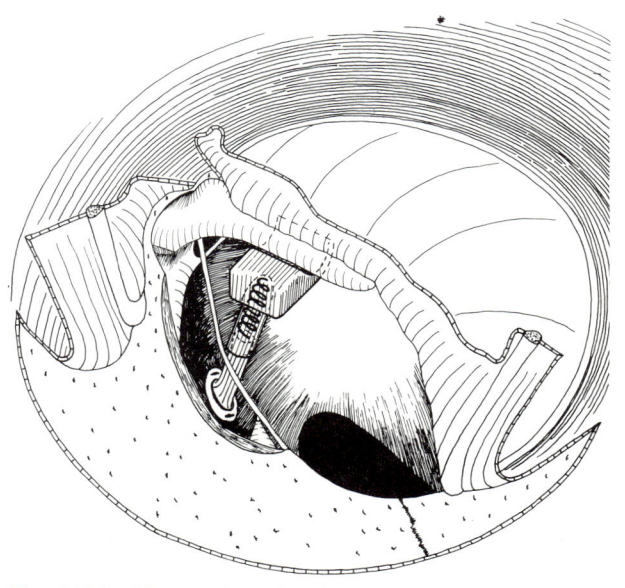

Fig. **1061 Magnan's titanium columella,** placed between the footplate and the malleus handle

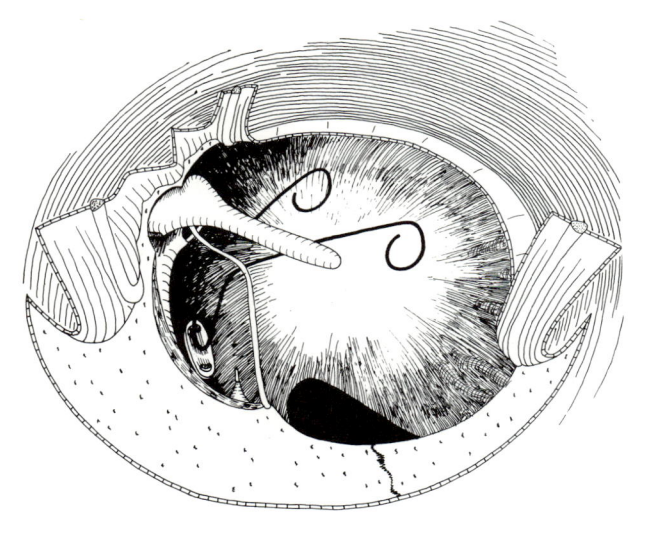

Fig. **1062 The Palva three-legged stainless-steel wire columella,** placed under the malleus handle in a case of total perforation

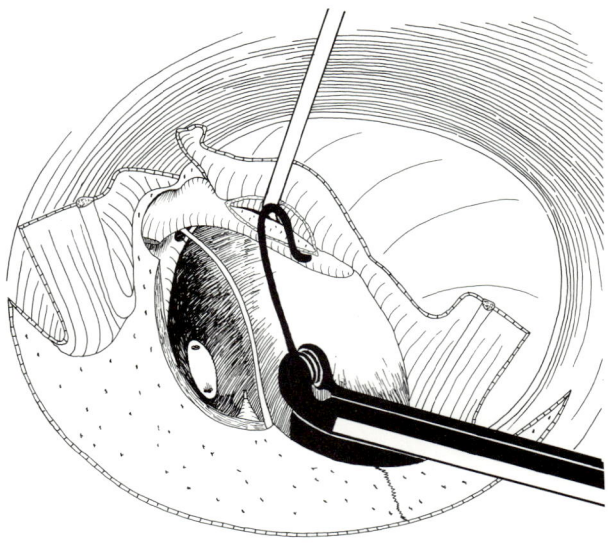

Fig. **1063 Placement of Sheehy's incus replacement prosthesis** (IRP). An incision is made on the posterior aspect of the malleus handle, and the periosteum is elevated from the lateral aspect of the malleus handle. The IRP prosthesis in inserted into the groove between the drum and the malleus handle

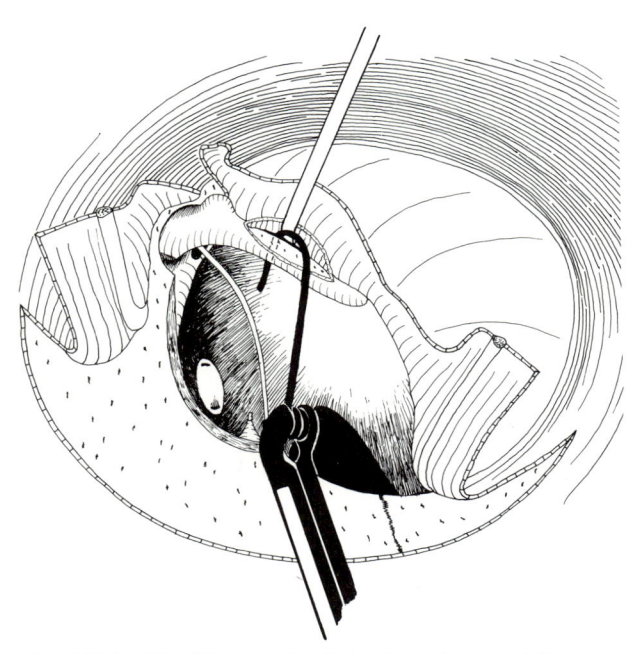

Fig. **1064** The IRP prosthesis is placed around the malleus handle

(Fig. **1064**), and the wire is fixed using a rugine (Fig. **1065**). Usually, a 6.25-mm long IRP prosthesis is used for the columella. The loop of the IRPprosthesis is placed on the footplate, and secured in position with small Gelfoam balls. The problems with IRP prostheses are that it is difficult to obtain the exact length of the columella, and its fixation to the footplate is insecure.

The new method, in which the wire is fixed through a hole made in the malleus handle (Hüttenbrink 1992b) has improved the wire methods considerably, both with columellae in a mobile footplate (Fig. **1066**) and with stapedectomy prostheses.

The gold wire antenna TORP (Pusalkar and Steinbach 1991) consists of a rectangular wire platform of 0.4 mm pure gold and a gold shaft running from the center of the platform rectangularly downward and ending in a thicker base (Fig. **852**). The base of the columella is placed on the footplate. The platform is covered with a tragal cartilage plate (Fig. **1067**). Pusalkar and Steinbach achieved surprisingly good hearing gains using the gold wire prostheses.

Fig. 1065 The wire of the IRP prosthesis is fixed to the malleus handle, and the prosthesis is adjusted ot the footplate

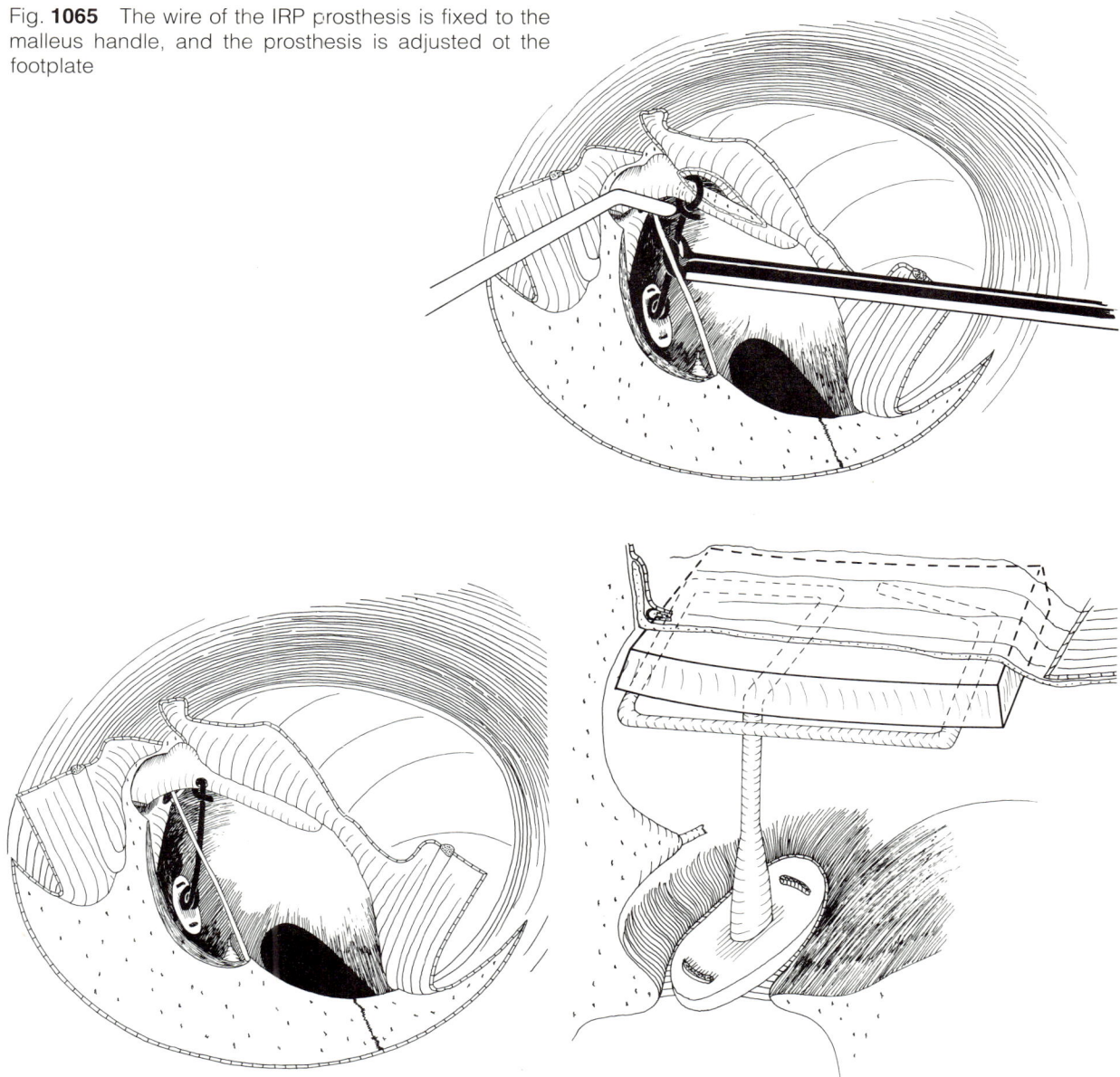

Fig. 1066 **The Hüttenbrink method of fixing a stainless-steel wire columella** with a ho e through the upper part of the malleus handle. The wire is placed through the hole and fixed

Fig. 1067 The gold wire antenna TORP (Pusalkar and Steinbach 1991). The base of the prosthesis is placed on the footplate. The wire platform is placed under the drum, and covered with cartilage plate

Compound columellae

One of the problems with the columella is the fixation of the shaft in the oval-window niche region, either through fibrous tissue or by new formation of bone at the facial nerve prominence. To avoid this problem, thin shafts with little or no tendency to produce fixation to their surroundings have been used. At the beginning of the tympanoplasty era, polyethylene and Teflon tubes and shafts, and later Plasti-Pore, Polycel, ceramics, and hydroxyapatite shafts, have been used.

Another problem is with the contact between the platform and the drum, causing extrusion of the prosthesis in ears with retraction of the eardrum. With platforms made of cartilage, there is no resorption; in platforms made of ossicles or cortical bone,

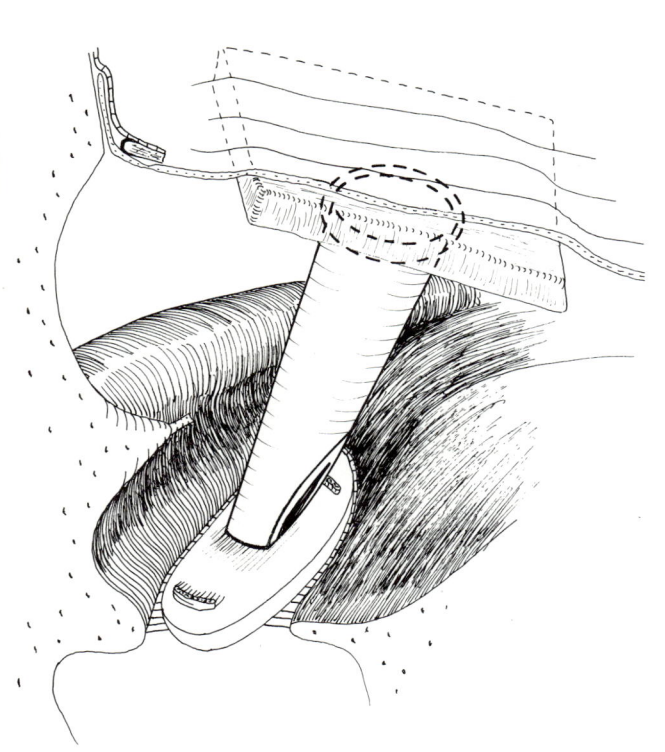

Fig. **1068** The first composite graft with a polyethylene strut and a piece of cortical bone

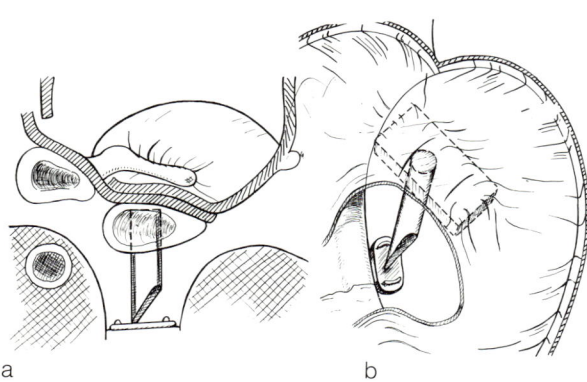

Fig. **1069a** A polyethylene strut–incus compound graft columella. **b** The polyethylene–cortical bone compound graft columella, used during the 1960s (Tos 1972)

some bone resorption takes place in ears with tubal dysfunction and drum retraction, but extrusions are less common than when the platform is made of the same material as the shaft, e.g., with synthetic biomaterials. A combination of a platform made of ossicles or cortical bone and a shaft made of synthetic materials has been used for compound graft columellae, particularly in ears with no malleus. The relatively large platform has broad contact with the ear drum, but is has never been proved that compound grafts are functionally better than simple columellae.

Platforms with ossicles and cortical bone; such as polyethylene tubes, were covered with pieces of cortical bone (Fig. **1068**) or bone chips placed on the head of the prostheses, which had rather small diameters, as early as the 1960s (Harrison 1969). The bone should partly prevent extrusion of the prosthesis, and partly enlarge the area of contact with the drum. In the late 1960s, the present author used compound grafts with Shea polyethylene stapedectomy struts and autogenous incus and cortical bone (Fig. **1069**), but the results were poorer in compound grafts compared with simple incus columellae (Tos 1969, Tos 1972).

Compound grafts with Teflon, Plasti-Pore, Polycel, and ceramics have been used mainly in connection with autogenous incus (Figs. **1070, 1071**). Better sound transmission to the footplate should be achieved by placing the Plasti-Pore shaft into the incus off center (Fig. **1072**), but again there are as yet no data to support this.

For compound grafts with cortical bone, the piece of bone has to be a 6×5–mm solid, compact bone at least 2 mm thick, to allow a hole to be drilled for the Teflon, Plasti-Pore, or other shafts. Harvesting a cortical bone graft for the compound columella cannot be carried out with hollow chisels, as the produce fractures. For compound grafts with cortical bone, the author has harvested cortical bone at the superior edge of the cavity by drilling a rectangular groove with a 0.5-mm cutting burr (Fig. **1073**). After the groove has been made deep enough using a 4-mm straight rhinoplasty chisel, a rectangular piece of cortical bone can be harvested. The edges of the bone are drilled smooth, and it is trimmed to the appropriate size. A hole is drilled into the bone, and a shaft is inserted.

The cortical compound graft can be placed in relation to the malleus handle in many ways. The placement can be similar to some of the interpositions illustrated in chapter 19 (p. 323–328). Usually, the cortical bone is a large platform facing the drum or the malleus handle, if it is present. When the malleus handle is present, it is preferable to

Columellae with Biocompatible Materials

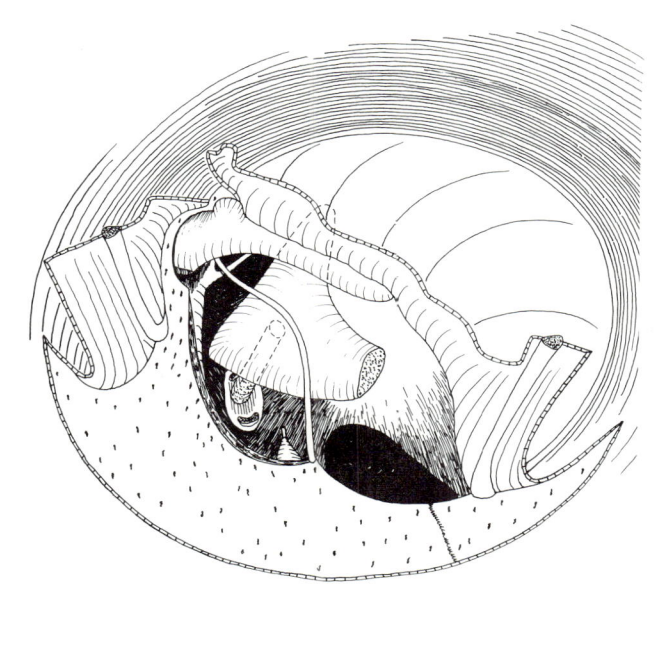

Fig. **1070** A Plasti-Pore–incus compound graft columella. The incus is placed with its short process under the malleus handle, and the long process is directed inferiorly

Fig. **1071** Side view of the Plasti-Pore–incus columella, with the short process placed under the malleus handle

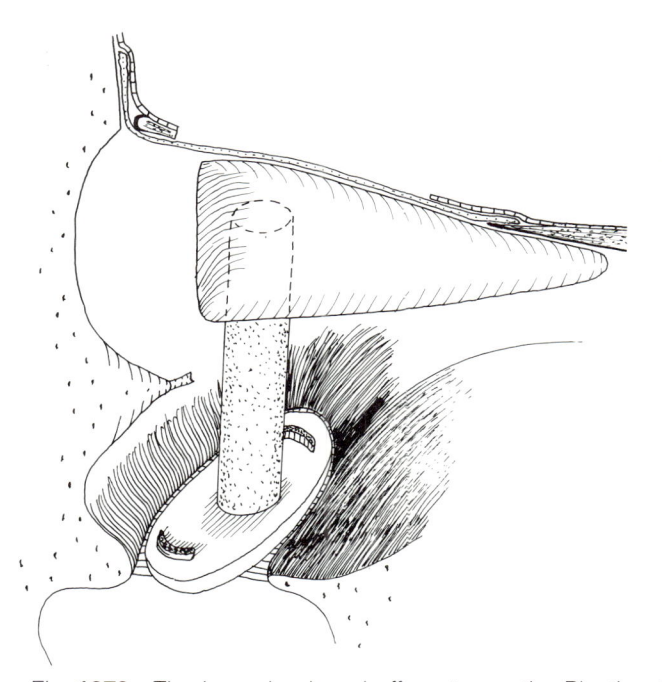

Fig. **1072** The incus is placed off-center on the Plasti-Pore strut in cases with a missing malleus handle

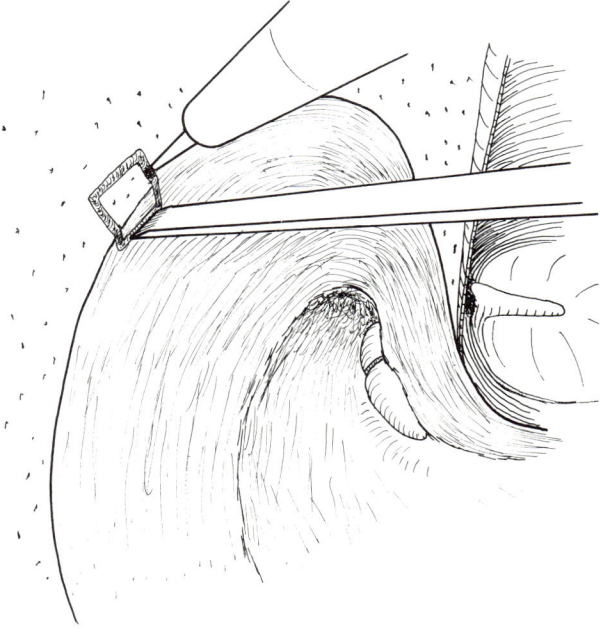

Fig. **1073** Harvesting of a compact piece of bone from the upper edge of the cavity to be used in construction of the compound grafts. A rectangular groove is drilled with a sharp burr, and the piece of bone is removed using a rhinoplasty chisel

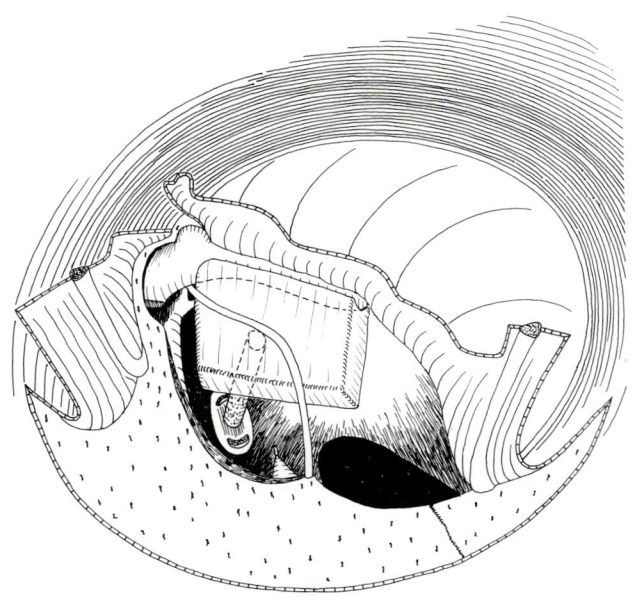

Fig. **1074** A cortical bone–Plasti-Pore compound graft. The cortical bone is placed along the malleus handle and a groove is made for the malleus handle along the side of it

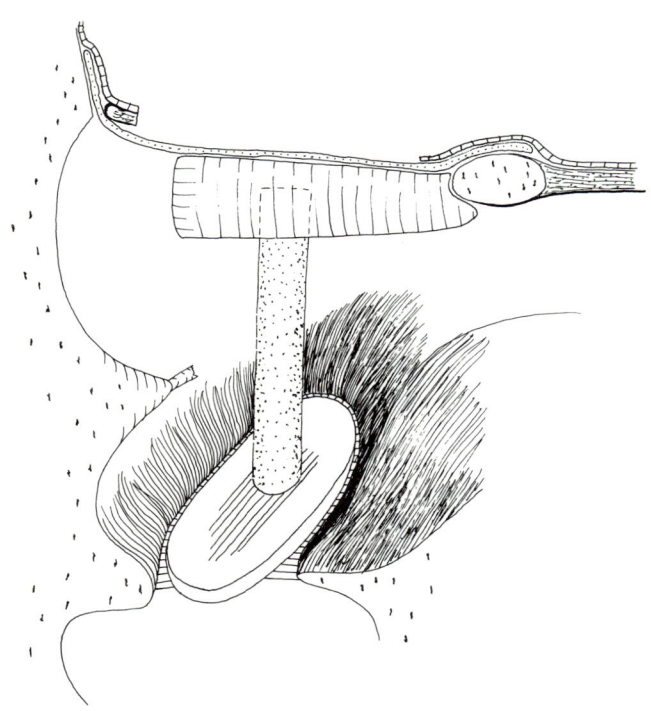

Fig. **1075** Side view of the cortical bone–Plasti-Pore compound graft columella. The cortical bone is placed at the level of the malleus handle, and has good contact with it

place a cortical bone platform parallel to the handle and drill a long groove for the malleus handle (Figs. **1074, 1075**). In this way, retraction of the drum, at least, can be prevented.

Bauer (1988) has created an elegant Polycel–bone compound columella (Fig. **1076**). A small hole is drilled into an accessible surface of the bone. Around the small central hole, a large circular groove is drilled. The depth of the groove determines the height of the piece of bone to be used for the compound graft. The Polycel cylinder is gently inserted into the hole. The piece of bone is chiseled away with a thin rhinoplasty chisel. The compound graft is placed on the footplate in a canal wall–down mastoidectomy with a missing malleus handle and stapedial arch. The graft is supported with Gelfoam balls and covered with fascia (Fig. **1077**). Schobel (1993) has used the same method independently.

Compound grafts with cartilage are shown above (pp. 287–288, 299–301) in connection with wire techniques and artificial prostheses. These grafts include Sheehy's covering of Plasti-Pore PORPS and TORPS with cartilage slices (Figs. **811–813**); the Jackson and Glasscock method of fixing the cartilage plate to the PORP or TORP (Fig. **815**) and a similar alternative (Fig. **816**); proposed cartilage covering of the Gerlach wire-basket interposition graft (Fig. **849**); and the suggested covering of the Palva two-legged prosthesis with cartilage (Fig. **852**), or with a bony plate, as indicated by Palva (Fig. **958**). Other methods include the covering of gold wires with tragal cartilage plates (Figs. **845–855, 1067**); the thumb touch technique with tragal cartilage plate in ears with a missing malleus handle (Figs. **951–955**); the Saraceno method of covering the Shea Plasti-Pore TORP (Figs. **1038, 1039**); the Moretz peg-top-TORP combined with tragal cartilage (Figs. **1044–1046**); and the Passali–Livi TORP with an allogenous septal cartilage platform and a teflon piston connection with a steel link (Fig. **1045 d**).

The Smyth T-cartilage wire prosthesis is a compound T-graft using allogenous septal cartilage and wire (Fig. **1078**). The wire is inserted through the prosthesis, plaited together as a columella, and placed on the footplate.

The Schobel cartilage-bed method of producing a compound perichondrium–cartilage–Plasti-Pore columella graft (Schobel 1993) is performed as follows. A large piece of tragal cartilage, with perichondrium attached on both sides, is harvested. The perichondrium is elevated on one side. A cartilage disk with a diameter of 6 mm is cut (Fig. **1079**). Using a thin sharp chisel or a scalpel,

Columellae with Biocompatible Materials 381

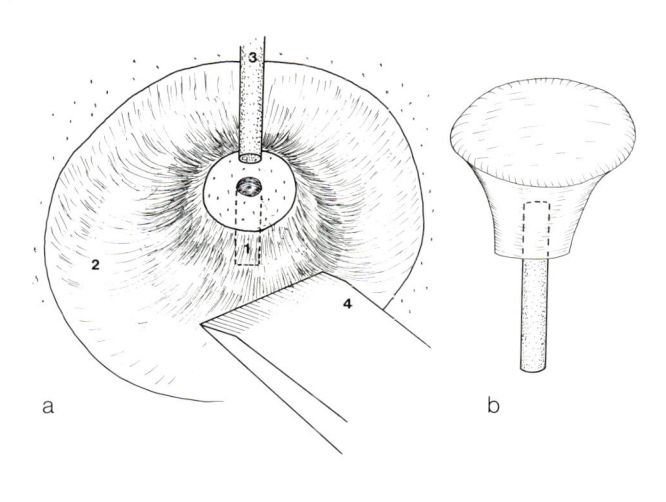

Fig. **1076a** Harvesting a piece of cortical bone for use as a compound graft with Polycel (Bauer). 1) A 0.5-mm hole is drilled into the cortical bone. 2) A large groove is drilled round the small hole with a cutting burr. 3) A Polycel strut is pushed into the small hole. 4) The piece of cortical bone is chiseled away using a thin rhinoplasty chisel. **b** The final shape of the Bauer compound graft columella

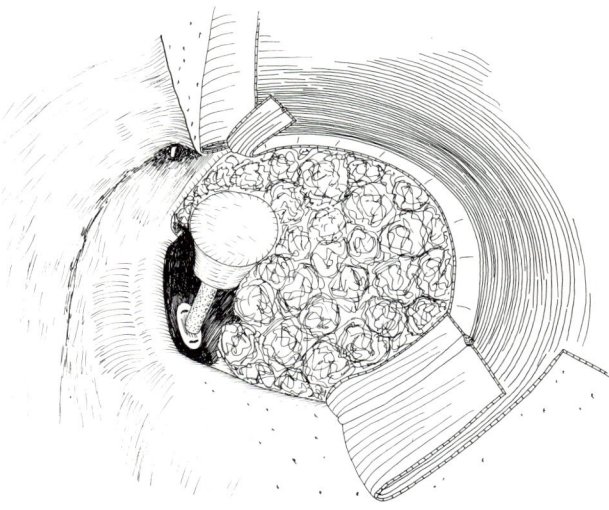

Fig. **1077 The Bauer compound graft columella-** placed on the footplate with no ossicles in a case with total perforation and canal wall–down mastoidectomy. The tympanic cavity is filled with Gelfoam, and is closed with an underlay fascia graft

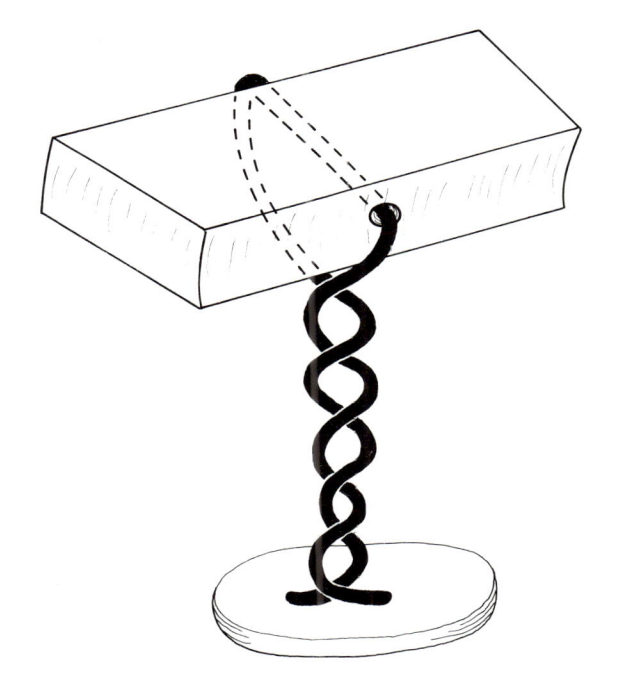

Fig. **1078 The Smyth compound columella,** made of tragal cartilage and a wire plaited together to form a columella shaft

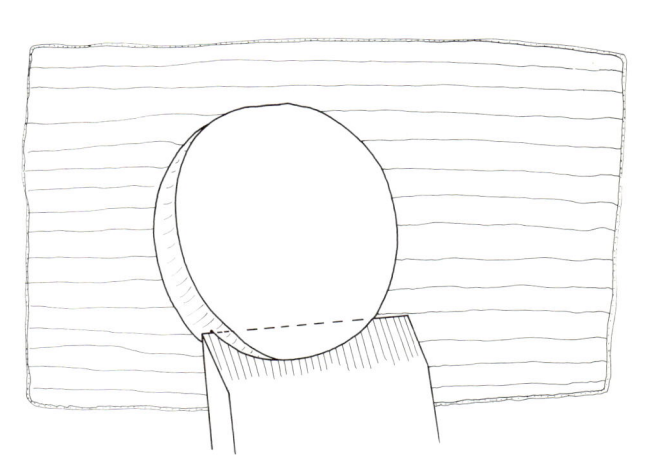

Fig. **1079 The Schobel compound tragal cartilage–perichondrium TORP.** After harvesting tragal cartilage, a 6-mm disk of cartilage is cut out. The disk is sliced horizontally with a thin chisel

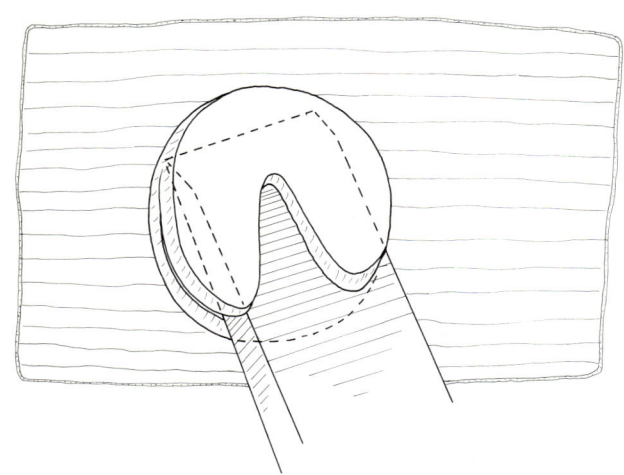

Fig. **1080** A slit is cut into the upper cartilage slice

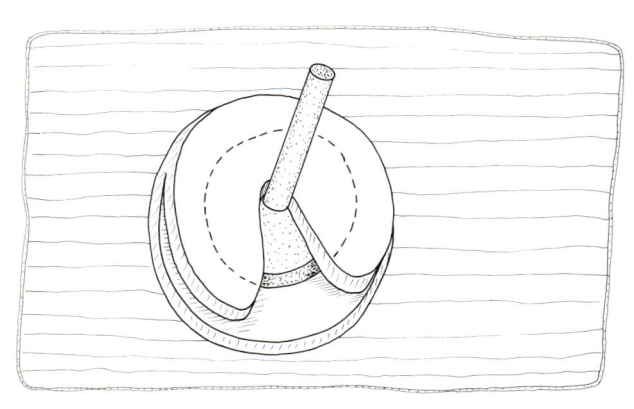

Fig. **1081** The platform of the Plasti-Pore TORP is placed between the two cartilage layers, which are still connected to each other on one part of the disk. The perichondrium is still attached on the outer cartilage layer, and the prosthesis is ready to be placed on the footplate

the cartilage disk is partly sliced horizontally (Fig. **1080**). After a slit has been made in the superficial cartilage slice (Fig. **1080**), the shaft of the TORP is placed in the center of the disk, and the platform is inserted between the two cartilage slices (Fig. **1081**). The attached perichondrium covers the perforations and the attic region.

The prognosis for type 3 tympanoplasty columellae is much poorer than with type 2 tympanoplasty interpositions. The hearing results are poorer, and the extrusion and reoperation rates are high. Columellae made of cortical bone and ossicles become fixed to their surrounding or are resorbed. Cartilage columellae are soft to begin with, and they become even softer due to fibrous degeneration and disappearance of the cartilage. The sound pressure transmission is therefore usually not very good with cartilage columellae. The problem with wire, especially IRP wire, is that its contact with, and anchorage on, the footplate is difficult. Finally, the problem with artificial grafts is that they frequently extrude and tilt, and the TORP becomes displaced. The most common extrusion mechanism is retraction of the drum, mainly between the platform and the posterosuperior bony annulus (Sanna et al. 1987) (Fig. **1082**), resulting in tilting of the prosthesis. After retraction of the drum under the platform and around the shaft, the platform will be displaced and extruded.

Compound grafts definitely delay extrusion, but their function is poorer than that of uncovered columellae. Tilting and fixation of compound grafts occurs in the same way as with uncovered platforms.

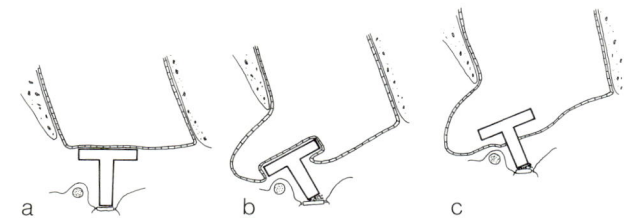

Fig. **1082** The most common mechanism of extrusion of a Plasti-Pore TORP in an intact canal-wall. **a** The TORP is nicely in place. **b** The drum has retracted on both sides of the TORP. The posterosuperior retraction pocket, towards the facial prominence, causes the prosthesis to tilt. **c** With further retraction around the shaft, the platform of the TORP is displaced and will be extruded

22 Type 4 and 5 Tympanoplasty

Type 4 tympanoplasty was the most common form of tympanoplasty performed by Wullstein (Fig. **687**). In contrast to the Wullstein period, from the late 1950s to the early 1970s, type 4 and type 5 tympanoplasties are nowadays seldom performed. The reason for this is mainly the popularity and dominance of the columella methods, which build up the tympanic cavity to produce a type 3 tympanoplasty, instead of performing a type 4 tympanoplasty with the cavum minor technique. The classic type 5 tympanoplasty—the fenestration of the lateral semicircular canal (Figs. **686, 687**)—has today been almost completely replaced by stapedectomies and stapedotomies.

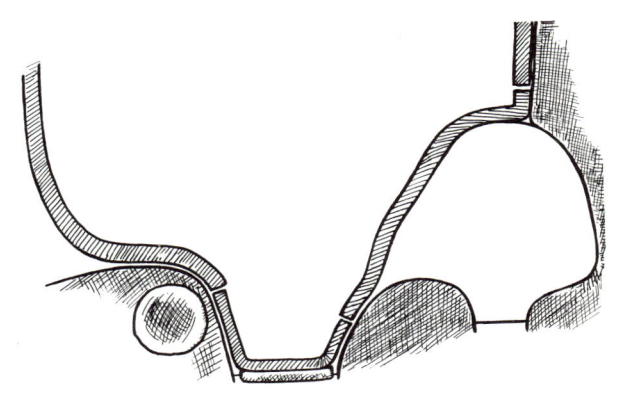

Fig. **1083** Type 4 tympanoplasty, with protection of the round-window niche and covering of the footplate and oval-window niche with the skin

Type 4 Tympanoplasty

The principle of type 4 tympanoplasty is to protect the round window from sound pressure. In tympanoplasty type 4, the sound pressure transformation mechanism is not built up; only the round window is protected. The sound pressure reaches the footplate directly, but it cannot reach the round window membrane. In this way, a pressure difference between the two windows is produced (Fig. **1083**). The oval-window niche communicates directly with the ear canal, and the round window communicates with the Eustachian tube via the air-filled cavum minor in the hypotympanum.

Theoretically, acoustic perception after this procedure can never be better than 25 dB, due to the absence of an impedance-matching mechanism. In practice, however, an acoustic perception of 40 dB in the speech frequencies must be considered a satisfactory result.

Type 4 Tympanoplasty Techniques

The precondition for type 4 tympanoplasty is a canal wall–down mastoidectomy situation, a patent Eustachian tube, and a mobile footplate, but otherwise no ossicles. The tympanic graft, usually fascia, is inserted into the hypotympanum over the round window lateral to the Eustachian tube opening. It is then laid against the promontory, leaving the oval window niche uncovered (Fig. **1083**). To ensure that the fascia graft takes on the promontory and at the edges of the oval window, the mucosa has to be scraped off and the bone denuded where the graft contacts the medial wall of the middle ear. The denuded bone should be roughened by passing the diamond burr over it. There are several methods of closing the hypotympanum and placing the fascia graft.

1) *Onlay grafting.* After a canal wall–down mastoidectomy, the mucosa from the mesotympanum, sinus tympani, and footplate, as well as part of the promontory and part of the facial nerve prominence, is removed, and the bone is denuded (Fig. **1084**). The ear-canal skin is incised 1 mm lateral to the annulus all the way round, and the epithelium is removed from the drum remnant and the annulus region, as well as the ear-canal skin close to the drum. The fascia placed on the annulus and fixed in the anterior tympanomeatal angle with Gelfoam balls. The fascia is then placed on the prominence of the tensor tympani muscle, the promontory, and the posterior ear-canal will (Fig. **1085**). The fascia graft is fixed to the promontory with small Gelfoam balls. A 3×3-mm Thiersch flap is placed on the footplate and the oval window niche, and adapted to the edges of the fascia. The skin also covers part of the facial nerve prominence. The Thiersch flap is fixed to the footplate with small Gelfoam balls, and carefully adapted around the oval window niche. Finally, the epithelial flaps are

22 Type 4 and 5 Tympanoplasty

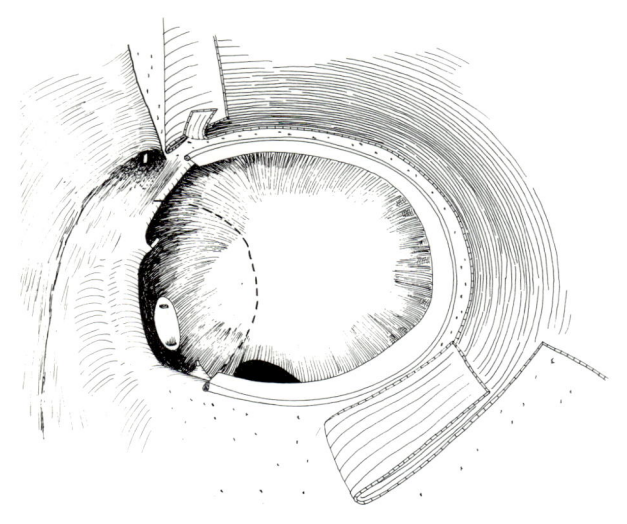

Fig. **1084** Type 4 tympanoplasty in a case with canal wall–down mastoidectomy, total perforation, and no ossicles. The dotted line indicates the border for removal of the mucosa in the mesotympanum. The ear-canal skin 1 mm lateral to the annulus is incised, and the epithelium from the drum remnant and annulus is removed

returned (Figs. **1086, 1087**). More fascia can also cover the rest of te cavity, depending on the techniques used for management of the mastoid cavity and ear-canal reconstruction.

2) *Intermediate fascia grafting.* After removal of the middle-ear mucosa around the oval window niche and the footplate, the epithelium from the drum remnant, annulus, and the most medial part of the ear-canal skin is elevated outward. (Fig. **1088**). The fascia is placed on the annulus, and the flaps are returned. They are fixed with Gelfoam balls all the way round the annulus. The fascia is fixed to the promontory with Gelfoam balls. The Thiersch flap is placed on the footplate and the oval window niche, and fixed with Gelfoam balls (Fig. **1089**), and the remaining epithelial flaps are returned.

3) *Underlay fascia grafting technique.* The mucosa is removed from around the ovel window niche and from the footplate. The mucosa under the fibrous annulus is detached or removed as far as the bone, using a curved elevator. The hypotympanum and tubal orifice are filled with Gelfoam in order to hold the fascia in place under the annulus. The fascia is placed under the annulus and carefully adapted to the denuded bone (Fig. **1090**). The Thiersch flap is placed on the footplate and the denuded bone of the oval window niche, and held in place with Gelfoam balls. The epithelial flaps are returned (Fig. **1091**).

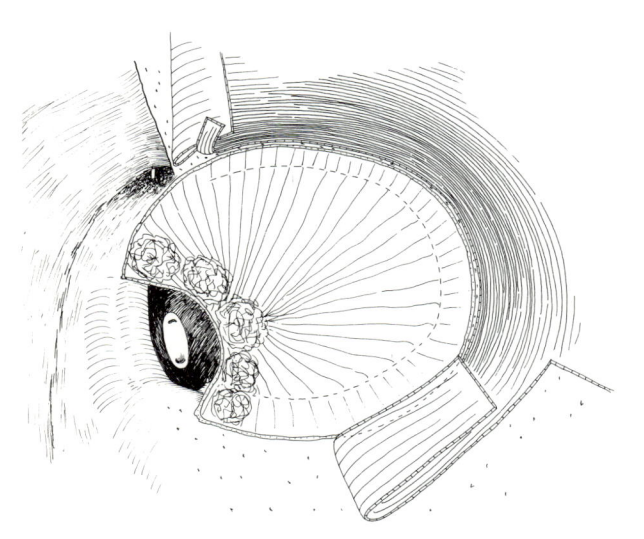

Fig. **1085** The fascia is placed on the drum remnant, the annulus, and the denuded bone. Superiorly, the fascia is placed on the prominence of the tensor tympani muscle and on the promontory. The fascia is fixed with Gelfoam balls

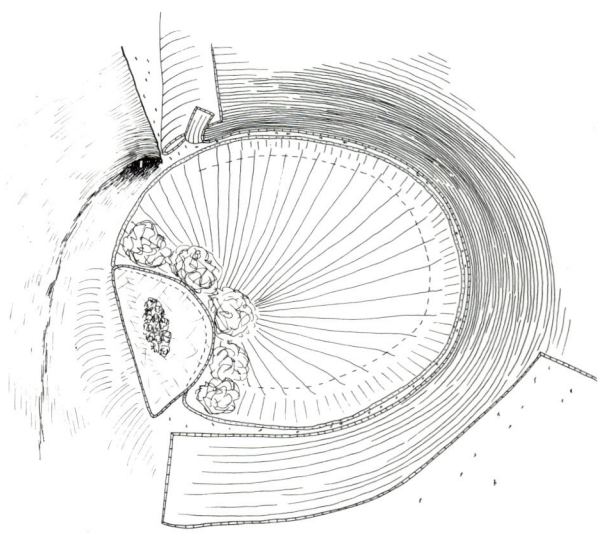

Fig. **1086** A Thiersch flap covers the round-window niche and the footplate. Small Gelfoam balls are placed on the footplate. The posterior skin flap is returned

Type 4 Tympanoplasty

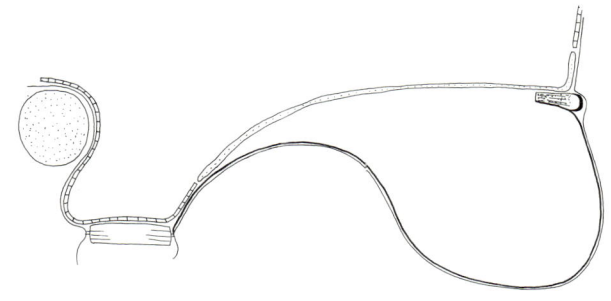

Fig. **1087** Side view of type 4 tympanoplasty with onlay fascia grafting. The fascia is placed on the annulus, the drum remnant, and the promontory. The Thiersch flap covers the facial nerve prominence, the footplate, and the oval window niche

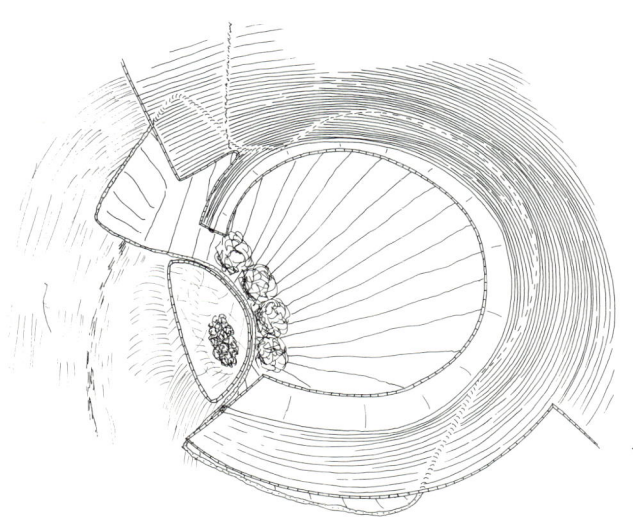

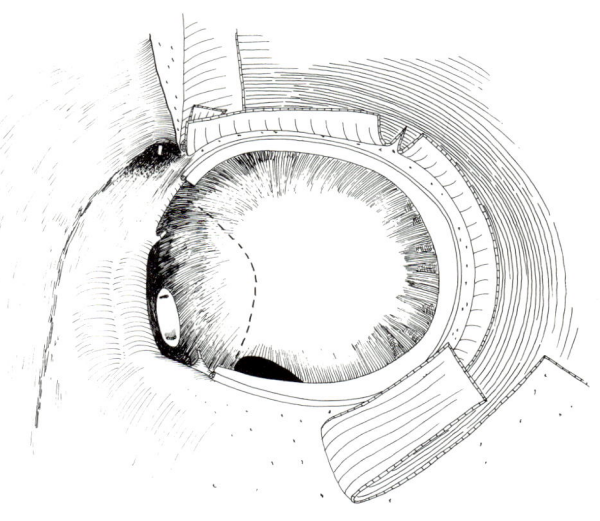

Fig. **1088** Intermediate fascia grafting in a case with canal wall–down mastoidectomy, total perforation, and no ossicles. The epithelium from the drum remnant and the annulus, as well as the skin, are elevated outward. The dotted line indicates the border for removal of the middle-ear mucosa around the oval-window niche

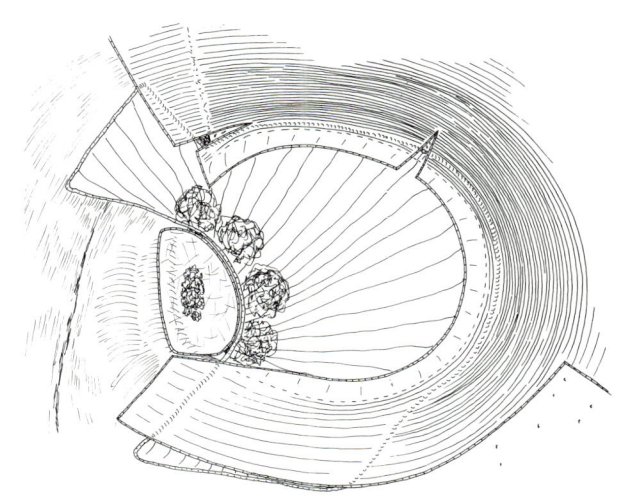

Fig. **1089** The fascia is placed on the drum remnant and the annulus, as well as on the denuded bone all the way round the annulus. The skin flaps are replaced. Superiorly, the fascia is fixed to the promontory. A Thiersch flap is placed on the footplate, the oval-window niche, and the facial prominence

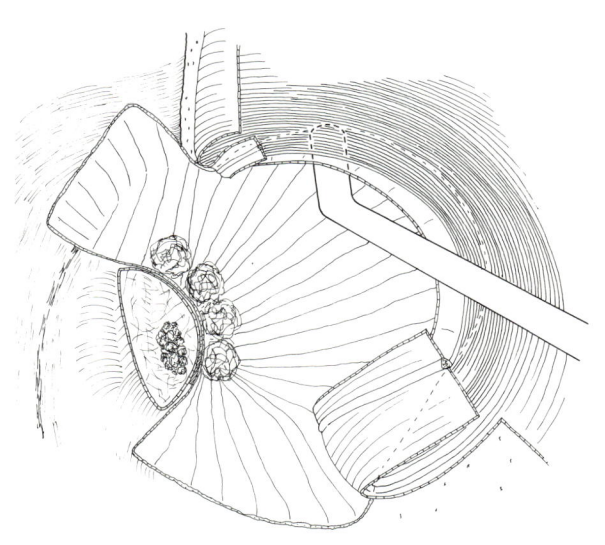

Fig. **1090** Type 4 tympanoplasty in a case with canal wall–down mastoidectomy, total perforation, and no ossicles, with underlay grafting of the fascia. The fascia is placed under the annulus and adapted to the denuded bone. Superiorly, the fascia is placed on the attic wall and on the promontory. A Thiersch flap covers the oval-window niche and the facial nerve prominence

◁ Fig. **1091** The epithelial flaps are replaced. The Thiersch flaps and the fascia are fixed with Gelfoam balls

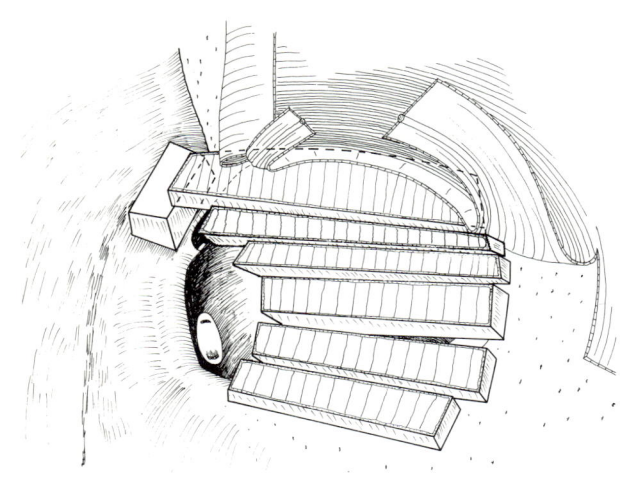

Fig. 1092 **The Heermann type 4 tympanoplasty technique** in a case with canal wall–down mastoidectomy, total perforation, and no ossicles. The ear-canal skin and the annulus are elevated. A piece of cartilage palisade is placed on the prominence of the tensor tympani muscle—an architrave. The most anterior palisade is placed underneath the bony annulus and on top of the architrave, and the subsequent cartilage palisades are placed inferiorly on the bony annulus and superiorly on the promontory

4) *The Heermann cartilage palisades technique.* As in the palisade myringoplasty technique (Figs. **627–633**), the most anterior palisade is placed under the bony annulus. A small piece of cartilage—an architrave—lies on the prominence or the tensor tympani muscle. The most anterior palisade is placed on the architrave. The following palisades are placed on the inferior bony annulus and the denuded part of the promontory, leaving the oval window niche open (Fig. **1092**). The epithelial flaps are replaced. Heermann (1991) does not carry out any additional covering of the cartilage palisades. The perichondrium left on the palisades should be enough to close the small holes between them.

Proctor (1969), analyzing the results of type 4 tympanoplasty in a total of 206 consecutive cases, found the average preoperative hearing to be 47.1 dB, with the postoperative hearing 43.3 dB. Social hearing at the 35-dB level was obtained in 33.5% of the patients. Hearing was improved by 10 dB or more in 37%, and deteriorated by 10 dB or more in 18%. The reason why treatment failed to provide patients with satisfactory were: hearing 1) inadequate Eustachian tube function; 2) a stiff annular ligament, causing inadequate mobility of the footplate; 3) insufficient mucosa in the hypotympanum in the round window niche; 5) reperforation of the tympanic membrane; 6) recurrent cholesteatoma; and 7) persistent suppuration. Compared with a radical operation with no reconstruction, the results of type 4 tympanoplasty were satisfactory.

The present author's experience in cholesteatoma treatment (Tos 1982) shows that type 4 tympanoplasty produced stable results, and the operation should be performed much more often than it is today. This would avoid the many reoperations that are necessary after unsuccessful columella techniques, which ultimately, in many cases, do not offer patients any hearing improvement.

Type 5 Tympanoplasty

Tympanoplasty type 5 is divided into types A and B (Figs. **686, 687**). Type A indicates fenestration of the lateral semicircular canal, which is today an extremely rare operation in otosclerosis surgery. Following previous radical surgery and fixation of the footplate, type 5 A tympanoplasty with fenestration of the lateral semicircular canal is also performed extremely rarely, if at all. The third indication is congenital atresia combined with severe deformities in the middle ear, but today a bone-anchored hearing aid is inserted in such cases instead of using a fenestration.

Type 5 A Tympanoplasty Techniques

The techniques of fenestration have been thoroughly described elsewhere (e.g., Shambaugh and Glasscock 1980, Wullstein and Wullstein 1990). The operation only will be mentioned briefly here.

After a previous radical operation and when the footplate is fixed, the skin incision goes over the facial ridge and around the lateral semicircular canal. The large tympanomeatal flap is elevated, exposing the entire lateral semicircular canal and the facial nerve (Fig. **1093**). The exact position of the lateral semicircular canal in relation to the facial nerve is determined. Using a diamond drill, the overall surface of the lateral semicircular canal is slightly drilled off, preserving the contours of the canal. Two techniques are used to open the semicircular canal:

1) *The cupula technique.* In this technique, two blue lines are formed along the horizontal canal. The dome of the cupula is left intact, so that it will not become too thin and fracture when the cupula is removed. By polishing with a diamond

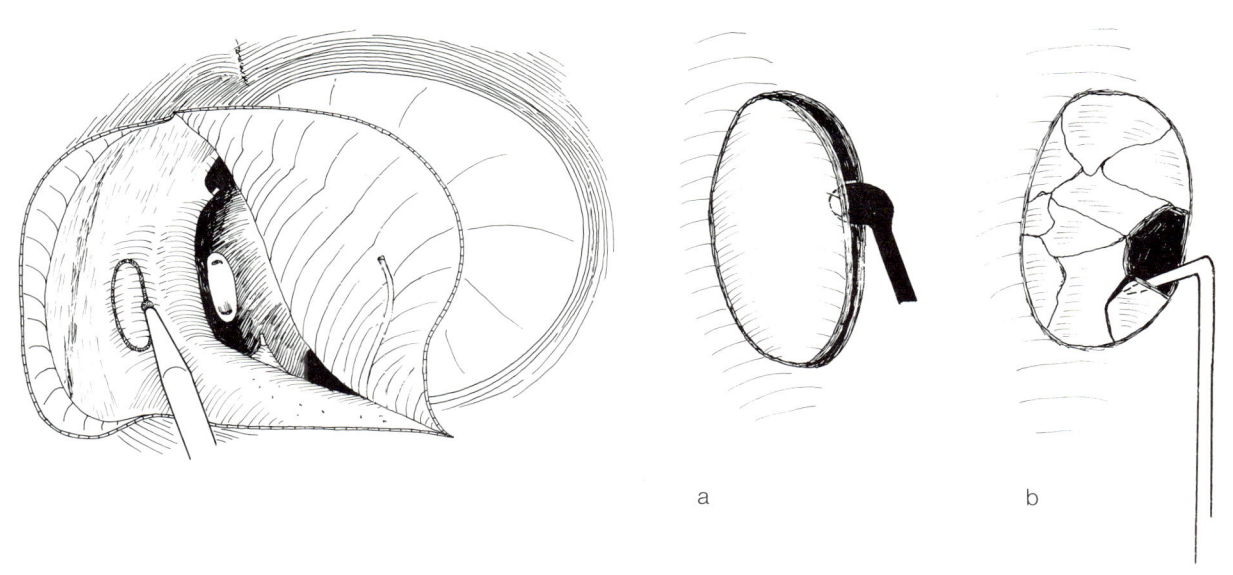

Fig. 1093 Fenestration of the lateral semicircular canal in a case with old radical cavities, and a tympanic cavity with a membrane, fixed footplate, and no ossicles. The tympanomeatal flap, including the epithelium from the attic and aditus, is elevated, and the footplate is exposed. With a small diamond drill, blue lines are drilled at the lateral semicircular canal

Fig. 1094 Fenestration of the lateral semicircular canal. **a** The cupula technique. The dome of the lateral semicircular canal is elevated after the blue lines are drilled around the dome. **b** The eggshell technique. The dome of the lateral semicircular canal is thinned flat, and the bone is removed piece by piece with a hook

burr the blue lines are formed (Fig. **1093**). With a special knife, a fracture is made in the labyrinth at the blue line, and the cupula is gently elevated and snapped off in one piece (Fig. **1094a**).

2) *The morcellation technique.* In the morcellation, or eggshell technique, a distinct cupula is not formed. The bone is removed in fragments after being drilled thin (Fig. **1094b**).

The tympanomeatal flap is returned, and carefully adapted to the operning on the lateral semicircular canal. The tympanomeatal flap is carefully packed around the whole of the lateral semicircular canal to attach the edges of the bone (Fig. **1095**).

Type 5 B Tympanoplasty Techniques

Tympanoplasty type 5 B refers to a stapedectomy in a previous radical cavity with no ossicles and a fixed footplate. Gacek (1973) introduced the term "modified tympanoplasty type 5," but Paparella (1967), Proctor (1969) and Sato (1969) earlier performed stapedectomy in cases with previous radical cavities. Gacek's technique was stapedectomy and filling of the oval-window niche with fatty tissue, as follows. An incision is performed along the posterior ear-canal wall, continuing over the lateral semicircular canal region and the facial nerve prominence (Fig. **1096**). The tympanomeatal flap is ele-

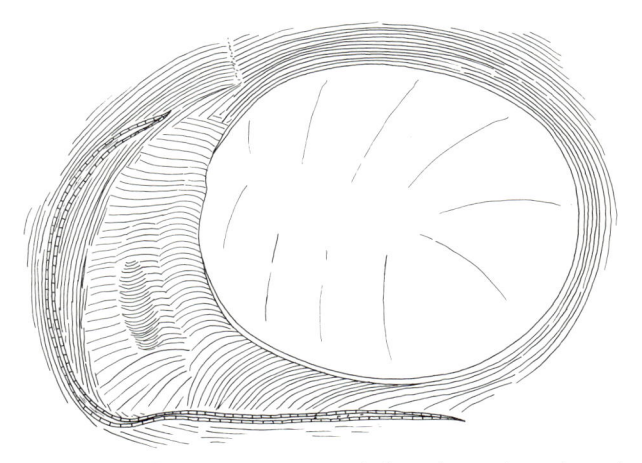

Fig. 1095 The tympanomeatal flap is replaced and carefully adapted around the opening of the lateral semicircular canal. It is packed with Gelfoam balls

vated, exposing the oval-window niche and the fixed footplate (Fig. **1097**). With a perforator, a hole is made in the center of the footplate, which is fractured, with the posterior and anterior halves being removed using a small hook. After the stapedectomy is complete the oval-window niche is filled with fatty tissue (Fig. **1098**). The tympanomeatal flap is returned and fixed with Gelfoam balls (Fig. **1099**).

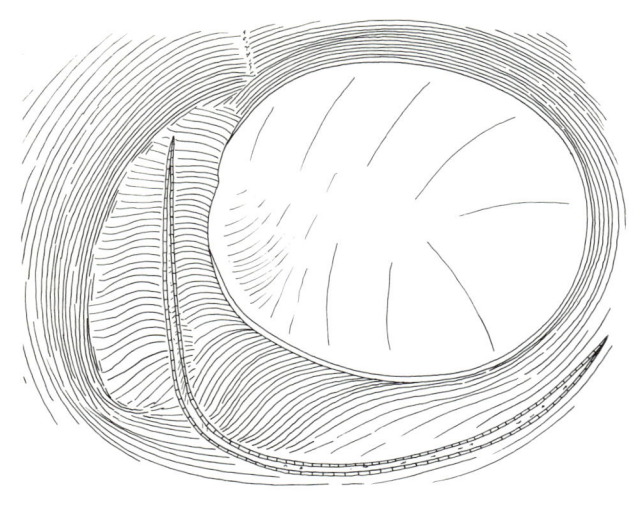

Fig. **1096** The incision for a type 5B tympanoplasty in a case with an old radical cavity, no ossicles, and a fixed footplate. The skin incision is made in the posterior ear canal over the # and lateral semicircular canal region

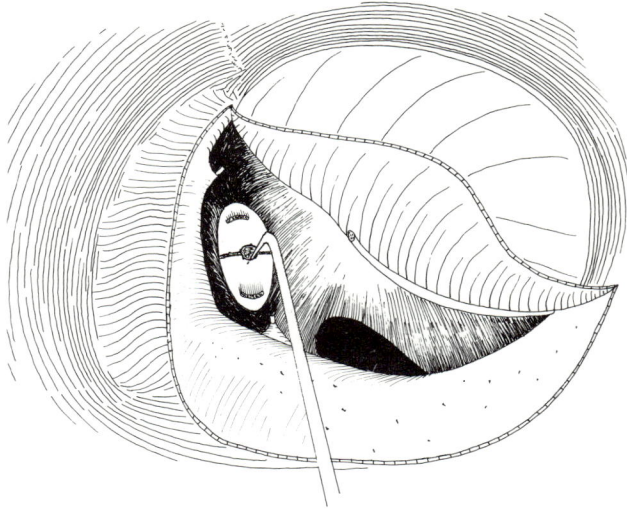

Fig. **1097** The tympanomeatal flap is elevated, and the footplate is exposed. A hole and a fracture are performed in the middle of the footplate, and the posterior half of the footplate is elevated

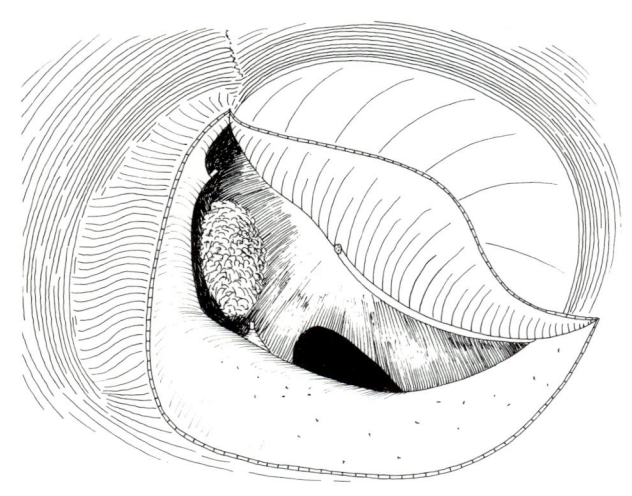

Fig. **1098** After stapedectomy, the round-window niche is filled with fatty tissue

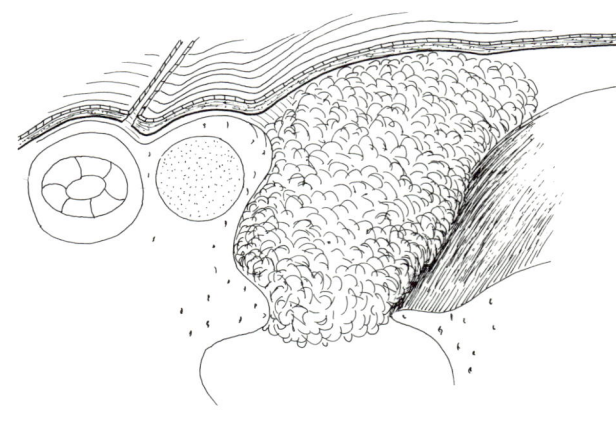

Fig. **1099** Side view of the round-window niche filled with fatty tissue. The epithelial membrane is replaced on the facial prominence

An alternative to Gacek's technique is to place an allogenous stapes onto a fascia (Fig. **1100**). In the same situation, with a radical cavity and a fixed footplate, the incision is made in the same way as shown in Figures **1096** and **1097**. After stapedectomy, a fascia, vein, or perichondrium covers the oval-window niche. An allogenous stapes with its footplate directed towards the drum is placed on the fascia. The niche is filled with Gelfoam, stabilizing the stapes and the fascia. The tympanomeatal flap is returned. In this situation, the footplate of the allogenous stapes is higher than the facial nerve prominence, and cannot fall into the vestibulum, but the packing should be done carefully, avoiding pressure on the drum. The author has used this method several times, with good functional results.

In another method of rebuilding an old radical cavity, the stapedectomy can be performed during a second stage. In the first stage, the tympanic cavity is reconstructed, the allogenous stapes is positioned, and an allogenous incus or a piece of tragal cartilage is placed on top of the stapes (Fig. **1101**). In the second stage, the footplate is removed, and the oval-window niche is covered with fascia. The allogenous stapes and incus are in place, and there is no risk that they will protrude into the vestibulum. If there is any risk of pressure on the vestibulum, the implanted incus can be removed, with only the stapes being be interposed, as shown in Figure **1100**.

Several other methods of rebuilding the tympanic cavity in the first stage and then performing stapedectomy in a second stage have been described in cases with previous radical cavity, no ossicles, and fixation of the footplate. These methods may also be classified as type 5 B tympanoplasty.

After conservative radical surgery with the malleus handle preserved and a fixed footplate, an incus replacement prosthesis (IRP) with stainless-steel wire can be inserted (Fig. **1102**). After removal of the footplate, the oval window is covered with fascia, and the IRP prosthesis is mounted on the malleus handle, as shown above Figs. **1063–1065**). This procedure is usually performed in canal wall–up mastoidectomy surgery. In canal wall–down mastoidectomy procedures, platinectomy can be performed in the second stage, and the steel-wire prosthesis can be mounted on the malleus handle during the first stage.

All methods of reconstructing the malleus handle can be included in the stapedotomy and stapedectomy procedures in cases with conservative radical surgery and a fixed stapes or footplate. These methods include transplantation of the drum–malleus allograft (Figs. **960, 961**), reconstruction of the malleus (Figs. **963–967**), and creation of a compound fascia–malleus graft, as described by Schiller (1979) (Figs. **968–973**).

There is a simple method of stapedectomy and reconstruction of the malleus using a cartilage palisade, as follows (Fig. **1103**). The tympanic cavity is opened, as indicated previously, by an incision over the ## and the facial nerve prominence. A piece of tragal cartilage is placed on the facial nerve prominence to increase the height of the tympanic cavity. Another tragal cartilage palisade is placed on the promontory and on the cartilage lying on the facial prominence. This cartilage functions as a malleus handle. After stapedectomy, a Schuknecht prosthesis with wire and fibrous tissue is used. It is placed in the oval-window niche, and the wire is tightened around the cartilage palisade (Fig. **1103**). The tympanomeatal graft is replaced. If the flap is

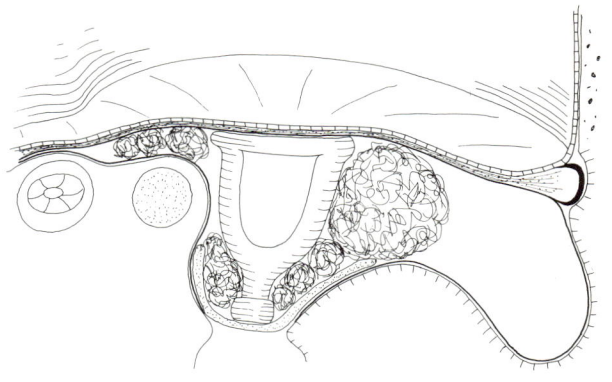

Fig. **1100** After stapedectomy, the niche is covered with fascia, and an allogenous stapes is placed between the fascia and the retracted drum, which is placed on the facial prominence in a case after canal wall–down mastoidectomy, with no ossicles and a fixed footplate

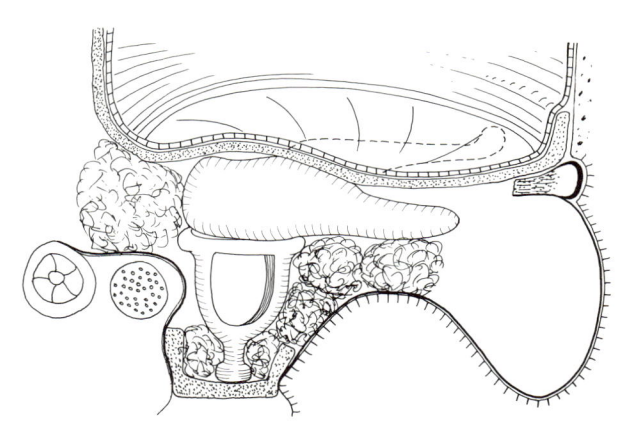

Fig. **1101** The stapes–incus assembly in a case with a rebuilt middle ear after a previous canal wall–down mastoidectomy, with no ossicles and a fixed footplate. The footplate is removed, and the oval-window niche is covered with fascia. The allogenous stapes is supported with Gelfoam balls

too short due to the placement of cartilage blocks in the attic, it can be strengthened by a fascia.

Many possibilities are still open in reconstructing the drum with the malleus handle, preparing for a stapedotomy or stapedectomy at a second stage. Among these are the new techniques practiced by Fisch, performing stapedotomy in apparently hopeless cases with chronic otitis media, after rebuilding a tympanic cavity, the drum, and the malleus in two stages.

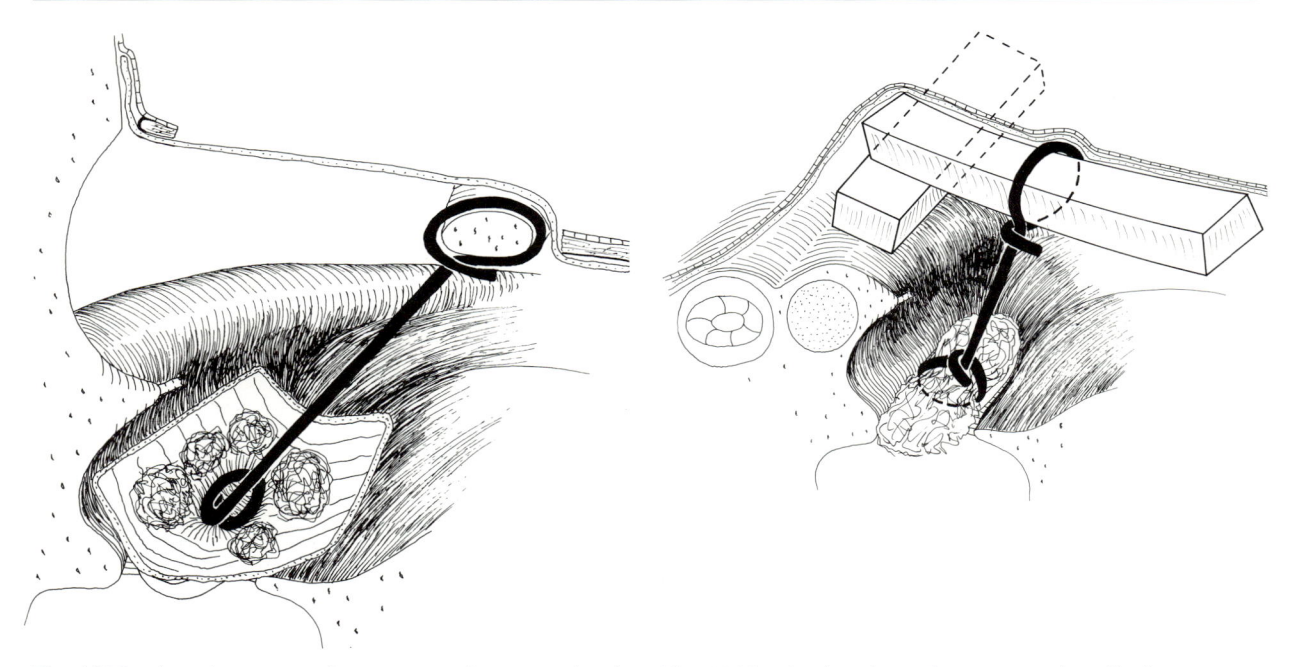

Fig. 1102 An incus replacement wire prosthesis mounted on the malleus handle, connecting the fascia covering in the oval-window niche with the malleus after stapedectomy. Small pieces of Gelfoam secure the anchorage of the prosthesis to the fascia

Fig. 1103 A situation after a canal wall–down mastoidectomy, with no ossicles and a fixed footplate. A platinectomy has been performed, and a Schuhknecht prosthesis is fixed to a cartilage palisade placed on the promontory and onto another piece of cartilage lying on the facial prominence. A membrane covering the tympanic cavity is strengthened with an underlay fascia graft

Packing the Ear Canal and the Cavity

The ear canal should be packed with Gelfoam balls moistened with antibiotics (ampicillin, tetracycline, or both). All the skin flaps and the fascia are fixed carefully with Gelfoam balls. After a layer of Gelfoam balls has been placed, small pieces of gauze moistened with a hydrocortisone–terramycin cream, are introduced. The pieces of gauze are 1–2 cm long, and form the second layer of packing. The last packing procedure in the ear canal involves using a long gauze moistened with the same cream to fill out the rest of the ear canal.

The packing is changed after three weeks, and patients are usually discharged one of two days after the operation. They return after a week for removal of the stitches, and on the 21st postoperative day, all the gauze is removed, although the Gelfoam balls are left in place. After the gauze has been removed, the Gelfoam balls out, and they are removed after about 14 days. At this point, the first audiogram test is carried out. The patient is followed up on an outpatient basis, with regular checkups 1, 3, 6, and 12 months after the operation. For research purposes, patients continue to receive follow-up attention after this as well, with regular re-evaluations.

References

Amedee RG, Mann WJ, Riechelmann H. Cartilage palisade tympanoplasty. Am J Otol 1989;10:447–50.

Andersen HC, Jepsen O, Ratjen E. Ossicular chain defects: prognosis and treatment. Acta Otolaryngol 1962;54(5):393–402.

Applebaum EL. Incudostapedial joint prosthesis, 1990 Catalog supplement, Smith & Nephew. Minneapolis: Richards Company, 1990.

Austin DF. Ossicular reconstruction. Arch Otolaryngol 1971;94:525–35.

Babighian G. Use of a glass inomer cement in otological surgery. J Laryngol Otol 1992;106:1–6.

Bailey HA. Methods of reconstruction in tympanoplasty, 2: maintenance of the anterior sulcus–tympanic membrane relationships in tympanoplastic surgery. Laryngoscope 1976;86:179–84.

Bauer M. Bone autograft for ossicular reconstruction. Arch Otolaryngol 1966;83:335–8.

Bauer M. Polycel–bone composite drum-to-footplate columella. Otolaryngol Head Neck Surg 1988;98:305–9.

Bellucci RJ. Tympanoplasty: the malleus stapes wire and total defect skin graft. Laryngoscope 1966;76:1439.

Bellucci RJ. Basic considerations for success in tympanoplasty. Arch Otolaryngol 1969;90:732–41.

Bellucci RJ. Dual classification of tympanoplasty. Laryngoscope 1973;83:1754–8.

Bennet RJ. Observations on drumhead repair in tympanoplastic surgery. J Laryngol 1971;85:745–72.

Betow K. Transplantationen von Trommelfell und Gehörknöchelkette. Klinische Erfahrungen bei der Verwendung von Homotransplantaten bei Tympanoplastiken. Berlin: de Gruyter 1970.

Birch DA. Preliminary communication: myringoplasty performed with a peritoneum homograft. J Laryngol 1961;75:922–3.

Black B. Development of a new TORP/PORP. J Otolaryngol Soc Austral 1987;6:58–9.

Black B. Design and development of a contoured ossicular replacement prosthesis: clinical trials of 125 cases. Am J Otol 1990;11:85–9.

Bocca E, Cis C, Zernotti E. L'impiego di liber di periostio nella timpanoplastica. Arch Ital Otol 1959;suppl 40:205–11.

Bondy G. Totalaufmeislung mit Erhaltung von Trommelfell und Gehörknöchelchen. Mschr Ohrenheilkd [Vienna] 1910;44:15.

Booth JB. Myringoplasty – factors affecting results: final report. J Laryngol Otol 1973;87:1039–84.

Brandow EC. Homograft tympanic membrane in myringoplasty. Trans Am Acad Ophthalmol Otolaryngol 1969;73:825–35.

Brandow EC. Homograft tympanic membrane myringoplasty. Arch Otolaryngol 1976;102:473–7.

Calcaterra TC. The window shade technique of tympanic membrane grafting. Laryngoscope 1972;82:45–9.

Caparosa R. An atlas of surgical anatomy and techniques of the temporal bone. Springfield: Thomas, 1972.

Chalat NI. Tympanic membrane transplant. Harper Hosp Bull [Detroit] 1964;22:27–34.

Chandler JR. The anterior canal wall bulge: indications and techniques for removal. Laryngoscope 1976;86:185–90.

Charachon R. La tympanoplastie. Presses Universitaires, Grenoble: 1990.

Charachon R, Roulleau P, Bremond G, et al. Les ossiculoplasties: état actuel. Paris: Arnette, 1987.

Claros-Domenech A. Cent tympanoplasties pratiquées à l'aide d'un greffe libre de membrane périostique. Rev Laryngol 1959;80:917.

Cole RA. Ossicular replacement with self-stabilizing presculptured homogenous cartilage. Arch Otolaryngol 1992;1108:561–2.

Cornish CB. Use of freeze-dried aortic valve homografts in aural surgery. Lancet 1965;i:943.

Cornish CB, Scott PJ. Freeze-dried heart valves as tympanic grafts. Arch Otolaryngol 1968;88:350–6.

Deguine C. Les ossiculoplasties: bilan et perspectives. Acta Otorhinolaryngol (Belg.) 1991;45:81–6.

Don A, Linthicum FH. The fate of cartilage grafts for ossicular reconstruction in tympanoplasty. Ann Otol Rhinol Laryngol 1975;84:187–93.

Elbrønd O. Defects of the auditory ossicles in ears with intact tympanic membrane. Acta Otolaryngol (Stockh.) 1970;suppl 264;1–51.

English GM, Hildyard VH, Hemenway WG, Davidson S. Autograft and homograft incus transpositions in chronic otitis media. Laryngoscope 1971;81:1434–47.

Everberg G, Henrichsen J, Gormsen J. Plasma coagulation in myringoplasty and fascialis transplantation. Lancet 1977;i:1257–8.

Everberg G, Gormsen J, Henrichsen J, Tos M. Plasma klot teknik ved myringoplastik. Dansk Otol Selsk Forh 1979/80;33.

Farrior BJ. Tympanoplasty in 3-D. 3 vols. Tampa, FL: American Academy of Ophthalmology and Otolaryngology, 1968.

Fisch U. Tympanoplasty and stapedectomy: a manual of techniques. Stuttgart: Thieme 1990.

Fleury P, Legent F, Lefebre C. Techniques chirurgicales de l'oreille Paris: Masson, 1974.

Forman FS. Corneal grafts in middle ear surgery: a preliminary report. Laryngoscope 1960;70:1691–8.

Frenckner P. Eine Operationsmethode zum plastischen Verschluß von Trommelfellperforationen. Acta Otolaryngol 1955;45:19–24.

Frootko NJ. Applying the language of transplantese to tympanoplasty. Acta Otolaryng (Belg.) 1985;39:374–6.

Gacek R. Results of modified type V tympanoplasty. Laryngoscope 1973;83:437–47.

Garcia-Ibanez E, Estrada O, Montenegro M, Rivas P. La miringoplastica endomeatica. Technica e risultati. Oto-Rino-Laringol 1986;36:27–30.

Gerlach H. Variationen einer Drahtspirale als Schalltransformation bei der Tympanoplastik. Z Laryngol Rhinol Otol 1971;50:543–8.

Gerlach H. Die Stepp-Plastik zur Erhaltung der Trommelfellebene. Arch Ohren Nasen Kehlkopfheilkd. 1972;202:662–6.

Gerlach H. Unsere Erfahrungen mit der Stepp-Plastik bei tympanoplastischen Operationen. Laryngol Rhinol Otol 1975;54:198–9.

Gersdorff MCH, Maisin JP. Hunting E. Comparative study of the clinical results obtained by means of Plasti-Pore and ceramic ossicular prosthesis and bone allografts. Am J Otol 1986;7:294–7.

Geyer G, Helms J. Reconstructive measures in middle ear and mastoid using a biocompatible cement: preliminary clinical experience. In: Heinke G, Soltesz U, Lee AJC, eds. Clinical implant materials. Amsterdam: Elsevier, 1990:529.

Gibb AG, Steward IA. Dentine as a material for ossicular reconstruction in tympanoplasty. Arch Otolaryngol 1972;96:346–9.

Giddings NA, Brackmann DE, Kwartler JA. Transcanal infracochlear approach to the petrous apex. Otolaryngol Head Neck Surg 1991;104:29–36.

Glaninger J, Neuhold R. Eine Methode zur Konservierung menschlicher Gehörknöchelchen. Mschr Ohrenheilkd Laryngol 1968;102:569–77.

Glasscock ME. Tympanic membrane grafting with fascia: overlay vs. undersurface technique. Laryngoscope 1973;83:754–70.

Glasscock ME. Ossicular chain reconstruction. Laryngoscope 1976;86:211–21.

Glasscock ME, House WF. Homograft reconstruction of the middle ear: a preliminary report. Laryngoscope 1968;78:1219–25.

Glasscock ME, Shea MC. Tragal cartilage as an ossicular substitute. Arch Otolaryngol 1967;86:308–17.

Glasscock ME, Sheehy JL. Tympanic membrane grafting with temporalis fascia: a report of four years' experience. Arch Otolaryngol 1967;86:391–402.

Glasscock ME, Jackson CG, Nissen AJ, Schwaber MK. Postauricular undersurface tympanic membrane grafting: a follow-up report. Laryngoscope 1982;92:718–27.

Glasscock ME, Jackson CB, Knox GW. Can acquired immunodeficiency syndrome and Creutzfeldt-Jakob disease be transmitted via otologic homografts? Arch Otolaryngol Head Neck Surg 1988;114:1252–5.

Goldenberg RA. Hydroxyapatite ossicular replacement prostheses: preliminary results. Laryngoscope 1990;100:693–700.

Goldenberg RA. Hydroxyapatite ossicular replacement prostheses: a four-year experience. Otolaryngol Head Neck Surg 1992;106:261–9.

Goodhill V. Tragal perichondrium oval window graft. Laryngoscope 1961;71:975–83.

Goodhill V. Tragal perichondrium and cartilage in tympanoplasty. Arch Otolaryngol 1967;85:480–91.

Goodhill V. Ear deseases, deafness and dizziness. New York: Harper and Row, 1978.

Goodhill V, Harris I, Brockman SJ. Tympanoplasty with perichondrial graft. Arch Otolaryngol 1964;79:131–7.

Gristwood RE. Riveting techniques in the grafting of tympanic membrane defects. J Otolaryng Soc Austral 1977;4:143–4.

Grote JJ. Long-term results with hydroxyapatite implants in ossiculoplasty. In: Tos M, Thomsen J, Peitersen E, eds. Cholesteatoma and mastoid Surgery. Amsterdam: Kugler, 1989:1178–81.

Grote JJ, Van Blitterswijk CA. Reconstruction of the posterior auditory canal wall with a hydroxypatite prosthesis. Ann Otol Rhinol Laryngol 1986;95(suppl 123):6–9.

Guilford FR. Tympanoplasty: use of prosthesis in conduction mechanism. Arch Otolaryngol 1964;80:80–6.

Guilford FR. Repositioning of the incus. Laryngoscope 1965;75:136–242.

Gundersen T. Reconstruction of the ossicular chain by incus prosthesis: a preliminary report. Acta Otolaryngol 1964;58:227–9.

Hall A, Rytzner C. Stapedectomy and auto-transplantation of ossicles. Acta Otolaryngol 1957;47:318–24.

Hall A, Rytzner C. Malleus–stapes transposition. Pract Oto-Rhino-Laryngol 1959;21:316–22.

Hamberger CA, Liden G. Transmeatale Myringostapediopexie bei Unterbrechung der Gehörknöchelchenkette. Arch Ohren Nasen Kehlkopfheilkd 1958;173:390.

Harrison WH. Prosthetics in tympanoplasty. Arch Otolaryngol 1960;71:437–42.

Harrison WH. Prosthesis versus patient's tissue in ossicular reconstruction. Laryngoscope 1969;79:60–84.

Heermann H. Trommelfellplastik mit Fasciengewebe von Musculus Temporalis nach Begradigung der vorderen Gehörgangswand. HNO 1961;9:136–7.

Heermann J. Surgery of the oval window in otosclerosis. J Laryngol Otol 1963;42:699–708.

Heermann J. Thirty years' autograft tragal and conchal cartilage perichondrium palisade tympanum-epitympanum-, antrum and mastoid plasties–13 000 cases. In: Charachon R, Garcia-Ibanez E, eds. Long-term results and indications in otology and otoneurosurgery. Amsterdam: Kugler,1991:159–64.

Heermann H, Heermann J. Endaurale Chirurgie/Endaural surgery. Munich: Urban & Schwarzenberg, 1964.

Heermann J, Heermann H, Kopstein E. Fascia and cartilage palisade tympanoplasty: nine years' experience. Arch Otolaryngol 1970;91:228–41.

Hildmann H, Steinbach E. Experimentelle Untersuchungen zur Verträglichkeit von Fascientransplantaten. Arch Ohren Nasen Kehlkopfheilkd 1970;196:133–6.

Hildmann H, Karger B, Steinbach E. Ossikeltransplantate zur Rekonstruktion der Schallübertragung im Mittelohr. Eine histologische Langzeituntersuchung. Laryngol Rhinol Otol 1992;71:5–10.

Holewinski J. A trial of covering the tympanic membrane with a corneal graft (preliminary report). Otolaryngol Pol 1958;12:349–50.

Hough JVD. Incudo-stapedial joint separation, etiology, treatment and significance. Laryngoscope 1959;69:644–64.

Hyldyard VH, English GM, De Blanc BG, et al. Stapes homograft: a report of four human cases. Arch Otolaryngol 1968;88:55–62.

Hüttenbrink KB. Die Mechanik und Funktion des Mittelohres, 2: Hörphysiologische Anmerkungen zu Mittelohroperationen. Laryngol Rhinol Otol 1992 a;71:552–7.

Hüttenbrink KB. Vorschläge zur Verbesserung der akustischen Qualität von Mittelohrprothesen. Arch Otorhinolaryngol 1992 b;(suppl 2):328–9.

Högset O, Bredberg G. Plaster of Paris. thermal properties and biocompatibility. A study of an alternative implant material for ear surgery. Acta Otolaryngol 1986;101:445–52.

Jackson GC, Glasscock ME, Schwaber MK, Nissen AJ, Christiansen SG, Smith PG. Ossicular chain reconstruction: the TORP and PORP in chronic ear disease. Laryngoscope 1983;93:981–6.

Jahnke K. Advances in middle ear surgery. Adv Otorhinolaryngol 1988;39:65–82.

Jahnke K. Neue Keramik-Implantate zur Rekonstruktion der Gehörknöchelchenkette. Laryngol Rhinol Otol 1992;71:1–4.

Jahnke K, Plester D. Praktische Hinweise zur Anwendung von Mittelohr-Implantaten aus Aluminiumoxid-Keramik. HNO 1980;28:115–18.

Jahnke K, Plester D. Bioinert ceramic implants in middle ear surgery. Ann Otol Rhinol Laryngol 1991;90:640–2.

Jahnke K, Swan IRC. Bioinert ceramic for ossicular chain reconstruction. In: Charachon R, Garcia-Ibanez E, eds. Long-term results and indications in otology and otoneurosurgery. Amsterdam: Kugler, 1991:197–201.

Jahnke K, Plester D, Heimke G. Aluminiumoxid-Keramik, ein bioinertes Material für die Mittelohrchirurgie. Arch Otorhinolaryngol 1979;223:373–6.

Jansen C. Die Erhaltung des äußeren Gehörganges bei der Radikaloperation und eine neue Art der Tympanoplastik. Zbl HNO 1962;74:36.

Jansen C. Cartilage tympanoplasty. Laryngoscope 1963; 73:1288–1302.

Jansen C. Homo- and heterogenous graft in reconstruction of the sound conduction system. Acta Oto-Rhino-Laryngol (Belg.) 24 1970;24:60–5.

Jongkees LB. Surgery of the mastoid and the petrous apex and of the intratemporal part of the facial nerve. In: Naumann HH, ed. Head and neck surgery, vol. 3; Ear. Stuttgart: Thieme, 1982:113–70.

Juers AL. Preservation of hearing in surgery for chronic ear disease. Laryngoscope 1954;64:235.

Juers AL. Myringostapediopexy. Arch Otolaryngol 1960;71:376–9.

Kartush IM. Kartush incus: stapes strut prosthesis. 1989 Catalog supplement, Smith & Nephew. Minneapolis: Richards Company, 1989.

Keller AP. Maintenance of the drumhead in tympanoplasty. Laryngoscope 1976;86:196–8.

Kley W. Fortschritte auf dem Gebiet der Hörverbesserung: Zur Tympanoplastik. Mschr Ohrenheilkd 1964;98:385–97.

Kley W. Frakturen und Luxationen der Gehörknöchelchenkette bei Schläfenbeinfrakturen. Z Laryngol Rhinol 1966;45:292–313.

Kley W. Surgical treatment of chronic otitis media and its immediate consequences. In: Naumann HH, ed. Head and neck surgery, vol. 3: Ear. Stuttgart: Thieme, 1982:171–265.

Kobrak HG. The middle ear. Chicago: University of Chicago Press, 1959.

Körner O. Über Gehörplastik, 3. Verh Dtsch Otol Ges 1894;1:110–25.

Körner O. Die eitrigen Erkrankungen des Schläfenbeins. Wiesbaden, Germany: Bergmann, 1899.

Krumpholz K. Tympanoplastik mit bindegewebigen Dobbeltransplantat. Mschr Ohrenheilkd 1969;103:413.

Kup W. Die 3-Schichten Plastik des Trommelfells unter Verwendung eines Hilfsimplantates aus lyophilisierter Dura. Arch Ohren Nasen Kehlkopfheilkd 1967;188:593–603.

Larsen P., Tos M. Ear polyps in posterior superior retraction pockets, Herodion. ORL 1992;54:328–33.

Lesinski SG. Homograft tympanoplasty in perspective. Laryngoscope 1983;93(suppl 32):1–37.

Lempert J. Fenestra nova ovalis: a new oval window for the improvement of hearing in cases of otosclerosis. Arch Otolaryngol 1941;34:880.

Maffei G, Zini C. Trapianti e impianti in otorinolaringoiatria. Sassari: Gallizzi, 1972.

Magnan J. Le cholestéatome (notions actuelles) [dissertation.] Marseilles: Universitiy of Marseilles, 1972.

Magnan J. [Personal communication] 1992.

Marquet J. Reconstructive microsurgery of the eardrum by means of a tympanic membrane homograft. Acta Otolaryngol 1966;62:459–64.

Marquet J. Human middle ear transplants. J Otolaryngol Otol 1971;85:523–39.

Matte U. Über Versuche mit Anheilung des Trommelfells an das Köpfchen des Steigbügels nach operativer Behandlung chronischer Mittelohreiterungen. Arch Ohrenheilkd 1901;53:96–9.

Mehmke S. Neue Wege der Tympanoplastik. Acta Otolaryngol 1961;61:23–34.

Miglets AW. Paparella MM, Saunders HN. Atlas of ear surgery. St. Louis: Mosby, 1986.

Miodonski J. Collumellisatio et mobilisatio ossiculorum auris mediae. Otolaryng Pol 1956;10:223–33.

Moon CN. Ossicular reconstruction in tympanoplasty: mobile stapes without crural arches, fixed stapes with and without crural arches. Laryngoscope 1976;86:223–36.

Morimitsu T. Illustrated ear surgery. Tokyo: Medical Illustration Co., 1991.

Nelson RA. Temporal bone surgical dissection manual. Los Angeles: House Ear Institute, 1983.

Nickel AL. The use of homologous vein grafts in otolaryngology. Laryngoscope 1963;73:919–25.

Oppenheimer P, Harrison WH. The missing lenticular process. Arch Otolaryngol 1963;78:143–50.

Ørtegren U. Trumhinneplastik. Forhandlinger i Svensk Otolaryngol Förening 1958–59.

Ørtegren U. Trumhinneplastik med fascia [dissertation.] Lund: University of Lund 1964.

Ørtegren U. Myringoplasty. Acta Otolaryngol (Stockh.) 1964;(suppl 139):1

Overbosch HC. Homograft myringoplasty with micro-sliced septal cartilage. Proc Otorhinolaryngol 1971;33:356–7.

Panse R. Stacke's Operationsmethode zur Freilegung der Mittelohrräume während des ersten Jahres ihrer Anwendung in der Ohrenklinik zu Halle. Arch Ohrenheilkd 1893;34:257.

Panis R, Haid T, Scheele J. Die Anwendung eines Fibriklebers zur Rekonstruktion der hinteren Gehörgangswand. Z Laryngol Rhinol 1978;58:400–3.

Panis R, Rettinger G. Verschluß von kleiner Rezidivperforation nach Tympanoplastik mit einem neuen Fibrinklebstoff. HNO 1979;27:413–15.

Palva T. Reconstruction of ear canal in surgery for chronic ear. Arch Otolaryngol 1962;75:329–34.

Palva T. A new approach to radical surgery of the chronic otitis media. Pract Otorhinolaryngol 1962;24:372–82.

Palva T. Reconstruction of ear canal and middle ear in chronic otitis. Acta Otolaryngol 1963;(suppl 188):228.

Palva T. Middle ear surgery in Northern Europe. Arch Otolaryngol 1963;78:363–70.

Palva T. Surgery of chronic ear without cavity: results in 130 cases with musculoperiosteal flap and fasciotympanoplasty. Arch Otolaryngol 1963;77:570–80.

Palva T. Surgery of the chronic ear. Eye Ear Nose Throat 1969;48:16–22.

Palva T, Palva A, Kärjä J. Myringoplasty. Ann Otol Rhinol Laryngol 1969;78:1074–80.

Palva T, Palva A, Kärjä J. Results with 2- or 3-legged wire columellization in chronic ear surgery. Ann Otol Rhinol Laryngol 1971;80:760–5.

Palva T, Ylikoski J, Mäkinen J. Use of lyophilized dura in aural surgery. Otorhinolaryngology 1978;40:129–38.

Paparella M. Management of the ossicles in tympanoplasty: consideration of techniques. Acta Otolaryngol 1967;65:81–92.

Passali D, Livi W. [Personal communication.] 1993.

Paulsen K. Einführung in die rekonstruktive Mikrochirurgie des Mittel- und Innenohres. Stuttgart: Schattauer, 1974.

Pennington CL. Fascia graft myringostapediopexy. Laryngoscope 1966;76:1459–73.

Pennington CL. Incus interposition techniques. Ann Otol Rhinol Laryngol 1973;82:516–31.

Pfaltz CR. Piffko P. Substitution of the stapedial arch by free cartilage grafts. Arch Otolaryngol 1968;87:24–33.

Pfaltz CR, Pfaltz R, Schmidt P. Reconstructive surgery in chronic otitis media: statistical analyzing of long-term results. Otorhinolaryngology 1975;37:257–70.

Péré P. Erfahrungen mit der Palisadentechnik zum Trommelfellverschluß. Z Laryngol Rhinol Otol 1989;68:569–70.

Perkins R. Homograft tympanic membrane with suture sling. Laryngoscope 1970;80:1100–7.

Plester D. Skin and mucous membrane grafts in middle ear surgery. Arch Otolaryngol 1960;72:718–21.

Plester D. Myringoplasty methods. Arch Otolaryngol 1963;78:310–16.

Plester D, Hildmann H, Steinbach E. Atlas der Ohrchirurgie. Stuttgart: Kohlhammer, 1989.

Popper O. Periosteal flap grafts in mastoid operations. Afr Med J 1935;9:77.

Portmann M. Tympanoplasty. Arch Otolaryngol 1963;78:2–19.

Portmann M. The ear and temporal bone. New York: Masson, 1979.

Preobrazhenski YB. The employment of preserved dura mater grafts in tympanoplasty. Vestn Otorinolaringol 1961;23:60.

Proctor B. Some observations on types III and IV tympanoplasty. Otolaryngol Clin N Am 1969;16:107–30.

Pulec JL, Sheehy JL. Ossicular chain reconstruction. Laryngoscope 1973;83:448–65.

Pusalkar AG, Steinbach E. Gold implants in middle ear reconstruction surgery. In: Yanagihara N, Suzuki J, eds. Transplants and implants in otology, vol. 2. Amsterdam: Kugler, 1991:111–13.

Reck R. Bioactive glass ceramic in ear surgery: animal experiments and clinical results. Laryngoscope 1984;94:(suppl 33)1–54.

Reck R. Clinical findings in cholesteatomatous surgery. In: Tos M, Thomsen J, Peitersen E, eds. Cholesteatoma and mastoid surgery. Amsterdam: Kugler, 1989:1169–81.

Ringenberg JC. Fat graft tympanoplasty. Laryngoscope 1962;72:188–92.

Rosen S. Mobilization of the stapes to restore hearing. N Y J Med 1953;53:2650.

Roulleau P, Gomulinski L. François M. Les tympanoplasties. Paris: Wagram, 1984.

Rubinstein M, Sadé J, Korine E. Malleolostapedial transposition in middle ear surgery. Arch Otolaryngol 1962;76:323–8.

Sadé J. Secretory otitis media and its sequelae. Edinburgh: Churchill Livingstone, 1979.

Sadé J. Ossiculoplasty bone and couplers. In: Babighian G, Vedman JE, eds. Transplants and implants in otology. Amsterdam: Kugler, 1987:119–28.

Sadé J, Berco E. Atelectasis and secretory otitis media. Ann Otol Rhinol Laryngol 1976;85(suppl 25):66–72.

Sale CS. Myringoplasty with subcutaneous tissue graft. Arch Otolaryngol 1969;89:494–8.

Salen B. Myringoplasty using septum cartilage. Acta Otolaryngol 1963;(suppl 188):82–91.

Sanna M, Gamoletti R, Magnani M, Bacciu S, Zini C. Enhanced biofunctionality of Plasti-Pore ossicular prosthesis with the use of homologous cartilage. Am Otol 1982;4:138–41.

Saraceno AC, Gray WC, Blanchard CL. Use of tragal cartilage with the total ossicular replacement prosthesis. Arch Otolaryngol 1978;104:213–14.

Sato R. Type IV tympanoplasty: results after stapedectomy. Acta Otolaryngol 1969;70:248–53.

Saunders WH, Paparella MM. Atlas of ear surgery. St. Louis: Mosby, 1971.

Schiller A. Middle ear reconstruction by malleo-myringoplasty. J Laryngol Otol 1979;93:1063–73.

Schobel H. Probleme der Wiederherstellungschirurgie nach Otitis media. Mschr Ohrenheilkd 1965;99:503–12.

Schobel H. Personal experience in the development of ossiculoplasty. In: Nakano K, ed. Cholesteatoma and mastoid surgery. Amsterdam: Kugler, 1993.

Schuring AG, Lippy WH, Ziv M. An incus replacement prosthesis: the ossicle cup. Arch Otolaryngol 1978;104:439–41.

Shambaugh G, Glasscock ME. Surgery of the ear. 3rd ed. Philadelphia: Saunders, 1980.

Shea C, Glasscock ME. Tragal cartilage as an ossicular substitute. Arch Otolaryngol 1967;80:308–17.

Shea JJ, Jr. Fenestration of oval window. Ann Otol Rhinol Laryngol 1958;67:932–51.

Shea JJ, Jr. Vein graft closure of eardrum perforations. Arch Otolaryngol 1960;72:445–7.

Shea J. Plastipore ossicular replacement prosthesis. Laryngoscope 1976;86:239–40.

Shea JJ, Emmett JR. Biocompatible ossicular implants. Arch Otolaryngol 1978;104:191–6.

Shea JJ, Homsy CA. The use of Proplast in otologic surgery. Laryngoscope 1974;84:1835–41.

Shea JJ, Moretz WH. Peg tip fixation of Plastipore-TORP. Otolaryngol Head Neck Surg 1989;93:279–80.

Sheehy JL. Tympanic membrane grafting: early and long-term results. Laryngoscope 1964;74:985.

Sheehy JL. Ossicular problems in tympanoplasty. Arch Otolaryngol 1965;81:115–22.

Sheehy JL. The intact canal wall technique in management of aural cholesteatoma. J Laryngol 1970;84:1–31.

Sheehy JL. Tympanoplasty with mastoidectomy: a re-evaluation. Laryngoscope 1970;80:1212–30.

Sheehy JL. Surgery of chronic otitis media. In: English GM. ed. Otolaryngology. Vol. 2 Hagerstown: Harper and Row, 1972:1–86.

Sheehy JL. Surgery for chronic otitis media. In: English, GM. Otolaryngology. 2nd ed. Vol. 1. Philadelphia: Lippincott, 1990:1–86.

Sheehy JL, Glasscock ME. Tympanic membrane grafting with temporalis fascia. Arch Otolaryngol 1967;86:391–402.

Shinkawa A, Sakai M. Ossicular reconstruction with ceramic prosthesis in cholesteatoma surgery. In: Yanagihara N, Suzuki J, eds. Transplants and implants in otology. Amsterdam: Kugler, 1992:117–22.

Siedentop KH, Brown C. Type III polyethylene columella tympanoplasty. Arch Otolaryngol 1966;83:560–5.

Smyth GDL. Chronic ear disease. Edinburgh: Churchill Livingstone, 1980.

Smyth GDL. Five year report on PORPs and TORPs. Arch Otolaryngol Head Neck Surg 1982;90:343–6.

Smyth GDL, Kerr AG. Homologous graft for ossicular reconstruction in tympanoplasty. Laryngoscope 1967;77:330–6.

Smyth GDL, Kerr AG, Goodey RJ. Curent thoughts on combined approach tympanoplasty, 2: Restoration of the sound transformer mechanism. J Laryngol Otol 1971;85:417–30.

Spencer TJ. The use of tragal cartilage in ossicular reconstruction. Laryngoscope 1976;86:224–9.

Stacke L. Über eine Methode der Plastik zur Deckung der bei der operativen Freilegung der Mittelohrräume entlösten Knochenfläche. Verh Dtsch Otol Ges 1895;2:83–91.

Steinbach E, Pusalkar A. Long-term histological fate in ossicular reconstruction. J Laryngol Otol 1981;95:1031–9.

Steinbach E, Karger B, Hildmann H. Zur Verwendung von Knorpeltransplantaten in der Mittelohrchirurgie. Eine histologische Langzeituntersuchung von Knorpelinterponaten. Laryngol Rhinol Otol 1992;71:11–14.

Storrs LA. Myringoplasty with use of fascia graft. Arch Otolaryngol 1961;74:45–9.

Strauss P, Pult P, Kurzeja A, Isselstein M, Mach P. Verbessert Human Fibrinkleber die Ergebnisse der Tympanoplastik? Z Laryngol Rhinol Otol 1984;63:615–17.

Surdille M. New technique in the surgical treatment of severe and progressive deafness from otosclerosis. Bull N Y Acad Med 1937;13:673.

Suzuki JI. Complications of ear surgery, immediate and delayed. In: Alberty PW, Ruben RJ, eds. Otologic medicine and surgery. Vol. 2. Edinburgh: Churchill Livingstone, 1988:1363–87.

Szpunar J. Biological reconstruction of the ossicular chain. Arch Otolaryngol 1967;86:79–307.

Tabb HG. Closure of perforations by vein grafts: a preliminary report of twenty cases. Laryngoscope 1960; 70:271–86.

Tabor JR. Methods of ossiculoplasty. Springfield: Thomas, 1971.

Theissing G, Theissing J. Kurze HNO-Operationslehre für Ärzte und Studierende, Vol. 2 Stuttgart: Thieme, 1975.

Tobeck A. Steigbügel Verstorbener als Steigbügelersatz bei der Otosklerosoperation. Z Laryngol Rhinol Otol 1962;41:31–41.

Tolsdorff P. Perichondrium cartilage composite grafts in tympanoplasty. In: Charachon R, Garcia-Ibanez E, eds. Long-term results and indications in otology and otoneurosurgery. Amsterdam: Kugler, 153–8.

Tos M. Tympanoplastik ved kronisk suppurativ otitis media. Ugeskr Læger 1969;131:1385–92.

Tos M. Kirurgisk behanding af hørendsættelsen. Metoder, resultater og indikationer ved høreforbedrende operationer. Mskr Prakt Læger 1972:51–67.

Tos M. Tympanoplasty in partial defects of the stapedial arch. J Otol Laryngol 1975;89:249–57.

Tos M. Homograft stapes–incus assembly: a new ossiculoplasty. Arch Otolaryngol 1978 a;104:119–21.

Tos M. Homograft stapes in middle ear surgery. Clin Otolaryngol 1978 b;3:263–268.

Tos M. Operative Therapie bei Otitis mit Erhaltung der Hinteren Gehörgangswand (intact wall technique). HNO 1978 c;26:217–23.

Tos M. Pathology of the ossicular chain in various chronic middle ear disease. J Otol Rhinol Laryngol 1979;93:769–80.

Tos M. Obliterative otitis media. J Otol Rhinol Laryngol 1979;93:569–73.

Tos M. Stability of myringoplasty based on late results. Otorhinolaryngology 1980;42:171–81.

Tos M. Relationship between secretory otitis in childhood and chronic otitis and its sequelae in adults. J Laryng Otol 95 1981;95:1011–22.

Tos M. Modification of combined-approach tympanoplasty in attic cholesteatoma. Arch Otolaryngol 1982;108:772–8.

Tos M. Short- and long-term results with ossiculoplasty in cholesteatomatous ears. In: Sadé J, ed. Cholesteatoma and mastoid surgery. Amsterdam: Kugler, 1982:547–58.

Tos M. Sequelae following secretory otitis and their relationship to chronic otitis and cholesteatoma. In: English GM, ed. Otolaryngology, Vol. I. Philadelphia: Lippincott, 1990:1–30.

Tos M, Arndal H. Tympanoplasty in missing malleus handle. Am J Otol [submitted] 1992.

Tos M, Lau T. Long-term hearing results in cholesteatoma. In: Charachon R, Garcia-Ibanez E, eds. Long-term results and indications in otology and otoneurosurgery. Amsterdam: Kugler, 1991:89–94.

Tos M, Lau T. Long-term hearing results of, and indication for, different techniques in cholesteatoma surgery. In: Charachon R, Garcia-Ibanez E, eds. Long-term results and indications in otology and otoneurosurgery. Amsterdam: Kugler, 1991:95–8.

Tos M, Paulsen G. Changes of pars tensa after secretory otitis. Otorhinolaryngol 1979;41:313–28.

Tos M, Thomsen J. Cerebrospinal fluid leak after translabyrinthine surgery for acoustic neuromas. Laryngoscope 1985;95:351–4.

Tos M, Lau T, Plate S. Sensorineural hearing loss following chronic ear surgery. Ann Otol Rhinol Laryngol 1984;93:403–9.

Tos M, Stangerup SE, Holm-Jensen S, Sørensen CH. Spontaneous course of secretory otitis and changes of the ear drum. Arch Otolaryngol 1984;110:281–9.

Tos M, Everberg G, Henrichsen J. Autologous tissue seal in myringoplasty. Laryngoscope 1987;97:370–1.

Trombetta A. Perforations of tympanic membrane and tympanoplasty: closure by pericardium–a preliminary report of 9 cases. Arch Otolaryngol 1963;77:81–4.

Turner JL. Hearing results in malleostapediopexy. Arch Otolaryngol 1969;89:83–7.

Utech H. Über diagnostische und therapeutische Möglichkeiten der Tympanotomie bei Schallleitungsstörungen. Laryngol Rhinol 1959;38:212–21.

Utech H. Über die Verwendung von Knorpelgewebe bei Tympanoplastik und Stapeschirurgie. NHO 1961;9:232.

Van Blitterswijk CA, Grote JJ. Biological performance of ceramics during infection and inflammation. CRC Crit Rev Biocompatibility 1989;5:23–83.

Vizkelety T, Kovács F, Bodo G. Ossiculoplasty in case of intact stapes. In: Tos M, Thomsen J, Peitersen E, eds. Cholesteatoma and mastoid surgery. Amsterdam: Kugler, 1989:1157–9.

Wayoff M, Chobaut JC, Deguine C, et al. Les greffes du tympan. Paris: Arnette, 1990.

Wehrs RE. The homograft tympanic membrane after 12 years. Ann Otol Rhinol Laryngol 1982;91:533–7.

Wehrs RE. 1987.

Wehrs RE. Incus replacement prosthesis of hydroxyapatite in middle ear reconstruction. Am J Otol 1989;10:181–2.

Wolfermann A. Reconstructive surgery of the middle ear. New York: Grune and Stratton, 1971.

Wullstein HL. Operationen am Mittelohr mit Hilfe des freien Spaltlappentransplantates. Arch Ohren Nasen Kehlkopfheilkd 1952;161:422–35.

Wullstein HL. Past and future of tympanoplasty. Arch Otolaryngol 1963;78:371–85.

Wullstein HL. Operationen zur Verbesserung des Gehöres. Grundlagen und Methoden. Stuttgart: Thieme, 1968.

Wullstein HL, Wullstein S. Tympanoplasty: osteoplastic epitympanotomy. Stuttgart: Thieme, 1990.

Wullstein S. Osteoplastic epitympanotomy. Ann Otol Rhinol Laryngol 1974;83:663–9.

Yamamoto E. Alumina-ceramics (Bioceram) as columella materials in ossicular reconstruction. Pract Otol (Kyoto) 1982;74:2731–8.

Yamamoto E. Aluminium oxide ceramic ossicular replacement prosthesis. Ann Otol Rhinol Laryngol 1985;94:149–52.

Yamamoto E. Ceramic implants in middle ear surgery. In: Babighian G, Veldman JE, eds. Transplants and implants in otology. Amsterdam: Kugler, 1988:269–76.

Yamamoto E, Michitako I, Morinaka S. Use of micro-sliced homograft cartilage plates in tympanoplasty. Acta Otolaryngol (Stockh) 1985;(suppl 419):123–4.

Yanagihara N, Saiki T, Yamanaka E, Gyo K. Use of hydroxyapatite in ossiculoplasty. In: Babighian G, Veldman JE, eds. Transplants and implants in otology. Amsterdam: Kugler, 1988:277–384.

Yuasa R, Suetake M, Kaneko Y, Kambayashi J. A new simple myringoplasty with fibrin glue. In: Yanagihara N, Suzuki J, eds. Transplants and implants in otology, 2. Amsterdam: Kugler, 1992:207–10.

Zini C. Homotransplantation de dent en tympanoplastie. Rev Laryngol 1970;91:258–61.

Zini C. [Personal communication.] 1992.

Zini C, Sanna M, Bacciu S, Delagu P, Gamoletti R, Scandellari R. Molded tympanic heterograft: an eight-year experience. Am J Otol 1985;6:253–6.

Zini C, Sheehy JL, Sanna M. Microsurgery of cholesteatoma of the middle ear. Milan: Ghedini, 1993.

Zöllner F. Die Radikaloperation, mit besonderen Bezug auf die Hörfunktion. Z Laryngol Rhinol 1951;30:104.

Zöllner F. Die Schalleitungsplastiken, 1. Acta Otolaryngol 1954;44:370.

Zöllner F. Eingriffe bei Gehörgangs- und Mittelohrmißbildung. Acta Otolaryng 1954;44:517–24.

Zöllner F. Hörverbessernde Operationen bei entzündlich bedingten Mittelohrveränderungen. Arch Ohren Nasen Kehlkopfheilkd 1957;171:1–62.

Zöllner F. Tympanoplasty. In: Coates G, Schenck HP, Miller MV, eds. Otolaryngology. Vol. 1. Hagerstown: Prior, 1959.

Zöllner F. Technik der Formung einer Columella aus Knochen. Z Laryngol Rhinol 1960;39:536–40.

Index

A

Acquired immune deficiency syndrome, see AIDS
Aditotomy 85–86
AIDS risk 126, 151, 236
   allogenous ear drum 236
   allogenous fibrin glue 151
   allogenous grafts 126
Air-bone gap closure, mean, in cholesteatoma 253
Allogenous costal cartilage prosthesis 282–283
Allogenous dentin 284, 367
   columella 367
   prosthesis 284
Allogenous drum-malleus graft 340–343
   tympanoplasty with missing malleus handle 340–342
Allogenous ear drum 126–127, 229–236
   AIDS risk 236
   dissection 229–231
      transcranial route 229–231
      transmeatal route 229–231
   in total perforation with intact malleus 231–236
   transplantation 229–236
      Brandow's method 231–232
      Marquet's method 234–236
      Perkins' method 233–234
Allogenous fibrin glue 149–151
   AIDS risk 151
   Duploject system 150–151
   viral hepatitis B risk 151
Allogenous grafts 126–127
   AIDS risk 126
   allogenous ear drum 126–127
   lyophilized dura 127
Allogenous stapes, tympanoplasty type 2 277
Allograft drum, see also allogenous ear drum
   AIDS risk 236
   middle-sized perforations 231
   small perforations 231
   total perforations with intact malleus 231–236
Anesthesia 7–10
   general 10
   local 7
      Jonkees technique 9–10
      Plester's technique 8
      techniques 8
      Wullstein's technique 9
Annulus, elevation 51
Antenna prosthesis 300–301
Anterior approach 68–69
   Goodhill's technique 63, 68–69
   Popper's technique 68–69
   position of surgeon 63

Anterior atticotympanotomy 70, 253
Anterior tympanotomy 81–82
   incisions 81
Antibacterial agents 4
Antibiotics 4–5
Apoceram T-columella 374
Apoceram-P-type prosthesis 293
Applebaum's hydroxyapatite incudostapedial joint prosthesis 311
Atticotomy 84, 86
Atticotympanotomy
   anterior 70, 253
   posterior 70, 253
Austin's malleus-stapes assembly 275
Austin's off-centered TORP 369
Autogenous fibrin glue 149–150
Autogenous grafts 88–126
   conchal cartilage 102–110
   conchal perichondrium 102–110
   ear-canal skin 120–123
   fascia lata 120
   fatty tissue 117–118
   heterotopic skin 124–126
   periosteum 111
   subcutaneous tissue 119
   temporalis muscle fascia 88–96
   tragal perichondrium 97–101
   vein grafts 116
Autogenous incus
   use in interposition tympanoplasty type 2 245

B

Babighian's technique, for reshaping long process 315–316
Babighian's telescopic prosthesis 298
Babighian's telescopic TORP 375
Bauer's compound graft columella 381
Bell prosthesis 300–301
Belluchi's malleostapediopexy 320–321
Bioactive ceramics, in tympanoplasty type 2 292–297
Bioceram 289
   CORP-P prosthesis 291
   CORP-T columella 371–372
Biocompatible materials
   for columellae 368–382
   in tympanoplasty type 2 285–301
Bioglass 292
Bioinert ceramic prosthesis 289–292
Black's oval T-prosthesis 372
Black's prosthesis 293
Black's spanner prosthesis 295, 297
Black's spanner strut 374–375
Bony prominence, removal 217, 225
Brackmann's modified TORP 369–370

Brandow's method, allogenous drum transplantation 231–232

C

Calcium phosphate 293–297
   ceramic prostheses in tympanoplasty type 2 293
Canal skin, elevation 50
   lateral displacement 18
   removal 23, 29, 41
Cartilage, allogenous, in tympanoplasty type 2 277–284
   autogenous, in tympanoplasty type 2 277–284
   columellae 362–367
   conchal, see conchal cartilage
   costal, see costal cartilage
   plates, in disrupted ossicular chain 338–339
      interposition 336–338
      slicing technique 212–213
   septal, see septal cartilage
   tragal, see tragal cartilage
   use in myringoplasty 208–216
Causse's TORP 369
Ceramic ossicular replacement prosthesis – partial (CORP-P) 291
   Bioceram T-columella 371–372
   Yamamoto's prosthesis 291
Ceramic prosthesis(es)
   calcium phosphate 293–297
   glass 292–293
   in tympanoplasty type 2 289–297
Ceramic(s), bioactive 292–297
   bioinert 289–292
   columellae 371–374
Ceravital 292, 372
   columellae 372
Cholesteatoma(s) 2–3
   attic 2
   disruption of incudostapedial joint 252
   congenital 2
   ear canal 2–3
   hidden 70
   iatrogenic 3
   incidence 243
   inclusion 2
   mean air-bone gap closure 253
   posttraumatic 2
   recurrent 2–3
   residual 2–3
   sinus 2
   tensa retraction 2, 77
Circumferential incision, lack of 50
Cole's allogenous costal cartilage columella 367
Cole's technique for harvesting costal cartilage 282–283
Columella(e), see also prosthesis(es) 348–382

Collumella(e)
  allogenous costal cartilage 366–367
  allogenous dentin 367
  allogenous incus 354–356
  allogenous malleus 357–358
  allogenous stapes 358–362
  Apoceram T-shaped 374
  autogenous incus 350–353
  autogenous malleus 357–358
  Bioceram CORP-T 371–372
  of biocompatible materials 368–382
  cartilage 362–367
  ceramic 371–374
  Ceravital 372
  Cole's allogenous costal cartilage 367
  compound 377–382
    Bauer's 381
    cortical bone-Plasti-Pore 380
    cortical bone-Polycell 380–381
    cortical bone-polyethylene 378
    incus-Plasti-Pore 379
    incus-polyethylene 378
    Schobel's tragal cartilage-perichondrium TORP 381
    septal cartilage-wire 380–381
    Smyth's 380–381
  conchal cartilage 362–364
  cortical bone 356–357
  dense hydroxyapatite 372–374
  Fluoroplastic 368
  Frialite 371–372
  glass ionomer cement 374
  Glasscock's tragal cartilage strut 364
  Goodhill's tragal cartilage-perichondrium compound T-shaped 363–364
  Guilford's Teflon 368
  hybrid, hydroxyapatite-Fluoroplast 373
    hydroxyapatite-Plasti-Pore 373
  Jansen's T-cartilage 365
  malleable Polycell 369–371
  metallic 374–375
  metallic wire 375–376
  Palva three-legged 375–376
  Plasti-Pore 368–369
  polyethylene 368
  porous plastic 368–369
  Proplast 368
  Smyth's L-shaped 365
  Smyth's septal cartilage 365
  stainless steel wire, Hüttenbrink's fixation method 376–377
  Tabor's Teflon footplate-malleus 368
  Teflon 368
  tragal cartilage 362–364
  in tympanoplasty type 3, with stapes absent 348–382
  variations in placement 348–367
  Zini's costal cartilage 366–367
Computed tomography 2
Conchal cartilage
  columella 362–364
  endaural approach 109–110
  graft material 102–110
  incisions for graft harvest 102
  plates 212
  resection lines 108–109
  retroauricular incision 103–108
  separate posterior incision 102
Conchal perichondrium
  graft material 102–110
  incisions for graft harvest 102
Control windows 70
CORP-P, see ceramic ossicular replacement prosthesis
Cortical bone
  columella 356–357
  compound columellae 378–381
    cortical bone-Plasti-Pore 380
    cortical bone-Polycell 380–381
    cortical bone-polyethylene 378
  prosthesis 275
    L-shaped 275–276
  shaping of, tympanoplasty type 2 273–277
Costal cartilage 282–283, 366–367
  allogenous columella 366–367
  allogenous prostheses 282–283
  Cole's allogenous 367
  harvesting 282–283
  Cole's technique for harvesting 282–283
  use for allogenous prostheses 282–283
Cupula technique
  tympanoplasty type 5A 386–387

D

Dentin, allogenous 284, 367
  columellae 367
  prostheses 284
Discharge
  conservative treatment 4
  constant 3
  intermittent 3
  surgical treatment 5
Discrimination score 2
Drum epithelium, removal 139–141
Drum-malleus allograft 340–343
Drum perforation(s)
  anterior 128, 152–162, 157–164, 184–186, 194–196, 200–201
    onlay techniques
      with epithelial flaps 157–164
      with removal of epithelium 152–153
    posterior tympanotomy 200–201
    underlay techniques
      with large tympanomeatal flaps 194–196
      without tympanomeatal flaps 184–186
  classifications 128
  dissection of edges 135–139
  dry, causes 128–132
  excision of edges 133–135
  incidence 244
  inferior 128, 153–155, 164–169, 186–188, 192–194, 196–198
    onlay techniques
      with epithelial flaps 164–169
      with removal of epithelium 153–155
    swing-door technique 192–194
    underlay techniques
      with large tympanomeatal flaps 196–198
      without tympanomeatal flaps 186–188
  middle-sized, allograft drum 231
  onlay sandwich technique 181–183
  pathogenetic aspects 128–132
  posterior 128, 156–157, 179–180, 188–190, 199–200
    onlay techniques
      with epithelial flaps 179–180
      with removal of epithelium 156–157
    swing-door technique 188–190
    underlay techniques
      with large tympanomeatal flaps 199–200
  small, allograft drum 231
  subtotal 128
  total 128
    combined perichondrium-cartilage grafts 210–212
    Goodhill's method 208–209
    myringoplasty 331–334
    onlay technique
      with epithelial flaps 169–179
      with removal of epithelium 155–156
    swing-door technique 190–192
    thumb touch technique 338
    underlay techniques 332
      total elevation of fibrous annulus 202–205
    use of perichondrium 208–209
    with intact malleus, allogenous transplantation 231–236
  underlay technique with tympanomeatal flaps 188–201
Drum-remnant, elevation 51
  epithelium elevation (Morimitsu technique) 50
  epithelium management 139
  fixation of underlay graft 144–149
Dry ear, constantly 3
Duploject system 150–151
Dura, lyophilized, allogenous graft material 126–127

E

Ear canal 217–228
  curved, endaural approach 226–228
    with ear speculum 217–224
  myringoplasty 217–228
  retroauricular approach 225–226
  Sheehy's skin removal technique 228
  skin 18, 23, 29, 41, 50, 120–123
    autogenous graft material 120–123
      harvesting 121
    elevation 50
    lateral displacement 18
    removal 23, 29, 41
    terminology of incisions 6
    use in myringoplasty 121–123
Ear drum, see also drum
  allogenous graft material 126–127
  allogenous transplantation 229–236
    Brandow's method 231–232
    Marquet's method 234–236
    Perkins' method 233–234

perforation, *see* drum perforation(s)
speculum 11–14
   fixed 11–13
   Holmgreen-Plester 11
   nonexpanding 11
   selfretaining 11
Eggshell technique, tympanoplasty type 5A 387
Endaural approach 11–33, 90–94, 217–228
   curved ear canal 226–228
      with ear speculum 217–224
   disadvantages 15
   intercartilaginous incisions 15–19
   temporalis muscle fascia grafts 90–94
   Wolfermann's modification 30
Eosinophilic granuloma 4
Epithelial flaps 141
   disadvantages 141–142
Epithelium, removal, in onlay techniques 152–157
Epitympanotomy, osteoplastic 63–67
Eustachian tube orifice, polyps 4

F

Farrior's classification of tympanoplasty 240
Farrior's incision 28–33, 93, 110
Farrior's technique, retroauricular approach 41–42
Fascia grafting
   intermediate, tympanoplasty type 4 384
   underlay, tympanoplasty type 4 384–385
Fascia lata
   autogenous graft material 120
      harvesting 120
Fatty tissue
   autogenous graft material 117–118
      harvesting 117–118
   in myringoplasty 118
Fenestration, lateral semicircular canal 386
Fibrin glue 149–151
   allogenous 150–151
      AIDS risk 151
      viral hepatitis B risk 151
   autogenous 149–150
   in tympanoplasty 149–151
Fibrous annulus
   total elevation in total perforation 202–205
Fisch's off-centered TORP 369
Fisch's technique, retroauricular approach 39–40
Fistula, of semicircular canal 2
Flap(s)
   epithelial 141
      anterosuperior 157
      disadvantages 141–142
      use in onlay techniques 157–180
   Körner's 108–109
   laterally-based 45
      skin 20
   malleus 157–158
   Panse's 22–23
   superolaterally-based 44

Surdille's 20, 22–23
tympanomeatal 18
   large 20
      use in underlay techniques 194–201
   management 45–49
   small 18
      use in underlay technique 188–201
Fleury's incision 93
Fluoroplastic, columellae 368
   compound columellae 373
      hydroxyapatite-Fluoroplast 373
      Shea's hydroxyapatite-Fluoroplast TORP 373
Forceps, Sheehy ossicle-holding 267
Frialite 289, 371–372
   columellae 371–372

G

Gerlach's wire-basket prosthesis 298–299
Glass ceramics, prosthesis in tympanoplasty type 2 292–293
Glass ionomer cement
   columellae 374
   prosthesis 297–298
Glasscock's prosthesis 326
Glasscock's technique, combined perichondrium-cartilage grafts 210–212
Glasscock's tragal cartilage prosthesis 280
Glasscock's tragal cartilage strut columella 364
Glomus jugulare tumors 77
Glucocorticosteroids 4
Gold prosthesis 300–301
Gold wire antenna TORP 376–377
Goldenberg's hydroxyapatite TORP 373
Goldenberg's hydroxyapatite-Plasti-Pore prosthesis 327
Goldenberg's incus-stapes prosthesis 372–373
Goldenberg's prosthesis 295–297
Goodhill's method
   use of perichondrium in total perforation 208–209
Goodhill's technique, anterior approach 63, 68–69
Goodhill's tragal cartilage strut 363
Goodhill's tragal cartilage-perichondrium compound T-columella 363–364
Graft(s)
   combined perichondrium-cartilage 210–212
      Glasscock's technique 210–212
Graft material(s)
   allogenous 126–127
      ear drum 126–127
   autogenous 88–126
   conchal cartilage 102–110
   conchal perichondrium 102–110
   ear-canal skin 120–123
   fascia lata 120
   fatty tissue 117–118
   heterotopic skin 124–126
   lyophilized dura 127

   middle ear reconstruction 88–127
   periosteum 111–116
   subcutaneous tissue 119
   temporalis muscle fascia 88–96
   terminology 88
   tragal perichondrium 97–101
   vein 116
   xenogenous 127
Granuloma, eosinophilic 4
Grote's prosthesis 293–294, 374
   hydroxyapatite L-shaped 374
Guilford's Teflon columella 368

H

Hand-Schüller-Christian disease 4
Heermann's A and B incisions 15–21, 92
Heermann's annulus-stapes cartilage plate 281
Heermann's B incision 109
Heermann's C incision 24, 93
Heermann's cartilage palisades technique, tympanoplasty type 4 386
Heermann's L-shaped cartilage annulus-tensor tympani plate 366
Heermann's palisade cartilage tympanoplasty 214–216
Hepatitis B, viral, risk from allogenous fibrin glue 151
Herodium 4
Heterotopic skin 124–126
Holmgreen-Plester ear speculum 11
Horse-rider prosthesis 278
Hubbard's footplate-malleus strut 369–370
Hüttenbrink's malleostapediopexy 322
Hüttenbrink's method, fixation of stainless steel wire columella 376–377
Hydroxyapatite
   Applebaum's incudostapedial joint prosthesis 311
   dense, for columellae 372–374
   Goldenberg's hydroxyapatite TORP 373
   Goldenberg's hydroxyapatite-Plasti-Pore prosthesis 327
   Grote's
   hydroxyapatite L-shaped prosthesis 374
   hybrid columellae 373
      hydroxyapatite-Fluoroplast 373
      hydroxyapatite-Plasti-Pore 373
   Kartush's incus-stapes prosthesis 374
   prostheses in tympanoplasty type 2 293
   Shea's hydroxyapatite-Fluoroplast TORP 373
   Yanagihara's prosthesis 293
Hypotympanotomy 77–81
Hystoacryl 149

I

Incision(s)
   for anterior tympanotomy 81
   circumferential, omission of 50
   for conchal cartilage graft harvest 102

Incision(s)
  for conchal perichondrium graft harvest 102
  Farrior's 28
  Heermann's A and B 15–21, 92
  Heermann's B 109
  Heermann's C 24, 93
  for inferior tympanotomy 75
  intercartilaginous 6
    Heermann's A and B 15–19
  lateral circumferential 35
    circular 6
  lateral radial 6
  Lempert's 26–27
  medial circumferential 6, 42
  medial radial 6
  Portmann's posterosuperior 51–53
  posterior, separate, for conchal cartilage graft 102
  for posterior tympanotomy 70–71
  posterosuperior 51
  radial conchal 6
  retroauricular 34
    for conchal cartilage graft 103–108
  retroauricular flap 55–59
  retroauricular fold 35
  Rosen's 18–19, 70–71
  Shambaugh's 25
  superior, for osteoplastic epitympanotomy 64
  for superior tympanotomy 83
Incudostapedial joint
  disruption in tympanoplasty type 2 249–251
Incudostapediopexy 308–319
  with bone and cartilage 308–314
  with ionomer cement 314–316
  Mehmke's wire 316–317
  with wires 316
Incus
  extraction, in tympanoplasty type 2 245–248
  interposition 334–335
    with retracted malleus 260–264
    in tympanoplasty type 2 254–264
  shaping of, in tympanoplasty type 2 265–270
Incus columella
  allogenous 354–356
  autogenous 350–353
Incus prosthesis
  placement 270
Incus remnant
  grooves in 316, 318
  holes in 316, 318
Incus replacement prosthesis (IRP) 242
  stainless steel wire 375–377
Indications, middle ear surgery 2–6
Inferior tympanotomy 70, 75–81
  incisions 75
Interposition(s)
  of cartilage plates 336–338
  of incus 334–335
  in tympanoplasty type 2 245–254
  of various prosthesis 340
Intracranial complications 2
Ionomer cement
  fixation of pexis wires 318–319
  use in incudostapediopexy 314–316
IRP, see incus replacement prosthesis

J

Jansen's short T-prosthesis 277–278
Jansen's T-cartilage columella 365
Jansen's T-shaped allogenous septal cartilage prosthesis 363
Jonkees technique, local anesthesia 9–10

K

Kartush prosthesis 293
  incus-stapes, hydroxyapatite 374
Kraus modified Schuring ossicular implant 326, 329

L

Lempert's incision 26–27, 93, 110
Lyophilized dura 126–127

M

Macor 292
Magnan titanium columella 374–375
Magnan titanium PORP prosthesis 298
Magnan titanium TORP prosthesis 298
Malleomyringoplasty 344–345
Malleoplasty, of defective malleus handle 342–343
Malleoplatinopexy 242
Malleostapedial transposition
  in tympanoplasty type 2 302–305
Malleostapediopexy 320–322
  Belluchi's 320–321
  Hüttenbrink's 322
Malleus
  retracted, incus interposition 260–264
Malleus columella
  allogenous 357–358
  autogenous 357–358
Malleus handle
  absent, tympanoplasty 330–347
  allograft 342–343
  defective, malleoplasty 342–343
  preservation 346–347
Malleus head
  shaping of, tympanoplasty type 2 271–272
Malleus replacement prosthesis 344–345
  Schiller's technique 344
Malleus-stapes assembly, Austin's 275
Marquet's method, allogenous drum transplantation 234–236
Mastoid-process periosteum 111–112
  graft material 111–112
  harvest 111–112
Mastoidectomy, canal wall-up 5
  retroauricular cortical 273
  skin incision 55
Meatoplasty, Portmann's 109
Mehmke's wire incudostapediopexy 316–317
Metal columellae 374–376
Metal prostheses
  in tympanoplasty type 2 298–301
Metallic wire for columellae 375–376
Microslicing, of septal cartilage 212–213
Middle ear
  inspection 70
  mucosa 4
    appearance in otomicroscopy 4
  surgery, indications 2–6
    position of surgeon 63
    preoperative management 2–6
  surgical approaches 5–6
Morcellation technique
  tympanoplasty type 5A 387
Moretz peg-top TORP 370–371
Morimitsu's technique
  drum-remnant epithelium elevation 50
Mucosa, middle ear 4
  appearance in otomicroscopy 4
Myringoincudopexy 130, 240, 245, 249, 305–307
Myringoplasty(ies) 5, 87ff., 128ff.
  classification of techniques 132
  in curved ear canal 217–228
  definition 128
  with ear-canal skin 121–123
  fatty tissue grafts 118
  general principles of technique 133–149
  graft materials 88–127
  onlay techniques 132, 152–183
  Plester's technique 121
  total drum perforation 331–334
  underlay techniques 133, 184–207
  use of cartilage 208–216
  use of perichondrium 208–216
Myringosclerosis 5, 129
Myringostapediopexy 130, 240–242, 245, 323–324
  transcanal 323–324

N

Neuroma, acoustic 2
Noncholesteatomatous conditions
  indications for surgery 5

O

Onlay grafting
  tympanoplasty type 4 383–384
Onlay sandwich technique 181–183
Onlay technique(s) 152–183
  with epithelial flaps 157–180
    anterior perforation 157–164
    inferior perforation 164–169
    posterior perforation 179–180
    total perforation 169–179
  myringoplasty 132
  onlay sandwich technique 181–183
  with removal of epithelium 152–157
    anterior perforation 152–153
    inferior perforation 153–155
    posterior perforation 156–157
    total perforation 155–156
  three-flap, with perichondrium 208–209
Ossicular chain
  disrupted, cartilage plates in 338–339

Index

disruption of 252–254, 334–335
  intact, disruption, tympanoplasty type 2 252–254
  pathology, incidence 243–244
Ossicular defects, incidence 330
Ossicular implant, Kraus modified Schuring 326, 329
Ossicular wiring 254
Ossiculoplasty 238
Osteoplastic epitympanotomy 63–67
Osteoplastic tympanotomy, superior incision 64
Otitis
  adhesive, incidence 243
  granulating, incidence 243
  noncholesteatomatous chronic 3–5
  obliterative 5
Otitis media
  adhesive 5
  chronic granulating 3, 5
  chronic purulent 3, 5
  chronic suppurative 3, 5
Otomicroscopy 2
  middle ear mucosa 4
Otosclerosis
  disruption of incudostapedial joint 252

P

Palisade cartilage tympanoplasty (Heermann) 214–216
Palva's swing-door technique, retroauricular approach 38
Palva's three-legged columella 375–376
Palva's three-legged wire prosthesis 300
Palva's two-legged wire prosthesis 300–301, 340
Pars tensa
  abnormalities 132
  anatomy 128
  atrophy 129
Partial ossicular replacement prosthesis (PORP) 283–284, 286–293
  Magnan titanium PORP prosthesis 298
  Shea's off-center PORP 293
Passali-Livi TORP 370–371
Pathogenesis, of drum perforations 128–132
Patient positioning 12
Perforations, *see* drum perforations
Perichondrium
  conchal, *see* conchal perichondrium
  tragal, *see* tragal perichondrium
  use in myringoplasty 208–216
  use in total perforation 208–209
Periosteum 111–116
  autogenous graft material 111–116
  endaural approach for harvesting 114–116
  mastoid-process 111–112
    graft material 111
  as mesthelial graft 111
  temporal squama 112–114
Perkins' method, allogenous drum transplantation 233–234
Pexis 245, 305–324

classification 305
  in tympanoplasty type 2 245, 305–324
  wires, fixation with ionomer cement 318–319
Plasti-Pore
  compound columellae 380
    cortical bone-Plasti-Pore 380
    incus-Plasti-Pore 380
  columellae 368–369
  Goldenberg's hydroxyapatite-Plasti-Pore prosthesis 327
  hybrid columellae 373
    hydroxyapatite-Plasti-Pore 373
  prosthesis, in tympanoplasty type 2 286–287
Platinectomy 238–239
Plester's myringoplasty 121
Plester's technique, local anesthesia 8
  retroauricular approach 35–36
Polycell 369–371, 380–381
  compound columellae 380–381
    cortical bone-Polycell 380–381
  malleable, for columellae 369–371
  peg-stem total ossicular prosthesis 370–371
  prostheses in tympanoplasty type 2 286–287
Polyethylene
  columellae 368
  compound columellae 378
    cortical-bone-polyethylene 378
    incus-polyethylene 378
  prostheses in tympanoplasty type 2 285–286
  Shea's polyethylene stapes strut 368
Polyps, attic 4
  aural 4
  Eustachian tube orifice 4
Popper's technique, anterior approach 68–69
Porous plastic
  columellae 368–369
  prostheses tympanoplasty type 2 286–288
PORP, *see* partial ossicular replacement prosthesis
Portmann's incision, posterosuperior 51–53
Portmann's meatoplasty 109
Posterior atticotympanotomy 70, 253
Posterior tympanotomy 70–74
  incisions 70–71
  Rosen incision 70–71
Posterior vascular strip technique (Sheehy) 60–62
Posterosuperior incision 51–53
Preoperative management 2–6
Preoperative sedation 7
Proplast, columellae 368
  Shea's Proplast columella 368
Prosthesis(es), *see also* columella(e)
  allogenous costal cartilage 282–283
  allogenous dentin 284
  antenna 300–301
  Apoceram-P-type 293
  Applebaum's hydroxyapatite incudostapedial joint 311
  Austin's off-centered TORP 369
  Babighian's telescopic 298
  bell 300–301

bioactive ceramics, in tympanoplasty type 2 292–297
Black's 293
Black's oval T-shaped 372
Black's spanner 295, 297
Brackmann's modified TORP 369–370
Causse's TORP 369
ceramic materials 289–297
  in tympanoplasty type 2 289–297
cortical bone 275
Fisch's off-centered TORP 369
Gerlach's wire-basket 298–299
glass ionomer cement 297–298
Glasscock's 326
Glasscock's tragal cartilage 280
gold 300–301
Goldenberg's 295–297
Goldenberg's hydroxyapatite-Plasti-Pore 327
Goldenberg's incus-stapes 372–373
Goodhill's tragal cartilage strut 363
Grote's 293–294
Grote's hydroxyapatite L-shaped 374
Heermann's L-shaped cartilage annulus-tensor tympani plate 366
horse-rider type 278
Hubbard's footplate-malleus strut 369–370
incus, placement 270
interposition 340
Jansen's short T-type 277–278
Jansen's T-shaped allogenous septal cartilage 363
Kartush's 293
Kartush's incus-stapes, hydroxyapatite 374–375
Magnan titanium PORP 298
Magnan titanium TORP 298
malleus replacement 344–345
  Schiller's technique 344
metal, in tympanoplasty type 2 298–301
Moretz peg-top TORP 370–371
Palva's three-legged wire 300
Palva's two-legged wire 300–301, 340
partial ossicular replacement 283–284
Passali-Livi TORP 370–371
Polycel peg-stem total ossicular 370–371
polyethylene 285–286
porous plastic 286–288
Sadé's long tripod 314
Sadé's small tripod 314
Schuring's combined 329
semi-incus 269
Shea's 293
Shea's off-center PORP 293
Sheehy's incus replacement prosthesis 375–377
Smyth's boomerang septal cartilage strut 365
Spencer's tragal cartilage 310–311, 313
synthetic biomaterials 285–286
Teflon 285–286
tilt-top TORP 368
titanium 298

Index

Prosthesis(es)
  Utech riding cartilage type 326
  Wehrs incus 294–295
  Wehrs incus-stapes 372–373
  Yamamoto's partial ceramic ossicular replacement 291
  Yanagihara's hydroxyapatite 293
  Zini's T-shaped allogenous costal cartilage 283–284

R

Resection lines, for conchal cartilage 108–109
Retroauricular approach 34–62
  curved ear canal 225–226
  Farrior technique 41–42
  Fisch technique 39–40
  Palva's swing-door technique 38
  Plester technique 35–36
  position of surgeon 63
  posterior vascular strip technique 60–62
  temporalis muscle fascia grafts 95–96
  Wullstein-Kley technique 42–43
Rosen's incision
  for posterior tympanoplasty 70–71

S

Sadé's long tripod prosthesis 314
Sadé's small tripod prosthesis 314
Saraceno's technique
  fixing tragal cartilage to Plasti-Pore TORP 369
Schiller's technique
  malleus replacement prosthesis 344
Schuring's combined prosthesis 329
Semi-incus prosthesis 269
Sensorineural hearing loss, asymmetric 2
Septal cartilage
  Jansen's T-shaped prosthesis 363
  microspliced 212–213
  Smyth's boomerang strut 363
  Smyth's prosthesis 363
  wire prosthesis 380–381
Shambaugh's incision 25, 93, 110
Shea's hydroxyapatite-Fluoroplast TORP 373
Shea's off-center PORP 293
Shea's Plasti-Pore columella 368
Shea's polyethylene stapes strut 368
Shea's Proplast columella 368
Shea's prosthesis 293
Sheehy's incus replacement prosthesis 375–377
Sheehy's ossicle-holding forceps 267
Sheehy's skin removal approach, curved ear canal 228
Sheehy's technique, posterior vascular strip 60–62
Skin, heterotopic 124–126
Skin grafts 124–126
  full-thickness 124–125
  heterotopic skin 124
  split-skin 125–126
Smyth's boomerang septal cartilage strut 365
Smyth's compound columella 380–381
Smyth's L-columella 365
Smyth's septal cartilage columellae 365
Speculum holder, Richards 12
  Schuknecht's 11
  Treace 12
Speculum, see ear speculum
Speech reception threshold 2
Spencer's tragal cartilage prosthesis 310–311, 313
Stapedial arch 325–329
  defects 325
  partial defects, tympanoplasty 325–329
Stapes
  allogenous, tympanoplasty type 2 277
  columella, allogenous 358–362
  surgery 15
Subcutaneous tissue
  as autogenous graft material 119
  harvesting 119
Superior approach 63–67
  incisions 64
  position of surgeon 63
Superior tympanotomy 83–86
  aditotomy 85–86
  atticotomy 84, 86
  incisions 83
Surgeon
  positions for middle ear surgery 63
    anterior approach 63
    retroauricular approach 63
    superior approach 63
Surgical approaches 5–6
  anterior approach 5
  endaural approach 5
  retroauricular approach 5
  superior approach 5
Swing-door technique 38, 188–194
  inferior drum perforation 192–194
  Palva's, retroauricular approach 38
  posterior drum perforation 188–190
  total drum perforation 190–192
  underlay technique 188–194
Synthetic biomaterials
  in tympanoplasty type 2 285–286

T

Tabor's Teflon footplate-malleus columella 368
Teflon
  columellae 368
  Guilford's columella 368
  prostheses in tympanoplasty type 2 285–286
  Tabor's footplate-malleus columella 368
Temporal squama periosteum 112–114
  as graft material 112–114
  harvesting 112–114
Temporalis muscle fascia
  for autogenous grafts 88–96
  borders 89
  cross-section 89
  dried 92
  endaural approach 90–94
  fiber direction 89
  harvesting tips 89–90
  retroauricular approach 95–96
  wet 92
Terminology, canal-skin incisions 6
Three-flap onlay technique
  with perichondrium 208–209
  with fascia 169–174
Thumb touch technique 212, 338
  total perforation 338
Tilt-top TORP 368
Tisseel 150
Tissucol 150
Titanium prosthesis 298
TORP, see total ossicular replacement prosthesis
Tos's three flap onley technique 169–174
Total ossicular replacement prosthesis (TORP) 288
  Austin's off-centered 369
  Babighian's telescopic 375
  Brackmann's modified 369–370
  Causse's 369
  Fisch's off-centered 369
  gold wire antenna 376–377
  Goldenberg's hydroxyapatite 373
  Magnan titanium 298
  Moretz peg-top 370–371
  Passali-Livi 370–371
  Shea's hydroxyapatite-Fluoroplast 373
  Schobel's tragal cartilage-perichondrium 381
  tilt-top 368
Tragal cartilage 97
  columella 362–364
  Glasscock's prosthesis 280
  Glasscock's strut 364
  Goodhill's strut 363
  Goodhill's T-shaped columella 363–364
  incision for removal 97
  plates 212
  reinsertion 100
  Saraceno's fixing technique 369
  Schobel's TORP 381
  Spencer's prosthesis 310–311, 313
Tragal perichondrium 211
  for autogenous grafts 97–101
  hemigraft 97
  total graft 97
Transcanal approach 11
Transcanal myringostapediopexy 323–324
Transmeatal approach 11
Transposition
  malleostapedial 302–305
  malleus head to stapes head 303–305
  malleus neck to stapes head 302–303
  in tympanoplasty type 2 245, 302–305
Trauma, of middle ear 2
Tricalcium phosphate
  prostheses in tympanoplasty type 2 293
Tumors, glomus jugulare 77
Tympanoplasty 2
  classification 238–240

Farrior's classification 240
general 238–244
with missing malleus handle 330–347
   allogenous drum-malleus graft 340–342
palisade cartilage 214–216
in partial defects of stapedial arch 325–329
use of fibrin glue 149–151
Wullstein's classification 240–241
Tympanoplasty type 1 238–239
Tympanoplasty type 2 238–239
   allogenous stapes 277
   bioactive ceramic prosthesis 292–297
   type 2, with biocompatible materials 285–301
   disruption of incudostapedial joint 249–252
   disruption of intact ossicular chain 252–254
   extraction of incus 245–248
   glass ceramic prosthesis 292–293
   interposition 245
      of incus 254–264
   pexis 245, 305–324
   shaping cortical bone 273–277
   shaping incus 265–270
   shaping malleus head 271–272
   stapes present 245–284
   transposition 245, 302–305
   use of allogenous cartilage 277–284
   use of autogenous cartilage 277–284
   use of autogenous incus 245
Tympanoplasty type 3 238–239
   with stapes absent 348–382
      prognosis with columellae 348
Tympanoplasty type 4 238–239, 383–386
   Heermann's cartilage palisades technique 386
   intermediate fascia grafting 384
   onlay grafting 383–384
   techniques 383–386
   underlay fascia grafting 384–385
Tympanoplasty type 5 386–390
Tympanoplasty type 5A 238–239
   cupula technique 386–387
   eggshell technique 387
   morcellation technique 387
   techniques 386–387
Tympanoplasty type 5B 238–239
   techniques 387–390
Tympanosclerosis 5
Tympanotomy(ies) 70–87
   anterior 70, 81–82
      incisions 81
   classification 70
   exploratory 70
   inferior 70, 75–81
      incisions 75
   posterior 70–74, 200–201
      anterior perforation 200–201
      incisions 70–71
   superior 70
      incisions 83

U

Underlay graft(s)
   fixation under drum remnant 144–149
   total drum perforation 332
   Yuasa's method 150–151
Underlay sandwich techniques 205–207
Underlay techniques 184–207
   myringoplasty 133
   posterior tympanotomy in anterior perforation 200–201
   sandwich technique 205–207
   swing-door technique 188–194
      inferior perforation 192–194
      posterior perforation 188–190
      total perforation 190–192
   total elevation of fibrous annulus 202–205
      total perforation 202–205
   with large tympanomeatal flaps 194–201
      anterior perforations 194–196
      inferior perforations 196–198
      posterior perforations 199–200
   with tympanomeatal flaps 188–201
      swing-door technique 188–194
   without tympanomeatal flaps 184–188
      anterior perforation 184–186
      inferior perforation 186–188
Utech riding cartilage prosthesis 326

V

Vascular strips
   anterior 30
   inferior 29
   superior 31
Vein graft(s) 116–117
   autogenous 116
   harvesting 116–117
Viral hepatitis, risk from allogenous fibrin glue 151

W

Wehrs incus prosthesis 294–295
Wehrs incus-stapes prosthesis 372–373
Wire
   fixation with ionomer cement in pexis 318–319
   Gerlach's wire-basket prosthesis 298–299
   gold, antenna TORP 376–377
   Mehmke's incudostapediopexy 316–317
   metallic 375–376
      for columellae 375–376
   Palva's three-legged prosthesis 300
   Palva's two-legged prosthesis 300–301, 340
   stainless steel, Hüttenbrink's fixation method 376–377
      incus replacement prosthesis 242
   use in incudostapediopexy 316

Wolfermann's modification, endaural approach 30
Wullstein-Kley technique, retroauricular approach 42–43
Wullstein's classification of tympanoplasty 240–241
Wullstein's technique, local anesthesia 9

X

Xenogenous grafts 127

Y

Yamamoto's CORP-P 291
Yanagihara's hydroxyapatite prosthesis 293
Yuasa's method, underlay graft 150–151

Z

Zini's costal cartilage columella 366–367
Zini's T-shaped allogenous costal cartilage prosthesis 283–284